OXFORD MEDICAL PUBLICATIONS

Tropical gastroenterology

Tropical gastroenterology

G. C. COOK
M.D., D.Sc., F.R.C.P., F.R.A.C.P.
Professor of Medicine and Chairman of Clinical Sciences, The University of Papua New Guinea. Formerly, Medical Specialist, Royal Nigerian Army; Lecturer in Medicine, Makerere University, Uganda; Professor of Medicine, the Universities of Zambia, Lusaka and Riyadh, Saudi Arabia.

OXFORD
OXFORD UNIVERSITY PRESS
NEW YORK DELHI
1980

Oxford University Press, Walton Street, Oxford OX2 6DP

OXFORD LONDON GLASGOW
NEW YORK TORONTO MELBOURNE WELLINGTON
KUALA LUMPUR SINGAPORE HONG KONG TOKYO
DELHI BOMBAY CALCUTTA MADRAS KARACHI
NAIROBI DAR ES SALAAM CAPE TOWN

British Library Cataloguing in Publication Data

Cook, G C
Tropical gastroenterology. – (Oxford medical publications).
1. Digestive organs – Diseases
2. Tropical medicine
I. Title II. Series
616.3'00913 RC802 79-41545

ISBN 0-19-261228-X

Phototypeset in V.I.P. Times by
Western Printing Services Ltd, Bristol

Printed in Great Britain
at the University Press, Oxford
by Eric Buckley
Printer to the University

Preface

I have written this book because I have for several years felt that a text devoted to tropical gastroenterology was long overdue. I have endeavoured to write first for the clinician and clinical student working in the tropics, who is engaged with gastroenterological problems, which form a substantial part of a subject for long known as 'tropical medicine'. Secondly, I have written for the physician working in a temperate climate, who with the vast increase in rapid population movement is seeing more and more patients with gastroenterological diseases, some of which he has not even heard of, which have been acquired in tropical countries.

I have been guided by much personal knowledge and experience gained from some twelve years in tropical countries. Most of that time has been spent in academic posts in third-world universities and medical schools: two years (1960–2) at Lagos, Nigeria; two years (1965–7) at Makerere University, Uganda; five years (1969–74) at The University of Zambia; one year (1964–5) at Riyadh University, Saudi Arabia; and two years (1978–80) at The University of Papua New Guinea.

The longer one spends in tropical countries the more one appreciates that 'tropical medicine' is a non-entity. Medicine is basically the same the world over, but with some geographical and ethnological variations. Disease patterns depend not so much on ambient temperature as on public health standards and socioeconomic conditions. Much of the medicine in the third world of 1980 is precisely the same as that which existed in the United Kingdom and other 'developed' countries in the eighteenth and nineteenth centuries. Ideally therefore, demands for a book such as this should have a limited duration, as health standards in the third world improve.

For much of internal medicine in the tropics therefore, western texts are sufficient. However, there are a number of diseases which assume a greater importance in third world countries, and which are not dealt with to an adequate depth in such works; many of them carry a vast morbidity and mortality. I have attempted to cover them in greater detail. I have not however tried to cover again all that is contained in well-known texts on gastroenterology and liver disease, such as those written by Sir Francis Avery Jones and his colleagues, and Professor Dame Sheila Sherlock, respectively.

During the last few years some important advances have been made in the field of tropical gastroenterology. Work on absorption has led to the greatly improved management of cholera and other acute diarrhoeal diseases. Demonstration of bacterial colonization of the small intestine in postinfective tropical malabsorption ('tropical sprue'), and recognition of the importance of clostridial toxins in jejunitis necroticans ('pig bel' disease), necrotizing colitis, and antibiotic-associated colitis are other examples. In the field of hepatology, work on HB_sAg and alpha-feto-protein has advanced substantially our understanding of cirrhosis and hepatoma in the tropics.

Comparison of incidence rates of many diseases in various parts of the world must surely hold the key to their aetiology; large intestinal cancer, non-specific ulcerative colitis, and Crohn's disease, are three examples.

There will doubtless be omissions from this text because my personal knowledge of the third world contains deficiencies.

If my readers have suggestions for inclusion of other diseases should a further edition become desirable or possible or if they have any other criticism of a constructive or destructive nature, I shall be most grateful if they will write to me.

I am extremely grateful to Mrs Raka Natera for typing the whole of the manuscript, including the drafts from my long-hand; she has been exceedingly tolerant and generous with her time. I am also indebted to Doctor J. K. A. Clezy, Professor L. W. Deubert, and Doctor D. S. Pryor for reading and criticizing some of the chapters. I am grateful also to Doctors G. H. Aiken and J. C. Muirden for providing some of the pathology illustrations and radiographs, respectively. Finally I should like to thank the staff of Oxford Medical Publications for their help and kindness during the preparation of this work.

Port Moresby,
Papua New Guinea

G. C. Cook

Contents

Section 1 : Upper gastrointestinal tract

Section 2 : The liver and biliary system

Secion 6 : The large intestine

Section 1 : Upper gastrointestinal tract

1

The mouth, jaws, and salivary glands

Because it is one of the few accessible parts of the gastrointestinal tract, and because most gastrointestinal investigations are not easy to perform in tropical countries, a full examination of the mouth is often extremely rewarding (Tyldesley, 1969). A systematic inspection with a spatula and a good light is essential.

Oral diseases are extremely important in a tropical context; when the mouth is diseased, eating becomes difficult and a poor nutritional status may be worsened.

1.1. The lips, tongue, and buccal mucosa

1.1.1. Pigmentation of fungiform papillae of the tongue

This condition is a result of melanin deposition in the papillae of the tongue. It increases with age in many dark-skinned people. About 26 per cent of children in east Africa are affected, and it seems to be completely unassociated with malnutrition (Beet, 1948); the condition is present in about 50 per cent of adult Africans (Raper, 1948).

1.1.2. Viral infections

Virus infections involving the mouth and fauces are common in tropical countries. The sore throat associated with infectious mononucleosis is rarely encountered. Oral manifestations of smallpox are no longer seen.

Herpes simplex. Herpes simplex infection involving the lips (herpes labialis), tongue, buccal mucosa, and palate is common in children in tropical countries, especially those with kwashiorkor and measles, in whom a severe stomatitis may also occur. Herpes simplex is an important aetiological agent in cancrum oris (see below). It is often associated with pneumococcal lobar pneumonia and acute malaria. Vesicles of 3–5 mm diameter contain clear fluid at first and then become pustular. Permanent scarring is unusual. Multinucleated giant cells can be identified in smears stained with Geimsa. A specific herpes antiserum and an indirect immunofluorescent technique on cell scrapings can be used to make a rapid diagnosis (Gardner, McQuillin, Black, and Richardson, 1968). Rising antibody titres, and neutralization and compliment fixation tests are valuable in diagnosis.

Enteroviruses. Various members of this group—poliomyelitis, Coxsackie, Echo, and Reo viruses—may produce vesicular stomatitis and herpangina.

Behçet's syndrome. Oral ulceration is present in nearly 100 per cent of patients with this syndrome which is common in the Middle east, Cyprus, and Japan (James, 1979).

1.1.3. Bacterial infections

Acute infection. Such infections are common. Acute tonsillitis with recurrent sore throats is a frequent problem and may be associated with acute rheumatic fever; however it is the chronic manifestations of that disease which are encountered more often than the acute condition. A common practice in some parts of Africa is to remove the uvula (uvulectomy); sepsis, haemorrhage, and gross scarring may result.

Tuberculosis. This disease is not common in the oral cavity. Ulceration of the tongue and buccal mucosa may be secondary to pulmonary tuberculosis. It may consist of a solitary lesion or be part of the widespread disease; mode of infection is not known, but is probably haematogenous. The lesions may be proliferative, granulomatous, or ulcerated (Wilkinson, 1972; Laws, 1976; Rao, Satyanarayana, Sundareshwar, and Reddy, 1977). Presentation may be with a single patch, which has an appearance not unlike lichen planus (Tyldesley, 1978). Tuberculoma of the tongue is an unusual event.

Syphilis. This is a rare infection of the oral cavity. Intraoral chancres are rare. Condylomata may be present on the lips. Oral ulcers can occur in the secondary disease.

Yaws. The primary sore of this infection, caused by *Treponema pertenue*, may appear on the lips. The disease has now been eliminated from most tropical countries.

Leprosy. Oral lesions are unusual, but lepromas, small tumour-like masses, may appear on the tongue, lips, or hard palate.

Sulphonamides, which are widely used in the treatment of shigellosis (bacillary dysentery) (Chapter 24) occasionally give rise to the Stevens–Johnson syndrome in which there is extensive ulceration of the buccal and genital mucosa, and in addition erythema multiforme; the syndrome also occurs after virus and bacterial infections, and other therapeutic agents.

1.1.4. Mycotic infections

Moniliasis (Candidiasis). This is caused by *Candida albicans* and is extremely common in children. It causes white plaques on the oral mucosa often known as 'thrush'. Although usually a localized disease it may extend to the lungs with a fatal outcome. It seems probable that some of the oral changes described in tropical sprue in the nineteenth and early twentieth centuries were due to this organism (see below). It occurs especially in malnourished and debilitated patients and also after antibiotics, corticosteroids, and immunosuppressive agents. Monilial infections respond to nystatin.

Histoplasmosis. This is principally a disease of the reticuloendothelial system, and is caused by *Histoplasma capsulatum*. It is present throughout the tropics and subtropics. The source of infection is usually the faeces of chickens, bats, dogs, and cats. Children are more often affected than adults. Primary lesions may occur on the lips and mucous membranes of the mouth; however the lungs are usually the most severely affected organs. The fungus can be demonstrated in smears stained with Giemsa. A compliment-fixation test or mouse-culture technique may be used to confirm the diagnosis.

South American blastomycosis. This disease, caused by *Paracoccidioides brasiliensis*, produces ulcerative granulomatous lesions of the buccal mucosa. It occurs frequently in Brazil and is seen in most South American countries (Peña, 1967). It is probably spread by twigs used for cleaning the teeth which are contaminated with the fungus. The granulomatous ulcers spread slowly but extensively, and regional lymph glands become involved. The yeast cells are seen in haematoxylin and eosin preparations of the pus and crusts from superficial lesions.

Coccidioidomycosis. *Coccidioides immitis* is the cause of this disease which is limited to southern America. Extensive ulceration of the lips and face, with secondary infection, is an unusual complication. Amphotericin B is the most effective proven form of treatment for the systemic mycoses (Wilcocks and Manson-Bahr, 1972).* Various other systemic fungal (mycotic) infections can cause lesions of the upper lip in parts of the tropics (Edington and Gilles, 1976). Subcutaneous phycomycosis caused by a species of *Basidiobolus*, and rhino-entomophthoromycosis caused by *Delacroixia coronata* (Chapter 2) occasionally involve the lips.

1.1.5. Malnutrition and deficiency disease

Oral changes in severe protein-calorie deficiency are multiple, but are usually dominated by one or more infections (see above) with added evidence of vitamin and iron deficiencies.

Hypochromic anaemia. In iron-deficiency (hypochromic) anaemia, which is extremely common in all parts of the third world and is usually caused by hookworm infection, smoothness and pallor of the tongue are common. However, the incidence rates of glossitis, stomatitis, and dysphagia are surprisingly low when the frequency of anaemia is taken into account.

Riboflavin and other B vitamin deficiencies. A deficiency of these vitamins produces cheilosis, a condition in which the lips are cracked, *angular stomatitis*, grey-white fissures at both angles of the mouth, and *glossitis*, a sore tongue which is often abnormally deep red in colour. These changes are very common in pellagra.

Scurvy. This is an uncommon disease in the tropics; even in areas with a long, dry season during which time there are few fresh vegetables and fruits, it is rarely seen. Produced by a lack of dietary ascorbic acid, it produces severe gingivitis and loosening of the teeth.

1.1.6. Tropical malabsorption (TM) ('tropical sprue')

Oral changes in tropical malabsorption (TM) seem to be much less usual today

* Recent evidence suggests that miconazole gives favourable results in various tropical mycotic infections including coccidioidomycosis and South American blastomycosis (*Lancet*, 1979).

than they were in the past (Cook, 1978). That is probably because cases seen today are not as long-standing or severe as many of those described in the classical reports. Severe cases of TM seen at present occur mainly in expatriates following holidays or tours in Asia. In most eighteenth and nineteenth century reports, aphthous ulceration involving the tongue and buccal mucous-membrane was considered to be very common in the 'white flux' and 'hill diarrhoea' (TM) (Cook, 1978) (Chapter 20). In describing the oral changes associated with TM, which dominated most early accounts of the disease, Hillary (1766) described 'little small pustules, or pimples, filled with a clear acrid lymph at the end and sides of the tongue, which gradually increase in number and slowly spread to other parts of the mouth; soon the thin skin slips off and the tongue looks red and a little inflamed, and is almost raw like a piece of raw flesh and is tender and sore'. Writing of the 'white flux', Martin (1856) described 'anaemic ulcerations (chronic aphthae) of the mucous digestive surface'. The term 'tropical sprue' was first used by Manson (1880) to describe TM; he adopted the term sprue from the Dutch word *spruw* which was then in use to describe oral aphthous ulceration in children. Good descriptions of the oral changes seen in sprue or psilosis, were given by Thin (1890; 1897). One hundred and one of 150 cases of 'tropical sprue' reported in London by Low (1928) had tongue lesions when first seen and 44 had other oral signs as well. In some of the 200 cases reported by Manson-Bahr and Willoughby (1930) buccal changes were considered to have preceded the diarrhoea. Rogers (1913) felt that the oral changes of the disease were dependent on the length of history of systemic symptoms. Bahr (1915) however felt that exactly similar aphthae to those seen in 'tropical sprue' occurred in normal Europeans; he considered that aphthous ulceration was sometimes associated with secondary infection, possibly monilial in origin, which was superimposed on a progressive nutritional deficit. Brown (1908) was of the opinion that the oral lesions were similar to those of 'thrush'. It is now clear that aphthous ulceration can occur after long-standing malabsorption of other causes; a high incidence has for example been reported in gluten-induced enteropathy (Ferguson, Basu, Asquith, and Cooke, 1975; Wray, Carmichael, Ferguson, Lee, and Russell, 1978).

Today those lesions are rarely seen except in very severe prolonged cases of TM. Painful, burning sensations of the tongue and oral mucosa are sometimes a problem in a severe case; small painful vesicular erosions may occasionally be seen. Rarely there may be a severe glossitis with atrophy of filiform papillae; the fungiform papillae often persist for some time, however, on the atrophic surface.

1.1.7. Oral submucous fibrosis (sclerosing stomatitis, atrophia idiopathica [trophica] mucosae oris)

This is a chronic disease of unknown aetiology which may affect any part of the oral cavity (Joshi, 1953; Lal, 1953; Pindborg, 1965); a slow onset of fibro-elastosis of the submucous tissues with epithelial atrophy occurs. Leukoplakia is frequently associated with it. The condition is probably premalignant (Paymaster, 1956; Pindborg, 1965; Pindborg, Mehta, Gupta, and Daftary, 1968). Most reports are from India, or concern Indians resident in east Africa

(Wright, 1976). Descriptions of the disease have also been made from Nepal, Sri Lanka, Malaysia, Thailand, south Vietnam, and Papua New Guinea (Barnes and Duke, 1975). The chewing of chillies (*Capsicum annum*), possibly in the presence of low dietary A, B, or C vitamins might be aetiologically important (Wahi, Kapur, Luthra, and Srivastava, 1966), but that is not proven.

Most patients are in the 20 to 40 year age group; there are no sex or social-class differences in incidence rates. Presentation is with painful vesicles in the oral mucosa, which later becomes blanched and opaque. The soft palate, uvula, and anterior pillars of the fauces are usually involved; the lower lip and floor of the mouth may be affected. Distribution is symmetrical; white fibrous bands run in a vertical direction. The ultimate result is a loss of elasticity in the oral mucosa, accompanied by trismus. Hyalinized collagen in the submucosa with atrophy of the mucosa are constant features. In the early stages, eosinophils, and later an inflammatory exudate of lymphocytes and plasma cells, are present; at a late stage, obliteration of blood vessels also occurs.

Various forms of treatment have been tried. Surgery should probably be avoided because it tends to increase fibrosis. Administration of fibrinolysins, gold, and vitamins A and E have failed to produce improvement. Corticosteroids may give temporary relief. Consumption of chillies should be discontinued and mechanical irritants within the mouth removed. Vitamin B complex may be of value. Regular review should be undertaken so that a possible carcinoma can be recognized at an early stage.

1.1.8. Onyalai

In this condition, haemorrhagic bullae appear in the oral mucosa; it is a disease of children and young adults. East, central, and southern Africa are the areas from which it has been reported. The condition results from thrombocytopenia.

Megakaryocytes are present in normal or increased numbers in the bone marrow but the platelet lifespan is reduced (Lurie, Katz, Ludwin, Seftel, and Metz, 1969). There may be sequestration of platelets in the spleen, in which case splenectomy will induce a remission. Corticosteroids are of value.

Efforts to find a factor responsible for the thrombocytopenia have so far proved unrewarding; toxic and infective agents could be responsible.

Petechial haemorrhages may be seen in other haemorrhagic conditions and also bacterial endocarditis and septicaemic states; they are very difficult to see on the skin of dark-skinned people.

1.1.9. Oral tumours

Basal-cell carcinoma. The lips may be affected by this tumour. It is usually a disease of Europeans living in tropical countries. The high incidence in them is due to frequent exposure to powerful sun-light.

Carcinoma of the mouth. This is a squamous-cell carcinoma which arises in the buccal mucosa. This tumour is closely associated with chewing and smoking habits (Jafarey and Zaidi, 1976); it is common in Pakistan, India, Sri Lanka, Malaysia, Papua New Guinea, Indonesia, Brazil, and the Caribbean. In Papua

New Guinea (Atkinson, Chester, Smyth, and Ten Seldam, 1964; Cooke, 1969), Thailand (Tansurat, 1961), and in certain parts of India, oral carcinoma has been causally associated with the lime chewed with betel nut (*Areca catechu*).* When tobacco is added to betel nut and lime, the carcinogenic effect is apparently enhanced. Because it is usually spat out after being well chewed, there should not be an increased risk of carcinoma of the oesophagus or stomach. In Papua New Guinea, the tumour is common in coastal areas but it is rare in the highlands where betel nut is used to a much lesser extent (Wagner and Shepherd, 1976). During a ten-year period, 1958–67, oral cancer was responsible for 15·8 per cent of all malignancies reported to the Papua New Guinea tumour registry (Cooke, 1969).

In Bihar, a squamous-cell cancer ('Khaini cancer') which occurs between the lips and front teeth is associated with chewing tobacco leaf and lime; it is considered that vitamin A deficiency might be an important underlying aetiological factor.

In India, squamous-cell carcinoma of the hard palate occurs, in women especially, and is associated with smoking chutta (a coarse type of cheroot); the burning end of the cigarette is held inside the mouth. In Columbia, where the lighted end of the cigarette is usually also inside the mouth, oral carcinoma is similarly common. In areas where the quid is held under the tongue, carcinoma of the floor of the mouth may occur.This tumour seems to be uncommon in Africa (Davey, 1968) and most other parts of the tropics except those mentioned above (Edington and Gilles, 1976).

Early diagnosis is of paramount importance; 80 per cent of patients can be cured if the disease is treated early (Cugadasan, 1977).

Carcinoma of the tongue. Carcinoma of the anterior two-thirds of the tongue and the mandibular alveolar margins is common in some parts of the USSR where a mixture of tobacco, ash, oil, and lime ('nass') are chewed.

Burkitt's lymphoma of the buccal mucosa. The buccal mucosa, especially that of the palate, may be involved in children with Burkitt's lymphoma.

Epulides. These are very common tumours in Africa. The most usual one to be encountered is the firm, tough, 'healthy looking' fibrous variety (Davey, 1968), which is more common in women than men. There are no major differences from similar lesions in other parts of the world.

1.2. The gums and teeth

1.2.1. Cancrum oris

This is a gangrenous condition of the facial region, mainly the gums and cheeks, which is associated with Vincent's organism; widespread oral and facial deformities result. It may follow any acute systemic illness in malnourished people, especially children, in tropical countries. The disease is common throughout the third world; an account of 250 cases has been given by Tempest (1966) from Nigeria.

* The carcinogen might be one of the reduced pyridine alkaloids in betel nut (Ashby, Styles, and Boyland, 1979).

Children between two and five years are especially prone to the disease; adults in prisoner-of-war camps have also been affected (Dawson, 1945). Occasionally it complicates kwashiorkor (Trowell, Davies, and Dean, 1954). Three factors seems to be necessary for the disease to occur: (i) a predisposing debilitated state, which usually consists of severe undernutrition and anaemia; (ii) a specific mouth infection—fusiform bacilli and spirochaetes of Vincent's type play the dominant role; their presence in the slough is often obscured by secondary bacterial invaders, however; and (iii) a precipitating systemic illness, often measles or malaria. The disease may be complicated by broncho-pneumonia and lung abscess.

Cancrum oris probably begins as a gingival *Herpes simplex* infection which is invaded by *Borrelia vincenti* and *Fusiformis fusiformis* bacilli. These organisms can be demonstrated in smears from ulcerated lesions by Gram stain. *B. vincenti* is a spirochaete 5–10 μm in length; it is actively motile and Gram-negative. *F. fusiformis* is a cigar-shaped Gram-positive organism with a straight or slightly curved axis, and is 5–12 μm long. The gangrenous process spreads from an initial site, usually a carious or diseased tooth, to involve the gums, jaws, and cheeks. Thrombosis and gangrene of the cheek are followed by bacterial invasion of the slough. Osteomyelitis, with sequestrum formation of the jaw supervenes; that is followed by severe disfigurement. Gross deformities are more often seen now than before the introduction of antibiotics; most patients would formerly have died in the acute stage. Trismus may be a problem.

Histologically the striking feature is necrosis of tissues with a high concentration of organisms at the advancing edge of the lesion; granulation tissue and extensive fibrosis are present if healing takes place. Dark ground illumination and culture and animal inoculation are of value in diagnosis.

Prophylaxis consists of eliminating malnutrition in the area involved. Dental hygiene must be improved, and measles and malaria eradicated. Treatment in the acute phase of the disease consists of (i) a good protein, vitamin, and iron intake, (ii) an antibiotic for the specific mouth infection and accompanying bronchopneumonia (Jelliffe, 1953), and (iii) specific treatment for malaria or other systemic disease. Surgery is not indicated in the acute state; however, reconstructive surgery has much to offer later in this disease (Crockett, 1963; Davey, 1968). Facilities for plastic surgery are usually not available in third world countries.

Noma neonatorum. This is a gangrenous condition involving the lips, oral cavity, nose, and anal region of neonates. It is caused by *Pseudomonas aeruginosa* in young, and Fusospirochaetosis in older children (Ghosal, Sen Gupta, Mukherjee, Choudhury, Dutta, and Sarkar, 1978).

1.2.2. Dental and periodontal disease

Although periodontal disease is common throughout the third world, dental caries are less common in isolated rural areas (Trowell, 1960; Sinrod, 1965). However, with increasing 'westernization' and consumption of large amounts of refined sucrose, much more disease is appearing. In Papua New Guinea, the rate of dental caries seems to be related to the concentrations of certain trace elements in the soil and vegetables (Barmes, Adkins, and Schamschula, 1970). Periodontal disease predisposes to gingival inflammation, pyorrhoea, and loss of teeth. Both of those diseases have a common aetiology, i.e. dental plaque, and are thus preventable.

Infected tooth sockets and gums may give rise to systemic infections, with bacteraemia and resulting endocarditis; chronic rheumatic cardiac disease is very common in most tropical countries and bacterial endocarditis accounts for a substantial morbidity and mortality.

Dental fluorosis occurs in isolated areas of the tropics; it is common in Thailand (Leatherwood, Burnett, Chandravejjsmarn, and Sirikaya, 1965) and parts of India and China. It is characterized by mottled dental enamel and is due to an excessive intake of fluorine.

1.3. The jaws

1.3.1. Infections of the jaws

Tuberculosis. This is unusual. When it occurs, infection is either from the buccal cavity or by haematogenous spread.

Actinomycosis. This mycotic (fungal) disease is caused by *Actinomyces israelii* and *A. bovis* which are commensals in the oral cavity. The disease occasionally presents as a chronic suppurative process in the cervico-facial region ('lumpy jaw') from which numerous discharging sinuses may be present. The condition occasionally follows delayed healing of a tooth socket after dental extraction (Barnes, 1971). Characteristic 'sulphur granules' are found in the pus from an abscess; the organism can also be cultured. Penicillin is the treatment of choice.

1.3.2. Jaw tumours

Burkitt's lymphoma. The majority of jaw tumours in Africa, Papua New Guinea, and many other parts of the tropics are caused by Burkitt's lymphoma (Burkitt, 1958). Of 300 jaw tumours seen in Ibadan, Nigeria, 40 per cent were Burkitt's lymphomas. Tumours which present elsewhere in the world also occur in tropical countries, but there is no evidence of either an increased frequency or of a significant difference in their behaviour (Edington and Sheiham, 1966). Burkitt's lymphoma usually involves children; the peak incidence is at approximately 5–7 years. The geographical distribution is characteristic and seems to be related to climatic factors; it is rare in areas with a minimum mean temperature below 16°C and an annual rainfall of less than 50 cm (Burkitt, 1962 a, b, and c). A viral aetiology (the Epstein-Barr virus has been incriminated) with spread by a vector, possibly a mosquito, seems possible, although the causative nature of that association is not yet established (*Lancet*, 1978).

Jaw involvement is more common in young children and is unusual after 15 years of age. Jaw deposits can also occur after the initial deposits have occurred elsewhere in the body. Origin may be multifocal. It may involve both jaws on one or both sides; there may be four separate but simultaneous tumours. It begins in the marrow. The maxilla is involved more often than the mandible, and it usually first appears in relation to the molar and premolar teeth. Loosening of teeth is usually the first symptom; as the tumour grows teeth are displaced, one by one, and gross disfigurement occurs; secondary infection is common. Orbital involvement frequently occurs late in the disease.

The tumour appears macroscopically to be clearly demarcated from surrounding tissues; it is soft in consistency and yellowish-white with areas of necrosis and haemorrhage. Histological appearance is of a malignant lymphoma (O'Conor and Davies, 1960) which has certain specific features (Wright, 1963a and b; Burkitt and Wright, 1970). Sections show sheets of 'blast' cells with large round, oval or reniform nuclei and a narrow rim of cytoplasm, amongst which are scattered large histiocytes. Phase contrast and tissue culture techniques are available (Edington and Gilles, 1976). Radiology shows osteolytic lesions in the jaws; one of the earliest diagnostic features is the disappearance of the lamina dura which surrounds the unerupted teeth (Cockshott, 1965).

Treatment is with chemotherapeutic agents; methotrexate and cyclophosphamide are the most effective compounds (Oettgen, Burkitt, and Burchenal, 1963; Burkitt, Hutt, and Wright, 1965). With early tumours, complete clinical remission after two years or more is usual (Ngu, 1965); later in the disease, recurrence at other sites is common, and entirely new tumours may appear despite treatment.

Ameloblastoma (adamantinoma). Ameloblastoma is probably more common in most parts of Africa than in temperate areas of the world (Carayon, Reynaud, and Jousselin, 1961). It is a common cause of jaw tumours in Papua New Guinea (Cooke and Toohey, 1969). This is a locally malignant tumour, which does not metastasize; its precise nature is in some doubt.

The tumour usually presents at about 30 years of age and is twice as common in men compared with women; the lower jaw is more often affected than the upper. The history often dates back about six years. In Ibadan this tumour usually affects the anterior part of the mandible (Akinosi and Williams, 1968); that could be related to the increased incidence of periodontal disease and calculus deposition in Nigerians. The tumour is clinically firm or hard with a regular surface.

Teeth fall out one by one; pain is uncommon. Infection, which gains entry through the sockets of lost teeth, is followed by discharging sinuses either within the mouth or externally. Despite considerable discomfort and difficulty in eating, nutrition is usually well preserved.

The diagnosis is made from biopsy—histology and radiology. Histopathology shows nothing of particular note; solid and cystic types are recognized. In about 10 per cent of tumours, small amounts of melanin are present (Williams, 1967).

Treatment consists of surgical excision and involves removal of part or whole of the mandible.

Carcinoma of the para-nasal sinuses involving the jaw. This tumour seems to be more common in Africans than Europeans; it is not a common tumour in Papua New Guinea. In Johannesburg, Keen (1963) found that it accounted for 4 per cent of jaw tumours in Africans referred for radiotherapy, compared with 0·4 per cent in Europeans. As the tumour usually starts in the maxillary antrum in South Africa it seems likely that it is a result of snuff-taking. Snuff is made from *Aloe marlothii* which contains 3:4-benzpyrene, a known carcinogen; with a decrease in snuff-taking the incidence of the tumour has apparently declined.

Most are squamous-cell tumours which have reached an advanced stage by the time diagnosis is made. Radiotherapy gives the best chance of cure. In advanced cases, maxillectomy and intra-arterial chemotherapy may be tried.

1.4. The salivary glands

1.4.1. Simple hypertrophy

This is often seen in malnourished children, usually over 5 years (Trowell, 1960; Oduntan, 1972), and young adults; the diet usually contains a low protein and high carbohydrate content (Gillman, Gilbert, and Gillman, 1947). In a study of Nigerian children, the condition was shown to be more common in those from low income groups and from rural areas (Oduntan, 1972). It has been seen also in prisoner-of-war camps, and pellagrins, in Europe. It is sometimes associated with a severe *Ascaris lumbricoides* infection, and resolves after treatment of that disease (Murray, Murray, Murray, and Murray, 1978). It is also seen in association with chronic calcific pancreatic disease (Chapter 15). There is an association with alcoholic cirrhosis and achalasia of the cardia (Davey, 1968) (Chapter 3).

The aetiology is obscure. It might represent a functional hypertrophy in response to a high carbohydrate intake or nutritional surplus, after a prolonged period of malnutrition. Depression of cholinesterases, which occurs in malnourished infants, might favour increased parasympathetic activity and hyperfunction of the parotids. Endocrine factors have also been considered. In *severe* malnutrition, atrophy of the gland may be found. The parotids are most severely involved although the other salivary glands may also be affected.

Enlargement of the parotids is bilateral and painless (Farago, 1964). Biopsy shows hyperplasia with large numbers of secretory granules in the acinar cells (Salamon, 1958). Sialograms have been interpreted as indicating hypertrophy of the ductular and glandular systems. Davey (1968), however, considers results of sialography to be normal.

1.4.2. Infections of the salivary glands

Acute viral parotitis, caused by mumps, and acute pyogenic parotitis are common in tropical countries. Other inflammatory and non-inflammatory causes of parotid enlargement occur as in temperate zones.

Viral infections

Mumps. This virus disease is extremely common in tropical as well as temperate countries. Incubation period is 14–21 days. The disease is spread by droplet infection. There is an acute inflammation of the parotid glands with oedema and mononuclear infiltration. There is necrosis and monocyte, plasma cell, and histiocyte infiltration in the glandular stroma of the parotid gland; the epithelium may also be affected. There may be an associated acute pancreatitis (Chapter 15), meningo-encephalitis and cardiac and renal involvement.

Acute suppurative parotitis. Five strains of Coxsackie virus B-3 were isolated in an investigation on 34 patients with this condition at the Mulago Hospital, Kampala in 1968 (Mutanda, 1977).

Yellow fever. A parotitis may be present in yellow fever (Chapter 7).

Bacterial infections
Typhoid fever (salmonellosis). A parotitis occasionally occurs in *Salmonella typhi* infections; owing to secondary infection it may be a troublesome complication of the disease.

Shigellosis (bacillary dysentery). A parotitis has been described in this disease.

Parasitic infections
Cysticercosis. In *Taenia solium* infection (Chapter 19), cysticerci may be found in the parotid gland. It is doubtful however whether this has a clinical significance.

1.4.3. Salivary-gland tumours

Reports of salivary-gland tumours have been made from Nigeria (Edington and Sheiham, 1966), the Sudan (Hickey, 1956; El Hassan and Lynch, 1962) and South Africa (Schulenburg, 1954). There is no evidence that they are more common overall in Africa (Davies, Burkitt, and Dodge, 1964) than in other parts of the tropics. However, within Africa there are suggestions of striking differences in the site of origin. Tumours in the submandibular gland, lip, palate, and nose are five times more common in Africans compared with Europeans (Du Plessis, 1952); the reason for that is not understood.

Two-thirds or more of the tumours are in women of about 40 years of age. They are often symptomless, firm, deep in the mucosa, and sometimes pedunculated. The tumours are situated to one side of the midline, usually in the hard palate. Although they are slow-growing, half of the palate is frequently involved at presentation, and ulceration may also be present. Speech, mastication, and swallowing may be affected. Histologically there is nothing of particular note; the benign tumours are either cellular, mucinous, or a mixture of cellular and mucinous components. The incidence of malignant change is of the order of 20–30 per cent. Treatment is by diathermy excision; if it is benign the tumour usually shells out easily. Large tumours require maxillectomy.

Burkitt's lymphoma. Burkitt's lymphoma not infrequently involves the parotid and submandibular glands. The swellings are smooth, relatively painless, and rapidly growing.

Papillary cystadenoma lymphomatosum. The parotid is rarely involved in most groups indigenous to the tropics by *papillary cystadenoma lymphomatosum* (Warthim's tumour).

Malignant oncocytoma. A malignant oncocytoma (oxyphilic granular-cell tumour) of the parotid gland has been described in a Nigerian woman (Abioye, 1972).

References

ABIOYE, A. A. (1972). *E. Afr. med. J.,* **49,** 235.
AKINOSI, J. O. and WILLIAMS, A. O. (1968). *W. Afr. med. J.,* **17,** 45.
ASHBY, J., STYLES, J. A., and BOYLAND, E. (1979). *Lancet,* **1,** 112.
ATKINSON, L., CHESTER, I. C., SMYTH, F. G., and TEN SELDAM, R. E. J. (1964). *Cancer N.Y.,* **17,** 1289.
BAHR, P. H. (1915). *A report on researches on sprue in Ceylon.* 1912–1914. University Press, Cambridge.
BARMES, D. E., ADKINS, B. L., and SCHAMSCHULA, R. G. (1970). *Bull. Wld Hlth Org.,* **43,** 769.
BARNES, P. (1971). *Papua New Guin. med. J.,* **14,** 96.
—— and DUKE, P. (1975). *Papua New Guin. med. J.,* **18,** 66.
BEET, E. A. (1948). *E Afr. med. J.,* **25,** 433.
BROWN, W. C. (1908). *Sprue and its treatment.* John Bale, Sons and Danielsson, London.
BURKITT, D. (1958). *Br. J. Surg.,* **46,** 218.
—— (1962a). *Nature, Lond.,* **194,** 232.
—— (1962b). *Br. med. J.,* **2,** 1019.
—— (1962c). *Br. J. Cancer,* **16,** 379.
——, HUTT, M. S. R., and WRIGHT, D. H. (1965). *Cancer, N.Y.,* **18,** 399.
—— and WRIGHT, D. H. (1970). *Burkitt's lymphoma,* p. 82. Livingstone, Edinburgh and London.
CARAYON, A., REYNAUD, J., and JOUSSELIN, A. (1961). *Méd. trop.,* **21,** 835.
COCKSHOTT, W. P. (1965). *Br. J. Radiol.,* **38,** 172.
COOK, G. C. (1978). *Jl. R. Coll. Physns.,* **12,** 329.
COOKE, R. A. (1969). *Papua New Guin. med. J.,* **12,** 84.
—— and TOOHEY, J. (1969). *Papua New Guin. med. J.,* **12,** 18.
CROCKETT, D. J. (1963). *E. Afr. med. J.,* **40,** 552.
CUGADASAN, V. (1977). *Tropical Doctor,* **7,** 175.
DAVEY, W. W. (1968). *Companion to Surgery in Africa.* pp. 103, 148, and 174. Churchill Livingstone, Edinburgh, London, and New York.
DAVIES, J. N. P., BURKITT, D. P., and DODGE, O. G. (1964). *Cancer, N.Y.,* **17,** 1310.
DAWSON, J. (1945). *Br. dent. J.,* **79,** 151.
DU PLESSIS, D. J. (1952). *S. Afr. J. clin. Sci.,* **3,** 187.
EDINGTON, G. M. and GILLES, H. M. (1976). *Pathology in the tropics*; 2nd ed. pp. 268, 500, and 534. Edward Arnold, London.
—— and SHEIHAM, A. (1966). *Br. J. Cancer,* **20,** 425.
EL HASSAN, A. M. and LYNCH, J. B. (1962). *Sudan med. J.,* **1,** 3.
FARAGO, C. (1964). *Med. J. Aust.,* **2,** 218.
FERGUSON, R., BASU, M. J., ASQUITH, P., and COOKE, W. T. (1975). *Gut,* **16,** 393.
GARDNER, P. S., MCQUILLIN, J. BLACK, M. M., and RICHARDSON, J. (1968). *Br. med. J.,* **4,** 89.
GHOSAL, S. P., SEN GUPTA, P. C., MUKHERJEE, A. K., CHOUDHURY, M., DUTTA, N., and SARKAR, A. K. (1978). *Lancet,* **2,** 289.
GILLMAN, J., GILBERT, C., and GILLMAN, T. (1947). *S. Afr. J. med. Sci.,* **12,** 99.
HICKEY, B. B. (1956). *Br. J. Surg.,* **44,** 483.
HILLARY, W. (1766). *Observations on the changes of the air and the concomitant epidemical diseases, in the island of Barbadoes.* 2nd ed. p. 276. Hawes, Clarke and Collins, London.
JAFAREY, N. A. and ZAIDI, S. H. M. (1976). *Tropical Doctor,* **6,** 63.
JAMES, D. G. (1979). *New Engl. J. Med.,* **301,** 431.
JELLIFFE, D. B. (1953). *J. trop. Med. Hyg.,* **56,** 53.
JOSHI, S. G. (1953). *Indian J. Otolaryng.,* **4,** 1.

KEEN, P. (1963). *Clin. radiol.*, **14,** 250.
LAL, D. (1953). *J. all-India dent. Ass.*, **26,** 1.
Lancet (1978). **2,** 561.
—— (1979). **1,** 368.
LAWS, I. (1976). *Br. med. J.*, **2,** 45.
LEATHERWOOD, E. C., BURNETT, G. W., CHANDRAVEJJSMARN, R., and SIRIKAYA, P. (1965). *Am. J. publ. Hlth.*, **55,** 1792.
LOW, G. C. (1928). *Q. Jl. Med.*, **21,** 523.
LURIE, A., KATZ, J., LUDWIN, S. K., SEFTEL, H. C., and METZ, J. (1969). *Br. med. J.*, **4,** 146.
MANSON, P. (1880). *China. Imperial Maritime Customs II—Special Series No. 2. Medical Reports for the half year ended 31st March 1880.* 19th issue. p. 33. Statistical Department of the Inspectorate General, Shanghai.
MANSON-BAHR, P. and WILLOUGHBY, H. (1930). *Q. Jl. Med.*, **23,** 411.
MARTIN, J. R. (1856). *The influence of tropical climates on European constitutions.* p. 496. Churchill, London.
MURRAY, J., MURRAY, A., MURRAY, M., and MURRAY, C. (1978). *Am. J. clin. Nutr.*, **31,** 1363.
MUTANDA, L. N. (1977). *E. Afr. med. J.*, **54,** 266.
NGU, V. A. (1965). *Br. J. Cancer*, **19,** 101.
O'CONOR, G. T. and DAVIES, J. N. P. (1960). *J. Pediat.*, **56,** 526.
ODUNTAN, S. O. (1972). *E. Afr. med. J.*, **49,** 380.
OETTGEN, H. F., BURKITT, D., and BURCHENAL, J. H. (1963). *Cancer, N.Y.*, **16,** 616.
PAYMASTER, J. C. (1956). *Cancer, N.Y.*, **9,** 431.
PEÑA, C. E. (1967). *Am. J. clin. Path.*, **47,** 505.
PINDBORG, J. J. (1965). *Bull. Wld Hlth Org.*, **32,** 748.
——, MEHTA, F. S., GUPTA, P. C., and DAFTARY, D. K. (1968). *Br. J. Cancer*, **22,** 646.
RAO, T. V., SATYANARAYANA, C. V., SUNDARESHWAR, B., and REDDY, C. R. (1977). *J. oral Surg.*, **35,** 595.
RAPER, A. B. (1948). *E. Afr. med. J.*, **25,** 245.
ROGERS, L. (1913). *Dysenteries. Their differentiation and treatment.* p. 303. Oxford University Press, London.
SALAMON, T. (1958). *J. trop. Med. Hyg.*, **61,** 253.
SCHULENBURG, C. A. R. (1954). *S. Afr. med. J.*, **28,** 910.
SINROD, H. S. (1965). *Science, N. Y.*, **149,** 400.
TANSURAT, P. (1961). *Acta. Un. int. Cancr.*, **17,** 877.
TEMPEST, M. N. (1966). *Br. J. Surg.* **53,** 949.
THIN, G. (1890). *Br. med. J.*, **1,** 1357.
—— (1897). *Psilosis or 'sprue'. Its nature and treatment.* 2nd ed. Churchill, London.
TROWELL, H. C. (1960). *Non-infective disease in Africa.* pp. 193 and 196. Edward Arnold. London.
——, DAVIES, J. N. P. and DEAN, R. F. A. (1954). *Kwashiorkor.* pp. 24 and 64. Edward Arnold, London.
TYLDESLEY, W. R. (1969). *Oral diagnosis.* Pergamon Press, Oxford.
—— (1978). *Br. med. J.*, **2,** 928.
WAGNER, F. B. and SHEPHERD, A. (1976). *Papua New Guin. med. J.*, **19,** 156.
WAHI, P. N., KAPUR, V. L., LUTHRA, U. K., and SRIVASTAVA, M. C. (1966). *Bull. Wld Hlth Org.*, **35,** 793.
WILCOCKS, C. and MANSON-BAHR, P. E. C. (1972). *Manson's Tropical Diseases.* 17th ed. p. 664. Baillière Tindall, London.
WILKINSON, D. S. (1972). In *Textbook of Dermatology* (ed. A. J. Rook, D. S. Wilkinson and F. J. G. Ebling), 2nd ed. p. 622. Blackwell, Oxford.
WILLIAMS, A. O. (1967). *J. Path. Bact.*, **93,** 545.

WRAY, D., CARMICHAEL, H. A., FERGUSON, M. M., LEE, F. D., and RUSSELL, R. I. (1978). *Gut*, **19,** A439.
WRIGHT, D. H. (1963a). *Br. J. Cancer*, **17,** 50.
—— (1963b). *Int. Rev. exp. Path.*, **2,** 67.
WRIGHT, F. J. (1976). *E. Afr. med. J.*, **53,** 119.

2

The pharynx

SERIOUS disease involving the pharynx in tropical countries is dominated by nasopharyngeal carcinoma. However, a number of infections, many of them very common, must also be considered in order to present a comprehensive picture.

2.1. Pharyngeal infections

2.1.1. Viral infections

Acute coryza. The common cold is probably the most frequent cause of mild pharyngitis; it usually occurs during the prodromal phase and clears as the cold develops.

Infectious mononucleosis. Pharyngitis may be severe in this viral infection, which is clinically not often encountered in tropical countries. Infection seems to occur in early childhood and is largely asymptomatic.

Lassa fever. Severe pharyngeal involvement may occur in Lassa fever (Chapter 7). Any patient with a febrile illness contracted in West Africa, with a severe pharyngitis should be suspected of having this disease. White patches appear in the pharynx, soft palate, and tonsillar pillars. There may also be a cervical lymphadenopathy.

Rabies (hydrophobia). The major problem in rabies is an encephalitis. However, clonic spasm of the muscles of the pharynx (and larynx) prevent swallowing. That gives rise to hydrophobia, which is an important clinical feature of the disease.

2.1.2. Bacterial infections

Streptococcus pyogenes. Mild pharyngitis is common throughout the tropics, especially during the dry seasons. There may be a sore throat with pain on swallowing and a mild fever. A pharyngitis and enlarged cervical glands may be demonstrable. Although antibiotics are occasionally required, gargles and mouth washes are usually adequate. Acute rheumatic fever and glomerulonephritis are occasional sequelae.

Diphtheria. Pharyngeal diphtheria, due probably to the success of immunization campaigns, is far less common in developing countries than it used to be. Children are frequently immunized by cutaneous infection and that might be important in prophylaxis. However the disease does still occur in west Africa (Wyatt, 1974), and deaths are still occurring in Ibadan, Nigeria and Ghana.

Botulism. Caused by the exotoxin of *Clostridium botulinum* (Chapter 17), this disease may produce pharyngeal paralysis. The mortality rate is high.

Tuberculosis. Although rare, primary tuberculosis may occur in the nasopharynx (Martinson, 1963, 1967).

2.1.3. Mycotic infections

Moniliasis (Candidiasis). Invasion of the pharynx by *Candida albicans* is unusual, but can occur especially in malnourished and debilitated patients, and after antibiotics. It is associated with a high incidence of pulmonary infection and carries a high mortality rate.

Aspergillosis. The usual fungi (mycoses) of this group to affect man are *Aspergillus fumigatus* and *A. niger*. Pulmonary lesions with haematogenous spread from them to other organs give rise to the usual presentations (*Br. med. J.*, 1971). They can produce nasopharyngeal disease, associated with proptosis, especially in the Sudan.

Actinomycosis. This fungal disease caused by *Actinomyces israelii* and *A. bovis* rarely produces a chronic suppurative process in the nasopharynx; the organism is a commensal in the oral cavity.

Histoplasmosis. The pharynx is occasionally involved as a primary site of infection with *Histoplasma capsulatum* (Chapter 1).

Rhinosporidiosis. This is a mycotic disease caused by *Rhinosporidium seeberi*; it is common in India and Sri Lanka. Although the nasal cavity is most commonly involved, other mucosal surfaces, including the pharynx, are affected. It is characterized by granulomatous, hyperplastic, and polypoid lesions.

Rhino-entomophthoromycosis. This disease is caused by the fungus *Delacroixia coronata* (Martinson, 1963); it has been described in Nigeria, Jamaica, Kinshasa, Colombia, and Brazil. Although the nasal mucosa is the usual site of infection the pharynx may be involved.

2.1.4. Parasitic infections

Halzoun. An acute parasitic pharyngitis known as 'halzoun' occurs in the Middle east, especially in the Lebanon, and India. It is usually caused by eating the raw liver of a sheep or goat, which is infected with *Fasciola hepatica* (Chapter 14). It consists of an acute infection of the pharynx with young adult *F. hepatica*. *Linguatula serrata*, ingested in raw livers of domestic herbivores, has also been shown to cause the disease in the Lebanon (Schacher, Saab, Germanos, and Boustany, 1969). The fluke, *Isoparorchis hypselobagri*, ingested in raw bladders of catfish causes the condition in India. The leeches *Limnatis nilotica* (Watson and Kerim, 1956) and *Dinobdella ferox* (Keegan, Radke, and Murphy, 1970) can also cause a similar clinical picture. Clinically, there is severe pharyngeal pain, dysphagia, haemoptyses, and epistaxes; there may also be oedema of the face and neck, and aural symptoms.

2.2. Other inflammatory lesions of the pharynx

2.2.1. Scleroma (rhinoscleroma)

This specific disease of the upper respiratory tract usually affects the nasal passages; however the pharynx and also the larynx may be involved (Kafero, 1951; Ssali, 1972).

The disease is probably caused by *Klebsiella rhinoscleromatis*, but it has not been possible to transmit the disease in man. It is seen in south and central America, the USSR, and northern Africa. In Africa, it has been reported from Uganda, Zaire, Rwanda, Burundi, and Ghana. It is characteristically localized to limited areas and communities.

Scleroma is most commonly seen in young adults from 15 to 35 years of age; sex incidence is equal. Symptomatology depends largely on the location of the inflammation; nasal obstruction is common and dysphagia occurs when the pharynx is involved. Respiratory embarrassment may occur late in the disease.

There are specific histological appearances, which are dominated by a macrophage and plasma cell reaction; large foamy histiocytes (Mikulicz cells) are present and fibrosis is progressive. A swab or biopsy usually yields *K. rhinoscleromatis*, which is usually sensitive to streptomycin, chloramphenicol, tetracycline, and ampicillin.

Treatment consists of one of the antibiotics to which the organism is sensitive for up to two months; ampicillin 250–500 mg four-times daily has been successful in curing the disease after seven days. If there is extensive granulation tissue and fibrosis, surgery may be indicated.

2.2.2. Submucous fibrosis (sclerosing stomatitis, atrophia idiopathica [trophica] mucosae oris).

This condition (Chapter 1), although involving the mouth predominantly, can also affect the pharynx (Edington and Gilles, 1976). It is found predominantly in India and the Far east.

2.3. Pharyngeal tumours

2.3.1. Nasopharyngeal carcinoma (NPC)

This disease was first recognized in antiquity.Evidence of the tumour has been found in skulls in Ancient Egypt, and in Nubians and Iranians, some of which are 7000 years old (Clifford, 1972). This form of cancer has some most interesting epidemiological facets.

Distribution. In parts of China this is the commonest form of cancer (Digby, Fook and Che, 1941); in Canton it accounts for 57 per cent of all malignancies in men. That also applies to immigrant Chinese communities in several parts of the world. In some areas, however, the rate in Chinese born in China is significantly higher than in those born abroad. Moderately high rates have been reported from Thailand, Indonesia, Hawaii, California, and the Caribbean. The tumour is common in Hong Kong and Singapore, but rare in Korea and Japan.

In Africa, the disease was until recently thought to be rare; however, due largely to the work of Clifford (1965; 1970; 1972) the true incidence of the disease there has begun to emerge. In parts of Kenya, it is the commonest malignancy apart from hepatoma and oesophageal carcinoma; the disease is most common in Africans living in the higher and colder parts of Kenya, irrespective of their ethnic and tribal origins. The disease is also seen not infrequently in the Sudan, Uganda, Tanzania, and Malawi, and its frequency in west and north Africa seems to be higher than in European communities. It is however a rare tumour in South Africa. It is also unusual in Papua New Guinea, India, Sri Lanka, Japan, and America.

Aetiology. Principally because of the recognition of a very high incidence of the disease in the Chinese, and more recently in parts of Kenya, genetic factors have been carefully considered. Observations in both China and Kenya suggest that people with blood group A are relatively protected from nasopharyngeal cancer. However, observations that the place of birth influences the incidence rate in the Chinese suggests that if that has any significance at all, it can only be part of the story. Environmental factors have therefore been examined. The principal exogenous factors to be considered are carcinogenic chemicals, which are either inhaled or ingested, and viruses (*Lancet*, 1976). Attention has been concentrated on smoke in a domestic setting and especially on the use of grass or wood fires in poorly ventilated dwellings. Cooking in the highlands of Kenya is done indoors; a wood fire burns for much of the 24 hours and high concentrations of carcinogens have been detected. However in the Sudan where there is a hot, dry atmosphere that situation does not apply. It seems unlikely, furthermore, that inhalation of a chemical carcinogen is important in Hong Kong. Incense burning and snuff-taking (Zippin, Tekawa, Bragg, Watson, and Linden, 1962; Sturton, Wen, and Sturton, 1966) have been considered; snuff-taking is associated with an increased incidence of carcinoma of the maxillary sinus in southern Africa (Harrison, 1964). Workers exposed to hardwood dust probably also have an increased susceptibility to adenocarcinoma of the nasal cavity (*Br. med. J.*, 1968).

The role of ingested carcinogens is also not worked out. The Chinese eat large quantities of salted fish, which contains dimethyl and diethyl nitrosamine; however concentrations of those compounds are probably too low to be of significance. In the Chinese of Taiwan, trace elements have been suggested to be important in the pathogenesis of the tumour; high concentrations of environmental arsenic and nickel have been detected in the diet, soft coal used as fuel, house dust, and also in local tobacco. The possibility of vitamin A or carotene deficiency being aetiologically related is worthy of consideration; in experimental animals the epithelium of the upper respiratory tract is rendered sensitive to the effect of hydrocarbons by vitamin A deficiency. Studies in Kenya have in fact demonstrated low carotene concentrations in patients with nasopharyngeal carcinoma.

There is an extensive literature on the role of Epstein-Barr (EB) virus in the aetiology of nasopharyngeal carcinoma (*Lancet*, 1971). Consistently high titres of EB antibodies occur in NPC but not in other squamous-cell carcinomas of the mouth, pharynx, and upper respiratory tract (Klein, 1971). Furthermore, titres seem to vary with the stage of the disease and volume of tumour present; they also fall in remissions and in long-term survivors. However its role is by no means clear. In south China, the incidence rate of the tumour rises steeply in both sexes after the age of 20 years. Ho (1975, 1978) has suggested that the aetiology involves an interaction between a genetically determined sensitivity, early infection with EB virus, and consumption of a traditional preserved food by the southern Chinese. Salted fish contains a variety of volatile nitrosamines (see above) (Ho, Huang, and Fong, 1978); furthermore mutagenic activity was found in urine from rats fed with salted fish. There are also grounds for suspecting that adenoviruses 7 and 12 may play a part in causation of the disease.

In Kenya, men with nasopharyngeal carcinomas excrete higher amounts of urinary oestrogens and less 11-deoxy-17-oxosteroids compared with controls (Clifford and Bulbrook, 1966). It is possible that hormone status might sensitize the nasopharyngeal epithelium to the effects of an inhaled and/or ingested carcinogen. In experimental animals there is some evidence suggesting that oestrogen administration potentiates the carcinogenic effects of certain hydrocarbons.

Clinical. Peak age incidence is usually in the 40–60 year group, although it can occur at almost any age; all reports stress the male predominance. Because the site of the tumour is inconstant, symptomatology varies greatly (Clifford and Beecher, 1964). Most tumours are unilateral and arise in the lateral or supero-posterior walls of the nasopharynx; occasionally the anterior wall is involved and there may be widespread dissemination within the nasopharynx. From the viewpoint of the gastrointestinal tract, limitation of movement of the soft palate, due either to a tumour in the post-nasal space or to actual infiltration of the palate, or its musculature or nerves gives rise to most symptoms. Dysphagia is therefore an important symptom. Infiltration of the glossopharyngeal or vagus nerves is also associated with dysphagia. The pterygoid muscles or the motor branch of the third division of the third cranial nerve may be infiltrated by the tumour in the parapharyngeal space, and that may result in trismus. Other symptoms are related to encroachment of the tumour into the post-nasal space, with otological or ophthalmological involvement. Facial pain due to trigeminal involvement, or pain in the throat and pharynx due to glossopharyngeal involvement, are also not uncommon. The disease is usually advanced at presentation and large cervical node metastases are common (Clifford, 1972). Metastases to cervical glands, bones, lungs, and liver may also occur. Incidence of metastases is related more to the histological type than the site of the tumour: anaplastic or well-differentiated squamous carcinomas. Cranial nerve involvement is also common at presentation.

Investigation. In regions where the tumour is common, diagnosis can usually be made on the history alone. The tumour can then be seen and biopsied, using a nasopharyngoscope, and that is best done under general anaesthesia. Radiological examination of the skull and chest for erosions, invasion, and metastases is an important part of the assessment of the tumour; radiological evidence or erosion of the base of the skull was seen in 44 per cent of the cases described by

Clifford (1972). A lateral view of the skull may show a tumour in the posterior nasal space.

Pathology. Histological appearance varies greatly; it is usually a squamous-cell or an undifferentiated carcinoma. In 362 biopsies from patients with nasopharyngeal carcinoma reported by Clifford (1972), 71 per cent were anaplastic carcinomas and 11 per cent differentiated squamous carcinomas. Six per cent were reticulum cell sarcomas, 4 per cent adenocarcinomas, 4 per cent lymphosarcomas, and 4 per cent were unclassified. Lymphocytic infiltration is sometimes a marked feature.

Treatment. The only satisfactory treatment is radiotherapy; surgery has no place in the management of this tumour, for it is impossible to eradicate extensions of the growth into the para-pharyngeal space. The overall 5-year survival after radiotherapy in 1597 patients from 13 radiotherapy departments was 16 per cent (Clifford, 1972). Unfortunately radiotherapy is usually not available in the third world and, furthermore, transport of patients is very costly. In practice therefore it is usual to irradiate only those cases where a cure is felt possible. The remainder are given palliative chemotherapy. Cyclophosphamide 10 mg per kg bodyweight, intravenously, daily for three or four days or nitrogen mustard 0·5–1·0 mg per kg bodyweight, intravenously, are used. Agranulocytosis and thrombocytopenia are important toxic effects.

2.3.2. Hypopharyngeal carcinoma

A high frequency of hypopharyngeal carcinoma has been reported from northern Thailand. It is apparently caused by smoking a local form of cigar ('Keeyo') which contains Thai tobacco and chopped bark of the 'koi' tree (*Streblus asper*). There is also a high frequency of bronchial carcinoma in the same region (Menakanit, Muir, and Jain, 1971).

References

Br. med. J. (1968). **2,** 572.
—— (1971). **2,** 124.
CLIFFORD, P. (1965). *E. Afr. med. J.*, **42,** 260 and 373.
—— (1970). *Int. J. Cancer*, **5,** 287.
—— (1972). In *Medicine is a Tropical Environment* (ed. A. G. Shaper, J. W. Kibukamusoke, and M. S. R. Hutt). p. 174. British Medical Association, London.
—— and BEECHER, J. L. (1964) *Br. J. Cancer*, **18,** 25.
—— and BULBROOK, R. D. (1966). *Lancet*, **1,** 1228.
DIGBY, K. H., FOOK, W. L., and CHE, Y. T. (1941). *Br. J. Surg.*, **28,** 517.
EDINGTON, G. M. and GILLES, H. M. (1976). *Pathology in the tropics*. 2nd ed. p. 514. Edward Arnold, London.
HARRISON, D. F. N. (1964). *Br. med. J.*, **2,** 1649.
HO, H. C. (1975). *Jl. R. Coll. Surg. Edinb.*, **20,** 223.
HO, J. H. C. (1978). *Int. J. Radiat. Oncol. Biol. Phys.*, **4,** 181.
—— HUANG, D. P. and FONG, Y. Y. (1978). *Lancet*, **2,** 626.
KAFERO, E. D. (1951). *E. Afr. med. J.*, **28,** 315.
KEEGAN, H. L., RADKE, M. G., and MURPHY, D. A. (1970). *Am. J. trop. Med. Hyg.*, **19,** 1029.
KLEIN, G. (1971). *Postgrad. med. J.*, **47,** 141.

Lancet (1971). **1,** 218.
—— (1976). **2,** 1393.
MARTINSON, F. D. (1963). *J. Lar. Otol.*, **77,** 691.
—— (1967). *J. Lar. Otol.*, **81,** 229.
MENAKANIT, W., MUIR, C. S., and JAIN, D. K. (1971). *Br. J. Cancer*, **25,** 225.
SCHACHER, J. F., SAAB, S., GERMANOS, R., and BOUSTANY, N. (1969). *Trans. R. Soc. trop. Med. Hyg.*, **63,** 854.
SSALI, C. L. (1972). In *Medicine in a tropical environment* (ed. A. G. Shaper, J. W. Kibukamusoke and M. S. R. Hutt). p. 138. British Medical Association, London.
STURTON, S. D., WEN, H. L., and STURTON, O. G. (1966). *Cancer, N.Y.*, **19,** 1666.
WATSON, J. M. and KERIM, R. A. (1956). *J. trop. Med. Hyg.*, **59,** 147.
WYATT, G. B. (1974). *Tropical Doctor*, **4,** 110.
ZIPPIN, C., TEKAWA, I. S., BRAGG, K. U., WATSON, D. A., and LINDEN, G. (1962) *J. natn. Cancer Inst.*, **29,** 483.

3

The oesophagus

A MAJOR disease of some parts of the tropics, and one for which treatment is totally inadequate is oesophageal carcinoma. Its incidence is high in some, often very localized, areas; it is of great epidemiological interest but its cause is so far unknown. Oesophageal varices, secondary to portal hypertension, are frequently seen in all third world countries. Achalasia of the cardia, and stricture caused by swallowing corrosive agents are by no means uncommon, especially in parts of Africa. Foreign bodies are also a problem. In South America, Chagas' disease may give rise to mega-oesophagus.

Hiatus hernia and peptic oesophagitis seem to be unusual in most parts of the tropics, and certainly so in Africa. Although extemely common in some parts of Africa, thyroid enlargement, often of gross proportions rarely gives rise to severe dysphagia; when it does, the site of the obstructive symptoms is markedly higher than with oesophageal carcinoma.

3.1. Oesophageal trauma

3.1.1. Foreign bodies in the oesophagus

Near the great lakes of Africa and in coastal regions throughout the tropics, fish-bones may be swallowed with unpleasant consequences. The kola nut, common in west Africa, can be very difficult to remove from the oesophagus (Davey, 1968).

3.1.2. Corrosive stricture

Such lesions are common in Africa (Martinson, 1967). Young children and adults are mainly affected. The responsible agent varies in different parts of the continent (Davey, 1968); caustic soda (used for soap making), hydrochloric acid, sulphuric acid (for car batteries), nitric acid (in the goldsmith's trade), formic acid (used in the preparation of rubber), ammonia, potassium permanganate, lysol detergents, and hot tea have all been used (Martinson, 1978). They are taken either by accident or for suicidal or homicidal attempts, and in certain cases are used by local traditional practitioners. Johannesburg has an especially high incidence rate (Marchand, 1954; 1955a; 1955b).

Burns on the lips, tongue and palate are usually obvious. Although dysphagia may be present from the outset it may take several weeks for it to become manifest. Shock may be severe in the acute stage. In the acute stage also, perforation of the oesophagus or stomach, with formation of tracheo-oesophageal fistulae may occur. Bronchiectasis and lung abscess may result.

Many types of stricture can occur (Davey, 1968); the majority are in the lower one-third of the oesophagus. The extent of the lesion is best discovered by barium-swallow examination (Marchand, 1952), and may be very extensive involving most of the oesophagus. As healing occurs, granulation tissue, fibrosis and scarring occur.

In the acute stage, the corrosive must be neutralized with oral milk or olive oil. The shock is treated by giving intravenous fluids and pethidine. Hydration and nutrition can be maintained with a gastrostomy. Infection is prevented with antibiotics. Pulmonary complications are prevented by raising the foot of the bed. Once the stricture has formed, treatment is either by bouginage and dilatation, or by surgery—either gastropharyngostomy or pharyngocolostomy (Davey, 1968). A tube may be introduced through the stricture after adequate bouginage, through an incision in the neck (Leegard, 1945).

The stomach may also be involved, with resulting pyloric stenosis (Marks, Bank, Werbeloff, Farman, and Louw, 1963); that is characterized by delayed vomiting. Davey (1968) considers that alkalies produce predominantly oesophageal damage, whereas acids tend to be associated with severe pyloric damage.

3.1.3. Achalasia and reflux oesophagitis

Achalasia of the cardia is by no means rare in Africa (Badoe, 1966; Davey, 1968). Bilateral parotid hypertrophy (Chapter 1) is apparently frequently related to the disease in Ibadan, Nigeria; that is presumably associated with the resulting nutritional deficit.

A chest radiograph taken after a drink of water will give suggestive information in at least 50 per cent of cases; the mediastinum is widened and contains a fluid-level, and the gastric air bubble is absent. Achalasia-like deformities of the oesophagus due to carcinoma are also common and must be distinguished in most cases, by oesophagoscopy and biopsy.

Oesophagocardiomyotomy (Heller's operation) is the only curative procedure. Repeated oesophagoscopy and dilation may be used but in tropical countries the patient usually lives too far away to be able to attend for frequent treatment.

3.2. Carcinoma of the oesophagus (CO)

From a clinical viewpoint oesophageal carcinoma in the tropics is similar to that in the western world (Avery Jones, Gummer, and Lennard-Jones, 1968), apart from the fact that it is young men who are principally involved.

The incidence rate of oesophageal carcinoma varies greatly in different areas (Doll, 1967). Even in developed countries the differences in incidence rate are striking. For example in 1962, oesophageal cancer rates for men were 2.8 and 11.2 per 100 000 in Australia and France respectively; similarly, in women the respective rates were 0·9 and 5·5 in United States whites and in Finland (Oettlé, 1962). Apart from the marked geographical variations, a marked rise in incidence was noted in Africa after the second World War (Rose, 1965). Oettlé (1964) indicated that Cape Town, Bulawayo, Nairobi, and Mombasa were high-frequency areas. Burrell (1957) showed in East London that oesophageal cancer patients were clustered around *shebeens* (illicit spirit liquor stores).

In some parts of Africa the disease is exceedingly common; Kenya, eastern Zambia, and Malawi have the highest incidence rates. It accounts for very many hospital admissions. In the Transkei too, it has reached almost epidemic proportions (Burrell, 1957; 1962). It is however relatively unusual in west and north Africa.

It is also one of the commonest of tumours in China where its incidence rate differs in different provinces (Li, Kao, and Wu, 1962); although very common in Chinese living in Singapore, it is rarely seen in Chinese in Hawaii. It is a common tumour also in Chile, Assam, Jamaica, Curaçao, Brazil, Puerto Rico, Japan, Kazakhstan, and the USSR (Edington and Gilles, 1976).

It is usually a squamous carcinoma and involves the middle and lower part of the oesophagus. Smoking, alcohol, contamination of alcoholic drinks by asphalt, metal polish, and other toxins, and the ingestion of hot foods have all been suggested as aetiological agents.

3.2.1. Distribution of CO

The disease usually occurs in the middle and lower thirds of the oesophagus (Palmer, 1967); clinical diagnosis is usually reliable (Oettlé, 1962; Palmer, 1967), and radiology is virtually 100 per cent accurate. As the disease is well and easily recognized in the areas of the tropics where it is very common and known to carry a very bad prognosis, people usually die at home and reported frequency rates are doubtless too low (McGlashan, 1972); in addition many Africans are fatalists.

In several parts of the world the incidence of this malignancy is obviously unusually high, and can vary by as much as 300-fold in different countries (Doll, 1977; *Lancet*, 1978). Field studies show furthermore, that the epidemiological picture can alter very sharply over very short distances (*Lancet*, 1975). The highest rates are reported in eastern and southern regions of Africa, parts of Asia, and Curaçao, and parts of Brazil.

Africa. Sub-Saharan Africa was the first area to be investigated in detail. Several early reports referred to the high incidence rate of the disease in Kenya (Jarvis, 1935; Nevill, 1961; Linsell and Martyn, 1962; Whittaker, 1964).

Burrell (1957) working in South Africa considered that oesophageal carcinoma in Africans was associated with the brewing of illicit beer in old 44-gallon tar-drums which had originally contained asphalt and fuel-oil residues; however tar-drums are certainly not used throughout the whole of tropical Africa! In a large retrospective radiological study in Dar-es-Salaam, Tanzania, Grech (1965) found an incidence of 3 per cent for oesophageal carcinoma in 733 cases examined for dyspepsia. One case was in the upper one-third, 11 in the middle one-third and 10 in the lower one-third; they were usually squamous-cell carcinomas. The Transkei, parts of Zimbabwe Rhodesia, and western Kenya also have very high incidence rates; however it is unusual in west Africa (Ahmed and Cook, 1969; Cook, 1971; Cook and Burkitt, 1971; Warwick and Harington, 1973). In several high incidence areas there is evidence that the disease has become common only during the last 20 to 30 years. There is a marked local variation in incidence in different parts of east Africa (Hutt and Burkitt, 1965). Ahmed (1966) has given a detailed account of the geographical distribution of cancer within Kenya; the highest incidence rates are in west Kenya where it is the most common form of cancer (Edsmyr, Onyango, Tole and Willey, 1973), and around Mount Kenya. Diet, alcohol consumption, smoking habits, water supply, and soil composition were also investigated by Ahmed (1966) but no evidence of an aetiological agent was forthcoming. In a radiological study, Whittaker (1965) confirmed a high incidence in Nairobi.

Asia. In Central Asia, the epidemiology is best documented in the southern Caspian littoral (*Lancet*, 1973; 1978; Kmet and Mahboubi, 1972; Mahboubi, Kmet, Cook, Day, Ghadirian, and Salmasizadeh, 1973). In north-east Iran very high incidence rates have also been reported, especially in women (McGlashan, 1972). The people in the high-risk groups have a Turkic or Mongol origin and are agriculturalists; they may be either semi-nomadic pastoralists or settled subsistence farmers. Sheep and goats are the main livestock and the crops are wheat, barley, and cotton,

China. In and around the Taihang mountains of north China, oesophageal cancer has produced epidemics of dysphagia (*keh shih ping*), and is the commonest cause of death in some areas. In 1959 the prevalence rate was 379 per 100 000 with an annual mortality rate of 100–150 per 100 000 which has remained fairly steady over the years; in England and Wales the equivalent annual mortality rate is about 6 per 100 000 (*Lancet*, 1975).

Papua New Guinea. There is also a relatively high incidence in Papua New Guinea where the disease is common in both sexes (Muirden, 1976).

3.2.2 Aetiology of CO

There seems no doubt that the cause of the disease varies from area to area. In Europe and America alcohol and tobacco are common aetiological agents. An association between oesophageal carcinoma and alcohol was not confirmed in a study in the urban Bantu population of Johannesburg (Higginson, 1963); that author also felt that smoking was not an important factor in Africa. In both north-east Iran (Mahboubi *et al*, 1973) and the Transkei (Rose, 1973) the incidence of oesophageal carcinoma is very high in both sexes; in Iran, alcohol and tobacco clearly play a negligible role aetiologically (Joint IARC/Iran study group, 1977). In both of those areas, both sexes ingest mutagens. In north-east Iran, opium addiction is widespread; crude opium and opium dross (*sukhteh*) are eaten in large amounts. In one study, morphine was detected in the urine of 50 per cent of people over 35 years of age (Hewer, Rose, Ghadirian, Castegnaro, Malaveille, Bartsch, and Day, 1978). Poorer groups, who are at high risk from oesophageal carcinoma, take opium orally rather than by smoking it for economic reasons. In the Transkei, tobacco residues from the bowl or stem of the pipe are either eaten or chewed; smoking and the use of home-grown tobacco are the only environmental factors which can be associated with the high incidence of oesophageal carcinoma in both sexes (Rose,

1973). Samples of opium dross in north-east Iran, and tobacco-pipe residues in the Transkei, have been tested for mutagenic activity in strains of *Salmonella typhimurium* in the presence of rat liver microsomes (Hewer *et al*., 1978); all of the samples showed significant mutagenic activity. However, that study did not rule out the possibility of genetic factors also being involved.

Burrell, Roach, and Shadwell (1966) emphasized that soil-plant relationships were possible aetiological factors in the Transkei; deficiencies of molybdenum, copper, and manganese were common in the soil in high incidence areas. It was considered that that might lead to growth of plants less resistant to fungal infections. The possible role of zinc as a causative agent has also been raised (McGlashan, 1967). In central Africa a geographical pathology survey was made from the University of Zambia in 1965; data were collected from a network of 103 hospitals (McGlashan, 1968). There, the disease seemed to correlate geographically with the drinking of locally distilled spirit; whereas no oesophageal cancer was reported from areas where cassava is the staple food, the disease was common where maize was the staple (McGlashan and Bond, 1970). *Kachasu* is distilled from maize and sugar in local, crudely-made equipment (McGlashan, 1969); historically, it seems possible that that form of distillation was taken into south-central Africa along the Shire river valleys by the early Portuguese explorers. Although many samples of *Kachasu* were heavily contaminated with zinc and copper, the finding of small amounts of dimethyl-N-nitrosamine in some Zambian samples at a concentration of three parts per million, which is a level likely to prove pathogenic to man, was of considerable interest (McGlashan, Walters, and McLean, 1968); that compound can also cause liver and oesophageal cancer in experimental animals (Magee and Barnes, 1956; 1967). In other African countries also, including Ghana, Nigeria, Senegal, Kenya and Uganda, dimethyl-N-nitrosamine was found in illicitly distilled spirits (McGlashan, 1972); commercially bottled alcoholic spirits were shown to be free of that compound (McGlashan, Patterson, and Williams, 1970). Dimethylnitrosamine is present in the juice of *Solanum incanum*, which is an added component of African diets in South Africa (Du Plessis, Nunn and Roach, 1969).

A suggestion that formation of nitrosamines *in vivo*, with their subsequent excretion in saliva and gastric juice, might be important has not been confirmed (Lowenfels, Tuyns, Walker, and Roussel, 1978).

In north-east Iran, alcohol, tobacco, and local plants and herbs can be excluded, as can cooking techniques. Bread and tea are staples in the high incidence areas; there is also a low calorie and protein, vitamin A, riboflavin, and vitamin C intake. Morphine is both smoked and eaten in the high incidence areas. There is no evidence however of carcinogens in the bread and tea, although the grain is frequently contaminated by fungi. Overall, the restricted diet, and possibly the chronic morphine consumption, seem to be the most important factors in that area. Also in northern Iran, grape-vinegar is prepared by a fermentation process, which is apparently contaminated with dimethyl-N-nitrosamine. The women of the Turkoman tribe eat a mixture of raisins, crushed with pomegranate seeds and black peppercorns (*anarteen*) which too is contaminated with that compound (McGlashan, 1970). In the very high incidence areas in China, there is again no clearly discernable carcinogen. In that area however, domestic chickens also have gullet cancer (*Lancet*, 1975). That strongly suggests an environmental factor—either chemical or fungal.

In Sri Lanka, women are more often affected than men (Stephen and Uragoda, 1970); as in Iran that is an unusual sex ratio and it seems possible that betel nut chewing is aetiologically important.

There is evidence that concentrations of dimethyl-N-nitrosamine have been over-estimated by the methods used in some of the studies; the significance of that work should therefore be critically evaluated.

3.2.3 Presentation of CO

Mean age of presentation is in the fifth and sixth decades for male and females respectively; however young patients are often affected in the third decade. Dysphagia is the predominant symptom; it is progressive and ultimately prevents the swallowing of liquids. It is worthwhile to watch the patient while he drinks; undue noise and/or delay frequently indicate oesophageal stenosis. Epigastric pain as a presenting symptom occurs however at a surprisingly high frequency rate and attention may be directed away from the oesophagus (Davey, 1968). Retrosternal pain and an unproductive cough are other possible presenting symptoms. Weight loss which is often severe occurs as the disease progresses. It is often impossible on clinical and radiological grounds to distinguish the lesion from a carcinoma of the gastric fundus (Chapter 4).

3.2.4. Pathology of CO

The tumour is invariably a squamous-cell carcinoma; the thoracic portion of the oesophagus is primarily affected. The sites of the tumour are (Edington and Gilles, 1976): (i) cervical oesophagus (subcricoid, but above the sternal notch); (ii) thoracic oesophagus not involving the cardia; and (iii) distal oesophagus involving the cardia. If there is substantial gastric involvement, the tumour should be regarded as of gastric origin unless it can be shown to be a squamous-cell carcinoma. International agreement has been reached on the histological typing of oesophageal tumours (Oota and Sobin, 1977).

3.2.5. Investigation of CO

A barium-swallow is the major diagnostic technique (Whittaker, 1964); a sharp shelf-like effect is seen which distinguishes it from achalasia of the cardia (Fig. 3.1). The diagnosis can be confirmed by oesophagoscopy and biopsy, or by cytological diagnosis. In over 50 per cent of cases the diagnosis can be suspected from a plain chest radiograph (Levy, 1966a); there may be either changes in the mediastinum, e.g. a tumour mass, a dilated oesophagus or air in the oesophagus, or changes in the lung fields due to aspiration of swallowed material (Levy, 1966b). A simple brush-cytology method has been found to be of value in mass-screening, for the early detection of oesophageal carcinoma on the Caspian littoral (Dowlatshahi, Daneshbod and Mobarhan, 1978).

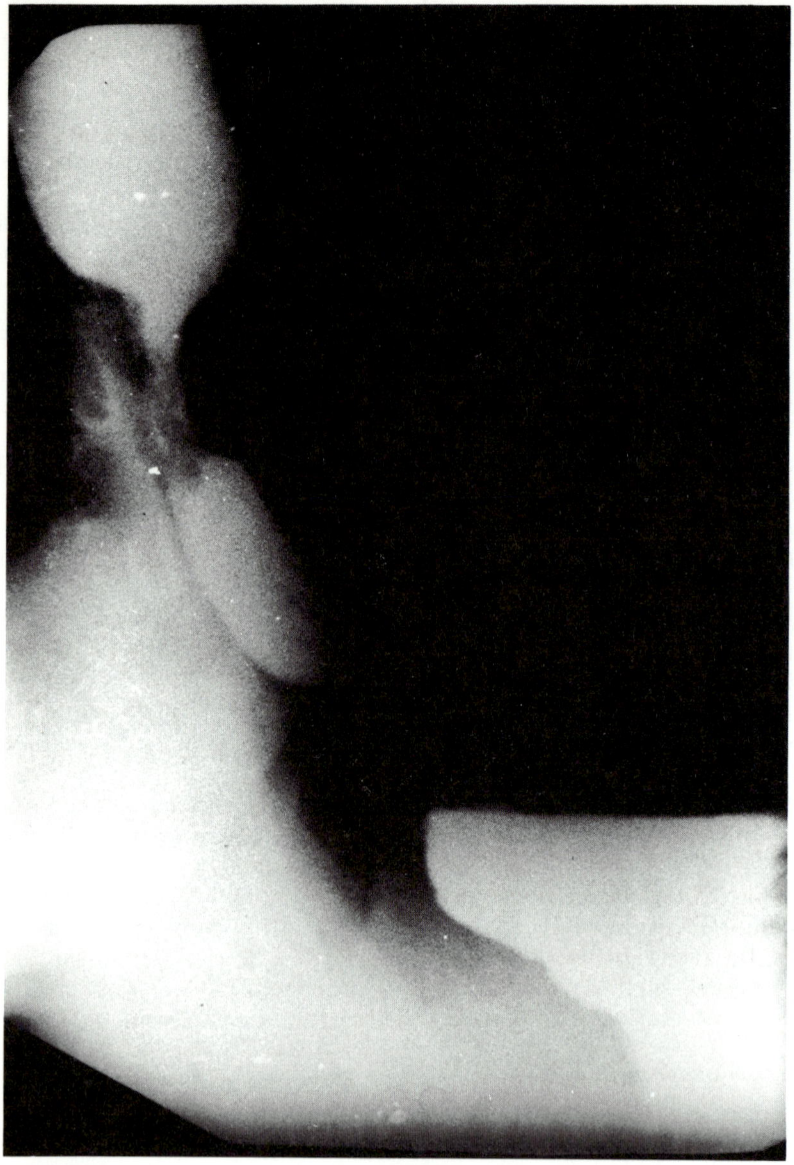

FIG. 3.1. Barium swallow in a 58-year-old Papua New Guinean woman who presented with epigastric pain and was subsequently admitted to hospital with a haematemesis. An oesophageal carcinoma was demonstrated at laparotomy.

3.2.6. Treatment of CO

If available, radiotherapy is the best form of treatment for proximal lesions (Edsmyr, Onyango, Tole, and Willey, 1973). Tumours of the lower half of the oesophagus can sometimes be treated successfully by resection and oesophagogastrostomy or by jejunal or colonic interpositions; the lesion is usually too far advanced in tropical countries, however, for such a procedure to be possible. A palliative procedure, which usually consists of passing a tube, orally, through the narrowed portion of the oesophagus, is usually the only form of treatment which is possible (MacArthur and Mercer, 1969; Takita, 1971; Palmer, 1973). Celestin's tubes tend however to block on an African diet (Davey, 1968) and on many bulky diets in tropical countries. Such tubes are often too short to pass through the long tubular growth. Gastrostomy improves nutrition but does not prolong survival; the inability of completely obstructed patients to swallow even saliva makes the operation of limited value. Cytotoxic agents have overall not been proved to be of value in the treatment of this tumour.

An initial favourable response has been claimed with intramuscular bleomycin (30 mg twice weekly for four weeks) given either alone or in conjunction with radiotherapy (Edsmyr, Knight, Miller, Nevill, Onyango, Bodo, and Levin, 1973).

3.3. Oesophageal varices

This is probably the commonest lesion affecting the oesophagus in most parts of the third world; the only real rival for a higher frequency rate is oesophageal carcinoma.

Although data are limited it seems probable that most gastrointestinal haemorrhage in Africa and Asia is due to bleeding oesophageal varices. Diagnosis is made by barium-swallow (Fig. 3.2) or oesophagoscopy. The causes of portal hypertension are listed in Chapter 11. There are no distinguishing features between oesophageal varices in tropical countries compared with those in the western world.

3.4. Infections of the oesophagus

3.4.1. Viral infections

Smallpox. Oesophageal lesions were relatively common in this disease when it frequently occurred in tropical countries; the lesions are similar to the cutaneous manifestations of the disease.

3.4.2. Bacterial infections

Bacterial infections of the oesophagus are rare. Occasionally tuberculosis and syphilis may produce oesophageal lesions (Morson and Dawson, 1972).

3.4.3. Mycotic infections

Moniliasis (candidiasis) is an occasional sequel to oral infection with that organism, especially in malnourished and debilitated people (Morson and Dawson, 1972). Fungi of the species, *Rhizopus, Absidia,* and *Mucor* can produce oesophageal lesions (usually predominantly ulceration), especially in malnourished children.

3.4.4. Parasitic infections

Chagas' oesophagitis. Mega-oesophagus may be a result of chronic *Trypanosoma cruzi* infection (Jung, 1959; Ferreira-Santos, 1961; Scherb and Arias, 1962).

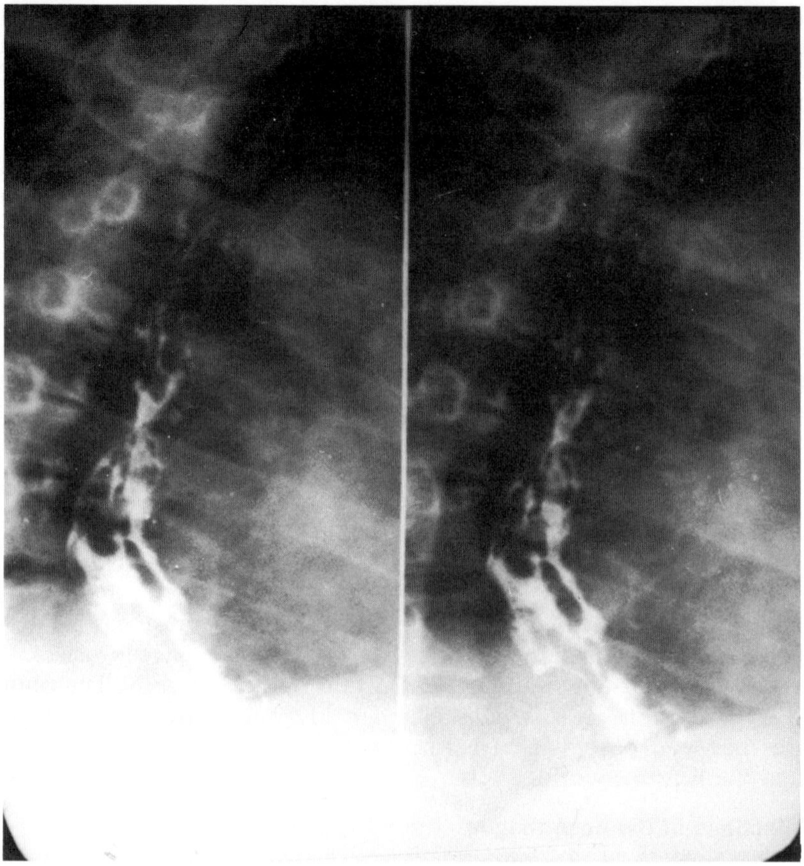

FIG. 3.2. Barium swallow in a 35-year-old Papua New Guinean man. Presentation was with haematemesis and melaena. A diagnosis of macronodular cirrhosis was made. A portacaval anastomosis was performed, but he died in hepatic coma shortly after operation.

The basic lesion is a degeneration of the intraluminal autonomic nervous plexuses secondary to the toxic action of the parasite. Extensive experimental studies have given support to the role played by *T. cruzi* in this lesion (Köberle, 1958). *T. cruzi* infections can be transmitted in blood from seemingly healthy donors; in São Paulo, Brazil, 2 per cent of donors may be infected (Edington and Gilles, 1976). It is thus of the utmost importance to screen donors in infected areas.

Dysphagia is the usual symptom.*

Chest radiographs show marked mediastinal widening after oral food or

* It has been seriously suggested that Charles Darwin contracted this disease during his travels to South America in *H.M.S. Beagle* (Adler, 1959). His frequent bouts of dysphagia, nausea and vomiting in subsequent years and the added possibility of myocardial disease made this a theoretical possibility in the minds of some medical historians. However, careful evaluation of Darwin's symptoms in later years does not apparently substantiate that possibility (Woodruff, 1968).

fluid. The grossly widened organ can be visualized on barium-swallow examination. This oesophageal lesion only occurs in the chronic form of the disease and it is very unusual to find parasites of *T. cruzi* in the peripheral blood. A compliment-fixation test may be positive in up to 95 per cent of cases; xenodiagnosis gives a variable positivity rate.

There is to date no satisfactory treatment for the disease. Mega-oesophagus is an irreversible lesion.

3.5. Miscellaneous conditions involving the oesophagus

3.5.1. Tropical malabsorption (TM)

Oesophageal lesions were previously common in this disease. However cases seen today are usually much more mild than in the past and significant abnormalities are probably now unusual (Cook, 1978). Hillary (1766) reported 'burning heat about the cardia, or upper mouth of the stomach' in TM. Oesophageal pain was emphasized by Manson-Bahr and Willoughby (1930). Morphological changes similar to those in the tongue and mouth were reported by Thin (1890), Brown (1908), Begg (1912), and Rogers (1913).

3.5.2. Paterson–Brown–Kelly syndrome and post-cricoid carcinoma

Both of these entities are uncommon despite the very high incidence of severe iron-deficiency anaemia in tropical countries. Similarly koilonychia is uncommon. The reason for that is unknown.

References

ADLER, S. (1959). *Nature, Lond.*, **184,** 1102.

AMHED, N. (1966). *E. Afr. med. J.*, **43,** 235.

—— and COOK, P. (1969). *Br. J. Cancer*, **23,** 302.

AVERY JONES, F., GUMMER, J. W. P., and LENNARD-JONES, J. E. (1968). *Clinical Gastroenterology*, 2nd ed. p. 343. Blackwell, Oxford and Edinburgh.

BADOE, E. A. (1966). *Ghana med. J.*, **5,** 17.

BEGG, C. (1912). *Sprue: its diagnosis and treatment.* Wright and Sons, Bristol.

BROWN, W. C. (1908). *Sprue and its treatment.* John Bale, Sons and Danielsson, London.

BURRELL, R. J. W. (1957). *S. Afr. med. J.*, **31,** 401.

—— (1962). *J. natn. Cancer Inst.*, **28,** 495.

——, ROACH, W. A., and SHADWELL, A. (1966). *J. natn. Cancer Inst.*, **36,** 201.

COOK, G. C. (1978). *Jl. R. Coll. Phycns.*, **12,** 329.

COOK, P. (1971). *Br. J. Cancer*, **25,** 853.

COOK, P. J. and BURKITT, D. P. (1971). *Br. med. Bull.*, **27,** 14.

DAVEY, W. W. (1968). *Companion to surgery in Africa.* p. 174. Livingstone, Edinburgh and London.

DOLL, R. (1967). *Prevention of cancer: pointers from epidemiology.* Nuffield Provincial Hospitals Trust, Oxford.

—— (1977). *Nature, Lond.*, **265,** 589.

DOWLATSHAHI, K., DANESHBOD, A., and MOBARHAN, S. (1978). *Lancet,* **1,** 125.

DU PLESSIS, L. S., NUNN, J. R., and ROACH, W. A. (1969). *Nature, Lond.*, **222,** 1198.

EDINGTON, G. M. and GILLES, H. M. (1976). *Pathology in the tropics.* 2nd ed. pp. 481, 536. Edward Arnold, London.

EDSMYR, F., KNIGHT, E. O. W., MILLER, J., NEVILL, G., ONYANGO, J., BODO, J., and LEVIN, A. (1973). *E. Afr. med. J.*, **50,** 449.

——, Onyango, J., Tole, N., and Willey, B. (1973). *E. Afr. med. J.*, **50,** 454.
Ferreira-Santos, R. (1961). *Am. J. dig. Dis.*, **6,** 700.
Grech, P. (1965). *E. Afr. med. J.*, **42,** 106.
Hewer, T., Rose, E., Ghadirian, P., Castegnaro, M., Malaveille, C., Bartsch, H., and Day, N. (1978). *Lancet*, **2,** 494.
Higginson, J. (1963). In *Geographical variations in observed frequencies of cancer of different sites* in *Cancer Progress.* (ed. R. W. Raven). p. 76. Butterworths, London.
Hillary, W. (1766). *Observations on the changes of the air and the concomitant epidemical diseases, in the island of Barbadoes.* 2nd ed. p. 276. Hawes, Clarke and Collins, London.
Hutt, M. S. R. and Burkitt, D. P. (1965). *Br. med. J.*, **2,** 719.
Jarvis, J. F. (1935). *E. Afr. med. J.*, **30,** 522.
Joint, I. A R. C./Iran study group (1977). *J. natn. Cancer Inst.*, **59,** 1127.
Jung, R. C. (1959). *Am. J. Gastroent.*, **32,** 311.
Kmet, J. and Mahboubi, E. (1972). *Science, N.Y.*, **175,** 846.
Köberle, F. (1958). *Gastroenterology*, **34,** 460.
Lancet (1973). **2,** 1365.
—— (1975). **1,** 1413.
—— (1978). **1,** 641.
Leegard, T. (1945). *J. Lar. Otol.,* **60,** 389.
Levy, J. I. (1966a). *S. Afr. J. Radiol.*, **4,** 1.
—— (1966b). *S. Afr. J. Radiol.*, **4,** 5.
Li, K. H., Kao, J. C., and Wu, Y. K. (1962). *China med. J.*, **81,** 489.
Linsell, C. A. and Martyn, R. (1962). *E. Afr. med. J.,* **39,** 642.
Lowenfels, A. B., Tuyns, A. J., Walker, E. A., and Roussel, A. (1978). *Gut*, 19, 199.
MacArthur, A. and Mercer, J. L. (1969). *Thorax*, **24,** 39.
McGlashan, N. D. (1967). *Lancet*, **1,** 578.
—— (1968). *Med. Jl. Zambia*, **2,** 17.
—— (1969). *Gut*, **10,** 643.
—— (1970). *Int. pathol.*, **11,** 50.
—— (1972). In *Medical geography.* (ed. N. D. McGlashan). p. 247. Methuen and Co, London.
—— and Bond, D. H. (1970). *Can. Geogr.*, **14,** 243.
——, Patterson, R. L. S. and Williams, A. A. (1970). *Lancet*, **2,** 1138.
——, Walters, C. L. and McLean, A. E. M. (1968). *Lancet*, **2,** 1017.
Magee, P. N. and Barnes, J. M. (1956). *Br. J. Cancer*, **10,** 114.
—— —— (1967). *Adv. Cancer Res.*, **10,** 163.
Mahboubi, E., Kmet, J., Cook, P. J., Day, N. E., Ghadirian, P., and Salmasizadeh, S. (1973). *Br. J. Cancer*, **28,** 197.
Manson-Bahr, P. and Willoughby, H. (1930). *Q. Jl. Med.*, **23,** 411.
Marchand, P. (1952). *Br. J. Radiol.*, **25,** 476.
—— (1954). *S. Afr. med. J.,* **28,** 415.
—— (1955a). *S. Afr. med. J.,* **29,** 195.
—— (1955b). *Thorax*, **10,** 171.
Marks, I. N., Bank, S., Werbeloff, L., Farman, J. and Louw, J. H. (1963). *Am. J. dig. Dis.*, **8,** 509.
Martinson, F. D. (1967). *J. Nig. med. Ass.*, **1,** 16.
—— (1978). *Tropical Doctor,* **8,** 123.
Morson, B. C. and Dawson, I. M. P. (1972). *Gastrointestinal pathology*. p. 19. Blackwell, Oxford, London, Edinburgh and Melbourne.
Muirden, J. C. (1976). *Papua New Guin. med. J.*, **19,** 149.
Nevill, G. (1961). *E. Afr. med. J.*, **38,** 515.
Oettlé, A. G. (1962). *S. Afr. Cancer Bull.*, **6,** 112.

—— (1964). *J. natn. Cancer Inst.*, **33,** 383.
OOTA, K. and SOBIN, L. H. (1977). *Histological typing of gastric and oesophageal tumours.* W.H.O., Geneva.
PALMER, E. D. (1973). *Am. J. Gastroent., N.Y.*, **59,** 487.
PALMER, P. E. S. (1967). *Natn. Cancer Inst. Monograph*, no. 25.
ROGERS, L. (1913). *Dysenteries. Their differentiation and treatment.* p. 303. Oxford University Press, London.
ROSE, E. F. (1965). *S. Afr. med. J.,* **39,** 1098.
—— (1973). *J. natn. Cancer Inst.*, **51,** 7.
SCHERB, J. and ARIAS, I. M. (1962). *Gastroenterology*, **43,** 212.
STEPHEN, S. J. and URAGODA, C. G. (1970). *Br. J. Cancer*, **24,** 11.
TAKITA, H. (1971). *N.Y. St. J. Med*, **71,** 2526.
THIN, G. (1890). *Br. med. J.*, **1,** 1357.
WARWICK, G. P. and HARINGTON. J. S. (1973). *Adv. Cancer Res.*, **17,** 82.
WHITTAKER, L. R. (1964). *E. Afr. med. J.*, **41,** 430.
—— (1965). *E. Afr. med. J.*, **43,** 336.
WOODRUFF, A. W. (1968). *Bull. N.Y. Acad. Med.*, **44,** 146.

4

The stomach and duodenum

DISEASES of the stomach are uncommon in Africa and most of Asia; there is some evidence for localized high incidence rates of benign gastric ulcer. Duodenal ulcer, contrary to reports a few years ago, is common in all parts of the tropics; there is limited evidence that it is more common in urban areas and that its incidence is increasing further. However, accurate incidence rates for diseases which are not immediately fatal are exceedingly difficult to obtain in most third-world countries. Both of those diseases can be expected to occur in Asian and African patients seen in the United Kingdom and the USA.

Other diseases of the stomach, when they occur, do not seem to have any significant differences from those in non-tropical countries (Avery Jones, Gummer, and Lennard-Jones, 1968; Morson and Dawson, 1972).

4.1. Gastric physiology

4.1.1. Gastric acid

Gastric acid production and secretion curves seem to be very similar for normal Nigerians (Rose, 1935; Tai da Rocha-Afodu and Adesola, 1976), Kenyans (Wasunna, Wakhisi, Anabwani, Mukuria, and Roy, 1973), Chinese (Fung, 1970), and Englishmen; stimulated acid output may be slightly lower in Nigerians.

However, in malnutrition, in children especially, basal-acid production is reduced (Gracey, Cullity, Suharjono, and Sunoto, 1977). Low gastric acid production has been incriminated in individual susceptibility to cholera and other acid-sensitive bacterial infections of the gastrointestinal tract (Nalin, Levine, Levine, Hoover, Bergquist, McLaughlin, Libonati, Alam, and Hornick, 1978); that study has clearly shown in American volunteers that hypochlorhydria predisposes to, and is not a result of cholera. Whereas beer increases acid production and decreases the likelihood of severe cholera and other acute diarrhoeal diseases, including travellers' diarrhoea, cannabis smoking reduces acid production and predisposes to invasion with acid-sensitive pathogens (Nalin, Levine, Rhead, Bergquist, Rennels, Hughes, O'Donnell, and Hornick, 1978).

Low gastric acid production has been recorded in tropical malabsorption (TM) (Chapter 20) in the presence of a varying degree of gastritis and mucosal atrophy; however, no relationship has been noted between acid concentrations and the severity of the gastric and intestinal lesions (Vaish, Sampathkumar,

Jacob, and Baker, 1965). It seems possible that individuals with depressed gastric acid production, in some possibly associated with an alcoholic gastritis, are prone to develop TM. There could also be a genetic factor involved.

In Nigerians with duodenal ulcer, free hydrochloric acid concentrations tend to be high (Konstam, 1955). High maximal gastric acid output was also found in patients with duodenal ulcer in Uganda (Dutt and Kajubi, 1972). Basal gastric acid output was found to be high in Ugandan university students with dyspepsia (Dutt, 1973).

4.1.2. Gastrin production

Fasting and postprandial plasma gastrin concentrations were estimated in 54 Ugandan adults, who had no evidence of gastrointestinal disease (Gjesing, 1975); the results were similar to those in normal people in other parts of the world. Plasma gastrin concentrations were measured in patients with hepatic schistosomiasis in Khartoum (Boulos, Okosdonossian, Elmunshid, ElMasri, Hassan, and Hobsley, 1978); there was no significant difference when compared with controls.

The Zollinger–Ellison syndrome is occasionally encountered; its features are the same as elsewhere.

4.2. Gastritis and widespread mucosal disease

4.2.1. Acute and chronic gastritis

Many patients in tropical countries present with epigastric pain (Braun, 1965). Undoubtedly gastritis accounts for some of them, but owing to the rarity of gastroscopic studies in tropical countries it is impossible at present to know the true situation (Wagner and Shepherd, 1976). Alcoholic gastritis seems to be common in many African countries.

Like corrosive oesophagitis, gastritis is seen fairly frequently in many African countries (Chapter 3). This may be either accidental or a suicide attempt (Marks, Bank, Werbeloff, Farman, and Louw, 1963). Hypertrophic gastropathy (Menetrier's disease) has been described in a 15-year-old Kikuyu boy in Kenya (Mwangemi, 1975); presentation was with severe anaemia. Due to its association with malignancy, laparotomy is indicated.

4.2.2. Addisonian pernicious anaemia

A true pernicious anaemia is uncommon in most tropical countries, possibly because all diseases of an autoimmune nature are rarely seen. It has however been reported in Asians (Jayaratnam, Seah, da Costa, Tan, and O'Brien, 1967) and Africans (Chuke, Traub, and Patel, 1972). Gastric atrophy and gastric resection can also give rise to inadequate amounts of intrinsic factor.

4.2.3. The stomach in tropical malabsorption (TM)

There is little precise knowledge on gastric structure or function in TM (see above). In severe cases it seems clear that changes are present which are similar to those in the mouth and oesophagus (Cook, 1978). Brown (1908) and Rogers (1913) referred to shallow ulcers and congested patches in the stomach in that condition.

4.2.4. Hiatus hernia and reflux oesophagitis

In east Africa, two radiological investigations have shown an extremely low incidence of hiatus hernia in Africans (Grech, 1965; Moore, 1967). In an analysis of 1023 barium meals at the Port Moresby General Hospital, Muirden (1976) found only two cases of hiatus hernia in Papua New Guineans. Those observations seem to agree with all workers in tropical countries, although it must be stressed that with limited radiological facilities and more acute problems, searches for hiatus hernia have probably not taken place at much depth. As more sophisticated life styles become more common and obesity becomes a real problem it seems highly likely that hiatus hernia will become far more common.

Reflux oesophagitis does not seem to be a great problem in tropical countries.

4.3. Specific infections of the stomach

4.3.1. Viral infections

Small pox. Gastric lesions similar to those seen on the skin were common in days gone by when smallpox was such a very common tropical infection.

4.3.2. Bacterial infections

Shigellosis (bacillary dysentery). Haemorrhagic lesions have been described in the stomach and duodenum in shigellosis.

Typhoid and paratyphoid fevers. The major lesions in these diseases involve the distal ileum. However, a much greater length of gastrointestinal tract may be involved. Ulcers have been reported as high as the stomach in paratyphoid B infections (Edington and Gilles, 1976).

Anthrax of the stomach. Anthrax, a disease caused by *Bacillus anthracis*, can cause acute small intestinal disease if insufficiently cooked, infected meat is eaten. Very rarely the stomach may be involved; a case of primary anthrax of the stomach with massive ascites has been described in an Iranian woman (Dutz, Saidi, and Kohout, 1970).

Relapsing fever. Haemorrhage from the stomach may occur in both tick-borne and louse-borne relapsing fevers (Chapter 7) as a result of thrombocytopenia.

Tuberculosis. Gastric involvement is a rare presentation of tuberculosis (El Masri, Boulos, and Malick, 1977). Gastrointestinal tuberculosis usually involves the ileocaecal region (Chapter 23).

Syphilis. This is a rare disease of the stomach (Morson and Dawson, 1972).

4.3.3. Mycotic infections

Moniliasis occasionally occurs, usually associated with an oesophageal infection (Morson and Dawson, 1972). Mucormycosis due to fungi of the species, *Rhizopus*, *Absidia*, and *Mucor* can produce gastric lesions, usually ulceration, especially in malnourished children.

4.3.4. Parasitic infections

Schistosomiasis. Occasionally ova of *Schistosoma mansoni, S. japonicum* and *S. haematobium*, produce pseudotubercle formation and scarring, and are seen in the stomach. Pyloric obstruction has been described in *S. japonicum* infections (Nai-Kuang and Pen-Ching, 1957).

Chagas' disease. Mega-oesophagus has been considered in Chapter 3. A rare complication of *Trypanosoma cruzi* infection is enlargement of the stomach which results from a disturbance of the myenteric plexus. The disease is a chronic manifestation of South American trypanosomiasis and a history of exposure there is necessary for a diagnosis of Chagas' disease of the stomach to be considered.

Eosinophilic granuloma of the pyloric antrum. This is a granulomatous condition of unknown cause which can affect almost any part of the small or large intestine; the commonest site is the pyloric antrum (Edington and Gilles, 1976). The most likely cause is an infection with either the nematode *Eustoma rotundatum* (Ashby, Appleton, and Dawson, 1964), or other parasites—the species differing in different parts of the world. Pathologically, there is diffuse or focal eosinophilic infiltration of the intestine. The lesions may be diffuse or localised; they may be polypoid. Ulceration is unusual.

Histologically there is a massive submucosal invasion with eosinophils; the muscularis may be invaded but not the serosa. The mucosa is usually left intact. Oedema and blood vessel congestion and lymphatic dilatation may be present and fragments of larvae may be identified. A peripheral eosinophilia may occur; macrocytic anaemia has occasionally been described before the onset of symptoms. Corticosteroids are said to be of value in management.

4.4. Gastric ulcer (GU)

4.4.1 Distribution and aetiology of GU

The incidence of this disease is much lower in all parts of the developing world than duodenal ulcer; in fact, although almost a rarity in some countries, it has been reported from all parts of Africa (Davey, 1968). It is possible that the disease is more uncommon in west than east Africa. When it does occur, there is really no significant difference in the disease from that in the western world. Impressions gained in the early years of the century have not changed and there can be no doubt of its low incidence rate. Most are prepyloric in position; nearly all show evidence of great chronicity with much fibrosis and narrowing of the lesser curvature. Gastric retention in the pyloric region (Balint and Spence, 1959) is common. Gastric ulcer involves men more than women and is a disease of the lower social strata; the majority of patients are in their fifth and sixth decades. Personal experience in Nigeria, Uganda, Zambia, and Saudi Arabia is consistent with most of the reports on the disease in tropical countries.

A low incidence of gastric ulcer was reported from Nigeria by Konstam (1954); during a nine-month period he did not see a single case at Ibadan. A radiological study by Barton and Cockshott (1961) from Ibadan also emphasized the rarity of gastric ulcers in west Africa. Nwokolo (1966) too has drawn attention to the rarity of gastric ulcer in southern Nigeria, and claimed that his article was the first to be devoted to that subject. At Ibadan, Nigeria, gastric ulcer is also very largely a disease associated with lower social strata (Amure and Elegbe, 1975). In western Uganda, where duodenal ulcer is common, gastric ulcer is also unusual. Taylor (1965) reported on five patients with the disease at Ankole; in three the ulcer was simple and in two it had penetrated the liver. In a post-mortem series at Kampala, over the period 1950 to 1961, a one per cent incidence of gastric ulcer was found; 63 cases were men and nine women (Taylor, 1965). Gastric ulcers have also been reported as being uncommon in Nairobi (Hansen and Daly, 1978); in that study, only 7·6 per cent of a series of cases admitted with acute gastrointestinal bleeding were shown with fibre-optic oesophagogastroduodenoscopy to have gastric ulcers.

In south India, the disease is apparently unusual.

Gastric ulcer seems however to be more common than would be expected in Papua New Guinea, especially the eastern highlands. In Goroka Base Hospital, 130 prepyloric and 90 lesser-curve ulcers were seen in a series of 317 patients with peptic ulcers during a three-year period (1973 to 1976) (Wagner and Shepherd, 1976). In a two-year period, Smith (1967) operated on 12 patients with gastric ulcer in the eastern highlands and Goroka, Shepherd (1975) operated on 128 patients with peptic ulcer disease, during a $3\frac{1}{2}$ year period, of whom at least 71 per cent had gastric ulcers; obstruction, haemorrhage, and perforation were the main indications for surgery. Also in Goroka, Wagner (1975) reported 194 patients with peptic ulcer in a 12-month period; there was a male predominance and 70 per cent had gastric ulcers. In a survey of 1023 barium meals carried out during a 30-month period at Port Moresby General Hospital, 27 cases of gastric ulcer were diagnosed, and that accounted for 15·5 per cent of abnormal investigations (Muirden, 1976); the disease was more common in men and was usually on the lesser curvature of the stomach.

4.4.2. Clinical aspects of GU

There are no significant differences from chronic gastric ulcer in western countries, apart from the fact that gastric retention seems to be more common, presumably a feature of chronicity. Pyloric obstruction must be distinguished from pyloric carcinoma, the effects of corrosives (Marks, Barb, Webeloff, Farman, and Louw, 1963) (Chapter 3), and compression by tuberculous glands around the superior mesenteric vessels, which can occlude the third part of the duodenum (Davey and Pearson, 1965). Nwokolo (1966) reported 36 cases between 1959 and 1964 in Nigeria; there were twice as many males and the peak age was between 40 and 60 years. Most were from unskilled or semi skilled groups. The mean duration of symptoms was 4·7 years. Pain was usually epigastric, and in 53 per cent was made worse by food; 81 per cent had had repeated vomiting at some time. Massive haemorrhage complicated 8 per cent and perforation 30 per cent; pyloric stenosis occurred in 30 per cent.

Investigations are as difficult as those for duodenal ulcer (see below) in many parts of the tropics. Only base hospitals and hospitals in major cities usually have X-ray equipment which is adequate for barium meal examinations, and few have personal experience of that technique. The feasibility of using a fibre-optic gastroscope in a 'bush hospital' has been evaluated (Wierman and Snyder, 1978); working in such a hospital in Rwanda, those authors found the procedure valuable and possible to carry out. It is nevertheless costly. Fig. 4.1 shows a large lesser curve gastric ulcer demonstrated on a barium meal.

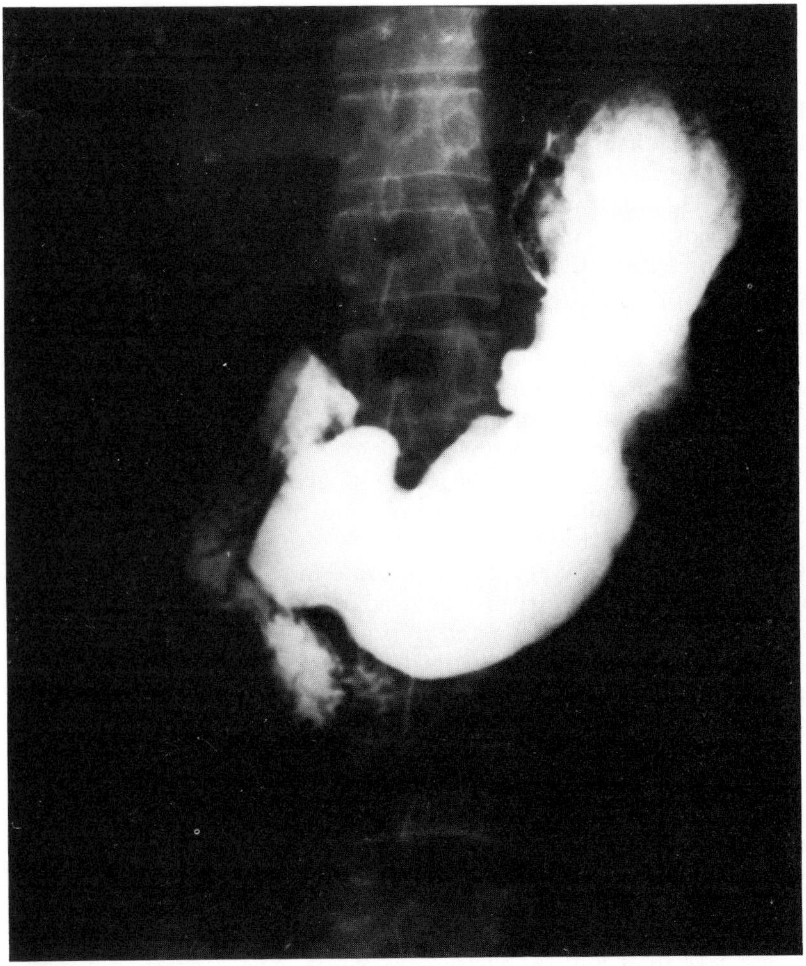

FIG. 4.1. Barium meal in a 54-year-old man from the Papua New Guinea highlands. A large lesser-curve ulcer is demonstrated. At surgery, the ulcer was shown to be benign and a Billroth-I gastrectomy was performed.

Carbenoxolone sodium ('Biogastrone') (Langman, 1968) is expensive and usually not readily available; if available it should be given orally, 100 mg thrice daily after meals for one week, and then 50 mg thrice daily until the ulcer has healed, i.e. some four to six weeks. Older less satisfactory therapeutic agents often have to be used, and regimes involving oral antacids and antispasmodics frequently provide symptomatic relief. It is always worthwhile to encourage cessation of smoking. Large quantities of milk in the diet are usually best avoided due to the very high incidence of adult hypolactasia in most parts of the tropics (Chapter 21). Complications of the disease usually require surgery.

4.5. Gastric carcinoma (GC)

4.5.1. Distribution and aetiology of GC

This is a less common tumour throughout the continents of Africa and Asia than it is in Europe; it is nevertheless widespread throughout the tropics. There are however considerable variations in incidence rates (Cook and Burkitt, 1971). It is, for example, more common in Ibadan, Nigeria where the frequency is 5·1 per cent of all malignancies (Edington and Maclean, 1965) than in Kampala, Uganda, and Maputo, Mozambique. In west Africa, the disease is generally not very common although there do seem to be local differences (Edington and Easmon, 1967). In Ghana, 67 cases were seen between 1956 and 65 at the Korle Bu Hospital, Accra (Badoe, 1966). In Nigeria, Blair (1923) did not see a case in 22 years, but Elmes and Baldwin (1947) found 22 cases in a retrospective analysis of 1000 pathological specimens sent to them from all over Nigeria, and Elebute, Ngu, Mainwaring, and Eruchalu (1963) described 86 patients with the disease at Ibadan between 1957 and 1961; in that series central and pyloric growths were most common, and the male : female ratio was 2·6 : 1·0. In northern Nigeria GC accounts for 2·4 per cent of all malignancies (Mabogunje, Subbuswamy, and Lawrie, 1978).

Davies (1959) reported that the disease was relatively common in Uganda, and that there was a very high incidence rate in the Kivu area. Differences in frequency at relatively short distances apart have been reported in Uganda (Templeton, 1973). In Rwanda and Burundi, and eastern Zaire it is said to be the commonest tumour in men; its frequency is also high around Mount Kilimanjaro. There is also a high frequency in parts of western Kenya and the West Lake province of Tanzania. It is an unusual cause of acute upper gastrointestinal bleeding in Nairobi, Kenya (Hansen and Daly, 1978), and that agrees with evidence from other endoscopy series; however those authors considered that gastric carcinoma was overall as great a problem in upper gastrointestinal bleeding as it is in the United Kingdom. In a large retrospective radiological study in Tanzania (733 cases), Grech (1965) found an incidence of 2·7 per cent for gastric carcinoma in patients X-rayed for dyspepsia.

Higginson and Oettlé (1960) reported that the incidence of gastric carcinoma was less than half in Africans in South Africa compared with USA negroes and whites, and Danish whites. In Johannesburg the hospital admission rate for gastric carcinoma in 1951 was 0·14 per 1000 in African patients and 0·86 per 1000 amongst Europeans (Charleswood and Frylinck, 1951). However UK migrants to South Africa seem to retain the gastric cancer rate experienced in Britain (McGlashan, 1972). There is a low rate in the Natal area.

In India, regional variations have been reported (Malhotra, 1967), but there and also in Singapore Chinese, the overall incidence is low.

Gastric carcinoma is one of the most common malignancies in Papua New

Guinea. Muirden (1967) found 14 cases of gastric carcinoma in Port Moresby, Papua New Guinea out of 1023 barium meals performed over a 30-month period; that accounted for eight per cent of abnormal investigations. In Madang, Braun (1965) found 17 gastric carinomas and 83 peptic ulcers in a 10-year period. The most frequent presentation is with pyloric obstruction (Wagner and Shepherd, 1976).

Methods for mapping morbidity and mortality rates for the disease in South Africa have been critically evaluated by McGlashan (1972); number of cases, or deaths, caused by the disease are usually compared with the number of people at risk in a given area. In a country with wide variations in population density, which is often the situation in the third world, that method inevitably leads to errors.

Apart from a significant relationship to blood group A, there seems to be no suggestion of a genetic or ethnic factor in the aetiology; like so many malignancies the cause doubtless lies in environmental factors. Relation to different dietary staples has been suggested, but not proved, in the aetiology in both India (Malhotra, 1967) and Uganda (Bijlsma, 1974). The carcinogenic effect of hydrocarbons in grilled or smoked meat or fish has been suggested as a factor in the western world and in Japan, where the disease is very common (Evans, Craven, Murphy, and Cleary, 1978), but there is little evidence. In Africa and Japan, pernicious anaemia is also uncommon.Alcohol, smoking, and vitamin A deficiency have all been suggested as significant factors, but none has been proved to be important.

4.5.2. Clinical aspects of GC

Clinically the disease behaves in a very similar way to that in the western world.

The male: female ratio is about 2:1 in most parts of Africa. Most tumours originate in the pyloric or prepyloric region.

The ulcerative form is most common, but polypoid and infiltrative types also occur. It is an adenocarcinoma—with a spectrum from well-differentiated to anaplastic. Differentiation between a large fundal carcinoma and a lower oesophageal carcinoma may be virtually impossible on clinical and radiological grounds. International histological typing of gastric tumours has been agreed (Oota and Sobin, 1977).

Two main groups are distinguishable (Lauren, 1965): the *intestinal* type, which is characterized by cells with a tendency to cohesion, and the formation of glandular structures and 'islands', and the *diffuse* type, where the cells separate and infiltrate individually. A higher rate of the former variety has been reported in areas where there is a high incidence rate of gastric carcinoma (Templeton, 1973). However, in northern Nigeria, which is a low incidence area (Mabogunje, *et al*., 1978), 65 specimens were classified using the criteria of Lauren (1965); 40 were intestinal, 16 diffuse, two mixed, and seven unclassifiable. That result was unexpected; furthermore those patients were mostly young, a fact which has also been thought to favour the diffuse lesion.

Fig. 4.2 shows a barium meal in a Papua New Guinean woman with a gastric carcinoma which involved the fundus and lower oesophagus.

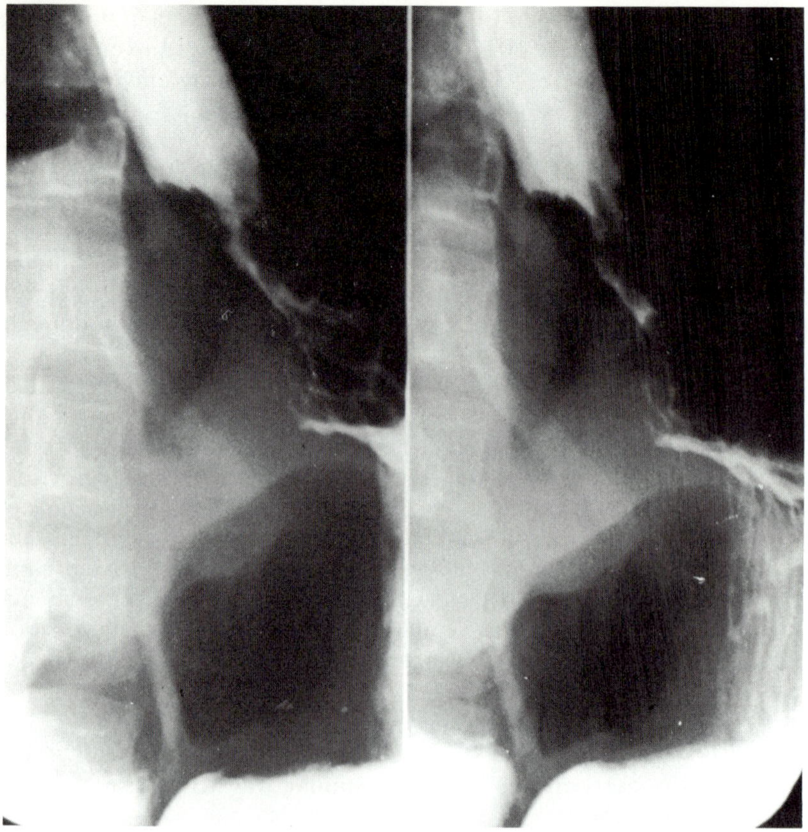

FIG. 4.2. Barium meal in a 50-year-old Papua New Guinean woman. A long stricture is demonstrated in the lower oesophagus and gastric fundus. Laparotomy confirmed that the lesion was malignant; histology showed an adenocarcinoma.

4.6. Other malignant conditions of the stomach

Disseminated tumours of the reticuloendothelial system—especially Burkitt's lymphoma—frequently affect the stomach (Edington and Easmon, 1967); haemorrhage may result. Owor (1977) has reported 40 cases of non-Burkitt's lymphoma of the gastrointestinal tract from Uganda; ten of them involved the stomach. Benign tumours do occur but appear to be no different in incidence or presentation compared with temperate zones (Edington and Gilles, 1976). Lymphoma of the stomach is occasionally seen in other tropical countries, including Papua New Guinea, but is probably no more common than in temperate regions.

4.7. Duodenal ulcer (DU)

4.7.1. Distribution of DU

The difficulties involved in mapping the prevalence of a disease like peptic ulcer which has a low mortality rate have been outlined (Tovey and Tunstall,

1975); hospitals in many parts of Africa and Asia are without radiology equipment and in many of those which have, the apparatus is inadequate for good barium-meal examinations. Those authors have concentrated on the incidence of major complications—pyloric stenosis, haemorrhage, and perforation—in attempting to map the disease. Even more difficult is the problem of comparing incidence rates over several decades; in both Africa and Asia there is some suggestive evidence that duodenal ulcer has become more common since the early years of the twentieth century (Trowell, 1960), but there are many inconsistencies (Tovey and Tunstall, 1975). For example, Bergsma reported 200 cases of peptic ulcer from Addis Ababa in 1931, Aitken commented on the high frequency of the disease in Lagos in 1933, and Roberts reported 44 cases of peptic ulcer at Kampala, Uganda in a two-year period in 1937.

As recently as the 1950s, duodenal ulcer was thought to be an uncommon disease in Africa (Davidson, 1954; *Br. med. J.*, 1959). The main problem was one of recognition and the figures did not reflect the true incidence of the disease; much epigastric pain, which is extremely common in all parts of Africa had undoubtedly been dismissed as being due to intestinal helminths. Reporting the true incidence of the disease depends on a satisfactory history (so very difficult to obtain in most parts of the developing world, where one is so dependent on interpreters) and good radiology facilities.

Africa. The situation in Africa at present seems to be as follows. In west Africa there is a high prevalence in the Cameroons, southern and eastern Nigeria, and probably Ghana. There are also high incidence rates in the Nile-Congo watershed, Rwanda, Burundi, eastern Zaire (Lake Kivu), western Tanzania and south-western Uganda, and the Ethiopian highlands.

In west Africa, Aitken (1933) reported on 48 patients with peptic ulcer over a three-year period; 47 had duodenal and one a gastric ulcer. Ellis (1948) operated on 120 patients in Lagos, Nigeria; he relied on careful history-taking, and did not have the help of radiology. In Ibadan, Konstam (1954) reported on 20 cases of the disease seen over a nine-month period; the ulcer was typically posterior and surrounded by fibrosis. He considered it a disease of the poorer classes. It was not uncommon there, he concluded; a view which was contrary to most previous opinion. A detailed report of radiologically proven post-bulbar ulcer was made by Barton and Cockshott (1961) from Ibadan; reviewing 595 barium meals in 1959 they found 263 duodenal and one gastric ulcer. Those cases were from one department over a one-year period and constituted about one-quarter of the cases of peptic ulcer there. They drew attention to the fact that it was the rural farmer who was usually affected. There was much fibrosis and stenosis which accounted for the rarity of perforation. Those authors considered duodenal ulcer to be as common there as in Britain. A further series was reported by Kolawole and Solanke (1973), also from Ibadan; most were on the anterosuperior portion of the duodenal bulb. Gastric outlet obstruction and choledochoduodenal fistulae were common complications; they considered that obstructive symptoms were frequently a result of oedema rather than fibrosis. In Ghana, 64 patients with peptic ulcer disease were seen in one hospital in Accra in a two-year period (Onori, 1959).

In east Africa, Connell (1937) found only five cases of duodenal ulcer in Tanzania during a 13-year period, while Vint (1937), in an autopsy study of 1800 cases in Kenya, did not find a single duodenal ulcer, and only one healed gastric ulcer; there were three gastric carcinomas. Miller (1966a and b) also considered that duodenal ulcer was unusual in east Africa. In reversing previous opinion (Braimbridge and Trowell, 1934; Vassalo, 1937; Wilkinson, 1957), Raper (1958) reported on 776 post-mortems between 1951 and 56 in Kampala, Uganda, and found peptic ulcers in 15·3 per cent of males and 4·7 per cent of females; the duodenal: gastric ratio was 6:1. Only five were diagnosed during life. Taylor (1965) also showed the disease to be far from uncommon in Uganda; of 44 patients operated for suggestive symptoms in Ankole, 22 had a simple duodenal ulcer; in eight this was complicated by stenosis, and in a further eight there was evidence of either penetration or stenosis. The ulcers were frequently multiple, and some of the most advanced were in young people. It was also the impression of that author that the highest incidence was in the tall, thin people of south-west Uganda—presumably the Hamites. Although there were stress features in some, most came from an unsophisticated, rural, cultivator background. Only three peptic ulcers were found in 1020 post-mortems at Kampala in 1949 (Ojiambo, 1965). However, over the next 10-year period, in 6768 post-mortems 141 (2 per cent) duodenal ulcers were found; 129 were in men and 12 in women (Taylor, 1965). Over a two-year period, Allbrook (1958) found 19 cases of peptic ulcer in a student population of 400 at Makerere University College. Also at Kampala, three peptic ulcers were found during 1020 autopsies over the period 1947 to 48 (*E. Afr. med. J.*, 1949). Shaper and Shaper (1958) however considered the disease to be fairly common in Kampala, Uganda. Working in Kampala from 1965 to 1967 there was no doubt that radiologically proven duodenal ulcer was a common disease, and was certainly not confined to urban populations; members of the Tutsi and Hima tribes who live largely on milk, and sit for much of their time watching cattle, often had the disease. Young adults and children were frequent sufferers. A high incidence was reported in mission hospitals in Rwanda and Burundi by Buxton (1954). Reports from Nairobi indicate that duodenal ulcer disease is not uncommon there (Khan, 1958; Whittaker, 1961; Ojiambo, 1965). Whittaker (1961; 1966) found 26 duodenal and four gastric ulcers in 15 months. Ojiambo (1965) studied 60 cases of radiologically proven disease during a 10-month period (1964–5); age range was three months to 70 years (mean 36 years) and there was no tribal grouping; 30 were unsophisticated country folk. Writing in 1966, Miller had no doubt of the growing incidence of the disease in Nairobi. Sixty ulcers were diagnosed every year at the Kenyatta National Hospital; stenosis was a frequent complication; the most widely employed surgical procedure was vagotomy with pyloroplasty. A high incidence in Nairobi was confirmed by Whittaker (1966); the ratio of duodenal to gastric ulcers was 12 : 1. Duodenal ulceration occurred just beyond the apex of the cap as in west Africa. In a recent study in Nairobi, on Kenyan children with abdominal pain, 11 of 20 who had barium examinations had changes consistent with duodenal ulcer disease (Cross, 1977); eight lived in Nairobi and the mean age was 10 years. In a study to determine the causes of dyspepsia in Dar-es-Salaam, Tanzania, Grech (1965) retrospectively reviewed 733 barium meals; 38 per cent showed an abnormality; the remainder were designated X-ray negative dyspepsia. Peptic ulcer was the most common lesion (26 per cent). The vast majority (170) were duodenal ulcers; 10 and 14 were pyloric and gastric, respectively.

At Bulawayo, Zimbabwe Rhodesia, 28 duodenal and six gastric ulcers were diagnosed in a six-month period in a radiological investigation (Baldachin and Palmer, 1959). In Salisbury, Zimbabwe Rhodesia, duodenal ulceration seems to be a predominantly urban disease and is far more common in men in the 29 to 39 age group, most of whom are unskilled workers (Friedlander and Gelfand, 1978). A five-year period in Lusaka, Zambia convinced me that the radiologically proven disease is common there in both urban and rural Africans; however, complications are unusual and stenosis is not a major problem. At the Baragwanath hospital, Johannesburg, 33 patients with the disease, three-quarters of which were duodenal, were seen in one year (Davey, 1968). In a 10-year period (1950 to 59), 100 Africans were admitted to the King Edward VIII Hospital in Durban, South Africa, with peptic ulcers; the duodenal: gastric ratio was 3·5 : 1·0 (Kark, 1961).

The belief strongly held earlier in this century that peptic ulcer was rare in Africans, in Africa, is now therefore firmly demolished. Whether or not there has been an increase in incidence with urbanization and 'westernization' is impossible to prove. It seems possible that there has been, but that is certainly not proven. Today the disease is common and very many patients presenting with epigastric discomfort (an extremely common presenting feature in any outpatient department in Africa), can be proved, if radiological facilities are available, to have a duodenal ulcer.

Asia. From India, Paterson and Hancock (1958) reported on 39 cases of duodenal ulceration in south India of whom 5 had post-bulbar ulcers; most came from agricultural communities. Hancock (1960) reported a personal series of 153 cases of duodenal ulcer and in a review of 527 consecutive barium meals considered that post-bulbar ulceration is a common condition in south India. Those reports also serve to emphasize the similarity between the disease in southern India and Nigeria (Konstam, 1954).

Papua New Guinea. The disease is common in Papua New Guinea (Muirden, 1976); during a 30-month period, radiological evidence of duodenal ulceration was found in 68 of 1023 barium meals at Port Moresby. In a three-year period 317 cases of peptic ulcer disease were admitted to Goroka Hospital in the eastern highlands; 81 were duodenal and 23 pyloroduodenal in position (Wagner and Shepherd, 1976). Overall, there was an 18 : 1 male : female sex ratio in that investigation.

4.7.2. Aetiology of DU

Genetic factors probably play a part in the incidence rate. In Uganda, there is no doubt that the disease is more common in the Hamitic tribes than the Bantu-speaking people. In Nigeria there are marked differences in incidence rates between people in the north and south of the country (Konstam, 1954). People with blood group 0, and non-secretors of A, B, and O blood group substances are prone to duodenal ulcers in Nigeria (Ball, 1962; Davey and Elebute, 1963).

Various dietary factors have been considered in an attempt to explain the proposed historical increase in incidence of the disease over the last three or four decades, together with the higher urban incidence rates in Asia and Africa (Tovey and Tunstall, 1975).

In southern India and Nigeria the diet is low in protein and high in carbohydrate; it is always bulky. The staples are rice and tapioca, yams and cassava respectively. Peppers and chillies have been suggested to be important in both Asia and Africa (Lewis and Aderoju, 1978); whereas there is limited evidence for that in south India, the duodenal ulcer rate is low in north Indians, Malayans, and Javanese where the consumption of spices is also high (Tovey and Tunstall, 1975). Thiamin and riboflavin deficiencies have been suggested as being important but that has never been proved. The currently fashionable high 'fibre' (Burkitt and Trowell, 1975), and refined carbohydrate (Cleave, 1974) hypotheses have inevitably been invoked, but there is no clear indication that either is relevant. There seems little to incriminate smoking, alcohol, or caffeine consumption. Stress and pace of living in urban areas have been blamed; however like the other factors examined there is no evidence at present. Ascariasis and hookworm disease also seem very unlikely to be relevant. In the West Indies, duodenal ulcer can occur as a complication of sickle-cell (SS) anaemia (Sergeant, Richards, Barbor, and Milner, 1968).

The disease is doubtless multifactorial, and at present there is no clear indication that any single factor is involved in the pathogenesis of this complex disease in any part of the third world.

4.7.3. Presentation of DU

In most respects presentation of the disease in the tropics is similar to that in western countries. The main difference relates to the high incidence of stenosis, probably a consequence of chronicity, and symptoms following that.

Epigastric pain is extremely common in many indigenous populations in tropical countries; it is important therefore that duodenal ulcers are not over-diagnosed. The cause of many such symptoms is unclear, but they frequently subside with antacids.

If pyloric stenosis occurs, there may be persistent vomiting leading to severe dehydration and weight loss, and hypokalaemic alkalosis.

In studies in Africa and India, all social classes seem to be affected, and the sex incidence always shows a higher rate in men. It should be remembered however that it is often especially difficult for women to get to hospital in rural Africa and Asia. Barton and Cockshott (1961) reported a 4·5:1 male: female ratio in Ibadan, Nigeria. The disease may occur at any time from infancy to the eighth decade, with a maximum incidence at about 30 years of age.

The history of epigastric pain, often worse at night, and nausea and vomiting is similar to that usually obtained in western countries; as gall-bladder disease is uncommon in Africa, duodenal ulcer is reasonably easy to diagnose. There is usually a long history of pain, occurring in bouts which become progressively more frequent; radiation to the back is common (Barton and Cockshott, 1961). In that study, 53 per cent had had haematemeses or melaena; although vomiting after meals was common, complete stenosis was very unusual. In a clinical study at Ibadan, Nigeria 300 cases of duodenal ulcer disease were reported (Amure, 1967). The presentation was on the whole similar to that in the western world, except that nausea and vomiting were more common in Nigeria. Post-bulbar ulcers were more common and accounted for about 5 per cent. In southern India, in a study of 153 cases of duodenal ulcer, results were similar to those from Africa (Hancock, 1960). Severe pain was usual and radiation to the back occurred in 37 per cent. Aggravation of pain by food, and relief by vomiting were frequent. Twenty-six gave a history of major bleeding. The very high incidence of stenosis (85 per cent) and gastric retention confirmed results of previous series from south India.

There is a suggestion that features of duodenal ulceration are different in rural and urban settings. In India, ulcers seem to have different characteristics (Somervell and Orr, 1936; Tovey, 1972; Tovey, 1975); in the cities the course is similar to that in western countries; in rural areas, however, ulcers tend to fibrose and are complicated by pyloric stenosis, while haemorrhage and perforation are rare. That is similar to experiences in Africa at Nairobi, Mombasa, Salisbury, Durban, and Johannesburg (Tovey and Tunstall, 1975); in those cities changes seem to have occurred fairly recently. In Papua New Guinea, personal experience suggests that there might be differences there also. However, these impressions must be viewed with caution because they could be explained by the fact that patients with stenosis as a complication can travel considerable distances to enter hospital and undergo surgery, whereas those with haemorrhage and perforation would die either at home, or before reaching hospital.

Epigastric tenderness and scarification marks acquired from a local medical practitioner are usually the only abnormal physical findings in an uncomplicated case.

It is therefore clear that in all parts of the third world, and especially in rural areas, stenosis is much more common than it is in the western world; there seems to be a great tendency for fibrosis to occur early, although the length of histories in the developing world are very difficult to be certain about. Interestingly, only 57 of 148 complications of peptic ulcer at Goroka Base Hospital in Papua New Guinea were due to obstruction (Wagner and Shepherd, 1976); that is a lower figure than in most tropical countries.

In a five-year period, Badoe (1972) saw 42 patients at the Korle Bu Hospital, Accra with pyloric obstruction; in 67 per cent this was caused by a chronic duodenal ulcer, in 24 per cent by carcinoma of the pyloric antrum, and in 5 per cent by prepyloric gastric ulcer. Ellis (1948) found pyloric obstruction in over 50 per cent of his patients. Visible peristalsis occurs and the stomach sometimes reaches gigantic proportions, extending from the diaphragm to the pelvis; occasionally, the ulcer mass is palpable. Davey (1968) describes three presentations: (i) in a patient with a typical duodenal ulcer history, signs of retention are discovered incidentally, (ii) there are few symptoms apart from abdominal distension and perhaps hiccough, and again examination reveals a grossly dilated stomach, and (iii) the extreme type where there is emaciation, dehydration and visible peristalsis in a gigantic stomach. The condition may also be associated with diarrhoea (Balint and Spence, 1959). Development of a fistula between the duodenum and biliary system has been reported from Nigeria (Lewis and Bohrer, 1969).

4.7.4. Pathology of DU

Although usually situated on the posterior wall of the upper part of the duodenum, the ulcer may be either anterior or posterior or both, or may 'saddle' the superior aspect of the first 2 cm of duodenum (Davey, 1968); the latter situation is common in both Ibadan, Nigeria and Nairobi, Kenya. There is usually much fibrosis and oedema, with thickening of the lesser omentum; adhesions may run from the serosal aspect of the ulcer to the neck of the gall-bladder. It is not clear whether the marked fibrous reaction is due to chronicity or has an ethnic basis in Africans, possibly being similar to keloid formation on the skin. The entire first part of the duodenum may feel, at operation, like an oedematous, fibrotic cartilaginous mass, and the head of the pancreas may also be involved. Obstruction is ultimately caused by oedema and reflex pylorospasm rather than a fibrotic narrowing of the duodenal lumen. The probable low incidence of perforation and haemorrhage may be due to the gross fibrotic reaction, and the unusual site of the ulcer, compared with most European cases (Davey, 1968).

4.7.5. Investigation of DU

Taylor (1965) working in western Uganda, relied on the history and presence of localized duodenal bulb tenderness for a clinical diagnosis. He also found two simple tests to be of value in diagnosis. Two or three glasses of water by mouth usually produced perceptible peristalsis, in the presence of marked pyloric stenosis. If that sign was negative, a stomach tube was inserted and a measured volume of water introduced; after 30 min the fluid was aspirated and the volume indicated the degree of stenosis. For peptic oesophagitis, instillation of N/10 HC1 and weak sodium bicarbonate into the distal oesophagus was recommended, and that relieved the symptoms in that situation. When radiology is not available, Davey (1968) has found the 'bed-rest test' of value; if pain has not been alleviated after four or five days of bed rest, the epigastric pain is not due to duodenal ulcer. Other investigations are ideally the same as those used in the western world. The main problem is that good radiology is often very difficult to obtain; portable X-ray units which are the rule in most rural hospitals are of no value for barium meals. Gas in the biliary tree, and the passage of barium into the bile ducts and pancreatic duct during a barium meal should be looked for; those signs are due to incompetence of the ampulla of Vater. Fistulous formation may also be visualized, and that too indicates a duodenal ulcer (Barton and Cockshott, 1961). Endoscopy is costly, and trained personnel experienced in its use are difficult to obtain. Although it is felt by some that fibre-optic gastroscopy is a feasible technique in a developing country, and is possibly superior to barium meals (Wierman and Snyder, 1978), that view is not shared by all (Tovey, 1978). The fractional test meal and Kay's augmented histamine test have been used in Africa, and give results similar to those in Europe (Ellis, 1934; Rose, 1935; Money and Cook, 1961). Testing for occult blood in the faeces is of very limited value due to the extremely high incidence of hookworm disease in all tropical countries.

Two investigations are of value in assessing the extent of stenosis. After a barium meal, if less than one third emptying has taken place in two hours, or half in three hours, the stenosis is significant. Also, volumes of 400 ml are aspirated from the stomach after an overnight (10 hour) fast.

4.7.6. Treatment of DU

Treatment of duodenal ulcers in the third world is usually limited by lack of effective therapeutic agents. Carbenoxolone sodium ('Duogastrone') and cimetidine are costly preparations and the local drug budget can rarely afford them. If available, 'Duogastrone' should be given as 50 mg four times daily before meals (swallowed intact) for six to 12 weeks (Amure, 1970; Davies and Reed, 1977). Although cimetidine offers good results if there is little fibrosis (Finkelstein and Isselbacher, 1978; *Lancet*, 1978) that compound is also too expensive for most third-world countries, For medical treatment, the older regimes of antacids and antispasmodics are frequently used. Smoking should be stopped. Salicylates and other gastric irritants should not be taken. Dietary restrictions are unnecessary, although frequent meals, if that is possible, diminish ulcer symptoms. Milk should not be encouraged to the extent that it is in the western world because adult hypolactasia is common and severe diarrhoea may ensue (Chapter 21). Bed rest is often difficult as hospitals are overloaded with more acute problems. Inevitably therefore, surgery is undertaken at an earlier stage in many cases. The ulcer is often very chronic and there is much fibrosis at presentation; chances of a cure with any form of medical treatment are in that case, remote. Also, many cases when first seen at hospital already have evidence of obstruction. Konstam (1954) considered that medical treatment offered little prospect of a lasting cure, but that good results were achieved with combined vagotomy and antrectomy, or pyloroplasty. In Ibadan, Nigeria Amure (1967) concluded that the immediate response to medical treatment is often good, but that post bulbar ulcers are sometimes highly refractory.

Due to the large bulk of the diet in western Uganda, Taylor (1965) considered that the more conservative surgical operations were desirable and that sub-total gastric resections were never indicated in the management of duodenal ulceration; that clearly applies also to most other parts of the tropics. He recommended vagotomy and drainage procedures; he considered that the nature of the duodenal pathology usually required a gastroenterostomy rather than a pyloroplasty. Davey (1968) was in agreement with those observations, and listed the following reasons: (i) the 'gastric reservoir' must never be interfered with, (ii) closure of the duodenal stump is usually impossible because it is oedematous and friable, (iii) results with vagotomy and drainage procedures in Ibadan were gratifying, and (iv) after those procedures, postoperative care is simple and intravenous fluids and nasogastric suction are rarely necessary.

Stomal ulcer can and does occur commonly in Africa, so for that reason gastrojejunostomy alone is not an acceptable operation (see below).

If retention is present, bed rest should precede operation. The oedema and spasm related to the ulcer subside on that regime; during that time the electrolyte balance, if disturbed, can also be corrected. If retention persists despite bed rest, Davey (1968) recommends a gastrojejunostomy under local anaesthesia and vagotomy at a later date.

4.8. Other complications of peptic ulcer disease

4.8.1. Upper gastrointestinal haemorrhage

All of the causes of gastrointestinal haemorrhage found in the western world also exist in the tropics (Miller, 1966b). However, the relative ratios seem to be different; oesophageal varices secondary to portal hypertension are very common and probably account for most cases (Chapter 11). The true incidence rates are extremely difficult to ascertain because many people die either at home, or before they can reach the nearest hospital or aid post.

Figures from Salisbury, Zimbabwe Rhodesia (Gelfand, 1965), and Johannesburg, South Africa (Grieve, Cooper, Fraser, Dubb, Gentin, Kavin, and Law, 1961) indicate that oesophageal varices are a more important cause than peptic ulcer or gastric carcinoma, although Davey (1968) considered from his own surgical experience at Ibadan, Nigeria that duodenal ulcer was the most common cause. In Nairobi, Kenya, the commonest cause of gastrointestinal haemorrhage may also be a bleeding duodenal ulcer (Carvalho and Ojiambo, 1974). In a further study, using fibre-optic oesophagogastroduodenoscopy, the precise site of bleeding was ascertained in 89 per cent of 66 patients in a prospective study; in 53 per cent duodenal ulcer was responsible for the haemorrhage (Hansen and Daly, 1978). At Goroka Base Hospital in the Papua New Guinea highlands, 64 of 148 complications of peptic ulcer disease were due to upper gastrointestinal haemorrhage (Wagner and Shepherd, 1976); in the same study there were only three admissions for bleeding oesophageal varices in a total of 124 admissions for liver and biliary disease.

The relative merits of endoscopy and radiology in the diagnosis of upper gastrointestinal haemorrhage have been investigated (Wilken, McGinn, Guyer, and Steer, 1976); overall a higher degree of accuracy was obtained using endoscopy, in that report.

Management of haemorrhage from a duodenal ulcer is as elsewhere. If the bleeding is uncontrollable due to erosion of a major vessel, Davey (1968) recommends opening the duodenum and under-running the bleeding vessel; this can be followed by a pyloroplasty or gastrojejunostomy, and vagotomy can be done either then, or at a later date. Perforation and periduodenal abscess occasionally occur and are treated as they are elsewhere.

Because of the difficulty of reaching hospital in the event of subsequent bleeds, surgery is undertaken at an earlier stage than is often the case in the western world.

4.8.2. *Perforation*

In western society, most cases of perforation result from duodenal or gastric ulcers. In most parts of the third world, those events are unusual i.e. gastric ulcer is uncommon, and duodenal ulcers become fibrotic and cause stenosis before obstruction. However, in Goroka Base Hospital in the eastern highlands of Papua New Guinea, 27 of 148 complications of peptic ulcer requiring surgery were perforations (Wagner and Shepherd, 1976). The commonest cause of perforation is usually typhoid fever (Chapter 22), where it occurs in the lower ileum. Amoebic colitis occasionally perforates (Chapter 25) but the event is usually a localized one. Very rarely a tuberculous ulcer perforates. Ascaris has been implicated in perforation (Chapter 19) but the evidence for this is not clear cut; ascaris tends to migrate to any opening, and that may take place after perforation has occurred (Amfon, 1963).

4.8.3. *Anastomotic ulcer*

In rural Burundi, 17 cases of anastomotic ulcer have been described in a 3·5-year period (Hamber and Von Bergen, 1972); the condition has hitherto been uncommon in Africa, possibly due to the preventive effect of the chronic stenosing pattern of peptic-ulcer. Those authors considered that the disease is probably increasing in incidence in that part of Africa.

References

AITKEN, A. B. (1933). *W. Afr. med. J.*, **6,** 63.
ALLBROOK, D. B. (1958). *E. Afr. med. J.*, **35,** 97.
AMFON, E. E. (1963). *Ghana med. J.*, **2,** 99.
AMURE, B. O. (1967). *Practitioner*, **199,** 330.
—— (1970). *Gut*, **11,** 171.
—— and ELEGBE, R. A. (1975). *W. Afr. med. J.*, **23,** 15.
ASHBY, B. S., APPLETON, P. J., and DAWSON, I. (1964). *Br. med. J.*, **1,** 1141.
AVERY JONES, F., GUMMER, J. W. P., and LENNARD-JONES, J. E. (1968). *Clinical Gastroenterology*. pp. 353 and 438. Blackwell, Oxford and Edinburgh.
BADOE, E. A. (1966). *W. Afr. med. J.*, **15,** 181.
—— (1972). *W. Afr. med. J.*, **21,** 154.
BALDACHIN, B. J. and PALMER, P. E. S. (1959). *Br. med. J.*, **2,** 304.
BALINT, J. A. and SPENCE, M. P. (1959). *Br. med. J.*, **1,** 890.
BALL, P. A. J. (1962). *Br. med. J.*, **2,** 948.
BARTON, C. J. and COCKSHOTT, W. P. (1961). *Br. J. Radiol.*, **34,** 216.
BERGSMA, S. (1931). *Archs intern. med.*, **47,** 144.
BIJLSMA, F. (1974). *Trop. geogr. med.*, **26,** 1.
BLAIR, M. C. (1923). *Br. med. J.*, **2,** 130.
BOULOS, P. B., OKOSDONOSSIAN, E. T., ELMUNSHID, H. A., ELMASRI, S. H., HASSAN, M. A., and HOBSLEY, M. (1978). *Gut,* **19,** 802.
BRAIMBRIDGE, C. V. and TROWELL, H. C. (1934). *E. Afr. med. J.,* **10,** 365.
BRAUN, T. G. (1965). *Papua New Guin. med. J.*, **8,** 83.
Br. med. J., (1959). **1,** 1462.
BROWN, W. C. (1908). *Sprue and its treatment.* John Bale, Sons and Danielsson, London.
BURKITT, D. P. and TROWELL, H. C. (1975). (editors) *Refined carbohydrate foods and disease.* Academic Press, London, New York, San Francisco.
BUXTON, K. L. (1954). *Lancet*, **2,** 1231.
CARVALHO, G. R. and OJIAMBO, H. P. (1974). *E. Afr. med. J.*, **51,** 63.

CHARLESWOOD, G. P. and FRYLINCK, R. (1951). *S. Afr. med. J.*, **25,** 551.
CHUKE, P. O., TRAUB, N. E. and PATEL, I. C. (1972). *E. Afr. med. J.*, **49,** 681.
CLEAVE, T. L. (1974). *The saccharine disease.* John Wright and Sons, Bristol.
CONNELL, W. K. (1937). *E. Afr. med. J.*, **14,** 89.
COOK, G. C. (1978). *Jl. R. Coll. Phycns.*, **12,** 329.
COOK, P. J. and BURKITT, D. P. (1971). *Br. med. Bull.*, **27,** 14.
CROSS, A. W. (1977). *E. Afr. med. J.*, **54,** 548.
DAVEY, W. W. (1968). *Companion to surgery in Africa.* p. 185. Livingstone, Edinburgh and London.
—— and ELEBUTE, E. A. (1963). *Gut*, **4,** 367.
—— and PEARSON, J. B. (1965). *Br. J. Surg.*, **52,** 189.
DAVIDSON, L. S. P. (1954). *Lancet,* **1,** 614.
DAVIES, J. N. P. (1959). *Modern Trends in Pathology.* (ed. D. H. Collins). p. 146. Butterworths, London.
DAVIES, W. A. and REED, P. I. (1977). *Gut*, **18,** 78.
DOGRA, J. R. (1940). *Indian J. med. Res.*, **28,** 481.
DUTT, B. (1973). *E. Afr. med. J.*, **50,** 125.
—— and KAJUBI, S. K. (1972). *E. Afr. med. J.*, **49,** 132.
DUTZ, W., SAIDI, F., and KOHOUT, E. (1970). *Gut*, **11,** 352.
E. Afr. med. J. (1949). **26,** 137.
EDINGTON, G. M. and EASMON, C. O. (1967). *Natn. Cancer Inst. Monogr.*, **25,** 17.
—— and GILLES, H. M. (1976). *Pathology in the tropics.* 2nd ed. pp. 323, 522 and 539. Edward Arnold, London.
—— and MACLEAN, C. M. U. (1965). *Br. J. Cancer*, **19,** 471.
ELEBUTE, E. A., NGU, V. A., MAINWARING, A. R. and ERUCHALU, R. C. (1963). *W. Afr. med. J.*, **12,** 11.
ELLIS, M. (1934). *W. Afr. med. J.*, **8,** 16.
—— (1948). *Br. J. Surg.*, **36,** 60.
ELMASRI, S. H., BOULOS, P. and MALICK, M. O. A. (1977). *E. Afr. med. J.*, **54,** 319.
ELMES, B. G. T. and BALDWIN, R. B. T. (1947). *Ann. trop. Med. Parasit.*, **41,** 321.
EVANS, D. M. D., CRAVEN, J. L., MURPHY, F. and CLEARY, B. K. (1978). *Gut*, **19,** 1.
FINKELSTEIN, W. and ISSELBACHER, K. J. (1978). *New Engl. J. Med.*, **299,** 992.
FRIEDLANDER, M. L. and GELFAND, M. (1978). *Tropical Doctor*, **8,** 205.
FUNG, W. P. (1970). *Gut*, **11,** 955.
GELFAND, M. (1965). *Cent. Afr. J. Med.,* **11,** 366.
GJESING, B. (1975). *E. Afr. med. J.,* **52,** 386.
GRACEY, M., CULLITY, G. J., SUHARJONO, and SUNOTO (1977). *Archs Dis. Childh.*, **52,** 325.
GRECH, P. (1965). *E. Afr. med. J.*, **42,** 106.
GRIEVE, M., COOPER, W., FRASER, B., DUBB, A., GENTIN, S. KAVIN, H. and LAW, I. (1961). *Gut*, **2,** 72.
HAMBER, G. and VON BERGEN, M. (1972). *E. Afr. med. J.*, **49,** 448.
HANCOCK, D. M. (1960). *Br. J. Surg.*, **48,** 128.
HANSEN, D. P. and DALY, D. S. (1978). *Am. J. trop. Med., Hyg.*, **27,** 197.
HIGGINSON, J. and OETTLÉ, A. G. (1960). *J. natn. Cancer Inst.*, **24,** 621.
JAYARATNAM, F. J., SEAH, C. S., DA COSTA, J. L., TAN, K. K. and O'BRIEN, W. (1967). *Br. Med. J.*, **3,** 18.
KARK, A. E. (1961). *Gut*, **2,** 363.
KAVIN, H. and LAW, I. (1961). *Gut*, **2,** 72.
KHAN, A. A. (1958). *E. Afr. med. J.*, **35,** 697.
KOLAWOLE, T. M. and SOLANKE, T. F. (1973). *Trop. geogr. Med.*, **25,** 325.
KONSTAM, P. G. (1954). *Lancet*, **2,** 1039.
—— (1955). *W. Afr. med. J.*, **4,** 203.
Lancet (1978). **2,** 1237.

LANGMAN, M. J. S. (1968). *Gut*, **9,** 5.
LAUREN, P. (1965). *Acta path. microbiol. scand.*, **64,** 31.
LEWIS, E. A. and BOHRER, S. P. (1969). *Gut*, **10,** 146.
—— and BOHRER, S. P. (1969). *Gut*, **10,** 146.
MCGLASHAN, N. D. (1972). In *Medical geography* (ed. N. D. McGlashan). p. 187. Methuen and Co., London.
MABOGUNJE, O. A., SUBBUSWAMY, S. G. and LAWRIE, J. H. (1978). *Gut*, **19,** 425.
MALHOTRA, S. L. (1967). *Gut*, **8,** 361.
MARKS, I. N., BANK, S., WERBELOFF, L., FARMAN, J. and LOUW, J. H. (1963). *Am. J. dig. Dis.*, **8,** 509.
MILLER, J. R. M. (1966a). *E. Afr. med. J.*, **43,** 259.
—— (1966b). *Am. J. dig. Dis.*, **14,** 755.
MONEY, G. L. and COOK, J. (1961). *E. Afr. med. J.*, **38,**105.
MOORE, E. W. (1967). *E. Afr. med. J.*, **44,** 513.
MORSON, B. C. and DAWSON, I. M. P. (1972). *Gastrointestinal pathology*. pp. 57 and 96. Blackwell, Oxford, London, Edinburgh and Melbourne.
MUIRDEN, J. C. (1976). *Papua New Guin. med. J.*, **19,** 149.
MWANGEMI, P. M. (1975). *E. Afr. med. J.*, **52,** 152.
NAI-KUANG, C. and PEN-CHING, C. (1957). *China med. J.*, **75,** 324.
NALIN, D. R., LEVINE, M. M., RHEAD, J., BERGQUIST, E., RENNELS, M., HUGHES, T., O'DONNELL, S., and HORNICK, R. B. (1978). *Lancet*, **2,** 859.
NALIN, D. R., LEVINE, R. J. LEVINE, M. M., HOOVER, D., BERGQUIST, E., MCLAUGHLIN, J., LIBONATI, J., ALAM, J., and HORNICK, R. B. (1978). *Lancet*, **2,** 856.
NWOKOLO, C. (1966). *W. Afr. med. J.,* **15,** 210.
OJIAMBO, H. P. (1965). *E. Afr. med. J.*, **42,** 629.
ONORI, E. (1959). *W. Afr. med. J.*, **8,** 84.
OOTA, K. and SOBIN, L. H. (1977). *Histological typing of gastric and oesophageal tumours.* W.H.O. Geneva.
OWOR, R. (1977). *E. Afr. med. J.*, **54,** 666.
PATERSON, D. E. and HANCOCK, D. M. (1958). *Br. J. Radiol.*, **31,** 660.
RAPER, A. B. (1958). *Trans. R. Soc. trop. Med. Hyg.*, **52,** 535.
ROBERTS, C. E. (1937). *E. Afr. med. J.*, **14,** 88.
ROGERS, L. (1913). *Dysenteries. Their differentiation and treatment.* p. 303. Oxford University Press, London.
ROSE, A. W. (1935). *W. Afr. med. J.*, **8,** 10.
SERGEANT, G. R., RICHARDS, R., BARBOR, P. R. H. and MILNER, P. F. (1968). *Br. med. J.*, **3,** 86.
SHAPER, A. G. and SHAPER, L. (1958). *E. Afr. med. J.*, **35,** 647.
SHEPHERD, A. (1975). *Papua New Guin. med. J.*, **18,** 43.
SMITH, F. (1967). *Papua New Guin. med. J.*, **10,** 25.
SOMERVELL, T. H. and ORR, I. M. (1936). *Br. J. Surg.*, **24,** 227.
TAI da ROCHA-AFODU, J. and ADESOLA, A. O. (1976). *E. Afr. med. J.*, **53,** 527.
TAYLOR, W. H. (1965). *E. Afr. med. J.*, **42,** 397.
TEMPLETON, A. C. (1973). *Recent results in Cancer research*, **41,** 40.
TOVEY, F. I. (1972). *Trop. geogr. Med.*, **24,** 107.
—— (1975). In *Refined Carbohydrate foods and disease* (ed. D. P. Burkitt and H. C. Trowell). p. 279. Academic Press, London.
—— (1978). *Tropical Doctor*, **8,** 112.
—— and TUNSTALL, M. (1975). *Gut*, **16,** 564.
TROWELL, H. C. (1960). *Non-infective disease in Africa*. p. 202. Edward Arnold, London.
VAISH, S. K., SAMPATHKUMAR., J., JACOB, R. and BAKER, S. J. (1965). *Gut,* **6,** 458.
VASSALO, S. M. (1937). *E. Afr. med. J.*, **14,** 83.
VINT, F. W. (1937). *E. Afr. med. J.*, **14,** 91.

WAGNER, F. (1975). *Papua New Guin. med. J.*, **18,** 45.
WAGNER, F. B. and SHEPHERD, A. (1976). *Papua New Guin. med. J.*, **19,** 156.
WASUNNA, A. E. O., WAKHISI, J., ANABWANI, G. M., MUKURIA, J. W. and ROY, A. D. (1973). *E. Afr. med. J.*, **50,** 444.
WHITTAKER, L. R. (1961). *E. Afr. med. J.*, **38,** 449.
—— (1966). *E. Afr. med. J.*, **43,** 336.
WIERMAN, J. and SNYDER, C. A. (1978). *Tropical Doctor*, **8,** 110.
WILKEN, B. J., MCGINN, F. P., GUYER, P. B. and STEER, H. W. (1976). *Papua New Guin. med. J.*, **19,** 163.
WILKINSON, J. (1957). *E. Afr. med. J.*, **34,** 627.

Section 2 : The liver and biliary system

5

The tropical liver: effect of chronic intestinal and reticuloendothelial infections

DISEASES of the liver in tropical countries can be divided roughly into those in which the reticuloendothelial and mesenchymal components—including the Kupffer cells, sinusoidal cells, portal venous radicles, and portal connective tissues—are predominantly involved, and those in which the hepatocytes and excretory pathways including the small and large bile-ducts are mainly involved (Hutt, 1971). The former group is characterized by intestinal infections, including schistosomiasis (Chapter 10) and malaria, and the latter by viral hepatitis, chronic hepatitis and cirrhosis (Chapters 7 and 8). In many of these conditions hepatic involvement is only part of a more generalized process.

Mild hepatomegaly is very common in most tropical countries. In Papua New Guinea, for example, some 15 per cent or more of the population (women more often than men) have significantly enlarged livers (Black, 1954; Peters, 1959; Schofield, 1962; Blackburn, Arter, Burchett, Murrell, Radford, Meehan, Ma, and McGovern, 1966) and the incidence increases with age. However, significant parenchymal damage is very unusual and the only demonstrable abnormality is a round-cell periportal infiltration sometimes associated with mild fibrosis. Kupffer-cell hyperplasia, nuclear pleomorphism in the hepatocytes, and dilatation of the central sinusoids and central vein are also seen. Those changes are associated with mildly elevated serum γ-globulin concentrations and *increased* clearance of bromsulphthalein (Arter, Stathers, Ma, Blackburn, and McGovern, 1968; Blackburn and Ma, 1972). Inflammation of the portal triads and fibrosis is however occasionally severe and portal hypertension may apparently be a sequel (McGovern and Kariks, 1966; Powell and McGovern, 1976).

The liver forms an extremely important line of defence (Nolan, 1978), and it is furthermore a very effective filtration system which protects the systemic circulation from numerous varied insults. Vast numbers of foreign substances are hurled at it in the portal blood: viruses, bacteria, ova, adult parasites, and antigens of many shapes and sizes (*Lancet*, 1978), to say nothing of the products of diet and nutrition. The role of endotoxins of enteric origin in the production of hepatic injury is not yet clear (Munford, 1978; Nolan and Leibowitz, 1978). The liver contains important elements of the reticuloendothelial system—Kupffer cells, lymphocytes, and plasma cells; many acute and chronic diseases prevalent in tropical countries exert a widespread influence on that system. Approximately 15 per cent of the cells within the liver lobule are in fact Kupffer cells (Gates, Henley, Pollard, Schmidt, and Schmidt, 1961); in carrying out their phagocytic and protective function they are, it seems, in danger of damaging adjacent hepatocytes. Those cells have been shown to be damaged by lysosomal enzymes liberated by Kupffer cells and macrophages (Ferluga and Allison, 1978). In mice, the clearance of particles from the blood by the liver is followed by a wave of mitoses in the hepatocytes, and this represents regeneration after acute hepatocellular damage (Bradfield and Wells, 1978). Mitoses and nuclear pleomorphism are thus very common in most liver-biopsy sections obtained in tropical countries. Associated with those appearances, 'stellate fibrosis', i.e. slender wisps of fibrous tissue radiating from the portal triads, but not connecting with each other, is frequently present (Fig. 5.1); that seems to have nothing to do, however, with cirrhosis.

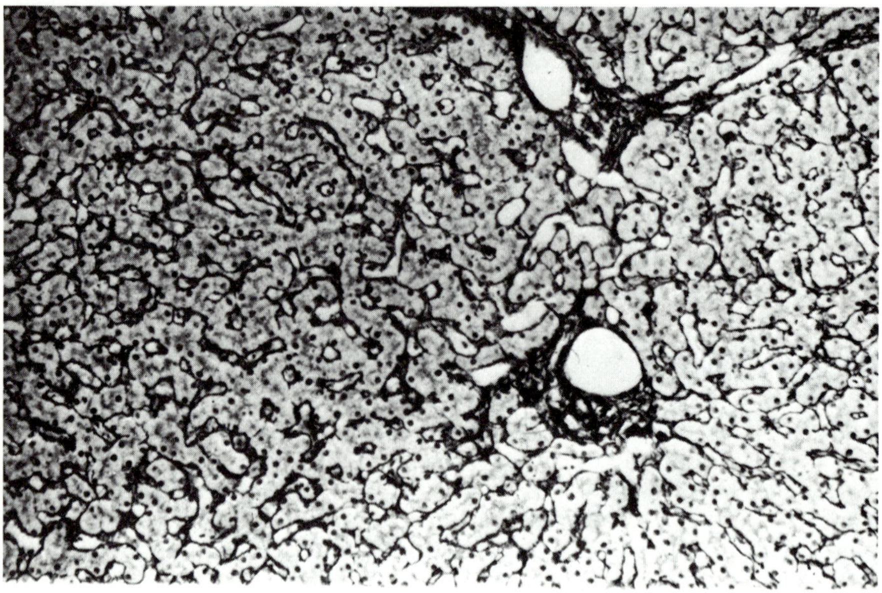

FIG. 5.1. Needle liver-biopsy section (reticulin stain) from a 12-year-old Ugandan child. There is an increase in fibrous tissue in the portal triads with extensions forming a 'stellate-fibrosis'; there is no evidence of cirrhosis or of distortion of the normal architecture. The portal areas contained a moderate round-cell infiltration.

Abnormal liver function and jaundice occur in pneumococcal lobar pneumonia (Chapter 6). Hepatocytes are damaged by circulating endotoxins produced by Gram-negative organisms. Occasionally the liver is invaded by viruses (Chapter 7) but rarely by bacteria (Nolan, 1978; Weinstein, 1978). If in fact bacteria do invade the liver the usual result is a pyogenic abscess (Chapter 12) rather than a hepatitis.

It is not surprising therefore that the liver, especially at the histological level, of the average inhabitant of a tropical country shows minor differences from that of a resident in a temperate country. In fact it might be anticipated that far more marked changes than are present would result.

5.1. Effect of chronic intestinal infections

5.1.1. Bacterial infections

The effect of intestinal bacterial infections on liver structure and function is difficult, at present, to evaluate accurately. It seems highly likely however that changes in the portal tracts, including the round-cell infiltration, and Kupffer-cell hyperplasia, which are very commonly seen in liver-biopsy specimens, are largely a result of such insults. In an *acute* intestinal infection, e.g. salmonellosis (typhoid fever), transient jaundice, and impaired hepatic function are frequently present (Chapter 22); Kupffer-cell hyperplasia and monocytic infiltration of the perisinusoidal and portal spaces, and foci of liver-cell necrosis can be demonstrated.

5.1.2. Helminthic infections

As with intestinal bacterial infections it is difficult to know at present what effect intestinal parasites, particularly the nematodes, which are exceedingly common in all tropical countries, have on liver structure and function.

Chronic inflammatory cells in the portal areas (lymphocytes and plasma cells) are very commonly seen in liver-biopsy specimens taken from people living in the tropics. The appearance is comparable with that seen in chronic persistent hepatitis (Becker, Scheuer, Baptista, and Sherlock, 1970). Because such changes are seen in patients in tropical countries where there is no malaria (Hutt, 1971) it seems most likely that intestinal helminths are partly, if not wholly, responsible.

Hepatomegaly may be present during the migratory phase of *Ascaris lumbricoides* (roundworm) infections (Chapter 19); focal areas of necrosis infiltrated with eosinophils and neutrophils can be demonstrated in liver-biopsies. Granulomatous lesions have also been described in liver sections during the migratory phase (Beaver and Danaraj, 1958). Larvae are rapidly destroyed and cannot usually be demonstrated in the lesions. The frequency of this course of events is impossible to assess because both ascariasis and hepatomegaly are extremely common in all tropical countries. Adult worms may be found in the liver, and have often ascended the biliary tree. Ova and fragments of adult worms may cause necrotic lesions surrounded by eosinophils and neutrophils; they are later replaced by chronic inflammatory cells, giant cells and fibroblasts. Such lesions can also be produced by *A. lumbricoides* ova alone (Khaleque and Alam, 1963); acute abscesses and haemorrhages may occur in addition (Rosenbaum and Johnston, 1966). The adult worms and ova rapidly disintegrate and are not detectable at a later stage.

In *Strongyloides stercoralis* infections (Chapter 20), hepatomegaly may be present during the migratory stage (Poltera, 1972; Nwokolo and Imohiosen, 1973). In severe infections the liver may be enlarged and congested, and small pinpoint, yellow granulomata present. If there is accompanying malabsorption and resultant malnutrition, fatty change may also be present. Larvae in addition to granulomas may be present in the hyperinfection syndrome (Chapter 20).

If there are eosinophils in the portal triads, early schistosomiasis (Chapter 10) should be suspected. Two of the most important parasitic infections of the intestinal tract are amoebiasis and schistosomiasis. They are principally diseases of the large intestine and are covered in Chapters 25 and 26, respectively; the liver lesions produced by those parasites are dealt with in Chapters 12 and 10 respectively.

5.2. Effect of chronic reticuloendothelial infections

5.2.1. Malaria

The part played by malaria in producing mild hepatomegaly in tropical populations is difficult to evaluate (see above). Black (1954) considered it important in Papua New Guinea and Walters and Waterlow (1954) felt it a contributory factor in the Gambia, but that conclusion has not been universally accepted (Bailey, 1966).

Endemic malaria produces changes in the reticuloendothelial components of the liver; the Kupffer cells, sinusoids, and portal triads. Damage to hepatocytes is most unusual; when it occurs it is probably a result of a complicating feature such as anoxia. Electron microscopy shows plasma membrane and mitochondrial damage (Rosen, Roycroft, Hano, and Barry, 1967). Cirrhosis is not a sequel of malaria infections. The changes in the livers of west Africans in areas of endemic malaria have been described (Edington and Gilles, 1976); mild hepatomegaly is very common in such populations and it seems probable that that is in part a result of malaria. In areas where malaria is hyper- or meso-endemic, three chronological phases of the disease can be defined: (i) during the first three to six months of life, passive maternal immunity produces a relative resistance to the disease, (ii) as the passive immunity wanes, the susceptible nonimmune child develops clinical manifestations of malaria and there is a considerable morbidity and mortality, and (iii) from the middle of the first decade onwards an increasing degree of immunity develops which is usually paralleled by an increase in malarial antibodies.

Phase ii is characterized by high parasitaemia and splenomegaly rates in populations at risk; in some individuals there is production of malarial pigment (Fig. 5.2) and premature red blood-cell destruction. There is hypertrophy and hyperplasia of macrophages in the liver and spleen; particulate matter and macromolecules are thus removed from the circulating blood. In this phase, liver-biopsy studies of children show an increasing percentage with large amounts of haemozoin pigment in the Kupffer cells throughout the liver lobule. Whereas lymphocytes occasionally occur in sinusoids they are not a prominent feature. Damage to hepatocytes is very unusual (Edington, 1954; Hutt, 1971). Sixty-five patients with primary attacks of *Plasmodium vivax* or *P. falciparum* were studied in Sri Lanka (Ramachandran and Perera, 1976). Thirty had splenomegaly and 23 hepatosplenomegaly. Thirty-seven (57 per cent) (35 had *P. vivax* and two *P. falciparum* infections) had a non-specific reactive hepatitis associated with hepatomegaly. Changes were similar in both *P. vivax* and *P. falciparum* infections. Kupffer-cell activity and malarial pigment were prominent in 90 and 80 per cent respectively. Portal tract infiltration was unusual. Ballooning and vacuolation of the hepatocytes, dilatation of centrilobular sinusoids, and sinusoidal lymphocytosis were seen in some. Granulo-

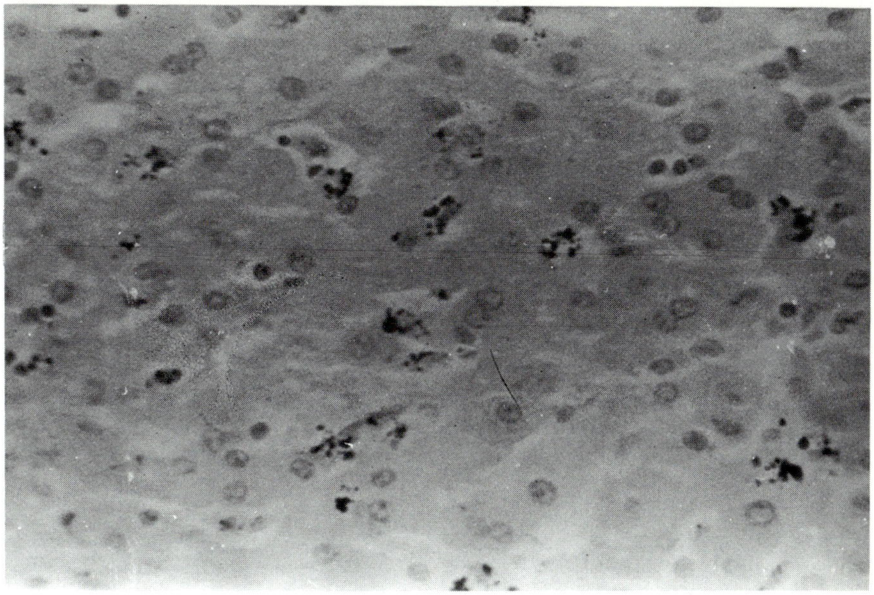

FIG. 5.2. Needle liver-biopsy section (haematoxylin and eosin) from a Papua New Guinean adult, showing heavy accumulations of malarial pigment.

matous lesions of varying size, which were most marked in the patients with hepatomegaly and jaundice, were seen in 50 per cent. Ten (15 per cent) of them (nine had a *P. vivax* and one a *P. falciparum* infection) had jaundice which was usually associated with hepatomegaly and that subsided with antimalarial treatment. Those investigators stressed that those hepatic changes which are seen very commonly in tropical populations, should be distinguished from viral hepatitis, hepatic amoebiasis, typhoid hepatitis, infectious mononucleosis, and Q fever.

As immunity develops (phase iii) there is a decreasing parasitaemia and splenomegaly rate in the general population, and individuals have lower parasite densities in the blood. Haemozoin production is simultaneously diminished, and subsequently stops. Liver-biopsy histology shows clearing of Kupffer-cell pigment; that starts in the central part of the liver lobule but ultimately takes place in the periportal areas also. Pigment is transported to the portal areas and is slowly absorbed as adulthood is reached; it is cleared by lymphatic drainage and can be found in the upper abdominal lymph nodes. This sequence of events is very similar to the clearing of iron from the reticuloendothelial system. Kupffer-cell hypertrophy and hyperplasia does not completely resolve however and is still present to some extent in adult life. As humoral antibodies develop in phase (iii) there is a variable proliferation of lymphoid and plasma cells in both liver and spleen. In a small proportion of cases hepatic sinusoidal lymphocytosis and splenic lymphocytosis become dense; these events usually occur together but in some there may be a poor correlation between sinusoidal lymphocytosis and splenomegaly. The combination of Kupffer-cell hyperplasia, hepatic sinusoidal lymphocytosis, and splenomegaly constitutes the *tropical splenomegaly syndrome* (TSS) (Leather, 1961; Powell and McGovern, 1976) (Chapter 16); patients with these very large spleens form the tail of a skewed normal distribution (Bruce-Chwatt, 1956; Shaper, 1969).

Hypergammaglobulinaemia in tropical countries, which affects most rural people is probably mainly a result of infections, especially malaria (Holmes, Stanier, and Thompson, 1955; McGregor and Gilles, 1960; Curtain, 1966).

There are other important primary infections of the reticuloendothelial system which involve the liver. The most important is probably leishmaniasis which is covered in Chapter 8. The systemic mycoses which also involve the reticuloendothelial system are also dealt with in that chapter.

5.3. Hepatic granulomas

Liver granulomas, which consist of lymphocytes, polymorphs, eosinophils, and giant-cells are by no means uncommon in tropical countries (Cook and Hutt, 1967; Vanier, Hutt, and Cook, 1968; Hutt, 1971). In many cases the cause is obscure. Probably the two most common diseases to produce them are schistosomiasis (Chapter 10) and tuberculosis. Tuberculous granulomata may be found in the absence of miliary tuberculosis and are characterized by necrosis with minimal cellular infiltration; they are not infrequently demonstrated incidentally in liver-biopsy specimens obtained for some entirely different reason. Brucellosis, leprosy (Chapter 8), toxocariasis, and strongyloidiasis (see above) are other conditions which may produce hepatic granulomata in tropical countries. In brucellosis, miliary granulomata are distributed throughout the reticuloendothelial system including the liver; they consist of epithelioid cells surrounded by lymphocytes, monocytes, and fibroblasts and giant cells may be present. Necrosis and suppuration may occur but there is never caseation. Although hepatitis is not a feature, centrilobular necrosis and extensive parenchymal destruction leading to cirrhosis has been described (Edington and Gilles, 1976); such events, if they occur, must however be exceedingly rare. Toxocariasis, caused by human infection with *Toxocara canis* and *T. catis* (which are dog and cat parasites, respectively), is common in many tropical countries. Larval infection of the human liver is common and granulomata formation takes place around the larvae. The importance of this disease in liver pathology in the tropics is not yet clear; it seems unlikely that it assumes a great significance. Microfilariae have also been implicated in granulomatous lesions in the liver parenchyma (Burganinon, 1937); the lobular pattern is preserved but the portal tracts are infiltrated, focally, with eosinophils. Such lesions may be seen in patients with tropical eosinophilia (eosinophilic lung) which is frequently caused by filariasis (Neva and Ottesen, 1978), but also by ascariasis, strongyloidiasis, schistosomiasis, and toxocariasis. There may be hepatomegaly and small white nodules may be seen in the liver tissue.

Sarcoidosis is a rare cause in west (Ogunlesi and Rankin, 1961; Cook and Carter, 1966) and east (Lobo, 1972) Africa, and that disease seems to be uncommon in most other parts of the tropics, including India, Singapore, the Philippines, Vietnam, Taiwan, and China (Present and Siltzbach, 1967).

In Q fever, a rickettsial zoonosis which is seen in sporadic and epidemic outbreaks in various parts of Africa (Babudieri, 1953; Collard and Udeozo, 1959; Guiot, 1964) and Saudi Arabia (Gelpi, 1966), granulomata are also seen in liver sections.

Frequently no cause can be found and despite extensive investigation, no clear aetiological agent is forthcoming.

References

Arter, W. J., Stathers, G. M., Ma M. H., Blackburn, C. R. B., and McGovern, V. J. (1968). *Trop. geogr. Med.*, **20**, 202.

Babudieri, B. (1953). *Monograph Ser. W.H.O.*, **19**, 157.

Bailey, K. V. (1966). *Med. J. Aust.*, **1**, 572.

Beaver, P. C. and Danaraj, T. J. (1958). *Am. J. trop. Med. Hyg.*, **7**, 100.

Becker, M. D., Scheuer, P. J., Baptista, A. and Sherlock, S. (1970). *Lancet*, **1**, 53.

Black, R. H. (1954). *Trans. R. Soc. trop. Med. Hyg.*, **48**, 226.

Blackburn, C. R. B., Arter, W. J., Burchett, P., Murrell, T., Radford, A., Meehan, K., Ma, M., and McGovern, V. J. (1966). *Papua New Guin. med. J.*, **9**, 21.

—— and Ma, M. H. (1972). *Papua New Guin. med. J.*, **15**, 84.

Bradfield, J. W. B. and Wells, M. (1978). *Lancet*, **2**, 836.

Bruce-Chwatt, L. J. (1956). *Bull. Wld Hlth Org.*, **15**, 513.

Burganinon, G. C. (1937). *Annls Soc. belge Méd. trop.*, **17**, 1.

Collard, P. and Udeozo, I. O. K. (1959). *W. Afr. med. J.*, **8**, 137.

Cook, G. C. and Carter, R. A. (1966). *Br. J. Dis. Chest.*, **60**, 23.

—— and Hutt, M. S. R. (1967). *Br. med. J.*, **3**, 454.

Curtain, C. C. (1966). *Papua New Guin. med. J.*, **9**, 145.

Edington, G. M. (1954). *Ann. trop. Med. Parasit.*, **48**, 300.

—— and Gilles, G. M. (1976). *Pathology in the tropics*. 2nd ed. pp. 10 and 330. Edward Arnold, London.

Ferluga, J. and Allison, A. C. (1978). *Lancet*, **2**, 610.

Gates, G. A., Henley, K. S., Pollard, H. M., Schmidt, E. and Schmidt, F. W. (1961). *J. Lab. clin. Med.*, **57**, 182.

Gelpi, A. P. (1966). *Am. J. trop. Med. Hyg.*, **15**, 785.

Guiot, G. (1964). *Méd. trop.*, **24**, 66.

Holmes, E. G., Stanier, M. W. and Thompson, M. D. (1955). *Trans. R. Soc. trop. Med. Hyg.*, **49**, 376.

Hutt, M. S. R. (1971). *Trans. R. Soc. trop. Med. Hyg.*, **65**, 273.

Khaleque, K. A. and Alam, K. S. (1963). *J. trop. Med. Hyg.*, **66**, 249.

Lancet (1978). **2**, 715.

Leather, H. M. (1961). *Br. med. J.*, **1**, 15.

Lobo, P. I. (1972). *E. Afr. med. J.*, **49**, 37.

McGovern, V. J. and Kariks, J. (1966). *Med. J. Aust.*, **2**, 441.

McGregor I. A. and Gilles, H. M. (1960). *Ann. trop. Med. Parasit.*, **54**, 275.

Munford, R. S. (1978). *Gastroenterology*, **75**, 532.

Neva, F. A. and Ottesen, E. A. (1978). *New Engl. J. Med.*, **298**, 1129.

Nolan, J. P. (1978). *New Engl. J. Med.*, **299**, 1069.

——, J. P. and Leibowitz, A. I. (1978). *Gastroenterology*, **75**, 445.

Nwokolo, C. and Imohiosen, E. A. E. (1973). *Br. med. J.*, **2**, 153.

Ogunlesi, T. O. and Rankin, T. B. (1961). *J. trop. Med. Hyg.*, **64**, 318.

Peters, W. (1959). *Trop. geogr. Med.*, **11**, 219.

Poltera, A. A. (1972). *Trans. R. Soc. trop. Med. Hyg.*, **66**, 520.

POWELL, K. C. and MCGOVERN, V. J. (1976). *Papua New Guin. med. J.*, **19,** 140.
PRESENT, D. H. and SILZBACH, L. E. (1967). *Am. Rev. resp. Dis.*, **95,** 285.
RAMACHANDRAN, S. and PERERA, M. V. F. (1976). *J. trop. Med. Hyg.*, **79,** 207.
ROSEN, S., ROYCROFT, D. W., HANO, J. E. and BARRY, K. G. (1967). *Archs Path.*, **83,** 271.
ROSENBAUM, J. M. and JOHNSTON, C. (1966). *Am. J. Dis. Child.*, **112,** 82.
SCHOFIELD, F. D. (1962). *Trans. R. Soc. trop. Med. Hyg.*, **56,** 60.
SHAPER, A. G. (1969). *Trans. R. Soc. trop. Med. Hyg.*, **63,** 206.
VANIER, T. M., HUTT, M. S. R. and COOK, G. C. (1968). *Br. med. J.*, **2,** 649.
WALTERS, J. and WATERLOW, J. C. (1954). *Spec. Rep. Ser. med. Res. Coun.* (Lond.), No. 285.
WEINSTEIN, L. (1978). *New Engl. J. Med.*, **299,** 1052.

6

Hepatic abnormalities associated with systemic bacterial infection

THIS form of jaundice has for long been recognized. Osler (1920) was aware that American negroes with lobar pneumonia were far more likely to become jaundiced than were white Americans. Trowell (1932) was aware that in Kenya, African patients with pneumonia frequently became jaundiced, and he considered (Trowell, 1960) that the hepatocytes were unduly vulnerable in Africans. Gelfand (1947), and Clain and Gelfand (1964) also reported a high incidence of jaundice in the presence of systemic bacterial infections, in Zimbabwe Rhodesia. Fifteen per cent of patients with pneumonia at the Mulago Hospital, Kampala are jaundiced (Shaper and Shaper, 1958). The jaundice is usually associated with pneumococcal or Klebsiella infections; although often severe at first it usually subsides rapidly within a few days.

Although the bacterial disease giving rise to jaundice is more often than not lobar pneumonia, any severe infection, including tropical pyomyositis and empyema (Eley, Hargreaves, and Lambert, 1965), may give a similar picture. Introduction of antibiotics has certainly not abolished the syndrome. The mechanism of the jaundice is obscure.

It is important that the condition is readily recognized in tropical countries, otherwise primary liver disease, usually viral hepatitis, may be diagnosed. Respiratory symptoms and signs may then be disregarded with disastrous results and the appropriate antibiotic treatment not started right away.

The incidence of the condition ranges from 3 to 26 per cent of patients with lobar pneumonia in different series (Zimmerman and Thomas, 1950; Tugwell and Williams, 1977).

There is no unanimity in the literature as to either the type or mechanism of this form of jaundice; in fact these probably vary in different areas. Hepatocellular jaundice, cholestasis, possibly associated with cholangitis, and excessive haemolysis, have all been suggested. Owing to the gross differences in the type of jaundice recorded in different reports it seems appropriate to deal with the various types separately.

6.1. Nature of the jaundice and hepatic dysfunction

6.1.1. Hepatocellular jaundice

In Ibadan, Nigeria, liver-biopsies from 11 adult Nigerians showed evidence of liver-cell damage with cloudy swelling of the parenchymal cells (Hall and Parry, 1963); in only one was there evidence of haemolysis. A greater portal infiltration with lymphocytes, plasma cells, and occasional polymorphs than is usual in Ibadan was reported. Occasional bile thrombi were observed in one of the two patients who died. There was no evidence of chronic liver disease. Similarly in Kampala, Uganda, of 21 patients studied 18 were considered to have evidence of a hepatitis (Kibukamusoke, Patel, and Hutt, 1964); one patient, who subsequently died, had evidence of cholestasis. There was no evidence of haemolysis. It was considered from that experience that the jaundice was due to a transient hepatitis with a cholestatic element, but without evidence of extensive liver-cell necrosis. There is sometimes a focal degeneration of hepatocytes, but usually necrosis can only be inferred from the presence of mitoses in the hepatocytes (Hutt, 1971). In Papua New Guinea also, jaundice seems to be predominantly hepatocellular in origin (Radford, Rhodes, and Matz, 1967); in a study of 27 cases, focal liver-cell death, usually without an inflammatory response, was usual. In three patients in that study, however, portal tract inflammatory infiltration was so marked that that together with the parenchymal cell necrosis made it impossible to distinguish the appearances from moderately severe viral hepatitis.

6.1.2. Intrahepatic cholestasis

Sixteen adult African men with lobar pneumonia and clinical jaundice were studied by Theron, Pepler, and Mekel (1972) at Pretoria, South Africa. Light microscopy showed swelling of the hepatocytes with narrowing and sometimes obliteration of hepatic sinusoids, but no evidence of cholestasis. However on electron microscopy there was dilatation of bile canaliculi with atrophy or disappearance of microvilli; also, deposition of hepatocellular bile pigment and evidence of a toxic liver injury was demonstrated by microsegregation of hepatocyte nucleoli, dilatation of rough endoplasmic reticulum, and increase in the numbers of free ribosomes and polysomes. Paracrystalline inclusions were seen in the mitochondria and there was an increase in fat-storing cells (lipocytes) during the acute phase. These changes were thought to represent a transient toxic liver injury with a marked cholestatic element. Evidence of mild cholestasis was occasionally seen in the Uganda study (Kibukamusoke, *et al.*, 1964). In eight patients with a variety of bacterial infections studied in Switzerland by Fahrländer, Huber, and Gloor (1964) electron microscopy showed marked intrahepatic cholestasis in the absence of injury to the hepatocytes. Other causes of intrahepatic cholestasis were excluded in that investigation.

6.1.3. Haemolytic jaundice

Twenty-eight Nigerians, most of them of Hausa or Fulani stock, were studied in Zaria, Nigeria by Tugwell and Williams (1977); they were compared with 70 patients with lobar pneumonia who were not jaundiced. Most had clear evidence of pneumococcal pneumonia, either from positive blood culture or by the demonstration of pneumococcal antigen in the blood or urine. Haemolysis which is a well known complication of glucose-6-phosphate dehydrogenase deficiency, was a dominant feature in that series. All had a raised reticulocyte count (mean 6·1 per cent; range 2 to 20 per cent); there was also an initial fall in the packed cell volume, and most had an excess of urobilinogen in the urine together with demonstrable iron in liver-biopsy specimens. The haemolysis was associated with glucose-6-phosphate dehydrogenase deficiency in 24 patients. More than half of the serum bilirubin was conjugated; serum alkaline phosphatase concentrations were mildly elevated in 10 of those patients. Light and electron microscopy showed changes consistent with haemolysis, although hepatocellular damage and cholestasis were also present (Williams, Tugwell, and Edington, 1976). There was no evidence of an immunological deficit in this group. The association between glucose-6-phosphate dehydrogenase deficiency, lobar pneumonia, and haemolysis has not been substantiated in another study (Parent, 1973).

6.1.4. Effect of systemic infection on biochemical tests of liver function in the absence of jaundice

In six patients with an infective process outside the liver, e.g. bacterial endocarditis or perinephric abscess, two or more of the enzymes: alkaline phosphatase, 5-nucleotidase, transaminases, and isocitric dehydrogenase, were raised (Neale, Caughey, Mollin, and Booth, 1966). Liver histology showed a non-specific reactive hepatitis with an increase of Kupffer cells and some portal infiltration; cultures of the biopsies were sterile. Four other patients with intrahepatic infections (either a pyogenic or amoebic liver abscess, or portal pylephlebitis) and raised serum B_{12} concentrations, had biochemical tests of liver function which were also abnormal; they were however indistinguishable from those in the patients with extra hepatic infections. The cause of the hepatic dysfunction was not investigated; direct bacterial invasion of the liver was considered unlikely and bacterial toxins were thought to be the probable cause. Using an intravenous galactose clearance test, it was not possible to detect an abnormality in seven patients with intra-abdominal sepsis who had abnormal liver-function tests (Royle, Kettlewell, Ilic, and Williamson, 1978); however, the rise in blood glucose was less after galactose than in a control group. Fever alone has, however, been shown to interfere with bromsulphthalein excretion (Hicks, Holt, Guerrant and Leavell, 1948).

6.1.5. Conclusions on the mechanism(s) of jaundice

It seems clear therefore that the jaundice associated with systemic bacterial infections has a complex basis. While some evidence of mild hepatocellular necrosis is usual, cholestatic features are usually more pronounced; most serum bilirubin is conjugated in most reports, but the serum alkaline phosphatase is not usually markedly elevated. The report of Tugwell and Williams (1977), in which the importance of haemolysis is stressed, also indicates that cholestasis was a marked feature on electron microscopy. The incidence of haemolysis doubtless depends largely on the underlying incidence of glucose-6-phosphate dehydrogenase deficiency in the population being studied; this is relatively high in west Africans and American negroes.

It may very well be that there is an individual susceptibility to a bacterial toxin, and that that may have a genetic basis; whether there is a relationship between such a predisposition to the results of mild hepatotoxic agents and systemic infections, and the Gilbert and Dubin-Johnson syndromes (see below) is not yet clear. A suggestion that the disease is viral in origin, and that a latent infection is activated by the bacterial pneumonia (Kibukamusoke, *et al.*, 1964), has not been substantiated.

6.2. Clinical aspects of the jaundice of systemic infection

6.2.1. Presentation

The patient is usually acutely ill, with a high fever, up to 41°C. Men are more often affected than women. Elderly people are probably more prone to the disease. The right lower lobe is affected more often than other lobes (Radford, *et al.*, 1967; Tugwell and Williams, 1977); this might be because diminished movement of the right diaphragm predisposes to consolidation of the right lower lobe. The liver is usually enlarged and frequently tender. The depth of jaundice is very variable, but it may be deep with serum total bilirubin concentrations of up to 290 μmol per l and a conjugated level of 136 μmol per l in the series described by Hall and Parry (1963). Tugwell and Williams (1977) reported concentrations up to 332 μmol per l, with a conjugated component of 239 μmol per l, and Kibukamusoke, *et al.* (1964) a concentration of 462 μmol per l. The condition does not seem to influence the prognosis adversely and death in the presence of deep jaundice is unusual; one of 18 in the Uganda (Kibukamusoke, *et al.*, 1964), and 2 of 11 in one of the Nigeria (Hall and Parry, 1963) series died. Pyrexia seems to continue for longer after antibiotic treatment is started, compared with patients with lobar pneumonia who are not jaundiced. Although the serum bilirubin occasionally reaches very high levels it is usually not, however, markedly elevated; the concentration was greater than 171 μmol per l (10 mg per dl) in three (n = 11), five (n = eight), four (n = 21), and two (n = 28) patients in the reports by Hall and Parry (1963), Fahrländer, *et al.* (1964), Kibukamusoke, *et al.* (1964), and Tugwell and Williams (1977), respectively. In the majority of patients most bilirubin is in the conjugated form. Serum alkaline phosphatase concentrations were elevated in 2, 6, 2, and 10 patients in those reports, respectively. Most patients have mildly raised serum transaminase concentrations, but it is very unusual for them to be grossly elevated (Kibukamusoke, *et al.*, 1964; Tugwell and Williams, 1977).

6.2.2. Differential diagnosis

It is extremely important that jaundice in the presence of lobar pneumonia, and other infections, is distinguished from viral hepatitis. If the condition is borne in mind, there is usually clear evidence of a bacterial infection and serum transaminases are probably never as markedly elevated as they are in early viral hepatitis. Other causes of acute hepatic injury with jaundice (Chapter 7) should also be excluded.

The enlarged tender liver with clinical evidence of pathology at the right lung base may make the distinction from hepatic amoebiasis (Chapter 12) difficult. However, jaundice is unusual in amoebic liver disease and the only abnormality in liver function tests, which is relatively consistent is a raised serum alkaline phosphatase concentration.

Pneumonia occurring in a patient with underlying chronic liver disease, including cirrhosis may also pose a diagnostic problem.

6.3. Other forms of jaundice precipitated by systemic infection

6.3.1. Gilbert's syndrome

In this condition (Gilbert and Lereboullet, 1901), there is an intermittent elevation of serum unconjugated bilirubin; deepening of jaundice often occurs after systemic infections. It seems to be common in Jewish people. When the bilirubin is elevated, mild generalized symptoms, malaise, nausea, and liver discomfort, are present (Foulk, Butt, Owen, Whitcomb, and Mason, 1959). The main importance of the syndrome is to recognize it and not mistake it for viral hepatitis or some more serious form of jaundice. Although there is some evidence that this is an inherited condition, the mode of transmission of which has been suggested to be a Mendelian autosomal dominant with incomplete penetrance and variability of expression, that is not proved. When serum bilirubin concentrations in a normal group of people are plotted they form a unimodal distribution and it seems likely that people with an elevated unconjugated bilirubin (Gilbert's syndrome) are normal but at the upper end of the normal distribution curve for serum bilirubin (Bailey, Robinson, and Dawson, 1977).

6.3.2. The Dubin–Johnson and Rotor syndromes

In these syndromes there is a high concentration of conjugated bilirubin (*Lancet*, 1978). In the Dubin–Johnson syndrome (Dubin and Johnson, 1954), there is a dark pigment in the liver, giving aspiration liver-biopsies a blackish appearance; that is not the case with the Rotor syndrome which was first described in the Philippines (Rotor, Manahan, and Florentin, 1948). Although the jaundice is cholestatic in type, there is no pruritis, and serum alkaline phosphatase concentrations are normal. The abnormality in bile excretion is probably the same in both syndromes but it is not yet certain what that is. The bromsulphthalein excretion curve is characteristic, with a secondary peak at 90 to 180 minutes.

The Dubin–Johnson syndrome seems to be more common than expected in the Madang district of Papua New Guinea (Vaughan, 1969; Vaughan, Marubbio, Maddocks, and Cooke, 1970); there is no evidence that it occurs in Africa, and many thousands of liver-biopsies have been examined there. The Rotor syndrome, too, seems to be unusually common in Papua New Guinea (Vaughan, 1969).

References

Bailey, A., Robinson, D., and Dawson, A. M. (1977) *Lancet*, **1,** 931.

Clain, D. and Gelfand, M. (1964). *Cent. Afr. J. Med.*, **10,** 217.

Dubin, I. N. and Johnson, F. B. (1954). *Medicine, Baltimore*, **33,**155.

Eley, A., Hargreaves, T., and Lambert, H. P. (1965). *Br. med. J.*, **2,** 75.

Fahrländer, H., Huber, F., and Gloor, F. (1964). *Gastroenterology*, **47,** 590.

Foulk, W. T., Butt, H. R , Owen, C. A., Whitcomb, F. F., and Mason, H. L. (1959). *Medicine, Baltimore*, **38,** 25.

Gelfand, M. (1947). *J. trop. Med. Hyg.*, **50,** 15.

GILBERT, A. and LEREBOULLET, P. (1901). *Sem. méd.*, **21,** 241.
HALL, E. W. and PARRY, E. H. O. (1963). *Trans. R. Soc. trop. Med. Hyg.*, **57,** 206.
HICKS, M. H., HOLT, H. P., GUERRANT, J. L. and LEAVELL, B. S. (1948). *J. clin. Invest.*, **27,** 580.
HUTT, M. S. R. (1971). *Trans. R. Soc. trop. Med. Hyg.*, **65,** 273.
KIBUKAMUSOKE, J. W., PATEL, K. M. and HUTT, M. S. R. (1964). *E. Afr. med. J.*, **41,** 203.
Lancet (1978). **2,** 926.
NEALE, G., CAUGHEY, D. E., MOLLIN, D. L. and BOOTH, C. C. (1966). *Br. med. J.*, **1,** 382.
OSLER, W. (1920). *The principles and practice of medicine.* Appleton, New York.
PARENT, M. A. (1973). *Lancet*, **2,** 155.
RADFORD, A. J., RHODES, F. A., and MATZ, L. R. (1967). *Med. J. Aust.*, **2,** 678.
ROTOR, A. B., MANAHAN, L., and FLORENTIN, A. (1948). *Acta med. philipp.*, **5,** 37.
ROYLE, G. KETTLEWELL, M. G. W., ILIC, V., and WILLIAMSON, D. H. (1978). *Clin. Sci. molec. Med.*, **55,** 199.
SHAPER, A. G. and SHAPER, L. (1958). *E. Afr. med. J.*, **35,** 647.
THERON, J. J., PEPLER, W. J., and MEKEL, R. C. P. M. (1972). *J. Path.*, **106,** 113.
TROWELL, H. C. (1932). *Kenya E. Afr. med. J.*, **9,** 258 and 294.
—— (1960). *Non-infective disease in Africa.* p. 26. Edward Arnold, London.
TUGWELL, P. and WILLIAMS, A. O. (1977). *Q. Jl. Med.*, **46,** 97.
VAUGHAN, J. P. (1969). *Papua New Guin. med. J.*, **12,** 128.
——, MARUBBIO, A. T., MADDOCKS, I., and COOKE, R. A. (1970). *Trans. R. Soc. trop. Med. Hyg.*, **64,** 287.
WILLIAMS, A. O., TUGWELL, P. and EDINGTON, G. M. (1976). *Archs Path.*, **100,** 25.
ZIMMERMAN, H. J. and THOMAS, L. J. (1950). *J. Lab. clin. Med.*, **35,** 556.

7

Acute hepatic injury of viral, bacterial, and parasitic origin

7.1. Viral hepatitis

THIS is a clinical syndrome, associated with a number of viral infections (WHO, 1975). Epidemic, infectious hepatitis (*type A hepatitis*) is usually caused by a viral infection of the gastrointestinal tract. Serum hepatitis is in most cases, produced by a virus which can now be easily detected by a marker antigen (HB_sAg) in blood (*type B hepatitis*). A variety of other virus infections, all of which produce an approximately similar clinical picture, are also grouped under this heading, at least temporarily.

Hepatitis B surface antigen (HB_sAg) (Blumberg, Alter, and Visnich, 1965) is present in the serum in type B hepatitis, and serological tests are now available to diagnose type A infections. When types A and B are accounted for by serological analyses, a group is left which has been designated non-A, non-B (type C) hepatitis.

Viral hepatitis is not usually considered as a 'tropical disease'. However, it is extremely important in all tropical countries and often carries a substantial mortality rate (Hutt, 1971; Powell and McGovern, 1976).

In Africa and Asia it is endemic, with occasional epidemics (Morrow, Smetana, Sai, and Edgcomb, 1968). In 1963, for example, there was a large epidemic at Madi, Uganda, and in 1964 and 1965 a similar one occurred at Karamoja where it was probably introduced by Sudanese refugees (Sood, Hulley, and Hutt, 1966); subsequent outbreaks occurred at Karamoja, Soroti and Kigezi.

This disease is an important health hazard for travellers, and especially European 'overlanders' during their hitchhikes or bus journeys across Asia (*Br. med. J.*, 1977); India, Pakistan, Afghanistan, and Nepal seem to be particularly severely infected areas. Mediterranean countries, including Israel, also have hepatitis rates which are substantially greater than those in the UK and other northern European countries.

7.1.1. Aetiology

Hepatitis A. The virus-like particles of this agent measure 27 nm in diameter and are present in the faeces in the acute phase of hepatitis A infections; those particles are often coated with antibody, which is present in convalescent serum. Serological tests for this agent are now available, but are so far less widely used than those for HB_sAg.

Hepatitis B. The antigen HB_sAg was first detected in the serum of an Australian aboriginal during serological investigations designed to detect inherited susceptibility to various diseases (Blumberg, *et al.*, 1965; Blumberg, 1972); it was subsequently known as Australia, or hepatitis-associated antigen. It was soon shown to be common in Pacific and Asian communities but very uncommon in the American population. The surface antigen is now known as HB_sAg and is a marker for infection with the hepatitis B virus (Zuzarte and Kasili, 1978).

Serum in virus B infections contains three distinct morphological entities: (i) small pleomorphic spherical particles, some 20 to 22 nm in diameter (Almeida, 1971), (ii) tubular forms of varying length with a constant diameter of 20 nm, and frequently containing a terminal bulbous swelling, and (iii) double-shelled spheroidal 'Dane particles' of 42 nm diameter (Dane, Cameron, and Briggs, 1970), with a core measuring 27 nm in diameter. The Dane particle carries HB_sAg on its surface and HB_cAg in its core; HB_sAg is also carried by the 20 nm particles. Antibody to hepatitis B (anti-HB_s) appears after the acute infection has subsided; in some tropical countries it is present in up to 30 per cent of the population (Anthony, Vogel, Sadikali, Barker, and Peterson, 1972).

Non-A, non-B hepatitis. Following the introduction of sensitive tests to detect types A and B hepatitis, it has now become clear that there is a further entity (or entities), non-A, non-B (type C) which is (are) also important in producing viral hepatitis (Dienstag, Alaama, Mosley, Redeker, and Purcell, 1977; Alter, Purcell, Holland, and Popper, 1978; *Br. med. J.*, 1978; Tabor, Gerety, Drucker, Seeff, Hoofnagle, Jackson, April, Barker, and Pineda-Tamondong, 1978). It is spread by both parenteral and oral routes, and a chronic carrier state can exist. Overall it seems likely that non-A, non-B hepatitis is not a homogeneous entity but encompasses a number of viral agents; it might in fact account for more cases of viral hepatitis than either the type A or type B virus.

7.1.2. Incidence and mode of infection

The incidence rate of the disease in the tropics is probably higher than in most temperate zones, and there is evidence to suggest higher morbidity and mortality rates (Hutt, 1971). It is clearly highly probable that only a very small minority of cases are seen in hospital; the true incidence and mortality rates are thus quite unknown. The increasing use of injections by both qualified and unqualified practitioners, and of blood-transfusions suggests that the disease is likely to become even more common. Evidence of that has come from a study by Maynard, Sadikali, Anthony, and Barker (1970); of 20 cases of clinical viral hepatitis, 12 had HB_sAg in their serum; three of 143 controls and 15 of 49 cases of cirrhosis also had positive results. Often it is not possible to screen all blood donors for HB_sAg and even if it were it would be impossible to reject all positive people as donors, so great is the need for blood. In western countries however where there is a very low positivity rate for HB_sAg great care should be taken in selection of donors from tropical countries (*Lancet*, 1973).

Hepatitis A (incubation period 2–6 weeks) is a considerable risk to the traveller and is usually transmitted by the orofaecal route, either directly, by contact with an infected individual, or indirectly, by drinking contaminated water. Areas where sanitation is poor are associated with an increased risk. The disease has a worldwide distribution, and occurs in epidemics. Spread by the intravenous route is, however, also possible. In the winter of 1955–6, 29 000 cases of this disease occurred in Delhi, India, during a seven-week period, after the main water supply of the city had been contaminated with sewage. Swimming pools have been responsible for some outbreaks. Raw shellfish and clams may also be important. Pregnant women seem to have a higher mortality rate than the non-pregnant (see below).

Hepatitis B (incubation period 6–26 weeks) is common in most tropical countries and in those, the carrier rate for HB_sAg is frequently high (Eke, 1976). In an investigation of viral hepatitis in Dar-es-Salaam, Tanzania, 82 per cent of patients had HB_sAg in the serum during the first week of the illness (Nantulya, Lindqvist, and Spencer, 1975); in the second week and after the third week 46 and 22 per cent, respectively, were positive. Corresponding figures during the illness from Kenya (Bagshawe, Parker, and Jindani, 1971), Uganda (Sadikali, 1972), and Ghana (Morrow, Sai, and Barker, 1971; Foli, Christian, and Swaniker, 1974) were 54, 62, 94, and 62 per cent, respectively.

Survival of hepatitis B virus is ensured by the reservoir of persistent carriers, of which there are estimated to be 120–175 million in the world. The prevalence of carriers in northern Europe and north America is less than 0·1 per cent, and in central and eastern Europe up to five per cent. In southern Europe and the countries bordering the Mediterranean, and in some parts of Africa and Asia up to 20 per cent of the population are carriers (Blumberg, Sutnick, and London, 1970; Prince, 1970; Bagshawe and Nganda, 1973).

Studies in Africa, Asia, and the Pacific islands have all given high rates. For example, approximately 20 per cent of serum samples from young asymptomatic people in the Philippines (Blumberg, Melartin, Guinto, and Lechat, 1970) and 9 per cent of those in Papua New Guinea (Simons, Binns, Malcolm and Yap, 1972) give positive results.

A high incidence of HB_sAg has been shown in Nigerian children (Williams, Fabiyi, Williams, Gupta, O'Connor, and Greenwood, 1973); the mode of infection is however not clear. Those with persistent antigenaemia tend to have evidence of acute and chronic liver disease.

The risk of virus hepatitis B infection not only from blood transfusions (Woodfield, 1977; Grady, 1978) but also from contaminated syringes has been stressed by many, including Zuckerman (1978); that route is possible even if needles are changed after each injection when a multidose syringe is being used. Spread may be by droplet infection, for the antigen is found in saliva. HB_sAg can be transmitted by mosquitoes in Nigeria, Kenya, and Uganda (Prince, Metselaar, Kakuko, Mukwaya, Ling, and Overby, 1972; Smith, Ogunba, and Francis, 1972; Brotman, Prince, and Godfrey, 1973; Wills, Saimot, Brochard, Blumberg, London, Dechene, and Millman, 1976) although that has not been confirmed in experimental studies in chimpanzees (Berquist, Maynard, Francy, Sheller, and Schable, 1976). Scarification, tattooing, circumcision, and possible carriage by parasites which penetrate the skin, have all been suggested as being important. HB_sAg can also be present in the faeces and the faeco-oral route may be more important in the tropics than in temperate countries (Morrow, *et al.*, 1971), although overall the parenteral route is probably the more important. Sexual contacts are also a source of transmission; the disease can clearly be spread venereally (Heathcote and Sherlock, 1974). In Papua New Guinea, babies sometimes have anti-HB_s in their cord serum, but not HB_sAg (Woodfield, 1972).

HB_sAg usually disappears from the serum after 6–12 weeks of convalescence; if it persists chronic liver disease may ensue (Chapter 8). In Uganda for example, it is present in a significantly higher proportion of patients with cirrhosis and hepatoma than controls (Vogel, Anthony and Sadikali, 1972).

Patients with hepatic schistosomiasis are often persistent carriers for HB_sAg (Lyra, Rebouças, and Andrade, 1976); furthermore, those carriers have more clinical signs of chronic liver disease and liver-biopsy sections show more chronic inflammation in the portal areas than in non-carriers.

Non-A, non-B hepatitis (incubation period 18–100 days) is usually transmitted by blood (Meyers, Dienstag, Purcell, Thomas, and Holmes, 1977; Hoofnagle, Gerety, Tabor, Feinstone, Barker, and Purcell, 1977).

7.1.3. Clinical presentation

The clinical presentation of viral hepatitis is described in standard texts (Sherlock, 1975). The prodromal phase with anorexia, nausea, fever, pain behind the eyes, and aversion to smoking is widely known; these symptoms are followed by darkening of the urine, jaundice, and upper abdominal discomfort. In some a cholestatic element gives rise to pale stools and pruritis. The whole illness usually lasts from two to three weeks. Several clinical courses are recognizable and they can all be caused by A, B, or non-A, non-B viruses: (i) acute icteric, (ii) acute non-icteric, (iii) relapsing, (iv) subacute ('bridging' hepatitis) (Boyer and Klatskin, 1970), (v) prolonged cholestatic, and (vi) fulminant. In addition, the post-hepatitis syndrome (Sherlock, 1975) is a genuine entity. Whatever the virus, the clinical picture is similar with the exception that virus B tends to produce a more severe illness and more chronic sequelae, compared with the others. Type B can also produce a 'serum-sickness' like syndrome in the initial stages of the disease (Graves, 1843); urticaria, maculopapular and erythematous rashes, arthralgia, and angioneurotic oedema may be present; these are due to circulating immune complexes of HB_sAg, HB antibody and complement (Alpert, Isselbacher, and Schur, 1971). There is also a reduction in the serum concentration of the C 3 component of complement.

The fact that viral hepatitis is a generalized disease which involves not only the liver but also the gastrointestinal tract, kidneys, and blood should be borne in mind (Conrad, Schwartz, and Young, 1964).

Virus A tends to cause disease in younger age groups, has a shorter incubation period, and generally runs a more benign course; it is also less likely to progress to active chronic hepatitis, chronic persistent hepatitis, and cirrhosis (Rakela, Redeker, Edwards, Decker, Overby, and Mosley, 1978).

The clinical course of the non-A, non-B virus, although usually more mild, is similar to that produced by the hepatitis B virus. That disease has been implicated in 15 cases of fulminant hepatitis, half of whom died (Rakela, Mosley, and Redeker, 1975); it can also give rise to active chronic hepatitis, chronic persistent hepatitis, and cirrhosis (Knodell, Conrad, and Ishak, 1977).

The disease may apparently be more severe in glucose-6-phosphate dehydrogenase deficient patients (Morrow, *et al.*, 1968). Evidence of haemolysis may be present.

Herpes simplex, rubella, and cytomegalovirus can also all produce an acute hepatitis especially in neonates. After multiple transfusions, Epstein-Barr virus, and cytomegalovirus are other responsible agents.

The jaundice of acute bacterial infections (Chapter 6) must be distinguished from viral hepatitis; there is usually clinical evidence of a severe infection and diagnosis is in most cases straightforward.

Both hepatic amoebiasis and typhoid fever may be associated with liver involvement; although deep jaundice is unusual in both, a tender liver is a feature, especially in the former condition (Chapter 12).

All other causes of acute hepatic damage, mentioned later in this chapter should be borne in mind.

Hepatic insults caused by therapeutic agents and toxins, sometimes a result of treatment by local 'medicine men' should be considered in the differential diagnosis. If therapeutic agents as used in the western world are responsible for some cases that is overshadowed by the vast number of cases of viral hepatitis; the exact role of local 'medicines' in the pathogenesis of liver injury is impossible to ascertain.

Hepatomegaly and abnormal liver-function tests are common in homozygous (SS) sickle-cell disease; that may be mistaken for viral hepatitis.

There are numerous causes of acute haemolysis in tropical countries and they must be differentiated from hepatitis as a cause of jaundice. The various haemoglobinopathies, the thalassaemias, glucose-6-phosphate dehydrogenase deficiency, acute malaria ('blackwater fever'), and various bacterial infections (especially lobar pneumonia) (Chapter 6) being some of them. Acute haemolytic anaemia may also be caused by viral infections (Choremis, Kattamis, Kyriazakou, and Gavriilidou, 1966) including viral hepatitis itself (Morrow, *et al.*, 1968) especially in the presence of glucose-6-phosphate deficiency. Malaria may also produce severe haemolysis in the presence of glucose-6-phosphate dehydrogenase deficiency (Devakul, Garby, and Harinasuta, 1966).

7.1.4. Fulminant viral hepatitis

This grave complication of viral hepatitis can follow type A, type B, and non-A, non-B hepatitis. It is very common in some parts of the tropics, including Africa (Himsworth, 1950). In Uganda it is not unusual to have several cases in hospital at one time with this complication, which has a 50–100 per cent mortality rate; however throughout Africa, there are great differences in incidence. For example in Zambia it is not nearly so common as in Uganda and Nigeria; it is almost a rarity in Papua New Guinea. In Nigeria, the condition is more common in women than men (Edington and Gilles, 1976); 4·4 and 0·8 per cent of post-mortems following viral hepatitis are in women and men, respectively. The clinical features of 18 women seen over an eight-year period at University College Hospital, Ibadan, with acute massive necrosis have been described (Ojo, Francis, and Onifade, 1971). The condition also carries a high mortality rate in India (Phatak and Patil, 1956). Whether undernutrition predisposes to a fatal outcome is unknown; a study in Nigeria in which groups of well-nourished and under-nourished people were observed in a single viral hepatitis epidemic suggested that that might be a factor. Fulminant hepatitis is also more common in pregnancy, although toxic herbal medicines may play a part in that. Hormonal, immunological, or dietary (Himsworth, 1950) factors may be involved. In a report from Addis Ababa, Ethiopia, 30 of 84 pregnant and 12 of 64 non-pregnant women developed fulminant hepatitis, most commonly in the third trimester (Tsega, 1976); mortality occurred in 19 and 7 respectively ($P < 0{\cdot}05$). Complications of the pregnancy and foetal death were also common.

Clinically there may be a change of personality in a usually deeply jaundiced patient; aggressive behaviour and episodes of mania are common. Although deepening jaundice is usual, death may occur in a severe case before jaundice develops. Persistent vomiting, and sometimes fever and foetor hepatis develop. There may also be a flapping tremor. Tendon reflexes may be hyperactive. The liver size decreases and the edge cannot be felt on abdominal examination. A bleeding diathesis and renal failure are usual in the terminal stages. The duration and depth of coma does not correlate with the severity of necrosis seen in liver-biopsy sections (Horney and Galambos, 1977).

Electroencephalographic changes are usual. Serum bilirubin and transaminases and other liver function tests are of no value in assessing the prognosis; the prothrombin ratio seems to be the best indicator of prognosis (Cook and Sherlock, 1965; Rake, Flute, Pannell, Shilkin, and Williams, 1973). There is usually an associated hypoglycaemia and the serum urea concentration is diminished.

Death is usually caused by cardiac or respiratory failure, cerebral oedema, septicaemia, renal failure, hypoglycaemia, or pancreatitis; usually several (or most) of those are responsible. No methods are available to distinguish this entity from fulminant hepatic failure associated with therapeutic agents (Cook and Sherlock, 1965).

7.1.5. Other sequelae of infection

About 10 per cent of patients with type B infections still have HB_sAg in the blood after six months, and the antigen may persist thereafter. Two courses are possible: (i) normal structure and function of the liver continue (the true 'carrier state'), or (ii) a chronic hepatitis (Chapter 8) develops, and macronodular cirrhosis and ultimately hepatoma may subsequently complicate that disease (Dudley, Scheuer, and Sherlock, 1972) (Chapter 9). Non-A non-B hepatitis can also be associated with the 'carrier state' and chronic hepatitis.

Type A hepatitis probably does not proceed to chronic hepatitis (Rakela, *et al.*, 1978; Sherlock, 1978); follow-up studies have failed to show evidence of a 'carrier state' or chronic hepatitis. In the USA 60 to 70 per cent of normal adults have antibodies to type A virus.

There is little doubt that viral hepatitis is the main cause for most cases of cirrhosis (usually of the macronodular type) seen in the tropics, although longitudinal studies in epidemics do not suggest that progression is common (Chuttani, Sidhu, Wig, Gupta, and Ramalingaswami, 1966). It is possible that in malnourished people, the disease more often progresses to cirrhosis.

Overall, there is no doubt that many cases of cirrhosis in the tropics are associated with this disease (Steiner and Davies, 1957); active chronic hepatitis, which is common in Uganda (Hutt, 1971) is also related. It must be emphasized however that there are a limited number of ways in which the liver can respond to injury due to different aetiological agents (Cook, 1965; Bulkley, Heizer, Goldfinger, Isselbacher, and Schulman, 1970).

7.1.6. Pathology

Pathological changes in tropical countries are similar in every way to those seen in temperate areas. The hepatocytes vary in size and there is marked ballooning and feathery degeneration; their nuclei are often bi- and multinucleated. The nucleoli are enlarged. Eosinophilic necrosis is most marked in the central zones. Rounded eosinophilic structures may be seen in the sinusoids. There is a focal infiltration of histiocytes, lymphocytes, and plasma cells with occasional eosinophils and neutrophils; portal tracts contain a similar infiltrate. There may be collapse and consolidation of reticulin in the central and periportal areas. Bile stasis may be prominent. Lipofuscin may be present in the Kupffer cells. Haemosiderin may also be present.

Fig. 7.1 shows the histology in an aspiration liver-biopsy from a patient with acute viral hepatitis.

In fulminant hepatitis, the course may be so rapid that jaundice is absent at death, although that is unusual. A severe bleeding diathesis is common, associated with disseminated intravascular coagulation. The liver is small, yellow and of soft consistency, with a wrinkled capsule. The cut surface shows patchy areas of red, yellow and brownish-green tissue representing areas of collapse, necrosis, and surviving liver tissue, respectively (Fig. 7.2). There may be an associated pancreatitis and myocarditis; necrosis of the proximal renal tubules is usual.

Histology in fulminant hepatitis shows massive liver-cell necrosis; those changes are usually most severe in the left lobe. All of the parenchymal cells are affected; they are swollen, granular, and devoid of nuclei. The intralobular capillary walls are affected. A rim of surviving hepatocytes may surround the portal tracts. There is little cellular infiltration. If survival occurs, which is unusual, areas of collapse disappear and there is proliferation of fibrous tissue and bile-ducts; greyish-white scars result and hyperplasia of surviving hepatocytes produces nodule-formation. In some areas the lobular pattern is maintained. If recovery occurs it is not entirely clear what happens to the liver histology; it seems likely that some patients recover completely, but some undoubtedly go on to a macronodular cirrhosis. There is certainly a risk of

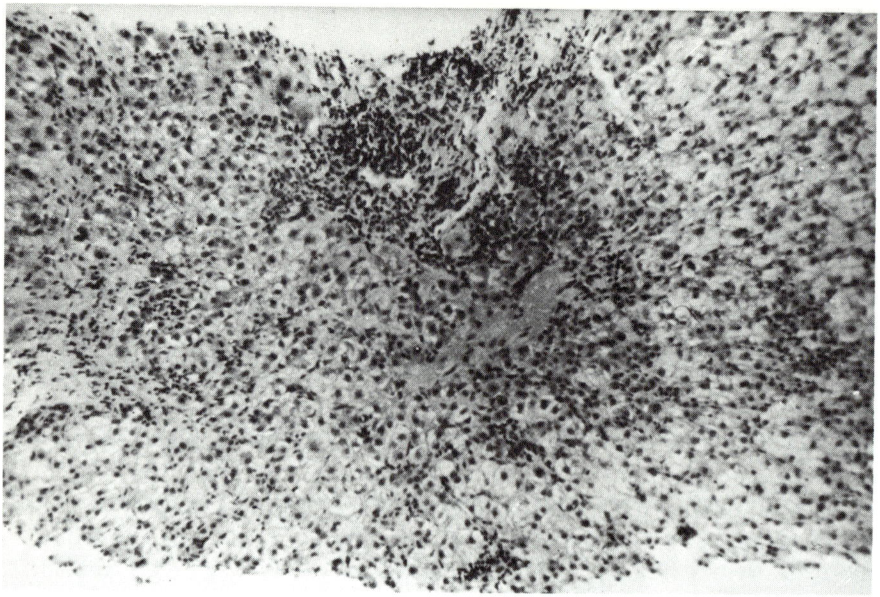

FIG. 7.1. Needle liver-biopsy section (haematoxylin and eosin) from a Papua New Guinean woman with viral hepatitis. Serum HB_sAg was negative. The clinical course was straightforward and uncomplicated.

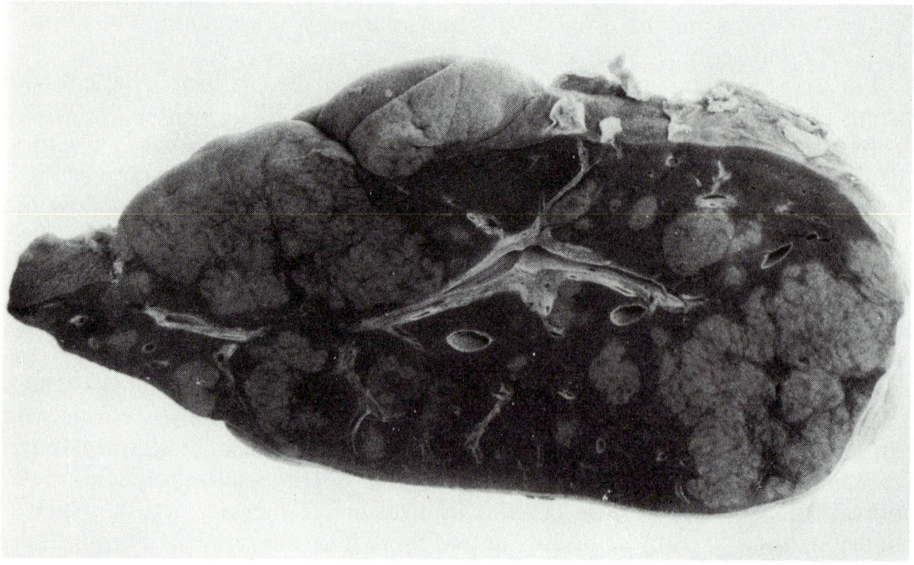

FIG. 7.2. Cut surface of the liver of a 20-year-old Australian aboriginal woman. The history was of jaundice and progressive malaise following a mild febrile illness some two or three weeks before. She had given birth to a healthy infant six months previously. Following admission to hospital, she lapsed into hepatic coma and died shortly afterwards. The liver was small and the section shows large pale areas of necrosis; there are also areas of relatively normal liver tissue.

developing active chronic hepatitis (Chapter 8) (Horney and Galambos, 1977); in that study, three of nine patients who had repeat liver-biopsies after recovery showed evidence of chronic complications.

7.1.7. *Investigation*

Biochemical disturbances occur early in the disease. Bilirubin in the urine appears before onset of clinical jaundice. Serum bilirubin, transaminases, and alkaline phosphatase concentrations are raised to varying degrees; the alkaline phosphatase rarely exceeds 30 King Armstrong units per dl. The prothrombin time is prolonged in severe cases and does not respond completely to vitamin K injections. Leucopenia and lymphopenia occur early in the disease; Coombs' positive haemolytic anaemia is a rare complication. It has been suggested that a rise in IgM is more common in type A hepatitis; a rise in serum total and IgM globulins takes place in both type A and type B.

In type B hepatitis, the virion (virus particle) appears in the plasma and has been called the Dane particle; it is produced in the cytoplasm of the hepatocyte, and is responsible for the HB_sAg reaction. Both core and '*e*' antigen appear in the serum later (Eleftheriou, Thomas, Heathcote, and Sherlock, 1975). About one month after exposure, *e* antigen (HB_eAg) (Magnius and Espmark, 1972) may be detected in the serum, but only transiently, unless continued infectivity and progressive liver disease are to ensue. Like core antigen, *e* antigen is localized in the hepatocyte nuclei; though sometimes present simultaneously, they are not identical (Arnold, Nielsen, Hardt, and Meyer zum Büschenfelde, 1977). Clinical hepatitis usually develops some two months after exposure, and the anti-core antigen appears shortly after the transaminases rise; however antibody to HB_sAg does not develop until about six months after exposure (Melnick, Dreesman, and Hollinger, 1976). Continued presence of HB_eAg in the serum is associated not only with progressive hepatic disease in the individual but probably renders him more infectious. Because patients with raised HB_eAg usually have evidence of progressive hepatic disease, demonstration of raised serum transaminases in a subject with HB_sAg seems to be of value in determining infectivity (Barbara, Mijovic, Cleghorn, Tedder, and Briggs, 1978).

Virus A particles appear in the faeces during the late incubation period of the disease and disappear a few days after development of jaundice. Antibody to virus A can now easily be detected (Moritsugu, Dienstag, Valdesuso, Wong, Wagner, Routenberg, and Purcell, 1976), but the methods are not yet in routine use.

Non-A, non-B (type C) hepatitis is diagnosed by exclusion of type A, type B, and other viruses. The HC antigen is not present in all cases of non-A, non-B hepatitis (Shirachi, Shiraishi, Tateda, Kikuchi, and Ishida, 1978), which indicates that there are more unidentified viruses that can cause the clinical syndrome of viral hepatitis.

7.1.8. *Treatment*

Indications for prophylaxis. Gamma-globulin is of proven efficacy in type A hepatitis (Pollock and Reid, 1969; Woodson and Clinton, 1969; *Co-operative study*, 1971), and might also confer some protection from type B hepatitis. It seems to be of value also in non-A, non-B hepatitis. For type B hepatitis, hyperimmune globulin containing high titres of anti-HB_s is probably better then gamma-globulin. However, more needs to be known about tourist hepatitis before this becomes a routine prerequisite for travellers.

Approximately 50 per cent of the one million annual Swedish tourists to Mediterranean countries obtain gamma-globulin prophylaxis before they set out (Iwarson and Stenqvist, 1976). Between 1965–74 there were 112 cases of 'tourist hepatitis' of whom 20 per cent were HB_sAg positive; only five of them had received prophylaxis. Those authors estimated that the incidence of hepatitis in tourists not given gamma-globulin was approximately 1 in 3000.

Because many healthy people, especially in the lower socioeconomic groups, have antibody to hepatitis A, and the proportion rises with increasing age, gammaglobulin should be reserved ideally for those without immunity. Unfortunately however tests for hepatitis A antibody are not yet widely available. At present gamma-globulin should only be given to visitors to the tropics—Africa, Asia, and the Far east where not only is the disease highly endemic but public health standards are frequently abysmally low.

Management of the straightforward case. This does not differ from the management in a temperate area and has been clearly described by Sherlock (1978). Bed rest during the icteric phase and avoidance of alcohol for six months are probably important. Commonsense grounds suggest that two hepatic insults are worse than one, but there is no clear proof that alcohol deprivation either hastens recovery or prevents the development of chronic complications. A normal diet should be given throughout; fat free diets are not indicated although fat may be poorly tolerated during the acute phase. Corticosteroids are not indicated; although they lessen the depth of jaundice and depress the serum transaminases, there is no evidence that they influence histology. The low infectivity of virus A hepatitis means that such patients can be nursed in ordinary hospital wards without a great danger of crossinfection; this is consistent with much clinical experience in the past, which now has a scientific basis.

Management of fulminant hepatitis. No treatment is of any real value in this very serious disease. Many methods of treatment have been used, largely as means of hepatic support, until regeneration of the hepatocytes occurs, but unsuccessfully; they include corticosteroids, exchange blood-transfusions, use of cross-circulation with a donor patient, extracorporeal perfusion with a baboon or pig liver, and hepatic transplant (Sherlock, 1975). Acute gastrointestinal haemorrhage, often a very difficult problem in management, may be controlled with cimetidine (Macdougall, Bailey, and Williams, 1977; Finkelstein and Isselbacher, 1978). The management of this disease is exceedingly depressing.

7.2. Other acute viral diseases involving the liver

Although not nearly as common as viral hepatitis, there are several other viral infections involving the liver which are also of great importance in a tropical context (Zuckerman, 1970), thus emphasizing the importance of not diagnosing every case of jaundice of acute onset as viral hepatitis.

7.2.1. *Yellow fever*

Yellow fever is caused by a group B arbovirus which is transmitted by mosquitoes (*Aëdes aegypti, A. africanus*, and *Haemagogus* species); it is characterized by fever, jaundice, a haemorrhagic diathesis, and albuminuria.

The endemic areas are tropical Africa and south America; occasional epidemics occur in, for example, the Sudan and Ethiopia (Sérié, 1963), Senegal (Chambon and Wone, 1967), and Nigeria (Monath, Lee, Wilson, Fagbami, and Tomori, 1974; Lee, Monath, Tomori, Fagbami, and Wilson, 1974).

Urban and *jungle* forms of the disease are recognized; the latter may be endemic or epizootic, and monkeys and other non-human primates are important in the epidemiology (Monath and Kemp, 1973). The urban form has a man-mosquito-man cycle.

Following a bite by an infected mosquito, the virus is passed to the regional lymph-glands; after replication there, a viraemia follows. The onset is sudden. The organs principally involved are the liver, kidney, and reticuloendothelial system. There may be petechial haemorrhages in the skin, and a bleeding diathesis which may include haematemesis and melaena; that is due to an effect of the virus on the capillary endothelium, associated with a prothrombin deficiency (see below). Severe liver involvement, with a rapidly progressive jaundice and hypoglycaemic attacks, is common. Albuminuria is present, as a result of acute tubular necrosis which occurs early in the disease; anuria, uraemia, coma, and death may follow. Cardiac involvement accounts for a bradycardia relative to the degree of pyrexia.

If death occurs in the first six days of infection, it is usually a result of hepatic failure; the second most usual cause is renal involvement. Pneumonia, cardiac involvement, parotitis, adrenal cortical necrosis, cutaneous infections, and renal abscesses may complicate the disease. If recovery occurs there is lasting immunity.

The liver is yellow and soft at post-mortem. Mid-zonal necrosis of the hepatocytes is the characteristic histological lesion; however almost the complete lobule may be involved, with a mere rim of hepatocytes around the portal tracts and centrilobular veins surviving. Patchy eosinophilic hyaline necrosis of the hepatocytes occurs, with disappearance of the nucleus, leaving behind a dense acidophilic mass, the Councilman body. Fatty change, ballooning, and feathery degeneration of hepatocytes are also usual. Kupffer cells may contain iron pigment and traces of lipofuscin. Liver architecture remains intact and cirrhosis is probably not a sequel to this disease. Bile-duct proliferation, bile retention, and a cellular inflammatory reaction are most unusual. After approximately two weeks of the disease, liver-biopsy histology shows a non-specific hepatitis with eosinophilic and ochre bodies in the sinusoids (Francis, Moore, Edington, and Smith, 1972).

The kidneys are swollen with cortical pallor and medullary congestion. Changes in the epithelial cells of the proximal tubules vary from fatty change to coagulation necrosis; basophilic concretions and products of haemoglobin destruction may appear as casts in the tubules.

An initial leucocytosis is followed by a leucopenia and lymphopenia. Serum transaminases are raised and prothrombin time markedly prolonged. Albuminuria is present, often with haemoglobinuria.

The virus may be isolated from blood by intracerebral mouse inoculation up to the fourth day of the disease (MacNamara, 1954); a rising titre of serum antibodies may be detected. Neutralization, complement-fixation and haemagglutination inhibition tests are also of value; the rise in HI, CF, and N antibodies is greater than for other group B arboviruses.

Liver-biopsy histology with virus isolation (Anderson and Wattley, 1955) is of value if the prothrombin time allows the procedure; in fatal cases, post-mortem liver histology with virus isolation is diagnostic.

7.2.2. Lassa fever, and Marburg and Ebola diseases

Lassa fever. This virus disease has undoubtedly been present, and has probably been widespread in west Africa for a long time (Gilles and Keane, 1977; Keane and Gilles, 1977). It was however first documented at Lassa, north-western Nigeria, in 1969 (Frame, Baldwin, Gocke, and Troup, 1970). There was a further outbreak at Jos, Nigeria in 1970 (Troup, White, Fom, and Carey, 1970). Subsequent outbreaks have occurred in Liberia (*Br. med. J.*, 1972) and Sierra Leone (Keane and Gilles, 1977). Early reports of this disease suggested an extremely high mortality rate; in the Sierra Leone outbreak however the figure was 15.6 per cent (Gilles and Keane, 1977). There are currently no reports of the disease originating from anywhere except west Africa. Lassa fever is now a notifiable disease in the UK (*Lancet*, 1976).

The causative agent is a member of the arena virus group (Buckley and Casals, 1970; Buckley, Casals, and Downs, 1970).

The mode of transmission is not clear. A common rodent in west Africa, *Mastomys natalensis*, is certainly responsible for a reservoir of infection, but the importance of rodent-to-man transfer is not yet clear (*Lancet*, 1974). It seems probable that man-to-man infection, possibly via the respiratory tract might occur. The incubation period is about one week.

High fever, a sore throat with a severe pharyngitis, and white patches in the pharynx (Chapter 2), soft palate, and tonsils, with cervical lymphadenopathy and headache are prominent features (White, 1972; Monath, 1974); epigastric pain and tenderness, diarrhoea, vomiting, cough, and a bleeding tendency may all be present. Although the liver is involved, jaundice is unusual. Myocarditis, pleural effusions and renal failure have been described.

Various grades of severity of the disease from a mild illness, which is sometimes asymptomatic, to a grave disease with a high mortality rate have been recorded. Death usually occurs on, or about, the tenth day of the disease.

Pathologically, findings are similar to those caused by type B arboviruses, including yellow fever. The liver is severely involved (Edington and White, 1972); there are focal areas of eosinophilic necrosis of the hepatocytes which contain lipochrome pigment, but there is no inflammatory exudate (Edington and Gilles, 1976). The liver sinusoids contain eosinophilic and brownish (ochre) bodies comparable to those seen in yellow fever (Villela, 1942). All parts of the lobule are randomly affected and fatty change and inclusion bodies are not seen. Portal tracts are normal apart from a mild cellular infiltration.

There is no ductular proliferation and efferent veins are normal. Eosinophilic necrosis in the absence of bile retention, cellular infiltration, and ochre bodies in liver biopsy specimens should suggest Lassa fever.

The intestine is grossly oedematous at post-mortem with small haemorrhages and a mild submucosal lymphocytic infiltration. Spleen, lungs, myocardium, and kidneys are also affected, and there may be a haemorrhagic diathesis. Circulating antigen-antibody complexes may damage the capillaries giving rise to increased permeability and haemorrhage.

There may be a leucopenia and a thrombocytopenia. Liver function tests (especially raised serum transaminase concentrations) indicate parenchymal damage; the prothrombin time is prolonged. Albuminuria with urinary casts, and later renal failure, may occur. Virus can be isolated from blood early in the disease, and from tissues at post-mortem. The complement-fixation test becomes positive after two weeks; it is virtually always negative in patients who die of the disease (Carey, Kemp, White, Pinneo, Addy, Fom, Stroh, Casals, and Henderson, 1972).

Strict isolation is essential. Post-mortem studies and virus isolation procedures should be performed with the greatest caution. The only procedure which seems of value, and there is as yet no scientific evidence to support it, is injection of immune serum, i.e. serum from a patient who has recovered from the disease (Leifer, Gocke, and Bourne, 1970).

Marburg and Ebola diseases. The first report of Marburg disease came from Marburg and Frankfurt, West Germany in 1967 (Siegert, 1970; Martini and Siegert, 1971; Monath, 1974), and Belgrade, Yugoslavia. Laboratory workers who came into contact with blood, organs, or cell-cultures of a batch of African green monkeys (*Cercopithecus aethiops*) imported from Uganda, developed a severe illness which was followed by a substantial mortality. The next report of the disease came from Johannesburg, South Africa (Gear, *et al.*, 1975); a hitch-hiker developed the disease after a tour of Zimbabwe Rhodesia; he subsequently died of the disease and two contacts developed it. In 1976–7 there was an extensive outbreak, with a very substantial mortality in Zaire and southern Sudan; the virus there was antigenically distinct from that in the previous outbreaks, and was named Ebola (*Lancet*, 1977).

Incubation period is from three to nine days. There is prostration, headache, myalgia, vomiting, watery diarrhoea, conjunctivitis, and a characteristic rash; confusion, widespread haemorrhages, haematemeses, coma, and death ensue in severe cases (Monath, 1974).

Most organs of the body are involved and there is widespread focal necrosis (Martini, 1969). The liver shows areas of focal necrosis; in the vicinity of the necrotic areas, basophilic bodies (one to four nm in diameter) are present, both intra- and extracellularly. There may be a pancreatitis. The reticuloendothelial system is also markedly involved. Although the stomach and intestines often contain blood at post-mortem there is no obvious source for the bleeding.

There is usually a leucopenia and thrombocytopenia; abnormal lymphocytes, plasma cells, and pyrinophilic blast cells (immunocytes) are present in the peripheral blood. Serum bilirubin is usually normal but may be raised, and serum transaminases are markedly elevated; coagulation is usually relatively normal. Jaundice and a haemorrhagic diathesis indicate a bad prognosis. Guinea pigs can be inoculated, and the virus has been identified in them by electron-microscopy. The antigen can be detected by immunofluorescence in liver-biopsy sections. A complement-fixation test is being developed.

7.2.3. Infectious mononucleosis (glandular fever)

Liver involvement, occasionally with jaundice, is very common in infectious mononucleosis (Dunnet, 1963). The disease is probably caused by the Epstein-Barr (EB) virus (Henle, Henle, and Diehl, 1968; Niederman, McCollum, Henle, and Henle, 1968; Gerber, Hamre, Moy, and Rosenblum, 1968), which has been implicated in the causation of Burkitt's lymphoma (Epstein, Achong, and Barr, 1964). Antibodies to the EB virus are present however in a high proportion of most population groups.

The incubation period varies from a few days to several weeks. The portal of entry of the virus is probably the mouth; kissing has been suggested in some outbreaks. It is an unusual disease to be diagnosed in the third world (Diehl, Taylor, Parlin, Henle, and Henle, 1969), probably because it is submerged beneath many more dramatic conditions. It has been suggested that infection in developing countries usually occurs early in life, while maternal antibodies are still present; protection after infection is probably lifelong.

Liver involvement gives rise to a hepatitis which in severe cases can be difficult to distinguish from viral hepatitis. Hepatic necrosis and liver failure is extremely rare, if in fact it ever occurs.

The reticuloendothelial system is principally involved and there is lymphadenopathy and splenomegaly. Myocarditis and neurological involvement with focal encephalomyelitis, a transverse myelitis or a Guillain-Barré type syndrome, are not uncommon.

A lymphocytosis with many abnormal cells ('glandular fever cells') is usual, although the lymphocyte count may be normal or even depressed. There is usually a mild thrombocytopenia. There may be a haemolytic anaemia. Serum transaminases are elevated in the majority of cases, to some extent or other, reflecting the hepatocellular damage. Heterophile antibodies, detected by the Paul-Bunnell test, and EB virus antibody can also be detected. Rheumatoid and antinuclear factors and a positive Wasserman reaction have been reported.

The liver shows periportal lymphocytic infiltration; the parenchymal changes are similar to those seen in viral hepatitis. Other causes of acute hepatitis, especially viral hepatitis should be considered, although marked lymphadenopathy is unusual in that disease. Cytomegalic inclusion disease and toxoplasmosis can be differentiated by complement-fixation tests. Adenovirus infections, brucellosis, typhoid fever, tuberculosis, trypanosomiasis, and leishmaniasis are other possible differential diagnoses.

7.2.3. Miscellaneous viral infections

Cytomegalovirus. Cytomegalic inclusion disease is most commonly seen in the neonate; it is rare in older children and adults, but is occasionally precipitated by cytotoxic and immunosuppressive agents (*Br. med. J.*, 1971a).

There is hepatomegaly with hepatitis and jaundice; focal necrosis can be demonstrated histologically. Fatal massive hepatic necrosis has been reported, but is rare (Shusterman, Frauenhoffer, and Kinsey, 1978). Splenomegaly, purpura, and thrombocytopenia are common. Neurological involvement, choroido-retinitis, optic atrophy, cerebral calcification, microcephaly, and mental retardation can also occur. Focal necrosis occurs in almost every organ.

Liver-biopsy may be diagnostic if there is a hepatitis. The virus may be isolated from urine, saliva, and other tissues. Cytomegalic cells, which are giant cells of 20–40 μm in diameter, with an enlarged nucleus containing a prominent inclusion body which is eosinophilic or basophilic, are found in the sputum and urine or salivary gland (and other tissues) at post-mortem.

Dengue fever. This group B arbovirus infection is widely spread throughout the tropics and causes a short, non-fatal febrile illness. A haemorrhagic form of the disease has become common in epidemic form in south-east Asia; it is most severe in children and has a very significant mortality (Bhamarapravati, Tuchinda, and Boonyapaknavik, 1967; Miles, 1978).

Focal hepatic necrosis occasionally occurs in Dengue fever; the virus may be isolated from liver tissue. Acidophilic bodies 8–12 μm in diameter may be seen free in the sinusoids (Nelson, 1960; Bhamarapravati *et al.*, 1967). The prothrombin time may be prolonged.

Kyasanur forest disease. A group B arbovirus causes this disease which occurs in Mysore State, India. Impaired liver function with degeneration of hepatocytes and prominence of the reticuloendothelial elements has also been reported (Chatterjea, Swarup, Pain, and Laxmana Rao, 1963). Gastrointestinal haemorrhage may be an important part of the clinical picture; the cause is however not clear. Virus can be isolated from many organs, including the liver.

Other arboviruses. Granular degeneration with oedema around the central vein may occur in these infections (Child, MacKenzie, Valverde, and Johnson, 1967). There is congestion and intestinal haemorrhage in the gastrointestinal tract.

Herpes simplex. Herpes simplex virus can cause a true hepatitis, with areas of necrosis, and intranuclear inclusions. The virus can be isolated from the liver. This manifestation of herpes simplex which is potentially lethal occurs usually, but not exclusively, in malnourished infants (Templeton, 1970; Edington and Gilles, 1976).

Chickenpox, smallpox, and measles. Focal hepatitis may be found in all of these diseases. However it is very rarely a predominant feature. Acute hepatic necrosis and death has been recorded in chickenpox (Knyvett, 1966).

Poliomyelitis. The importance of this disease is related to its effect on the anterior horn cells of the spinal cord and bulbar centres. The portal of entry however is usually the gastrointestinal tract. Liver sections may show focal necroses.

Lymphogranuloma venereum (Chapter 30). During the acute stage of this disease there may be widespread systemic involvement, including the liver.

Coxsackie. Coxsackie B virus, type 3, can cause a true hepatitis in adults (Sun and Smith, 1966). Coxsackie A Virus, type 4, has been isolated from a child with hepatitis (Morris, Elisberg, Pond, and Webb, 1962).

Q-fever. This is actually a rickettsial disease and the predominant clinical manifestations are pulmonary. However, hepatitis may dominate the picture and the disease may mimic viral hepatitis (Dupont, Hornick, Levin, Rapoport, and Woodward, 1971). Hepatocelluar necrosis with lymphocytic and eosinophilic infiltration may be present; ganulomas are also seen (Chapter 5).

7.3. Bacterial infections associated with acute hepatic injury

7.3.1. Leptospirosis (Weil's disease, spirochaetal jaundice, swamp fever, Japanese seven-day fever)

Leptospirosis is caused by spirochaetes of the *Leptospira* genus (Turner, 1973); there are many serotypes. *L. icterohaemorrhagiae* is the usual cause of the disease in man, although *L. bataviae* is common in south-east Asia and *L. grippotyphosa* is the usual agent in Thailand. Leptospiral infections seem to be common in the population of Papua New Guinea (Emanuel, 1959; Campbell, 1962). *L. canicola* occurs in dogs.

The disease occurs in damp, rat-infested areas and especially in sewerage workers; the organism enters via either wounds or mucous membranes exposed to the urine of the rat, dog, or pig, the carriers of the leptospira. The disease seems to be an occupational hazard of sugarcane labourers in Kenya (de Geus, Wolff, and Timmer, 1977).

The disease is an acute febrile one in which jaundice is the dominant clinical feature. Incubation period is approximately 10 days, which is followed by a septicaemic stage with jaundice, myalgia, and purpura which lasts about one week. During the second week symptoms and complications of acute renal failure ensue. This is followed by recovery or progressive uraemia in the third week.

The liver shows subcapsular and parenchymal haemorrhages. The hepatocytes are relatively intact. There may be focal or central necrosis with an infiltrate of mononuclear cells. There may also be bile stasis and fatty change. Spirochaetes are demonstrated in liver tissue by Levaditi's stain.

The renal lesion is prognostically far more important and is the usual cause of death; there is necrosis of the proximal renal tubules.

Haemorrhage involves many tissues and is due to capillary wall damage and not hepatic insufficiency. An endocarditis, pericarditis, and meningitis are sometimes present.

Liver function tests are very variable. A polymorphonuclear leucocytosis is present. Leptospira can be demonstrated in the blood and urine, and by culture and guinea-pig inoculation. There is albuminuria and evidence of tubular damage. Agglutinins, lysins, and complement-fixing antibodies appear towards the end of the first week of the disease and reach a maximum at approximately six weeks.

The treatment is penicillin at high dosage; however the evidence from animal experiments is that that agent must be given very early in the disease. In man, diagnosis is rarely made early on and the value of penicillin must remain *sub judice* (Edwards and Domm, 1960; Kocen, 1962).

7.3.2. Typhoid fever

Salmonellosis (typhoid fever). Hepatic involvement is a relatively frequent complication of typhoid fever in some tropical areas (Chapter 22). Presentation of this complication of the disease may be similar to viral or toxic hepatitis, cholangitis, and even hepatic amoebiasis (Osler, 1899; Stuart and Pullen, 1946). In viral hepatitis, prodromata usually precede the icteric illness, there is marked anorexia and the fever disappears as the jaundice deepens. Presence of an enlarged tender liver and restricted movement of the diaphragm suggests amoebiasis (Chapter 12).

Liver-biopsy shows areas of focal necrosis with mild pericholangitis and cholangitis (Singh, Nair, Krishnasamy, Aurora, Chandrasekar, and Bisht, 1978). Typhoid nodules, consisting of small collections of macrophages and lymphocytes with or without central necrosis, are situated in the parenchyma of the outer one-third of the liver lobule; *Salmonella typhi* may occasionally be detected. Cloudy swelling and the presence of small fat globules may be seen in the hepatocytes. Typhoid abscesses and cholangitis are rare complications.

Hepatic involvement may also consist of suppurative pylephlebitis and liver abscesses (Osler, 1899).

7.3.3. Miscellaneous bacterial infections

Streptococcal hepatitis. Acute bacterial hepatitis can be a cause of prolonged 'pyrexia of undetermined origin'. A report of such a case in which the responsible organism was *Streptococcus viridans* has been made (Weinstein, 1978). Liver-biopsy specimens showed a non-specific hepatitis; most of the infiltrate was lymphocytic, and there was loss of hepatocytes. The only indication that the fever had an hepatic origin was a persistently raised serum alkaline phosphatase. The causative organism was isolated from serial liver-biopsy specimens and despite very extensive investigations no primary site, other than the liver, was found. Rapid recovery took place on penicillin treatment.

Gonococcal disease. The gonococcus may invade the liver parenchyma directly or cause toxic liver damage; it has a predilection for the capsule and produces a perihepatitis (the Fitz-Hugh–Curtis syndrome). It is often associated with gonococcal pelvic inflammatory disease (Nolan, 1978); the diagnosis should be suspected in young women with fever, right-upper quadrant pain, and a friction-rub over the liver.

Bartonellosis (Oroya fever). Oroya fever is an acute febrile illness caused by *Bartonella bacilliformis*, a Gram-negative coccobacillus, in which severe anaemia is a prominent feature; it carries a high mortality. The disease is confined to Peru, Colombia, and Equador and is transmitted to man by the bites of sand flies.

The liver and spleen are enlarged; centrilobular necrosis is present in the liver where there is also erythrophagocytosis by Kupffer cells.

Melioidosis. This disease is confined to south-east Asia, and in particular, Thailand. It also occurs in Papua New Guinea. Ingestion of water contaminated with the urine or faeces of various rodents infected with *Pseudomonas pseudomallei*, or direct entry through damaged skin (*Lancet*, 1970) give rise to infection.

Multiple abscesses are found in many organs; in the liver, numerous minute abscesses can be demonstrated.

Plague. This disease is caused by *Yersinia pestis*, which can occur in various forms—bubonic, pneumonic, and septicaemic.

The liver may be enlarged and congested; there may be fatty degeneration and small greyish nodules containing degenerate and necrotic parenchymal cells, polymorphonuclear leucocytes, and many bacilli.

The organism may be found either in direct smears or after culture and animal inoculation; fluorescent-antibody, complement-fixation, and haemagglutination techniques are also of value.

Tularaemia. *Pasteurella tularensis* is the cause of this disease which often results from infected undercooked meat or infected water (*Br. med. J.*, 1971b). There may be focal necroses in the liver.

Relapsing fever. There are two forms of this disease. Tick-borne relapsing fever is caused by *Borrelia duttoni* and the louse-borne form by *B. recurrentis*. The diseases occur in parts of India, Africa, and south America; the former type is also seen in the Middle-east.

The liver is enlarged and congested; areas of focal necrosis are present. Jaundice may be present and there is a widespread haemorrhagic tendency caused by a thrombocytopenia.

The causative organisms can be identified in the peripheral blood by dark-ground illumination; they may be cultured in laboratory animals. Wasserman reaction and the Weil-Felix test may be positive.

Both penicillin and tetracycline have given good results.

7.4. Parasitic infections associated with acute hepatic injury

Toxoplasmosis. In acute toxoplasmosis, focal necrotic lesions with an inflammatory infiltrate may be present in the liver. There may be hepatosplenomegaly (Fleck and Ludham, 1965). The disease is caused by *Toxoplasma gondii*. The disease is very common in the humid tropics including Singapore (Zaman and Goh, 1969). The mode of transmission is not well understood, but raw beef and pork are thought to be important. A number of serological tests are of value in diagnosis.

Trichiniasis (trichinellosis). This disease is caused by the nematode worm *Trichinella spiralis* (Most, 1978). During invasion by the larvae, virtually all organs of the body may be involved, including the liver and gall-bladder. Focal necroses with an intense eosinophilic infiltration are found in all infected tissues.

Filariasis. Filariae have been claimed to produce hepatic granulomata (Chapter 5). Numerous microfilariae of *Dipetalonema perstans* invading sinusoids, have been incriminated in the production of hepatomegaly and upper abdominal pain (Garratt, 1945).

Blackwater fever. In this condition which is associated with *Plasmodium falciparum* infections, there is a rapid acute haemolysis leading to haemoglobinuria. The cause is so far unknown although there seems to be some association with quinine administration. It must be differentiated from acute haemolysis in the presence of malaria in glucose-6-phosphate dehydrogenase deficient individuals.

The liver is yellow brown and there is evidence of centrilobular necrosis; there may be biliary stasis. Death does not occur as a result of the hepatic injury, but from renal tubular necrosis.

References

ALMEIDA, J. D. (1971). *Postgrad. med. J.*, **47**, 484.

ALPERT, E., ISSELBACHER, K. J., and SCHUR, P. H. (1971). *New Engl. J. Med.*, **285**, 185.

ALTER, H. J., PURCELL, R. H., HOLLAND, P. V., and POPPER, H. (1978). *Lancet*, **1**, 459.

ANDERSON, C. R. and WATTLEY, G. H. (1955). *Trans. R. Soc. trop. Med. Hyg.*, **49**, 580.

ANTHONY, P. P., VOGEL, C. L., SADIKALI, F., BARKER, L. F., and PETERSON, M. R. (1972). *Br. med. J.*, **1**, 403.

ARNOLD, W., NIELSEN, J. O., HARDT, F., and MEYER ZUM BÜSCHENFELDE, K. H. (1977). *Gut*, **18**, 994.

BAGSHAWE, A. and NGANDA, T. N. (1973). *Trans. R. Soc. trop. Med. Hyg.*, **67**, 663.

BAGSHAWE, A. F., PARKER, A. M., and JINDANI, A. (1971). *Br. med. J.*, **1**, 88.

BARBARA, J. A. J., MIJOVIC, V., CLEGHORN, T. E., TEDDER, R. S., and BRIGGS, M. (1978). *Br. med. J.*, **2**, 1600.

BERQUIST, K. R., MAYNARD, J. E., FRANCY, D. B., SHELLER, M. J., and SCHABLE, C. A. (1976). *Am. J. trop. Med. Hyg.*, **25**, 730.

BHAMARAPRAVATI, N., TUCHINDA, P., and BOONYAPAKNAVIK, V. (1967). *Ann. trop. Med. Parasit.*, **61**, 500.

BLUMBERG, B. S. (1972). *Papua New Guin. med. J.*, **15**, 68.

——, ALTER, H. J., and VISNICH, S. (1965). *J. Am. med. Ass.*, **191**, 541.

——, MELARTIN, L., GUINTO, R., and LECHAT, M. (1970). *J. Chron. Dis.*, **23**, 507.

——, SUTNICK, A. I., and LONDON, W. T. (1970). *Am. J. Med.*, **48**, 1.

BOYER, J. L. and KLATSKIN, G. (1970). *New Engl. J. Med.*, **283**, 1063.

Br. med. J. (1971a). **1**, 687.

—— (1971b). **4**, 4.

—— (1972). **4**, 253.

—— (1977). **1**, 189.

—— (1978). **1**, 942.

BROTMAN, B., PRINCE, A. M., and GODFREY, H. R. (1973). *Lancet*. **1**, 1305.

BUCKLEY, S. M. and CASALS, J. (1970). *Am. J. trop. Med. Hyg.*, **19**, 680.

——, —— and DOWNS, W. G. (1970). *Nature, Lond.*, **227**, 174.

BULKLEY, B. H., HEIZER, W. D., GOLDFINGER, S. E., ISSELBACHER, K. J., and SCHULMAN, N. R. (1970). *Lancet*, **2**, 1323.

CAMPBELL, C. H. (1962). *Papua New Guin. med. J.*, **6**, 5.

CAREY, D. E., KEMP, G. E., WHITE, H. A., PINNEO, L., ADDY, R. F., FOM, A. L. M. D., STROH, G., CASALS, J., and HENDERSON, B. E. (1972). *Trans. R. Soc. trop. Med. Hyg.*, **66**, 402.

CHAMBON, L. and WONE, I. (1967). *Bull. Wld Hlth Org.*, **36**, 113.

CHATTERJEA, J. B., SWARUP, S., PAIN, S. K., and LAXMANA RAO, R. (1963). *Indian J. med. Res.*, **51**, 419.

CHILD, P. L., MACKENZIE, R. B., VALVERDE, L. R., and JOHNSON, K. M. (1967). *Archs Path.*, **83,** 434.
CHOREMIS, C., KATTAMIS, C. A., KYRIAZAKOU, M., and GAVRIILIDOU, E. (1966). *Lancet*, **1,** 269.
CHUTTANI, H. K., SIDHU, A. S., WIG, K. L., GUPTA, D. N., and RAMALINGASWAMI, V. (1966). *Br. med. J.*, **2,** 676.
CONRAD, M. E., SCHWARTZ, F. D., and YOUNG, A. A. (1964). *Am. J. Med.*, **37,** 789.
COOK, G. C. (1965). *Active chronic hepatitis and its response to corticosteroid therapy*. M.D. thesis, University of London.
—— and SHERLOCK, S. (1965). *Lancet*, **1,** 175.
Co-operative study (1971). *Archs intern. Med.*, **128,** 723.
DANE, D. S., CAMERON, C. H., and BRIGGS, M. (1970). *Lancet*, **1,** 695.
DE GEUS, A., WOLFF, J. W., and TIMMER, V. E. A. (1977). *E. Afr. med. J.*, **54,** 115.
DEVAKUL, K., GARBY, L., and HARINASUTA, T. (1966). *Ann. trop. Med. Parasit.*, **60,** 432.
DIEHL, V., TAYLOR, J. R., PARLIN, J. A., HENLE, G., and HENLE, W. (1969). *E. Afr. med. J.*, **46,** 407.
DIENSTAG, J. L., ALAAMA, A., MOSLEY, J. W., REDEKER, A. G., and PURCELL, R. H. (1977). *Ann. intern. Med.*, **87,** 1.
DUDLEY, F. J., SHEUER, P. J., and SHERLOCK, S. (1972). *Lancet*, **2,** 1388.
DUNNET, W. N. (1963). *Br. med. J.*, **1,** 1187.
DUPONT, H. L., HORNICK, R. B., LEVIN, H. S., RAPOPORT, M. I., and WOODWARD, T. E. (1971). *Ann. intern. Med.*, **74,** 198.
EDINGTON, G. M. and GILLES, H. M. (1976). *Pathology in the tropics.* 2nd ed. pp. 229 and 254. Edward Arnold, London.
—— and WHITE, H. A. (1972). *Trans. R. Soc. trop. Med. Hyg.*, **66,** 381.
EDWARDS, G. A. and DOMM, B. M. (1960). *Medicine, Baltimore*, **39,** 117.
ELEFTHERIOU, N., THOMAS, H. C., HEATHCOTE, J., and SHERLOCK, S. (1975). *Lancet*, **2,** 1171.
EKE, R. A. (1976). *E. Afr. med. J.*, **53,** 534.
EMANUEL, M. L. (1959). *Papua New Guin. med. J.*, **3,** 76.
EPSTEIN, M. A., ACHONG, B. G., and BARR, Y. M. (1964). *Lancet*, **1,** 702.
FINKELSTEIN, W. and ISSELBACHER, K. J. (1978). *New Engl. J. Med.*, **299,** 992.
FLECK, D. G. and LUDHAM, G. B. (1965). *Br. med. J.*, **2,** 1239.
FOLI, A. K., CHRISTIAN, E. C. and SWANIKER, G. R. E. (1974). *Ghana med. J.*, **13,** 3.
FRAME, J. D., BALDWIN, J. M., GOCKE, D. J. and TROUP, J. M. (1970). *Am. J. trop. Med. Hyg.*, **19,** 670.
FRANCIS, T. I., MOORE, D. L., EDINGTON, G. M., and SMITH, J. A. (1972). *Bull. Wld Hlth Org.*, **46,** 659.
GARRATT, E. I. (1945). *Trans. R. Soc. trop. Med. Hyg.*, **38,** 287.
GEAR, J. S. S., CASSEL, G. A., GEAR, A. J., TRAPPLER, B., CLAUSEN, L., MEYERS, A. M., KEW, M. C., BOTHWELL, T. H., SHER, R., MILLER, G. B., SCHNEIDER, J., KOORNHOF, H. J., GOMPERTS, E. D., ISAÄCSON, M., and GEAR, J. H. S. (1975). *Br. med. J.*, **4,** 489.
GERBER, P., HAMRE, D., MOY, R. A., and ROSENBLUM, E. N. (1968). *Science, N.Y.*, **161,** 173.
GILLIES, H. M. and KEANE, E. (1977). *Q. Jl. Med.*, **46,** 562.
GRADY, G. F. (1978). *New Engl. J. Med.*, **298,** 1413.
GRAVES, R. J. (1843). *A system of clinical medicine*, p. 564. Fannin and Co., Dublin.
HEATHCOTE, J. and SHERLOCK, S. (1973). *Lancet*, **1,** 1468.
HENLE, G., HENLE, W., and DIEHL, V. (1968). *Proc. natn. acad. Sci. U.S.A.*, **59,** 94.
HIMSWORTH, H. P. (1950). *Lectures on the liver and its diseases*. 2nd ed. pp. 48, 78, Blackwell, Oxford.
HOOFNAGLE, J. H., GERETY, R. J., TABOR, E., FEINSTONE, S. M., BARKER, L. F., and PURCELL, R. H. (1977). *Ann. intern. Med.*, **87,** 14.
HORNEY, J. T. and GALAMBOS, J. T. (1977). *Gastroenterology*, **73,** 639.

Hutt, M. S. R. (1971). *Trans. R. Soc. trop. Med. Hyg.*, **65,** 273.
Iwarson, S. and Stenqvist, K. (1976). *Scand, J. Infect. Dis.*, **8,** 143.
Keane, E. and Gilles, H. M. (1977). *Br. med. J.*, **1,** 1399.
Knodell, R. G., Conrad, M. E., and Ishak, K. G. (1977). *Gastroenterology*, **72,** 902.
Knyvett, A. F. (1966). *Q. Jl. Med.*, **35,** 313.
Kocen, R. S. (1962). *Br. med. J.*, **1,** 1181.
Lancet (1970). **1,** 761.
—— (1973). **1,** 32.
—— (1974). **2,** 632.
—— (1976). **2,** 380.
—— (1977). **1,** 581.
Lee, V. H., Monath, T. P., Tomori, O., Fagbami, A., and Wilson, D. C. (1974). *Trans. R. Soc. trop. Med. Hyg.*, **68,** 39.
Leifer, E., Gocke, D. J., and Bourne, H. (1970). *Am. J. trop. Med. Hyg.*, **19,** 677.
Lyra, L. G., Rebouças, G., and Andrade, Z. A. (1976). Gastroenterology, **71,** 641.
MacDougall, B. R. D., Bailey, R. J., and Williams, R. (1977). *Lancet*, **1,** 617.
MacNamara, F. N. (1954). *Bull. Wld Hlth Org.*, **11,** 391.
Magnius, L. O. and Espmark, J. A. (1972). *J. Immunol.*, **109,** 1017.
Martini, G. (1969). *Trans. R. Soc. trop. Med. Hyg.*, **63,** 295.
—— and Sigert, R. (1971) (editors). *Marburg Virus Disease.* Springer-Verlag, New York.
Maynard, E. P., Sadikali, F., Anthony, P. P., and Barker, L. F. (1970). *Lancet*, **2,** 1326.
Melnick, J. L., Dreesman, G. R., and Hollinger, F. B. (1976). *J. infect. Dis.*, **133,** 210.
Meyers, J. D., Dienstag, J. L., Purcell, R. H., Thomas, E. D., and Holmes, K. K. (1977). *Ann. intern. Med.*, **87,** 57.
Miles, J. A. R. (1978). *Asian J. infect. Dis.*, **2,** 1.
Monath, T. P. (1974). *W.H.O. Chron.*, **28,** 212.
—— and Kemp, G. E. (1973). *Trop. geogr. Med.*, **25,** 28.
——, Lee, V. H., Wilson, D. C. Fagbami, A., and Tomori, O. (1974). *Trans. R. Soc. trop. Med. Hyg.*, **68,** 30.
Moritsugu, Y., Dienstag, J. L., Valdesuso, J., Wong, D. C., Wagner, J., Routenberg, J. A., and Purcell, R. H. (1976). *Infect. Immunol.*, **13,** 898.
Morris, J. A., Elisberg, B. L., Pond, W. L., and Webb, P. A. (1962). *New Engl. J. Med.*, **267,** 1230.
Morrow, R. H., Sai, F. T., and Barker, L. F. (1971). *Br. med. J.*, **4,** 389.
——, Smetana, H. F., Sai, F. T., and Edgcomb, J. H. (1968). *Ann. intern. Med.*, **68,** 1250.
Most, H. (1978). *New Engl. J. Med.*, **298,** 1178.
Nantulya, V. M., Lindqvist, K. J., and Spencer, S. (1975). *E. Afr. med. J.*, **52,** 430.
Nelson, E. R. (1960). *J. Pediat.*, **56,** 101.
Niederman, J. C., McCollum, R. W., Henle, G., and Henle, W. (1968). *J. Am. med. Ass.*, **203,** 205.
Nolan, J. P. (1978). *New Engl. J. Med.*, **299,** 1069.
Ojo, O. A., Francis, T. I., and Onifade, A. (1971). *W. Afr. med. J.*, **20,** 339.
Osler, W. (1899). *Johns Hopkins Hosp. Rep.*, **8,** 373.
Phatak, L. V. and Patil, K. A. (1956). *Indian J. med. Sci.*, **10,** 593.
Pollock, T. M. and Reid, D. (1969). *Lancet,* **1,** 281.
Powell, K. C. and McGovern, V. J. (1976). *Papua New Guin. med. J.*, **19,** 140.
Prince, A. M. (1970). *Am. J. trop. Med. Hyg.*, **19,** 872.
——, Metselaar, D., Kafuko, G. W., Mukwaya, L. G., Ling, C. M., and Overby, L. R. (1972). *Lancet*, **2,** 247.
Rake, M. O., Flute, P. T., Pannell, G., Shilkin, K. B., and Williams, R. (1973). *Gut*, **14,** 574.

RAKELA, J., MOSLEY J. W. and REDEKER, A. G. (1975). *Gastroenterology*, **69,** 854.
——, REDEKER, A. G., EDWARDS, V. M., DECKER, R., OVERBY, L. R., and MOSLEY, J. W. (1978). *Gastroenterology*, **74,** 879.
SADIKALI, F. (1972). *E. Afr. med. J.*, **49,** 783.
SCHUSTERMAN, N. H., FRAUENHOFFER, C., and KINSEY, M. D. (1978). *Ann. intern. Med.*, **88,** 810.
SÉRIÉ, C. (1963). *Ethiopian med. J.*, **1,** 206.
SHERLOCK, S. (1975). *Diseases of the Liver and Biliary System.* 5th ed. pp. 107, 305. Blackwell, Oxford, London, Edinburgh, and Melbourne.
—— (1978). *Jl. R. Soc. Med.*, **71,** 430.
SHIRACHI, R., SHIRAISHI, H., TATEDA, A., KIKUCHI, K., and ISHIDA, N. (1978). *Lancet*, **2,** 853.
SIEGERT, R. (1970). In *Modern Trends in Medical Virology* (ed. R. B. Heath and A. P. Waterson). p. 204. Butterworths, London.
SIMONS, M. J., BINNS, C. W., MALCOLM, L. A., and YAP, E. H. (1972). *Papua New Guin. med. J.*, **15,** 91.
SINGH, D. S., NAIR, P. N. R., KRISHNASAMY, S., AURORA, A. L., CHANDRESEKAR, S., and BISHT, D. B. (1978). *J. trop. Med. Hyg.*, **81,** 68.
SMITH, J. A., OGUNBA, E. O., and FRANCIS, T. I. (1972). *Nature, Lond.*, **237,** 231.
SOOD, V., HULLEY, W. S. C., and HUTT, M. S. R. (1966). *Makerere med. J.*, **10,** 46.
STEINER, P. E. and DAVIES, J. N. P. (1957). *Br. J. Cancer*, **11,** 523.
STUART, B. M. and PULLEN, R. L. (1946). *Archs intern. Med.*, **78,** 629.
SUN, N. C. and SMITH, V. M. (1966). *New Engl. J. Med.*, **274,** 190.
TABOR, E., GERETY, R. J., DRUCKER, J. A., SEEFF, L. B., HOOFNAGLE, J. H., JACKSON, D. R. APRIL, M., BARKER, L. F., and PINEDA-TAMONDONG, G. (1978). *Lancet*, **1,** 463.
TEMPLETON, A. C. (1970). *J. clin. Path.*, **23,** 24.
TROUP, J. M., WHITE, H. A., FOM, A. L. M. D., and CAREY, D. E. (1970). *Am. J. trop. Med. Hyg.*, **19,** 695.
TSEGA, E. (1976). *E. Afr. med. J.*, **53,** 270.
TURNER, L. H. (1973). *Br. med. J.*, **1,** 537.
VILLELA, E. (1942). *Archs Path.*, **31,** 665.
VOGEL, C. L. ANTHONY, P. P., and SADIKALI, F. (1972). *J. natn. Cancer Inst.*, **48,** 1583.
WEINSTEIN, L. (1978). *New Engl. J. Med.*, **299,** 1052.
WHITE, H. A. (1972). *Trans. R. Soc. trop. Med. Hyg.*, **66,** 390.
WHO (1975). *Tech. Rep. Ser. Wld Hlth Org.*, no. 570. WHO Geneva.
WILLIAMS, A. O., FABIYI, A., WILLIAMS, A. I. O., GUPTA, B., O'CONNOR, E. H., and GREENWOOD, B. M. (1973). *E. Afr. med. J.*, **50,** 521.
WILLS, W., SAIMOT, G., BROCHARD, C., BLUMBERG, B. S., LONDON, W. T., DECHENE, R., and MILLMAN, I. (1976). *Am. J. trop. Med. Hyg.*, **25,** 186.
WOODFIELD. D. G. (1972). *Br. med. J.*, **3,** 763.
—— (1977). *Trop. geogr. Med.*, **29,** 257.
WOODSON, R. D. and CLINTON, J. J. (1969). *J. Am. med. Ass.*, **209,** 1053.
ZAMAN, V. and GOH, T. K. (1969). *Trans. R. Soc. trop. Med. Hyg.*, **63,** 884.
ZUCKERMAN, A. J. (1970). *Virus diseases of the liver.* Butterworths, London.
—— (1978). *Br. med. J.*, **2,** 696.
ZUZARTE, J. C. and KASILI, E. G. (1978). *E. Afr. med. J.*, **55,** 346.

8

Chronic hepatic injury (excluding alcoholic liver disease)

Chronic liver disease in tropical countries amounts very largely to cirrhosis (usually of a macronodular type), schistosomal liver disease (Chapter 10), and hepatocellular carcinoma (Chapter 9). Although not easily recognized, many cases of chronic hepatitis, frequently active chronic hepatitis, are also to be found; difficulty in recognition is due to (i) the fact that many people in tropical countries have hepatosplenomegaly, probably largely a result of malaria and intestinal infections (Chapter 5) and (ii) cutaneous stigmata of liver disease are extremely difficult to recognize in dark skins.

The diagnosis of chronic hepatitis is a clinical one; *chronic persistent* and *active chronic* hepatitis (ACH) should be differentiated on the basis of the clinical picture in the presence of consistent biochemical and histological evidence. Although histology is a valuable investigation, it is not in itself adequate for a diagnosis; that conforms to the feelings of an international team of pathologists (International group, 1977). Cirrhosis occurs at a variable stage in the natural history of active chronic hepatitis; for that reason those workers prefer to refer to 'ACH with cirrhosis' and 'cirrhosis with features of ACH'. Subacute necrosis is a clinical entity; histologists prefer to term the histological changes 'bridging hepatic necrosis (BHN)', thus avoiding a temporal inference.

8.1. Active chronic hepatitis (ACH)

This disease is common in all parts of the tropics (Hutt, 1971; Powell and McGovern, 1976), but was first described by Waldenström (1950) in Sweden. Good (1956) was one of the first investigators to comment on the dense plasma-cell infiltration in the liver. Mackay, Taft, and Cowling (1956) reported a high incidence of the lupus erythematosus (LE)-cell phenomenon and referred to that entity as 'lupoid hepatitis'. Various terms have been applied to the condition, including plasma cell hepatitis, chronic liver disease of young women, lupoid hepatitis, and chronic active liver disease. The condition is now known to cover a group of conditions with heterogeneous aetiologies, characterized by the histological appearance of 'chronic aggressive' hepatitis (Cook, 1965). There is marked piecemeal necrosis of the periportal hepatocytes and a dense plasma-cell infiltration (International group, 1977) (Fig. 8.1). Lymphocytes cytotoxic to hepatocytes are present (Cochrane, Moussouros, Thompson, Eddleston, and Williams, 1976); they may be responsible for the periportal inflammation and necrosis. Differentiation from acute viral hepatitis is sometimes difficult on both clinical and histological grounds.

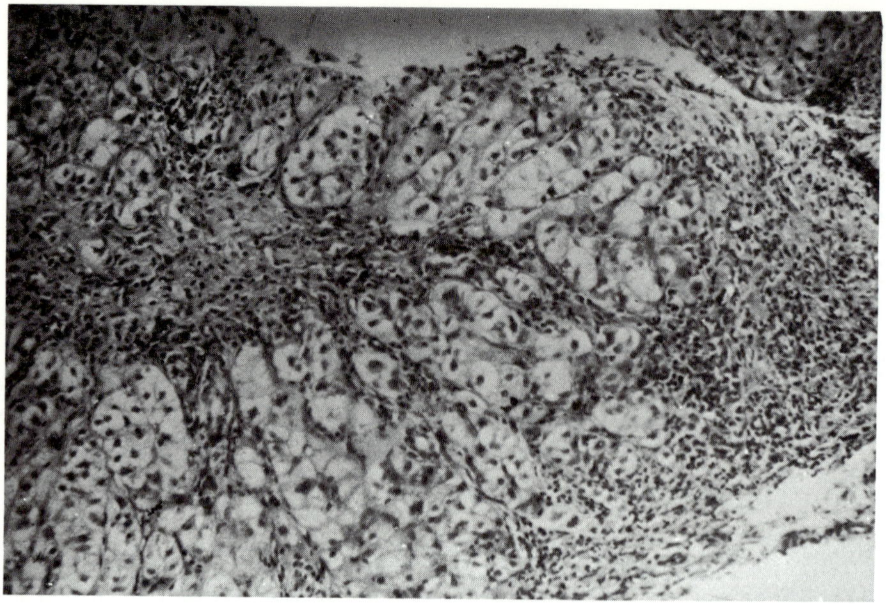

FIG. 8.1. Needle liver-biopsy section (haematoxylin and eosin) from a Ugandan woman with active chronic hepatitis; serum HB_sAg was negative. There is gross distortion of hepatic architecture with formation of typical 'rosettes' consisting of unhealthy hepatocytes. The infiltrate consists of plasma cells and lymphocytes. Cirrhosis was already present.

8.1.1. Aetiology of ACH

In some cases of virus B infection, HB_sAg and HB_eAg persist (Chapter 7) and that is probably responsible for the continuing hepatocyte damage; the incidence of this varies in different areas and occurs in 3 per cent of cases in Australia (Cooksley, Powell, Mistilis, Olsen, Mathews, and Mackay, 1972) and up to 51 per cent in Italy (Bianchi, *et al.*, 1972).

Non-A, non-B hepatitis can also proceed to ACH (Chapter 7).

Several aetiological agents are involved in ACH (Cook, 1965); the entity is merely the final common pathway resulting from diverse insults to the liver. As well as viral hepatitis, therapeutic agents may be responsible for the condition. The laxative, oxyphenisatin causes a condition biochemically, immunologically, and histologically identical to ACH (Reynolds, Peters, and Yamada, 1971), which resolves when the drug is discontinued. Methyldopa (Elkington, Schreiber, and Conn, 1969; Schweitzer and Peters, 1974), isoniazid (Maddrey and Boitnott, 1973), and nitrofurantoin (Lindberg, 1978) can all cause ACH; unfortunately the lesion is not always reversible on withdrawal of those agents. The end-result is macronodular cirrhosis.

Active chronic hepatitis may follow recovery from the acute phase of fulminant hepatitis (acute hepatic necrosis) (Chapter 7) (Horney and Galambos, 1977). It seems probable that schistosomiasis can also give rise to ACH.

The mechanism of continued hepatic damage in ACH is not clearly understood. It seems likely that cell-mediated autoimmune reactions are involved

(Cochrane, *et al.*, 1976). Patients with or without HB_sAg positive ACH show positive lymphocyte cytotoxicity for rabbit hepatocyte cultures which become negative after immunosuppressive treatment (Cochrane, Moussouros, Smith, Portmann, Eddleston, and Williams, 1978).

8.1.2. Presentation of ACH

Signs which suggest the onset of chronic hepatitis are: persistent jaundice of three months or more duration, development of cutaneous stigmata of liver disease, arthralgia, hepatosplenomegaly, persistently raised serum transaminases, and hyperglobulinaemia (mainly IgG) (Sherlock, 1975). Those abnormalities merge into the clinical picture associated with macronodular cirrhosis and portal hypertension (see below).

About 15 per cent of patients with ACH give a clear contact history with viral hepatitis (Cook, 1965). Other diseases under the heading of 'autoimmune diseases' such as rheumatoid arthritis, Hashimoto's disease of the thyroid, and non-specific ulcerative colitis have been associated with the condition, in temperate climates. Such diseases are unusual in most tropical countries—possibly because parasitic diseases, malaria in particular, have interfered with the immune response (Greenwood, Herrick, and Voller, 1970). About 15 per cent of cases in temperate areas have a positive lupus erythematosus (LE) cell test, although that has rarely been observed in the tropics. Antinuclear factor (ANF) is often present in the serum.

The course of the disease is variable, and depends largely on the length of time the 'active' picture lasts (either with or without corticosteroids), and the rate of progression of cirrhosis. Mortality is greatest in the first two or three years after diagnosis.

8.1.3. Pathology of ACH

The hepatocytes exhibit ballooning and much variation in size; there may be eosinophilic necrosis in some; there is characteristically 'rosette' formation (Scheuer, 1973; 1978). The portal tracts are heavily infiltrated with plasma cells, lymphocytes, and occasionally eosinophils and polymorphonuclear leucocytes. Development of fibrosis proceeds rapidly, and a well-developed macronodular cirrhosis is already present in the majority of patients when the diagnosis is first made.

8.1.4. Investigation of ACH

Serum bilirubin, transaminases, and total and gamma-globulin concentrations are raised; the degree of biochemical derangement is roughly proportional to the 'activity' of the histological picture. The raised gamma-globulin consists predominantly of IgG, although IgM is also elevated (Feizi, 1968). There is marked impairment of bromsulphthalein excretion (Cook, Velasco, and Sherlock, 1968). Lupus erythematosus cells may be present in the peripheral blood and bone marrow in a minority; serum antinuclear factor is often positive and in a minority the mitochondrial antibody is also present (although that occurs much more frequently in primary biliary cirrhosis which has not been reported from any tropical country as far as I am aware).

Needle biopsy of the liver shows the classical appearances of chronic aggressive hepatitis (see above). As portal hypertension develops, evidence of oesophageal varices and abnormalities in the splenovenogram become manifest.

8.1.5. Treatment of ACH

Controlled prospective trials of corticosteroids (Cook, Mulligan, and Sherlock, 1971; Soloway, Summerskill, Baggenstoss, Geall, Gitnick, Elveback, and Schoenfield, 1972; Murray-Lyon, Stern, and Williams, 1973) even though the design of some may not have been perfect (Wright, Seeff, Berk, Jones, and Plotz, 1977), have all demonstrated that mortality in ACH can be reduced by those agents. Immunosuppressive agents—6-mercaptopurine (Domeshek and Schwartz, 1960), azathioprine (Mistilis and Blackburn 1967), and chlorambucil (Phlippen, 1969)—also produce clinical and biochemical improvement. Soloway, *et al.* (1972) have indicated that a combination of 10 mg prednisone and 50 mg azathioprine daily is the safest regime; remissions can be induced by temporarily increasing the dosage (Schalm, Ammon and Summerskill, 1976). Careful follow-up is essential, and that is often very difficult to carry out in tropical countries. A decision must be reached as to whether the hazards of corticosteroids outweigh their advantages in primitive communities.

It seems likely that the response to treatment is less good in HB_sAg positive cases than in negative ones (Schalm, *et al.*, 1976; Meyer zum Büschenfelde, 1978); lymphocytes cytotoxic to hepatocytes persisted in 83 per cent of HB_sAg positive cases but in only 41 per cent of negative ones (Cochrane, *et al.*, 1978). The 'activity' of the disease at presentation may also determine the response to treatment. Thus the beneficial effects of corticosteroids reported by Cook *et al.* (1971) and Soloway, *et al.* (1972) may have been partly due to the fact that many of the cases were very active; that view is supported by evidence from Tygstrup and Juhl (1976). More controlled trials, in which the activity of the disease is very carefully taken into account, are urgently needed.

It is difficult to lay down hard and fast rules as to when immunosuppressive therapy should be started (*Lancet*, 1978a). However, low-dose prednisone and azathioprine regimes should probably be started in all patients with evidence of ACH in both liver-biopsy and biochemical tests of hepatic function. The decision as to whether to start corticosteroid therapy after two months of jaundice following an attack of viral hepatitis is a difficult one (*Lancet*, 1978a). If the condition is in fact ACH, then early treatment might assist in preventing the development of cirrhosis (though that is not proven); in a straightforward attack of acute hepatitis however, viral clearance could be hampered. A very high IgG and gammaglobulin together with the finding of ANF antibodies at high titre, point to a diagnosis of ACH. However very careful follow-up is essential.

Instead of prescribing immunosuppressive agents, a more logical method of dealing with this disease might be to boost the patient's innate immune response. In a limited uncontrolled study, 20 children with histologically proven active chronic hepatitis (19 were HB_sAg positive) were given weekly BCG injections (Brzosko, Debski, and Derecka, 1978); results after one year were encouraging; only nine had unchanged histology (in one the biopsy was normal, in three there was minimal evidence of hepatitis, and in seven others some improvement was noted). Although 12 were still HB_sAg positive, the serum SGPT had returned to normal in all of them. Results of a controlled trial of BCG in ACH will be of great interest (van Ypersele de Strihou and Pirson, 1978).

Human fibroblast interferon has been used in two patients with HB_sAg positive active chronic hepatitis (Kingham, *et al.*, 1978); a striking fall in core antibody titre and in DNA-binding antibody occurred which suggests that that line of treatment should be properly evaluated.

8.2. Chronic persistent hepatitis

This form of chronic hepatitis is usually benign, in contrast to active chronic hepatitis. Many cases seem to follow an acute attack of viral hepatitis, which smoulders on longer than usual. There is usually no abnormality on clinical examination, or there may be mild hepatomegaly with a tender liver edge. Most cases are detected on routine examination or when biochemical tests of liver function are carried out. There may be mildly elevated serum bilirubin and transaminase concentrations, and gamma-globulin is often mildly raised for months or years. Liver-biopsy histology shows expansion of the portal triads with an infiltration of lymphocytes and plasma cells (Becker, Scheuer, Baptista, and Sherlock, 1970; Scheuer, 1973).

This condition is histologically indistinguishable from the non-specific entity very commonly seen in tropical countries, in which the portal triads are expanded with plasma cells and lymphocytes (Chapter 5); in fact the dividing line between that condition and chronic persistent hepatitis is very indistinct. That entity is probably associated with intestinal parasitic disease and with repeated bacterial and virus infections of the intestine; biochemical tests of liver function are mostly normal, although serum globulin fraction may be elevated.

Most cases resolve over the course of a year or so although a minority develop active chronic hepatitis and ultimately cirrhosis.

Corticosteroid treatment depresses the serum bilirubin, transaminases, and globulin, but probably has no effect on histology; there are no controlled trials of corticosteroid therapy in this condition. Owing to their side-effects corticosteroids should not be given routinely.

8.3. Macronodular cirrhosis (MC)

Cirrhosis is a major problem in tropical medicine, and that disease is closely related to hepatoma (hepatocellular carcinoma). Most cirrhosis is of the macronodular ('post-necrotic') type.

On morphological grounds, there are two main types of cirrhosis; macro- and micronodular. The older terminology, 'portal' and 'post-necrotic' cirrhosis, is no longer acceptable; all cirrhosis is post-necrotic. Also, that classification does not help with the understanding of aetiology, because both types can, for example, be produced by alcohol. In macronodular cirrhosis, variable but generally large-sized hyperplastic liver nodules are separated by wide bands of fibrous tissue; that gives rise to a coarsely nodular and irregular surface. In micronodular cirrhosis, the nodules are smaller and their size is more constant; the surface appears finely nodular. Macroscopically the appearance of the liver varies considerably depending on its fat content which is usually high in alcoholic cirrhosis (Chapter 13).

Macronodular cirrhosis is a diffuse, pathological condition of the liver which is characterized by destruction of the normal architecture and with the formation of nodular hyperplasia and regeneration, and fibrosis; in simple fibrosis, hyperplasia of hepatocytes is not a feature. The condition is always preceded by intermittent or continuous degeneration of hepatocytes, with necrosis; the time scale of those events is very variable and probably depends on the aetiology.

8.3.1. Distribution of MC

Every doctor, nurse, or medical auxiliary who works in a third-world country is inevitably impressed at the very high incidence rate of cirrhosis, the bulk of which is of the macronodular type. The disease is very common in all African countries, and also in the Far east and Papua New Guinea. Throughout Africa cirrhosis is extremely common (Davies, Knowelden, and Wilson, 1965). A high incidence in Kenya was reported as long ago as 1930 by Vint. Most cirrhotic livers in Africa are of the macronodular type and severe fatty change is unusual. The situation in Papua New Guinea is similar (Cooke, 1968); macronodular cirrhosis is very common. This is a chronic condition and most sufferers do not present for medical treatment until late in the disease; many doubtless die at home without ever seeking medical attention. The true incidence rate is thus exceedingly difficult to obtain. Crude death rates compiled by the WHO (1976) do not differentiate between the various types of cirrhosis, and are not therefore awfully helpful; however high rates are recorded for Chile, Mexico, Austria, and France, while low rates are given for Egypt, Panama, the Philippines, Thailand, and Iran. Post-mortem figures from South Africa show similar rates for cirrhosis in African, 'cape-coloured', and white populations (Becker and Chatgidakis, 1961; Thompson, 1961).

8.3.2. Aetiology of MC

Cirrhosis occurs in a young age group in tropical countries; it is seen below the age of 20 years in Zimbabwe Rhodesia (Gelfand, 1961). It is more common in males by a ratio of approximately 3:1. Social class does not influence incidence rate. The most likely causative agents are the hepatitis viruses especially types B and non-A, non-B, which produce cirrhosis via active chronic hepatitis (ACH) (see above) (Cook, 1965); cirrhosis seems to be an unusual sequel to epidemics of type A viral hepatitis, e.g. New Delhi (Chuttani, Sidhu, Wig, Gupta, and Ramalingaswami, 1966), a fact which is perhaps surprising, but is consistent with the fact that hepatitis B, and the non-A, non-B viruses are aetiologically important. In Senegal, Camain (1957) considered that 15 per cent of patients with viral hepatitis eventually become cirrhotic. In Uganda, 12 of 20 patients with viral hepatitis had a positive HB_sAg; in cirrhosis 31 per cent were positive, whereas only 2 per cent of controls gave a positive result (Maynard, Sadikali, Anthony, and Barker, 1970). However there may also be other responsible factors; long-term clearance of immune complexes by Kupffer cells in the liver can cause zonal necrosis (Blackwell, 1965a) and cirrhosis (Blackwell, 1965b; Paronetto and Popper 1966). In fact the grossly increased Kupffer cell activity in tropical livers (Chapter 5) might put the surrounding hepatocytes at risk (Bradfield and Wells, 1978).

It seems extremely unlikely that protein malnutrition, even in its very severe form, kwashiorkor, is a predisposing factor in cirrhosis (Himsworth, 1950) (Chapter 13). However, the feeling that malnutrition plays a part is still prevalent, especially in Africa. Much cirrhosis in tropical countries is clearly not associated with an excessive alcohol intake; the incidence rate in all Islamic countries is high. In Saudi Arabia, alcohol (usually in the form of Scotch whisky) is widely consumed amongst the aristocracy, and undoubtedly some cirrhosis there has an alcoholic basis; however there is a great deal of cirrhosis in the Bedouin and Yemeni communities, which is not associated with either alcohol or schistosomiasis.

The role of parasites in the aetiology of cirrhosis is difficult to assess; however there is very little, if any, evidence that they play a significant role. Liver flukes produce dilatation of bile ducts, cholangitis, and malignant cholangiomas, but they do not cause cirrhosis. Although stellate fibrosis is occasionally seen in liver-biopsy specimens from patients with malaria (Chapter 5) there is no evidence of progression to cirrhosis. More likely parasites are *Schistosoma mansoni* and *S. japonicum*. Although they produce pipe-stem fibrosis and subsequently portal hypertension, they do not produce a true cirrhosis (Chapter 10). Also in areas where *S. mansoni* infection is very common, e.g. Brazil (Montenegro, da Silva, and Pontes, 1958), Puerto Rico (Martinez-Maldonado, Girod, and Ramirez de Arellano, 1965) and Egypt (Hashem, Zaki, and Hussein, 1961), cirrhosis does not seem to be a great problem. The presence of schistosomal ova in liver sections from patients with cirrhosis should not be taken as evidence of a causal relationship; the infection is almost certainly a coincidental finding.

Another group of agents which must be seriously considered are dietary toxins. The best known association between toxins and chronic liver disease occurs in Jamaica, where veno-occlusive disease is the result of ingestion of bush-teas containing *Senecio, Crotolaria*, and *Heliotropium* alkaloids (see below). Acute liver damage has been recorded after herbal medicines in South Africa (Neame and Pillay, 1964), various roots, and tubers eaten in times of famine in Zambia (Steyn, 1965), and after ingestion of wild yams (*Dioscorea rotundata*) in Malawi (Stevenson, 1962).

Mycotoxins should also be considered; however, evidence that they are causally associated with hepatoma is far stronger than in the case of macronodular cirrhosis (Chapter 9). There is no good evidence at present that macronodular cirrhosis is produced by a dietary toxin.

Although zinc and copper are increased, and molybdenum reduced in cirrhosis and hepatoma in South Africa (Butt and Higginson, 1957) there is no clear evidence to incriminate those or any other trace element in the aetiology of macronodular cirrhosis in the tropics.

8.3.3. Presentation of MC

Onset of symptoms may occur soon after a bout of hepatitis or it may be insidious (Sherlock, 1975). In addition to jaundice, cutaneous signs of liver disease may be present, but they are extremely difficult to detect in black and brown skinned people. There is a striking absence in most third-world countries of virtually all cutaneous stigmata of liver disease; spider naevi, clubbing, palmar erythema, liver nails, and alteration of hair distribution are rarely recorded. Purpura and petechiae are also very difficult, if not impossible, to detect in dark skins. Peripheral oedema, and subsequently ascites, may be present.

There may be gynaecomastia (Fig. 8.2) and loss of axillary and pubic hair, and testicular atrophy in men; failure of the damaged liver to detoxicate circulating oestrogens is thought to be responsible for those changes. Amenorrhoea is common in women.

Anaemia may be a prominent sign; it is caused by several factors, including decreased erythrocyte survival time, blood coagulation defects, gastrointestinal bleeding, and haemolysis. Leucopenia, thrombocytopenia, macrocytosis, and target cells may be present in the peripheral blood. Prothrombin deficiency may result from defective synthesis in the liver. Plasma fibrinolysins are often increased. High serum B_{12} concentrations are found in the serum, because that vitamin is usually stored in the liver.

Ascitic fluid accumulates in the peritoneal cavity with a protein content of 10 to 20 g per l, which is characteristic of a transudate. Gross ascites constitutes probably the most common clinical presentation of cirrhosis in third-world countries. Hypoalbuminaemia and increased aldosterone secretion, accompanied by reabsorption of sodium cause transudation of fluid through the capsule of the liver or the serosa of the gut and mesentery, to the abdominal cavity.

Portal hypertension is of a post-sinusoidal type (Chapter 11) resulting in splenomegaly, oesophageal varices, dilated inferior haemorrhoidal veins and also veins around the umbilicus (where a 'caput Medusae' is a rare finding) and the vestigeal vein in the ligamentum teres.

Associated features are relapsing pancreatitis, peptic ulcer disease, and gall-stones—but these are all rare in tropical countries; tuberculous peritonitis, which may complicate cirrhotic ascites, should always be excluded.

Death is usually due either to haemorrhage from oesophageal varices or hepatic coma. A silent bacterial peritonitis may occur (*Brit. med. J.*, 1964). Tuberculous peritonitis is a further cause of death.

8.3.4. Pathology of MC

The liver is reduced in size, but its normal shape is usually more or less retained. Regeneration nodules vary in size from a few millimetres to several centimetres and are cut off by bands of greyish-white fibrous tissue of irregular thickness (Fig. 8.3): they vary in colour from reddish-brown to green. Histologically, the liver consists of nodules of variable size, which are demarcated by bands of fibrous tissue of variable width. Lobular structures, e.g. central and portal tracts, can be recognized in some nodules. The fibrous tissue contains an excess

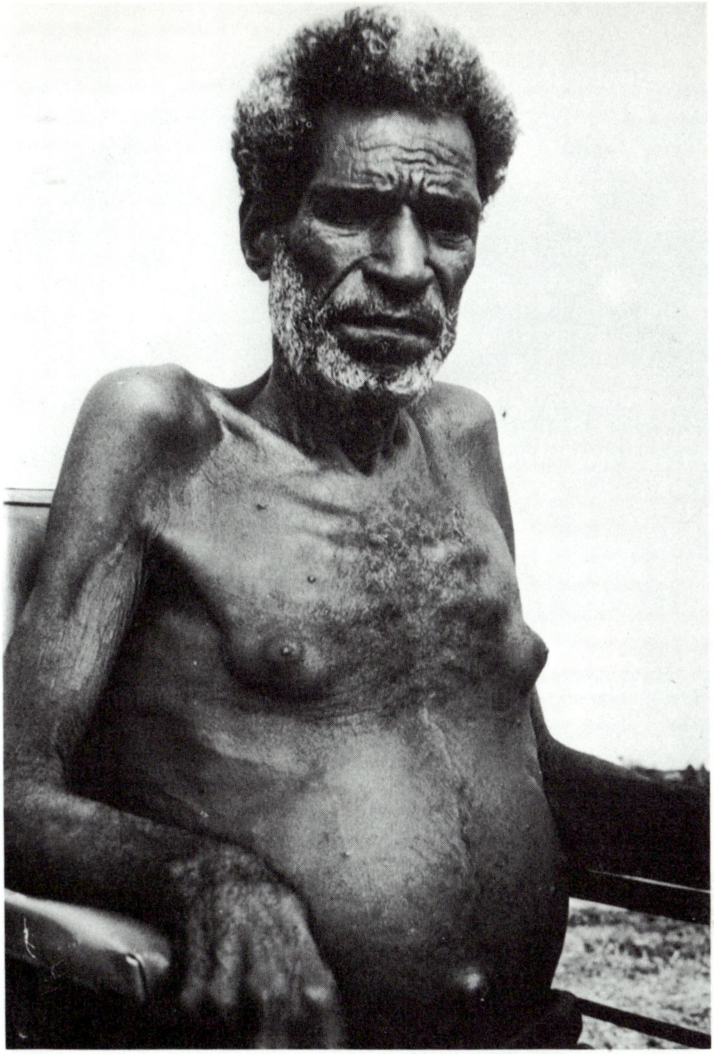

FIG. 8.2. A 60-year-old Papua New Guinean man with macronodular cirrhosis. Ascites and prominent veins on the anterior abdominal wall are shown, together with severe gynaecomastia.

of bile ducts, pseudoductules, vascular channels, histiocytes, and plasma cells. The liver cell cords are broadened, being two or more cells in width. There may be bile retention in the canaliculi, and Kupffer and parenchymal cells. Fat and haemosiderin are usually absent. Terminal haemorrhage from oesophageal varices results in widespread necrosis of some nodules.

There is confusion, on clinical grounds, between cirrhosis and the pipe-stem fibrosis which results from schistosomiasis (Forbes and Gelfand, 1962; Davey, 1968) (Chapter 10); clinically the two are similar, especially when portal hypertension has supervened. But, the histology is grossly different.

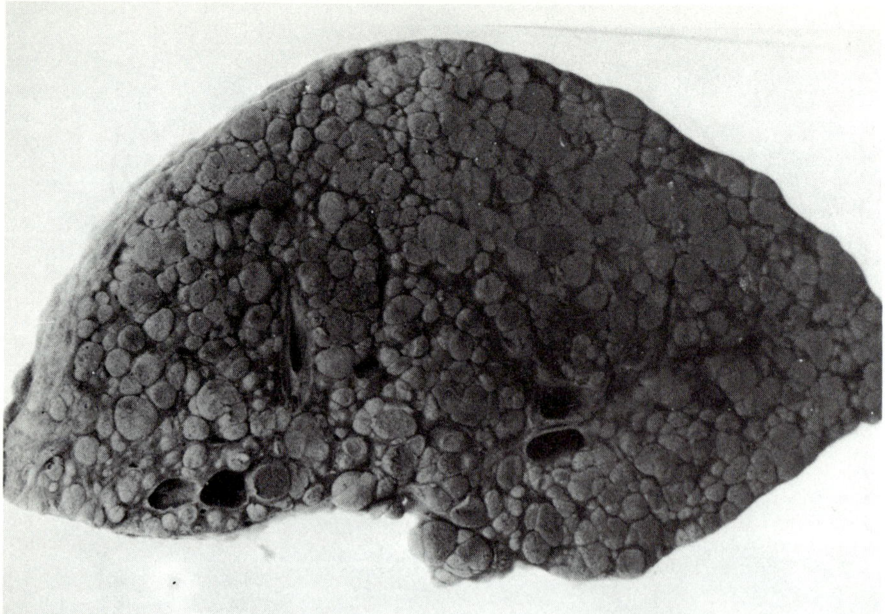

FIG. 8.3. Cut surface of the liver of a 17-year-old Papua New Guinean man. He was admitted to hospital with a short history of upper abdominal pain and jaundice; he died in hepatic coma a few days later. The section shows a coarse macronodular cirrhosis, which probably followed viral hepatitis; serum HB_sAg was not estimated.

8.3.5. Investigation of MC

Liver function tests should be performed. Serum bilirubin, transaminases, and alkaline phosphatase may be mildly elevated; the striking findings are depressed serum albumin and grossly elevated gamma-globulin concentrations. Bromsulphthalein excretion is impaired. Serum HB_sAg may be present at high concentration. Liver biopsy may be diagnostic; if cirrhosis is suspected a Vim-Silverman, rather than a Menghini needle, should be used to cut the hard liver tissue. Wedge biopsy at a limited laparotomy is rarely necessary for diagnosis. Splenovenography and hepatic vein catheterization will provide valuable haemodynamic information, if those techniques are available; both portal venous pressure and occluded suprahepatic vein pressure are elevated and that distinguishes the lesion from 'pipe-stem' fibrosis due to schistosomiasis. Peritoneoscopy has proved of great value in Nigeria in differentiating hepatic lesions (Davey, 1963).

A mild normocytic, normochromic anaemia is usually present; a macrocytic anaemia is unusual. If there is gastrointestinal bleeding a hypochromic anaemia may be present. Leucocyte and platelet counts are reduced. The prothrombin time is usually prolonged.

If prothrombin time and platelet count are reasonably normal, a liver-biopsy will usually clinch the diagnosis.

More refined techniques: splenovenography, scinti-scanning, etc., are rarely available in tropical countries.

8.3.6. Treatment of MC

With established cirrhosis, no treatment is available at present. It is important to ascertain whether a high degree of 'activity' is present. If so the predominant disease may be active chronic hepatitis with a rapidly progressive cirrhosis; corticosteroids may be of value in that situation (see above).

A good diet should be recommended, with alcohol restriction.

Treatment of hepatic failure and coma, which is partly due to a high blood ammonia concentration (Dawson, 1978) has been described by Sherlock (1975); dietary protein restriction with oral neomycin (1 g four-hourly) or lactulose (Chapter 11) (Conn, 1978) should be instituted. Onset of fluid retention and haemorrhage, due to portal hypertension, should be treated on their merits (Chapter 11).

Treatment of ascites is with diuretics; their effect is very often slow in tropical countries, due largely to the difficulty (or impossibility) of reducing salt intake. Frusemide ('Lasix') in a dose of 40 to 120 mg daily, orally, usually gives satisfactory results; that should preferably be given with spironolactone ('Aldactone') 100 mg daily. A recommendation that abdominal paracentesis is a valuable form of management in Papua New Guinea (Wagner and Shepherd, 1976) is unacceptable; by depleting the remaining protein reserves, and by disturbing the electrolyte balance, that procedure is dangerous. Ascites should be tapped (i) as an aid to diagnosis, and (ii) to relieve very tense fluid which is causing respiratory embarrassment.

As with advanced schistosomal liver disease, portacaval anastomosis has little place in management, due frequently to the advanced stage of the disease at diagnosis (Davey, 1968); serum bilirubin is usually greater than 26 μmol per l (1·5 mg per dl), serum albumin less than 30 mg per l, and there is usually some ascites.

8.4. Other forms of cirrhosis

8.4.1. Indian childhood cirrhosis (ICC)

Indian childhood cirrhosis is a great paediatric problem in India, especially in southern India, Calcutta, and the Punjab. The disease, which is usually diagnosed between 1·5 and 3 years of age, has a predilection for some ethnic groups and is commonly familial. The Brahmins, Kayasthas, Agrawals, Rajputs, and Sikhs, who are descended from the higher strata of Hindu society, are most commonly affected (Khanna, 1968; Majumdar, Kapoor, and Sharma, 1969). Children from vegetarian sects are frequently affected. ICC is usually more common in boys than girls, although in some series the sex ratio has approached unity. The mortality rate is very high.

Historically the disease has been recognized since 1000 BC, having been first described by Susruta.

ICC usually starts with mild vague symptoms, which include irritability and loss of appetite. The disease may run fulminant, acute, or subacute courses. In the more acute forms it may resemble viral hepatitis, whereas in the subacute type a gradual onset of jaundice and evidence of portal hypertension may be detected, as cirrhosis develops insidiously. Hepatosplenomegaly is a common presenting feature; jaundice and ascites occur later (Khanna, 1968;

Majumdar, *et al.*, 1969). Mortality rate is especially high in infancy. Older children frequently recover. Presentation rarely occurs in adult life. There is an increased incidence of peptic ulcer disease in both patients and relations (Sur and Bhatti, 1978). An increased incidence of diabetes mellitus has been reported. Asthma, Parkinsonism, and migraine are also more common.

Serum bilirubin and transaminases are elevated. Alkaline phosphatase is normal. Bromsulphthalein retention is increased. There is hypoalbuminaemia.

Histologically there is a progressive fibrosis with almost complete absence of regeneration. Groups of hepatocytes are separated and show severe degenerative changes (Patel, Parekh, and Chitale, 1974; Aikat, Bhattacharya, and Walia, 1974); there is variation in size with ballooning and large pale nuclei with enlarged nucleoli. Alcoholic hyaline is occasionally present, but there is no fatty change. Eosinophilic degeneration with a leucocytic infiltration may affect individual cells. Lipofuscin is occasionally present in the Kupffer cells. Giant cell transformation and bile stasis occur late in the disease. Portal tracts are infiltrated with lymphocytes, histiocytes, and occasional polymorphonuclear leucocytes. Fibrosis extends periportally, and progresses to a true cirrhosis which may be micro- (Smetana, Hadley, and Sirsat, 1961) or macro- (Achar, Raju, and Sriramachari, 1960) nodular. Malignant change is unusual.

Many possibilities have been considered in the aetiology of this disease (Sing, Jolly, and Kumar, 1961). Malnutrition is not a factor because most children with the condition come from upper-class families. Transplacentally transmitted hepatitis (Aikat and Sengupta, 1956), and hepatitis early in life (Chandra, 1970; Sundaravalli, 1971) have been considered. Chandra (1970) demonstrated positive HB_sAg in 6 per cent of 30 patients with ICC; serum immunoglobulins IgG, IgM, and IgA were raised, and smooth muscle antibody was present in 82 per cent. Autoimmunity has also received consideration (Prasad, 1962; Dixit and Gupta, 1970). Dietary aflatoxins have been suggested as a possible cause (Amla, Kumaris, and Murthy, 1970). Another suggestion is a low serum zinc concentration (Ghai and Vasuki, 1971).

Recently evidence that the disease results from an inherited disorder of tryptophan metabolism has been produced (Sur and Bhatti, 1978): that was demonstrated not only in patients, but also in parents and relations. Those authors concluded from a study of 29 families of patients with ICC, and 9 families with related disorders, that there is a basic deficiency of 3-hydroxyanthranilic oxidase with the subsequent accumulation of precursors of 3-hydroxyanthranilic acid on the tryptophan–niacin pathway. It was suggested that 'an autosomal dominant gene of intermediate dominance, with diminished expressivity and reduced penetrance in girls' was the most likely mode of inheritance.

It seems likely that there is an excess of copper within the hepatocytes in ICC. The hepatocytes contain orcein-staining deposits (Portmann, Tanner, Mowat, and Williams, 1978; Tanner, Portmann, Mowatt, and Williams, 1978), which are likely to represent increased copper-binding protein, similar to that in Wilson's disease (Salaspuro and Sipponen, 1976) (see below). In addition, renal tubular cells also contain the material; functional tubular abnormalities are known to occur in ICC (Saini, Dhatt, and Mehta, 1976; Dhatt, Gupta, and

Saini, 1968); both amino-acids and mono- and di-saccharides appear in the urine. Haemolytic anaemia, a feature of Wilson's disease, has also been reported in ICC (Gupta, Kalra, and Chaudri, 1975; Portmann, Tanner, Mowat, and Williams, 1978).

There is at present no known treatment. Sur and Bhatti (1978) have suggested that a low tryptophan diet with massive vitamin B_6 supplements might be the best way of arresting the disease.

8.4.2. Veno-occlusive disease (VOD)

Veno-occlusive disease (VOD) was first reported in the West Indies, but has also been demonstrated in north and South Africa, Jordan, and India (Gupta, Gupta, and Sharma, 1963). Al-Hasany and Mohamed (1970) have described a sudden outbreak of VOD in Iraq. In 1974 there was a large epidemic in Afghanistan (Mohabbat, Srivastava, Younos, Sediq, Merzad, and Aram, 1976). In 1975 a further outbreak, in which 42 per cent of 67 recorded cases died, occurred in the Sarguja district of India (Tandon, Tandon, Tandon, Narndranathan, and Joshi, 1976). It may be acute, subacute, or chronic and affects the central and sublobular hepatic veins. In the West Indies the disease accounts for some 30 per cent of cases of cirrhosis (Bras, Brooks, and Watler, 1961).

Presentation is usually with acute hepatomegaly and ascites; approximately 50 per cent recover, 20 per cent die in the acute stage, and the remainder develop chronic disease with portal hypertension (Stuart and Bras, 1957). The disease is most common in the one to six year age group. Sex incidence is equal; a familial incidence has been reported.

Differential diagnosis is from secondary thrombosis of the hepatic veins due to tumours or sepsis, and the Budd-Chiari syndrome (see below).

Central and sublobular hepatic veins show subendothelial oedema, intimal overgrowth of connective tissue, and narrowing and occlusion of the lumen. That is followed by centrizonal congestion, necrosis of hepatocytes, and fibrosis; those changes are similar to those in cardiac cirrhosis (see above), but are distinct from those of macro- (see above) and micro- (Chapter 11) nodular cirrhosis. Thrombosis of larger hepatic veins has been reported in this disease in South Africa (Selzer and Parker, 1951) and Egypt (Safouh and Shehata, 1965). It seems possible that *Senecio* alkaloids might be implicated in some cases of the *Budd-Chiari syndrome*—in which there is occlusion of the hepatic veins as they join the inferior vena cava (Selzer and Parker, 1951). Large doses of the alkaloids produce centrilobular liver damage, pulmonary oedema, and death in a few days. Survivors develop cirrhosis, and after repeated intermittent dosage giant-cell transformation of hepatocytes and hepatocellular carcinoma may occur. Women may secrete the toxic factor(s) in breast milk (Schoental, 1963; Schoental and Magee, 1959).

The disease is caused by 'bush-teas' containing pyrrolizidine-containing alkaloids (Hill, Stephenson, and Filshie, 1958; McLean, Bras, and György, 1964), especially *Crotalaria, Senecio*, and *Heliotropium*; toxicity is greater in young patients, and in males compared with females. In man, *senecio* alkaloids have long been known to be responsible for centrilobular hepatic lesions

(Willmot and Robertson, 1920; Selzer and Parker, 1951). VOD has been produced in *Macaca speciosa* monkeys by injecting monocrotaline (0·125 g per kg body weight) intraperitoneally (Allen, Carstens, and Katagiri, 1969). In other species senecio poisoning occurs in many parts of the world (Hill, 1960). In horses, a disease called 'jagsiekte' has been reported in horses in South Africa, and in northern Australia, 'Kimberley horse disease' can be produced by various species of *Crotalaria*; there is centrilobular necrosis and fibrosis of the liver (Gardiner, Royce, and Bokor, 1965).

8.4.3. Cardiac cirrhosis and chronic venous congestion

Persistent elevation of the hepatic venous pressure causes centrilobular congestion similar to that in veno-occlusive disease (VOD); that leads to centrilobular fibrosis, and a true cirrhosis.

Cardiomegaly of unknown aetiology is common in many parts of the tropics; it affects all ethnic groups and all ages. In long-standing cases hepatic congestion is marked. Progressive changes resulting in cirrhosis have been reported from South Africa (Gillanders, 1951) but that has not been confirmed in other parts of the tropics. In right-sided endomyocardial fibrosis, the liver is severely affected and there may be severe central congestion resulting in central fibrosis and cardiac cirrhosis. Small granulomata have been described in the liver in patients dying of endomyocardial fibrosis (Osunkoya, Carlisle, and Dawodu, 1972). There may be post-sinusoidal portal hypertension (Chapter 11). Oxygen desaturation of arterial blood may occur. Clinically there is a high jugular venous pressure, ascites, early finger clubbing, and arterial oxygen desaturation; in children stunting of growth may be prominent.

Constrictive pericarditis, often due to tuberculosis but also a long-term result of acute bacterial pericarditis, is not uncommon throughout the tropics. Hepatic fibrosis may be a result, but overall occurs much less commonly than in endomyocardial fibrosis (Edington and Gilles, 1976).

In beri-beri heart disease hepatomegaly is common, but severe liver disease and cirrhosis are unusual.

8.4.4. Iron overload (African siderosis)

Heavy deposits of iron are found in the absence of anaemia or haemolysis in the liver and viscera in several situations. The two main ones are (i) African siderosis, and (ii) haemochromatosis. Repeated blood-transfusions in patients with aplastic anaemia or other blood dyscrasias may produce a similar picture.

In long-standing haemolytic anaemia, due for example to sickle-cell disease and the severe forms of thalassaemia, heavy deposits of iron can be demonstrated. After repeated blood-transfusions in refractory anaemia, large amounts of iron may be found in the reticuloendothelial cells and later in the hepatocytes, pancreatic cells, and other organs.

The cause of iron accumulation in the liver and its importance in producing cirrhosis are not clear. African siderosis should not be confused with a mere iron excess in the Kupffer cells which can occur whenever there is a short red-cell survival, as in tropical splenomegaly (Chapter 16) and sickle-cell disease. In the majority of cases of siderosis, the excess iron is probably a result of an increased dietary intake of iron, but that may be influenced by other dietary factors. There is little, if any, clear evidence that iron is *per se* a precursor of cirrhosis. In chronic pancreatitis on the other hand, an excess of iron, and also fat in the liver, is a common finding in the tropics. At the Mulago hospital, Kampala, over 50 per cent of patients with chronic pancreatitis have an excess of iron in liver-biopsy sections (Hutt, 1971) (Chapter 15); the association of fat and iron in the liver is almost pathognomonic of that condition. There is an increased absorption of iron, and an impaired amino-acid absorption may have some bearing on the problem. In experimental animals excess iron absorption has been found after the pancreatic duct has been tied. However, even there cirrhosis does not seem to be a sequel.

Clinical. Men are affected more often than women; the sex difference is less marked after the menopause. The condition may be complicated by osteoporosis and vertebral collapse (Lorincz, Traub, Chuke, and Hussain, 1974).

Distribution. African siderosis is very common in South Africa (Gillman, Lamont, Hathorn, and Canham, 1957; Gillman, Canham, and Hathorn, 1958) and Zimbabwe Rhodesia (Gelfand, 1955). In South Africa, it is present in up to 80 per cent of the adult population (Gillman and Gillman, 1951; Higginson, Gerritson, and Walker, 1953); 70 per cent of Bantu men of 30 to 40 years have evidence of that (Bothwell and Isaacson, 1962). The distribution of iron in the hepatocytes depends partly on (i) the presence or absence of cirrhosis, and (ii) on the degree of overload; there is no evidence that cirrhosis is a direct result of iron overload. The condition has been reported from Ghana (Edington and Dodu, 1957). Although previously thought to be uncommon in Tanzania, Kenya, and Uganda (Davies, 1956); the condition now seems to be not uncommon in Uganda where it has a tribal basis (Hutt, 1971). In the nomadic Karamojong of the north-east, excess iron was present in 56 liver biopsy specimens examined over a two-year period, whereas during the same period only 18, 13, and 17 per cent of Ganda, Rwanda, and Ankole people had an excess; in most the liver architecture was normal and iron appeared as fine granules in the hepatocytes, being usually most marked around the portal areas. When large amounts were present in the hepatocytes, a considerable quantity was also present in the Kupffer cells and portal areas. Hutt (1971) considered that the condition in Uganda was similar to that in South Africa, and was due to a combination of dietary factors resulting in an overall excess iron absorption rate (Gillman, *et al.*, 1958). It now seems clear that the condition is more common in Uganda than hitherto suspected (Owor, 1974); 23 per cent of post-mortem livers at the Mulago Hospital, Kampala show evidence of hepatic haemosiderosis. Similarly in Zambia, a review of 482 liver biopsy-specimens showed a 25 per cent incidence of haemosiderosis (Lorincz, *et al.*, 1974). In Kenya, Foy and Kondi (1958) found the condition in two of three cases of megaloblastic anaemia. Fifty-one cases of Bantu siderosis were reported by Haddock (1965) from Dar-es-Salaam, Tanzania over a 10-year period; that represented about 10 per cent of liver-biopsies during that period.

Approximately half had histologically proved cirrhosis and 19 others had fibrosis but no definite evidence of cirrhosis; three of those with cirrhosis had a high alcohol intake. Upper abdominal pain was experienced by 11 of those without cirrhosis; four had had a heavy alcohol intake. All had hepatomegaly but only a minority had splenomegaly. Serum iron and iron binding capacity were both raised in the four cases studied. Skin biopsies showed an excess iron in the three cases examined. Cliff and Speight (1976) have also reported cases of haemosiderosis from Dar-es-Salaam, Tanzania; the condition is now recognized to be common there (Nhonoli, 1973) and seems to be associated with a high intake of locally-brewed liquor.

Aetiology. The cause of African siderosis is largely obscure. There is no doubt that iron intake is high in many of the areas where the disease is very common; iron pots are used for cooking. In laboratory animals, a high iron intake and either a predominantly maize diet, or one deficient in folic acid can produce the condition. Prolonged malnutrition with pancreatic damage and derangement of intracellular metabolism has been suggested. That anaemia in childhood conditions the mucosa to absorb excessive amounts of iron, is a further hypothetical mechanism. Various other hypotheses have also been suggested but none of them proven (Edington and Gilles, 1976). Gillman *et al.* (1958) considered that a deficient mealie diet combined with an excessive iron intake was the cause. Alcohol is a further possibility in some cases.

Pathology. There is considerable confusion as to whether the iron deposition is mainly in the hepatocytes or the reticuloendothelial system. In the liver, iron may be present in either of those sites, or both together; furthermore there may be large amounts of iron in hepatocytes, Kupffer cells, and portal tracts with or without cirrhosis. In Ghana, both the hepatocytes and reticuloendothelial system are involved (Edington, 1959). Heavy iron-deposits may be found in the duodenum and jejunum, spleen, and bone marrow but are unusual in the stomach, choroid plexus, pancreas, thyroid, skin, adrenals, and heart; that distribution is of value in differentiating the disease from haemochromatosis (Edington and Gilles, 1976).

The condition is common in patients with diabetes mellitus in South Africa (Seftel, Isaacson, and Bothwell, 1960) and Ghana (Dodu, 1958); 25 and 9 per cent of diabetics had the condition, respectively. Both acinar and islet cells of the pancreas contain pigment. It is difficult to be sure whether the pancreatic disease is the cause or result of iron overload. Because the cirrhosis is often micronodular in type and hepatoma is unusual, Edington and Gilles (1976) have suggested that that is probably a result of the iron overload, because most cirrhosis in Africa is macronodular and hepatoma is common. However it is possible that alcohol was the cause of both pancreatitis and micronodular cirrhosis.

Investigation. Plasma iron and iron-binding capacities are low or normal; in patients with large iron deposits in hepatocytes, Kupffer cells and portal tracts, in the presence of cirrhosis, high values comparable to those in haemochromatosis may be present.

Haemochromatosis. This disease is thought to be an inherited disorder of iron over-absorption transmitted by a Mendelian dominant (Williams, Scheuer, and Sherlock, 1962); excessive iron deposition takes place in the liver, pancreas, heart, and testes, and cirrhosis and diabetes mellitus result. The skin is pigmented due to melanin deposits. Because many patients with the condition are chronic alcoholics it is not clear whether this is truly a genetic disorder or whether it is part of a spectrum of disease (MacDonald and Mallory, 1960; MacDonald and Baumstag, 1964). The condition is worldwide in distribution and is more common in men than women.

Heavy iron deposits occur in the liver, pancreas, abdominal lymph nodes, heart, stomach, thyroid, and gastric glands; the iron is largely parenchymal in distribution. A micronodular cirrhosis and deposits of iron in the pancreas, with fibrosis and atrophy, are prominent features. Iron granules are also present in the enterocytes and macrophages of the lamina propria of the jejunum (Astaldi, Meardi, and Lisino, 1966).

Although there are obvious differences between African siderosis and haemochromatosis in their classical forms, Edington (1959) has claimed that in Ghana he was unable to differentiate some cases of siderosis from haemochromatosis. The situation in Tanzania seems to be similar (Nhonoli, 1973).

8.4.5. Wilson's disease (hepatolenticular degeneration)

Although not a common disease in the tropics, Wilson's disease is not often looked for. There seems however to be a relatively high incidence in Chinese people in Malaysia. It often presents without neurological symptoms and signs and may be difficult to differentiate from active chronic hepatitis. Presentation may be with cirrhosis, portal hypertension, and fulminant hepatitis. A high index of suspicion is required if early cases are not to be missed; if treatment with penicillamine is commenced early, results are good, but if there is delay in initiating treatment, the outlook is bad (*Br. med. J.*, 1978a). When suspected, the diagnosis can be confirmed by finding raised liver and urinary copper concentrations (Scott, Gollan, Samourian, and Sherlock, 1978).

8.4.6. Pericellular cirrhosis

Pericellular cirrhosis (diffuse interstitial cirrhosis) of unknown aetiology is found in adults in Mexico (Pérez-Tamayo, 1958); an association with tuberculosis has been suggested but not proved. Such a lesion is occasionally found in congenital syphilis, but a true cirrhosis is unusual; spirochaetes in that condition can be demonstrated by Levaditi's stain. A similar histological picture may occur in Indian childhood cirrhosis (ICC). In those cirrhoses individual hepatocytes are surrounded by cellular fibrous tissue which is infiltrated with histiocytes and lymphocytes.

8.4.7. Hereditary and neonatal causes of cirrhosis

Under this heading are a number of conditions which occasionally cause cirrhosis; they are not however especially important in tropical countries, and other texts (Sherlock, 1975) should be consulted. They include galactosaemia, type IV glycogen storage disease, fructose intolerance, congenital tyrosinosis, and mucoviscidosis (cystic fibrosis). The last condition seems to be particularly rare in the tropics; because there is an increased sodium chloride loss in the sweat, it seems probable that there has been a selective advantage against the gene in tropical countries. The recessive gene is present in about one in nine people in some western countries.

8.5. Other chronic diseases without an infective basis

8.5.1. Alpha$_1$ antitrypsin deficiency

The relative importance of alpha$_1$ antitrypsin deficiency in tropical countries is not yet known; however it seems to be rare in Africans (Fagerhol, 1976). This glycoprotein comprises 80 to 90 per cent of the serum α_1 globulin fraction; it is an inhibitor of trypsin and other proteases.

There are many variants of alpha$_1$ antitrypsin deficiency (Bearn, 1978; Morse, 1978); although clearly a genetically determined error of protein synthesis, it appears that environmental factors are necessary for it to produce overt abnormalities, for many fit people have very low concentrations of this protein.

The association between this deficiency state and liver disease was first described in children (Ganrot, Laurell, and Eriksson, 1967). Later work has clearly indicated an association between the condition and cirrhosis in adults (Gans, Sharp, and Tan, 1969; Sharp, Bridges, Krivit, and Freier, 1969; Berg and Eriksson, 1972; Cohen, Rubin, Echevarria, Sharp, and Teague, 1973).

Although the mechanism of liver damage is unclear at present it seems likely that in the presence of an hepatic insult (e.g. viral hepatitis or alcohol) individuals with a deficiency of alpha$_1$ antitrypsin have a reduced protective action within the liver against proteolytic enzymes.

The cirrhosis may be macro- or micronodular and may be accompanied by emphysema. Hepatocellular carcinoma may be a complication of the liver disease (Berg and Eriksson, 1972).

The diagnosis should be suspected in patients with both hepatic and pulmonary disease; confirmation of diagnosis is by measuring the concentration of alpha$_1$ antitrypsin in the serum.

No specific treatment is available at present; the complications of the cirrhosis and pulmonary disease must be treated on their merits.

8.5.2. Porphyria

There are marked geographical variations in the distribution of porphyria. In South Africa it is common in both Africans and white people. The disease is also common in Turkey. Acute intermittent porphyria has been reported from Kenya (Oomen, 1973); the overall incidence of the disease there is unknown.

Clinically, patients with porphyria may present as acute abdominal emergencies.

Abnormal porphyrins are produced in the liver or bone-marrow. If the bone-marrow is the origin, liver disease does not occur; the porphyrins responsible for the photosensitivity have an hepatic origin, however (Iber and Maddrey, 1965). There are four main types: (i) Porphyria variegata which is inherited by a Mendelian dominant gene and is common in South Africa, (ii) acute intermittent porphyria which is also inherited by a Mendelian dominant and is common in Sweden, (iii) porphyria cutanea tarda, which is often familial, and (iv) an acquired type, common in Turkey, which probably also has a familial basis. Fibrous changes in the liver, and cirrhosis, can occur in the first three types; in addition, haemosiderin is often present. Hepatic pathology does not occur in the fourth type.

Many patients with porphyria are chronic alcoholics. Patients with alcoholic liver disease occasionally have porphyrinuria, and it is often difficult to separate that from hepatic porphyria.

8.5.3. Sickle-cell disease (SS)

Hepatomegaly and impaired liver function tests are common in this disease (Hilkovitz and Jacobson, 1961); there may be a clinical picture similar to that in chronic hepatitis. Erythrophagocytosis of sickled cells by Kupffer cells is often present. In a 'crisis' the hepatic sinusoids are filled with sickled erythrocytes; obstruction to the blood flow by engorged Kupffer cells is common. There may be areas of focal necrosis with fibrosis; cirrhosis is common in the USA and west Africa (Edington and Gilles, 1976). Haemosiderosis may be marked and changes resulting from hypoxia in the hepatocytes are often present. In the USA, gallstones are common (Chapter 14) and cholestatic features may be present.

8.5.4. β-Thalassaemia major

Mild hepatomegaly is usual. There is anaemia and parenchymal and reticuloendothelial haemosiderosis. Hyperplasia of haemopoietic tissue and cirrhosis may complicate the disease.

8.5.5. Haemoglobin-H disease

This disease occurs in India, Indonesia, Burma, Thailand, and China, and also in Greeks and Italians. Recurrent attacks of jaundice and fever and splenomegaly may be present. Portal fibrosis and haemosiderosis of the periportal parenchymal cells is seen (Keng and Khoo, 1970).

8.5.6. Leukaemia

Leukaemias occur throughout the tropics but there is considerable evidence that they are less common than in temperate parts of the world (Edington and Gilles, 1976). In chronic lymphatic leukaemia, liver-biopsy specimens show marked lymphocytic infiltration of the sinusoids and portal tracts. The condition may be very difficult to differentiate from the tropical splenomegaly syndrome (TSS) (Chapter 16). Liver-biopsy appearances in the two conditions are very similar; the lymphocytes may be single, in rows, or clustered. Whether or not TSS can progress to lymphosarcoma is still not completely solved; if that sequence of events does occur it is rare.

8.6. Other chronic diseases caused by infections

8.6.1. Tuberculosis

Hepatic granulomata are very common in various forms of tuberculosis (Chapter 5); they usually heal without scarring but may calcify occasionally. Granulomata are frequently seen in liver-biopsies carried out in the investigation of 'pyrexia of undetermined origin' in tropical countries.

Tuberculomata (Chapter 12) and tuberculous abscess (Gracey, 1965) are unusual. Tuberculous cholangitis and pylephlebitis have been described.

There are not usually any signs or symptoms associated with the liver involvement; they are a result of the disease in other organs (Hersch, 1964; Korn, Kellow, Heller, Chomet, and Zimmerman, 1959), which is usually widespread and may be miliary with a very ill patient and a high pyrexia.

8.6.2. Leprosy

Hepatic involvement in all types of leprosy has been well documented (Agarwal, Maheshwar, Mittal, and Kumat, 1973; Karat, Job, and Rao, 1971), but especially in lepromatous leprosy. Hepatomegaly is sometimes present in patients with erythema nodosum leprosum. Although tests of liver function are frequently abnormal and there are granulomatous lesions in liver-biopsy specimens (Karat, *et al.*, 1971), clinical evidence of liver disease is very unusual. A high incidence of HB_sAg in lepromatous patients has been reported (Shwe and Zuckerman, 1972).

Browne (1964) has stressed that therapeutic agents used in the treatment of leprosy are probably responsible for some of the reported pathology.

In tuberculoid leprosy, tuberculoid follicles are often seen in the liver, either subserosally or in the portal tracts; they are not associated with symptoms. In lepromatous leprosy, the Kupffer cells proliferate and contain *Mycobacterium leprae*; they often persist there after the bacilli have cleared from the skin and nasal mucosa following treatment and may produce an important reservoir of infection. Miliary lepromata consisting of lepra cells and lymphocytes and plasma cells are found in the portal tracts, sinusoids and hepatic parenchyma. The liver may also be affected by secondary amyloidosis.

In a study of 42 asymptomatic children of leprosy patients, hepatic lesions were found in 47 per cent and acid-fast bacilli in 9·5 per cent (Mittal, Maheshwari, Saha, and Sharma, 1978); Kupffer cell hyperplasia, focal necrosis, granulomata, and portal tract infiltration were all encountered; however, as most of those changes are frequently seen in indigenous people in tropical countries their significance is difficult to interpret.

Similarly in the armadillo, experimental infections produce marked liver lesions (Job, Kirchheimer, and Sanchez, 1978); the initial lesion involves the Kupffer cells and later large collections of macrophages containing bacteria infiltrate the liver lobules; in late lesions the hepatocytes become foamy. In three of the lepromatoid livers, lesions compatible with erythema nodosum leprosum were seen.

8.6.3. Syphilis

Congenital syphilis of the liver no doubt occurs in tropical countries; that disease is fairly prevalent in some areas. However it is submerged beneath much other pathology at present.

In secondary syphilis, miliary granulomata may be present in the liver (Lee, Thornton, and Conn, 1971); jaundice and hepatitis are rare accompaniments, and should not be confused with viral hepatitis. Liver-biopsy sections show an infiltration with polymorphs and lymphocytes, with occasional centrizonal necrosis.

In the tertiary stage, single or multiple gummas (Symmers and Spain, 1946) may be present; they usually consist of a mass in the right lobe surrounded by fibrous tissue. Cirrhosis is never a sequel. The lesions regress over long periods of time after penicillin treatment.

8.6.4. Actinomycosis

The liver is occasionally the site of actinomycotic lesions, spread having taken place usually from the ileocaecal region via the portal venous system (Chapter 27). There may be multiple small abscesses and sinuses within the liver substance, caused by *Actinomyces israelii* or *A. bovis.*

8.6.5. Leishmaniasis (Kala-azar)

Visceral leishmaniasis (Kala-azar) is widely spread over much of the tropics, especially Africa, Asia (including the Mediterranean littoral), and southern America. The plains of the Ganges and Brahmaputra were especially notorious endemic areas, and since 1975, Bihar and Uttar Pradesh have been seriously involved (Sen Gupta, 1975). The disease is caused by *Leishmania donovani*, which usually requires an animal reservoir. Man is infected by the bite of sandflies of the Phlebotomus species. The disease may be epidemic.

Clinically the disease is characterized by fever, cachexia, anaemia, splenomegaly, and evidence of hypersplenism, leucopenia, and thrombocytopenia. There is hepatomegaly. Albuminuria is common. Hypoalbuminaemia is usually present; serum IgG and gamma-globulin concentrations are usually grossly elevated.

Leishmaniasis is a disease of the reticuloendothelial system; lymphatic tissues and the spleen are extensively involved. Splenomegaly is often gross, and there may be confusion, clinically, with the tropical splenomegaly syndrome (TSS) (Chapter 16). Hepatic pathology is characterized by mesenchymal and reticuloendothelial changes without severe involvement of hepatocytes.

Liver-biopsy specimens show hyperplastic Kupffer cells, and a round-cell infiltrate (usually consisting largely of plasma cells) in the sinusoids. The Kupffer cells may be stuffed with parasites (Leishman-Donovan bodies), which may also be present in histiocytes in the portal tracts. Lymphocytes and plasma cells are also found in the portal triads. The hepatocytes show non-specific changes and their glycogen content is diminished; the parasites are occasionally present in them (Meleney, 1925). An intralobular cirrhosis may be present, but that is an incidental finding.

An indirect fluorescent antibody test, splenic puncture, and bone-marrow examination are of value in diagnosis.

Treatment of the disease is difficult (*Br. med. J.,* 1978b). Sodium stibogluconate is not always effective, and amphotericin B and pentamidine are seriously toxic. An experimental technique incorporates antimony into liposomes which are preferentially taken up by reticuloendothelial cells, thus reaching the parasites at high concentration (Black, Watson, and Ward, 1977).

8.6.6. *African histoplasmosis*

This disease is caused by *Histoplasma duboisii* (Edington, 1971; Schwarz, 1971) and has been reported in Africa, south of the Sahara and north of Zimbabwe Rhodesia. Infection has been described in the baboon, but the mode of infection in man is unknown.

It may be a localized disease confined to the skin and regional lymph nodes, or can be a disseminated disease involving the abdominal viscera—especially the liver and spleen. The lungs are not usually affected.

The fungus cells stimulate production of histiocytes and giant cells. Fungal cells can be easily demonstrated in haematoxylin and eosin preparations.

8.6.7. *Cysticercosis*

Cysticerci, resulting from *Taenia solium* infection (Chapter 19), are occasionally found in the liver. It is doubtful however whether they have any clinical significance.

8.6.8. *Neonatal giant-cell hepatitis*

This disease is not uncommon in tropical countries (Edington and Gilles, 1976); it can be associated with congenital malformation of the bile-ducts, erythroblastosis foetalis, viral infections, and inborn-errors of metabolism (Smetana, Edlow, and Glunz, 1965). Toxoplasmosis, cytomegalic inclusion disease, herpes simplex (Bird, Ennis, Wort, and Gardner, 1963), virus hepatitis A, and rubella virus (Stern and Williams, 1966) have all been implicated in the pathogenesis.

8.7. Mechanism of hyperglobulinaemia in chronic hepatic disease

The mechanism of hyperglobulinaemia in liver disease, active chronic hepatitis in particular, has been reviewed by Triger and Wright (1973). All of the major immunoglobulin classes are involved, and the hyperglobulinaemia is due principally to increased synthesis, rather than decreased catabolism of gamma-globulin (Havens, Dickensheefs, Bierly, and Eberhard, 1953; 1954; Cohen, 1963). Defective sequestration of a wide variety of antigens by the Kupffer cells seems to be the most likely underlying mechanism. Failure of sequestration might be a direct result of damage to the Kupffer cells, saturation of the phagocytic properties of those cells by the breakdown products of tissue damage, or by-passing of the liver through the collateral circulation. The site of production of gamma-globulin is therefore probably in the spleen and lymph-nodes and not the liver; splenomegaly in chronic liver disease is presumably partly a result of that mechanism.

Certain dietary proteins (Triger, Alp, and Wright, 1972), intestinal bacteria (Triger *et al.*, 1972; Protell, Soloway, Martin, Schoenfield, and Summerskill, 1971; Bjørneboe, Prytz, and Ørskov, 1972) and other antigens (Walker, 1978) can produce elevated circulating antibody concentrations in patients with cirrhosis. High concentrations of dietary protein and gut flora, much of which retain the antigenic characteristics of the original protein, are absorbed from the small intestine into the portal system (*Lancet*, 1978b); there are two routes for absorption, (i) via the epithelium overlying the lymphoid nodules—Peyer's patches, tonsils, appendix, etc, and (ii) the columnar epithelium covering the villi. The portal blood is usually sterile, but in cirrhotic patients an *Escherichia coli* septicaemia occasionally occurs.

Increased antibody titres to *E. coli* have been demonstrated in patients after portacaval anastomoses (Bjørneboe *et al.*, 1972). In rats, both serum globulin and *E. coli* concentrations rise after similar operations (Triger and Wright, 1973).

It seems possible that mild degrees of liver damage impair the ability of the organ to detoxify gut-derived bacterial toxins which are usually innocuous; that may lead to further hepatic injury (Nolan and Leibowitz, 1978) as well as more widespread effects such as renal lesions (Nolan, 1975, 1978).

A hyper-reactive immune-state which occurs in active chronic hepatitis (ACH), is also a factor in the production of an excess of antibody.

References

Achar, S. T., Raju, V. B., and Sriramachari, S. (1960). *J. Pediat.*, **57,** 744.

Agarwal, S.C., Maheshwari, H. B., Mittal, M. M., and Komar, S. (1973). *Indian J. med. Res.*, **61,** 389.

Aiket, B.K., Bhattacharya, I., and Walia, B. N. (1974). *Indian J. med. Res.*, **62,** 953.

—— and Sengupta, K. P. (1956). *Indian J. med. Res.*, **10,** 169.

Al-Hasany, M. and Mohamed, A. S. (1970). *Archs Dis. Childh.*, **45,** 722.

Allen, J. R., Carstens, L. A., and Katagiri, G. J. (1969). *Archs Path.*, **87,** 279.

Amla, I., Kumari, S., and Murthy, V. S. (1970). *Indian J. Pediat.*, **7,** 262.

Astaldi, G., Meardi, G., and Lisino, T. (1966). *Blood*, **28,** 70.

Bearn, A. G. (1978). *Gut*, **19,** 470.

Becker, B. J. and Chatgidakis, C. B. (1961). *Acta Un. int. Cancr.*, **17,** 650.

Becker, M. D., Scheuer, P. J., Baptista, A., and Sherlock, S. (1970). *Lancet*, **1,** 53.

Berg, N. O. and Eriksson, S. (1972). *New Engl. J. Med.*, **287,** 1264.

Bianchi, P., Porro, C. B., Coltorti, M., Dardanoni, L., Blanco, C. D. V., Fagiolo, U., Farini, R., Menozzi, I., Naccarato, R., Pagliaro, L., Spanò, C., and Verme, G. (1972). *Gastroenterology*, **63,** 482.

Bird, T., Ennis, J. E., Wort, A. J., and Gardner, P. S. (1963). *J. clin. Path.*, **16,** 423.

Bjørneboe, M., Prytz, H., and Ørskov, F. (1972). *Lancet*, **1,** 58.

Black, C. D. V., Watson, G. L., and Ward, R. J. (1977). *Trans. R. Soc. trop. Med. Hyg.*, **71,** 550.

Blackwell, J. B. (1965a). *J. Path. Bact.*, **90,** 259.

—— (1965b). *J. Path. Bact.*, **90,** 245.

Bothwell, T. H. and Isaacson, C. (1962). *Br. med. J.*, **1,** 522.

Bradfield, J. W. B. and Wells, M. (1978). *Lancet*, **2,** 836.

Bras, G., Brooks, S. E. H., and Watler, D. C. (1961). *J. Path. Bact.*, **82,** 503.

Br. med. J. (1964). **2,** 774.

—— (1978a). **2,** 1384.

—— (1978b). **2,** 1179.

Browne, S. G. (1964). *W. Afr. med. J.*, **13,** 35.

Brzosko, W. J., Debski, R., and Derecka, K. (1978). *Lancet*, **2,** 311.

Butt, E. M. and Higginson, J. (1957). *Acta Un. int. Cancr.*, **13,** 599.

Camain, R. (1957). *Acta Un. int. Cancr.*, **13,** 617.

Chandra, R. K. (1970). *Lancet*, **1,** 537.

CHUTTANI, H. K., SIDHU, A. S., WIG, K. L., GUPTA, D. N., and RAMALINGASWAMI, V. (1966). *Br. med. J.*, **2,** 676.

CLIFF, J. L. and SPEIGHT, A. N. P. (1976). *E. Afr. med. J.*, **53,** 287.

COCHRANE, A. M. G., MOUSSOUROS, A., THOMPSON, A. D., EDDLESTON, A. L. W. F., and WILLIAMS, R. (1976). *Lancet*, **1,** 441.

COCHRANE, A. M. G., MOUSSOUROS, A., SMITH, A., PORTMANN, B., EDDLESTON, A. L. W. F., and WILLIAMS, R. (1978). *Gut*, **19,** 308.

COHEN, K. L., RUBIN, P. E., ECHEVARRIA, R. E., SHARP, H. L., and TEAGUE, P. O. (1973). *Ann. intern. Med.*, **78,** 227.

COHEN, S. (1963). *Br. med. Bull.*, **19,** 202.

CONN, H. O. (1978). *Gastroenterology*, **74,** 624.

COOK, G. C. (1965). *Active chronic hepatitis and its response to corticosteroid therapy*. M.D. Thesis, University of London.

——, MULLIGAN, R., and SHERLOCK, S. (1971). *Q. Jl. Med.*, **40,** 159.

——, VELASCO, M., and SHERLOCK, S. (1968). *Gut*, **9,** 270.

COOKE, R. A. (1968). *Papua New Guin. med. J.*, **11,** 7.

COOKSLEY, W. G. E., POWELL, L. W., MISTILIS, S. P., OLSEN, G., MATHEWS, J. D., and MACKAY, I. R. (1972). *Aust. N. Z. J. Med.*, **2,** 261.

DAVEY, W. W. (1963). *W. Afr. med. J.*, **12,** 275.

—— (1968). *Companion to surgery in Africa*. p. 201. Churchill Livingstone. Edinburgh, London and New York.

DAVIES, J. N. P. (1956). *E. Afr. med. J.*, **33,** 25.

——, KNOWELDEN, J. and WILSON, B. A. (1965). *J. natn. Cancer Inst.*, **35,** 789.

DAWSON, A. M. (1978). *Gut*, **19,** 504.

DHATT, P. S., GUPTA, H. L., and SAINI, A. S. (1968). *Indian J. med. Res.*, **56,** 39.

DIXIT, S. K. and GUPTA, R. C. (1970. *Indian J. Pediat.*, **17,** 324.

DODU, S. R. A. (1958). *Trans. R. Soc. trop. Med. Hyg.*, **52,** 425.

DOMESHEK, W. and SCHWARTZ, R. (1960). *Trans. Am. Ass. Physcns*, **73,** 113.

EDINGTON, G. M. (1959). *Cent. Afr. med. J.*, **5,** 186.

—— (1971). In *Human infection with fungi, actinomycetes and algae*. p. 139. Springer Verlag, New York.

—— and DODU, S. R. A. (1957). *Trans. R. Soc. trop. Med. Hyg.*, **51,** 429.

—— and GILLES, H. M. (1976). *Pathology in the tropics.* 2nd ed. pp. 383, 431, 472, and 570. Edward Arnold, London.

ELKINGTON, S. G., SCHREIBER, W. M., and CONN, H. O. (1969). *Circulation*, **40,** 589.

FAGERHOL, M. K. (1976). *Postgrad. med. J.*, **52,** suppl. 2, 73.

FEIZI, T. (1968). *Gut*, **9,** 193.

FORBES, J. I. and GELFAND, M. (1962). *Trans. R. Soc. trop. Med. Hyg.*, **56,** 305.

FOY, H. and KONDI, A. (1958). *Trans. R. Soc. trop. Med. Hyg.*, **52,** 46.

GANROT, P. O., LAURELL, C. B., and ERIKSSON, S. (1967). *Scand. J. clin. Lab. Invest.*, **19,** 205.

GANS, H., SHARP, H. L., and TAN, B. H. (1969). *Surgery Gynec. Obstet.*, **129,** 289.

GARDINER, M. R., ROYCE, R., and BOKOR, A. (1965). *J. Path. Bact.*, **89,** 43.

GELFAND, M. (1955). *Trans. R. Soc. trop. Med. Hyg.*, **49,** 370.

——, (1961). *Acta Un. int. Cancr.*, **17,** 604.

GHAI, O. P. and VASUKI, K. (1971). *Indian J. Pediat.*, **8,** 309.

GILLANDERS, A. D. (1951). *Br. Heart J.*, **13,** 177.

GILLMAN, J. and GILLMAN, T. (1951). *Perspectives in Human Malnutrition*. New York, Grune and Stratton.

GILLMAN, T., CANHAM, P. A. S., and HATHORN, M. (1958). *Lancet*, **2,** 557.

——, LAMONT, N. M., HATHORN, M., and CANHEM, P. A. S. (1957). *Lancet*, **2,** 173.

GOOD, R. A. (1956). *Am. J. Dis. Child.*, **92,** 508.

GRACEY, L. (1965). *Br. J. Surg.*, **52,** 442.

GREENWOOD, B. M., HERRICK, E. M., and VOLLER, A. (1970). *Proc. R. Soc. Med.*, **63,** 19.

GUPTA, P. S., GUPTA, G. D., and SHARMA, M. L. (1963). *Br. med. J.*, **1,** 1184.
GUPTA, S., KALRA, K., and CHAUDHRI, B. N. (1975). *Indian Pediatrics*, **12,** 1217.
HADDOCK, D. R. W. (1965). *E. Afr. med. J.*, **42,** 67.
HASHEM, M., ZAKI, S. A., and HUSSEIN, M. (1961). *J. Egypt med. Ass.*, **44,** 579.
HAVENS, W. P., DICKENSHEETS, J., BIERLY, J. N., and EBERHARD, T. P. (1953). *J. clin. Invest.*, **32,** 573.
——, ——, ——, and —— (1954). *J. Immun.*, **73,** 256.
HERSCH, C. (1964). *S. Afr. med. J.*, **39,** 587.
HIGGINSON, J., GERRITSON, T., and WALKER, A. R. P. (1953). *Am. J. Path.*, **29,** 779.
HILKOVITZ, G. and JACOBSON, A. (1961). *J. Lab. clin. Med.*, **57,** 856.
HILL, K. R. (1960). *Proc. R. Soc. Med.*, **53,** 281.
——, STEPHENSEN, C. F. and FILSHIE, I. (1958). *Lancet*, **1,** 623.
HIMSWORTH, H. P. (1950). *The liver and its diseases.* 2nd ed. pp. 48, 78. Blackwell, Oxford.
HORNEY, J. T. and GALAMBOS, J. T. (1977). *Gastroenterology*, 73, 639.
HUTT, M. S. R. (1971). *Trans. R. Soc. trop. Med. Hyg.*, **65,** 273.
IBER, F. L. and MADDREY, W. C. (1965). In *Progress in Liver Disease* (ed. H. Popper and F. Schaffner) **2,** 290. Heinemann, London.
International group (1977). *Lancet*, **2,** 914.
JOB, C. K., KIRCHHEIMER, W. F., and SANCHEZ, R. M. (1978). *Int. J. Lepr.*, **46,** 1.
KARAT, A. B. A., JOB, C. K., and RAO, P. S. S. (1971). *Br. med. J.*, **1,** 307.
KENG, C. B. and KHOO, T. K. (1970). *Gut*, **11,** 423.
KHANNA, K. K. (1968). *Indian J. Pediat.*, **35,** 285.
KINGHAM, J. G. C., GANGULY, N. K., SHAARI, Z. D., MENDELSON, R., MCGUIRE, M. J., HOLGATE, S. J., CARTWRIGHT, T., SCOTT, G. M., RICHARDS, B. M., and WRIGHT, R. (1978). *Gut*, **19,** 91.
KORN, R. J., KELLOW, W. F., HELLER, P., CHOMET, B., and ZIMMERMAN, H. J. (1959). *Am. J. Med.*, **27,** 60.
Lancet (1978a). **2,** 507.
—— (1978b). **2,** 715.
LEE, R. V., THORNTON, G. F., and CONN, H. O. (1971). *New Engl. J. Med.*, **284,** 1423.
LINDBERG, J. (1978). *Scand. J. infect. Dis.*, Suppl. 12.
Liver diseases Sub-committee (1955). *Indian J. med. Res.*, **43,** 723.
LORINCZ, G., TRAUB, N. E., CHUKE, P. O., and HUSSEIN, S. F. (1974). *E. Afr. med. J.*, **51,** 488.
MACDONALD, R. A. and BAUMSTAG, N. (1964). *Am. J. med. Sci.*, **247,** 649.
—— and MALLORY, G. K. (1960). *Archs intern. Med.*, **105,** 686.
MACKAY, I. R., TAFT, L. I. and COWLING, D. C. (1956). *Lancet*, **2,** 1323.
MCLEAN, E., BRAS, G., and GYÖRGY, P. (1964). *Br. J. exp. Path.*, **45,** 242.
MADDREY, W. C. and BOITNOTT, J. K. (1973). *Ann. intern. Med.*, **79,** 1.
MAJUMDAR, D. K., KAPOOR, V. K., and SHARMA, N. L. (1969). *Indian J. Pediat.*, **6,** 753.
MARTINEZ-MALDONADO, M., GIROD, C. E., and RAMIREZ DE ARELLANO, G. (1965). *Am. J. dig. Dis.*, **10,** 522.
MAYNARD, E. P., SADIKALI, F., ANTHONY, P. P., and BARKER, L. F. (1970). *Lancet*, **2,** 1326.
MELENEY, H. E. (1925). *Am. J. Path.*, **1,** 147.
MEYER ZUM BÜSCHENFELDE, K. H. (1978). In *Immune reactions in liver disease* (ed. A. L. W. F. Eddelston, J. C. P. Weber, and R. Williams). Pitman medical, Tunbridge Wells, England.
MITTAL, M. M., MAHESHWARI, H. B., SAHA, K., and SHARMA, R. (1978). *Int. J. Lepr.*, **46,** 42.
MISTILIS, S. P. and BLACKBURN, C. R. B. (1967). *Australas. Ann. Med.*, **16,** 305.
MOHABBAT, O., SRIVASTAVA, R. N., YOUNOS, M. S., SEDIQ, G. G., MERZAD, A. A., and ARAM, G. N. (1976). *Lancet*, **2,** 269.

MONTENEGRO, M. R., da SILVA, L. C., and PONTES, J. F. (1958). *Gastroenterology*, **34,** 1108.
MORSE, J. O. (1978). *New Engl. J. Med.*, **299,** 1045 and 1099.
MURRAY-LYON, I. M., STERN, R. B., and WILLIAMS, R. (1973). *Lancet*, **1,** 735.
NEAME, P. B. and PILLAY, V. K. G. (1964). *S. Afr. med. J.*, **38,** 729.
NHONOLI, A. M. (1973). *E. Afr. med. J.*, **50,** 229.
NOLAN, J. P. (1975). *Gastroenterology*, **69,** 1346.
—— (1978). *New Engl. J. Med.*, **299,** 1069.
—— and LEIBOWITZ, A. I. (1978). *Gastroenterology*, **75,** 445.
OOMEN, L. (1973). *E. Afr. med. J.*, **50,** 660.
OSUNKOYA, B. O., CARLISLE, R., and DAWODU, A. H. (1972). *Afr. J. med. Sci.*, **3,** 275.
OWOR, R. (1974). *E. Afr. med. J.*, **51,** 388.
PATEL, B. D., PAREKH, S. R., and CHITALE, A. R. (1974). *Indian J. Pediat.*, **11,** 19.
PARONETTO, F. and POPPER, H. (1966). *Am. J. Path.*, **49,** 1087.
PÉREZ-TAMAYO, R. (1958). *Am. J. clin. Path.*, **29,** 226.
PHLIPPEN, R. (1969). *Klin. Wschr.*, **47,** 524.
PORTMANN, B., TANNER, M. S., MOWAT, A. P. and WILLIAMS, R. (1978). *Lancet*, **1,** 1338.
POWELL, K. C. and MCGOVERN, V. J. (1976). *Papua New Guin. med. J.*, **19,** 140.
PRASAD, P. (1962). *Br. med. J.*, **2,** 1031.
PROTELL, R. L., SOLOWAY, R. D., MARTIN, W. J., SCHOENFIELD, L. J., and SUMMERSKILL, W, J. H. (1971). *Lancet*, **2,** 330.
REYNOLDS, T. B., PETERS, R. L., and YAMADA, S. (1971). *New Engl. J. Med.*, **285,** 813.
SAFOUH, M. and SHEHATA, A. H. (1965). *J. Pediat.*, **67,** 415.
SAINI, A. S., DHATT, P. S., and MEHTA, H. C. (1976). *Indian Pediatrics*, **13,** 713.
SALASPURO, M. and SIPPONEN, P. (1976). *Gut*, **17,** 787.
SCHALM, S. W., AMMON, H. V., and SUMMERSKILL, W. H. J. (1976). *Ann. clin. Res.*, **8,** 221.
SCHEUER, P. J. (1973). *Liver biopsy interpretation.* 2nd ed. Baillière, Tindall and Cassell, London.
—— (1978). *Gut*, **19,** 554.
SCHOENTAL, R. (1963). *Bull. Wld Hlth Org.*, **29,** 823.
—— and MAGEE, P. N. (1959). *J. Path. Bact.*, **78,** 471.
SCHWARZ, J. (1971). In *Human infection with fungi, actinomycetes and algae*. p. 139. Springer-Verlag, New York.
SCHWEITZER, I. L. and PETERS, R. L. (1974). *Gastroenterology*, **66,** 1203.
SCOTT, J., GOLLAN, J. L., SAMOURIAN, S., and SHERLOCK, S. (1978). *Gastroenterology*, **74,** 645.
SEFTEL, H. C., ISAACSON, C., and BOTHWELL, T. H. (1960). *S. Afr. J. med. Sci.*, **25,** 89.
SELZER, G. and PARKER, R. G. F. (1951). *Am. J. Path.*, **27,** 885.
SEN GUPTA, P. C. (1975). *J. Indian med. Ass.*, **65,** 89.
SHARP, H. L., BRIDGES, R. A., KRIVIT, W., and FREIER, E. F. (1969). *J. Lab. clin. Med.*, **73,** 934.
SHERLOCK, S. (1975). *Diseases of the liver and biliary system.* 5th ed. pp. 390 and 425. Blackwell, Oxford, London, Edinburgh and Melbourne.
SHWE, T. and ZUCKERMAN, A. J. (1972). *J. clin. Path.*, **25,** 401.
SING, A., JOLLY, S. S., and KUMAR, L. R. (1961). *Lancet*, **1,** 587.
SMETANA, H. F., EDLOW, J. B., and GLUNZ, P. R. (1965). *Archs Path.*, **80,** 553.
——, HADLEY, G. G. and SIRSAT, S. M. (1961). *Pediatrics, Springfield*, **28,** 107.
SOLOWAY, R. D., SUMMERSKILL, W. H. J., BAGGENSTOSS, A. H., GEALL, M. G., GITNICK, G. L., ELVEBACK, L. R., and SCHOENFIELD, L. J. (1972). *Gastroenterology*, **63,** 820.
STERN, H. and WILLIAMS, B. M. (1966). *Lancet*, **1,** 293.
STEVENSON, S. (1962). *Trans. R. Soc. trop. Med. Hyg.*, **56,** 438.
STEYN, D. G. (1965). *S. Afr. med. J.*, **39,** 344.
STUART, K. L. and BRAS, G. (1957). *Q. Jl. Med.*, **26,** 291.

SUNDARAVALLI, N. (1971). *Indian J. Pediat.*, **8,** 365.
SUR, A. M. and BHATTI, A. (1978). *Br. med. J.*, **2,** 529.
SUSRUTA SAMHITA (1952). *Uttar tantra*, 27, verse 15, Saraswati Pustakalaya, Kanpur, India.
SYMMERS, D. and SPAIN, D. M. (1946). *Archs Path.*, **42,** 64.
TANDON, B. N., TANDON, R. K., TANDON, H. D., NARNDRANATHAN, M., and JOSHI, Y. K. (1976). *Lancet*, **2,** 271.
TANNER, M. S., PORTMANN, B., MOWAT, A. P., and WILLIAMS, R. (1978). *Br. med. J.*, **2,** 928.
THOMPSON, J. G. (1961). *Acta Un. int. Cancr.*, **17,** 623.
TRIGER, D. R. and WRIGHT, R. (1973). *Lancet*, **1,** 1494.
——, ALP, M. H. and WRIGHT, R. (1972). *Lancet*, **1,** 60.
TROWELL, H. C. (1960). *Non-infective disease in Africa*, p. 29. Edward Arnold, London.
TYGSTRUP, N. and JUHL, E. (1976). In *chronic hepatitis* (ed. P. Gentilini, H. Popper, and U. Teodosi). p. 42. Basel.
VAN YPERSELE DE STRIHOU, C. and PIRSON, Y. (1978). *Lancet*, **2,** 836.
VINT, F. W. (1930). *Kenya E. Afr. med. J.*, **7,** 349.
WAGNER, F. B. and SHEPHERD, A. (1976). *Papua New Guin. med. J.* **19,** 156.
WALDENSTRÖM, J. (1950). *Leber, Blutproteine und Nahrungseweiss Stoffwechs; Sonderband 15.* p. 113. *Bad kissingen.*
WALKER, W. A. (1978). *Archs Dis Childh.*, **53,** 527.
WILLIAMS, R., SCHEUER, P. J., and SHERLOCK, S. (1962). *Q. Jl. Med.*, **31,** 249.
WILLMOT, F. C. and ROBERTSON, G. W. (1920). *Lancet*, **2,** 848.
WHO (1976). *World Health Statistics Annual*, 1, W.H.O., Geneva.
WRIGHT, E. C., SEEF, L. B., BERK, P. D., JONES, E. A., and PLOTZ, P. H. (1977). *Gastroenterology*, **73,** 1422.

9

Hepatocellular carcinoma (HCC) (hepatoma) and other hepatic malignancies

THE very high incidence of hepatocellular carcinoma (HCC), most commonly in young men, is one of the outstanding problems of medicine in tropical countries; in areas of high incidence, 50 to 80 per cent of cirrhotic livers undergo malignant change (Edington and Gilles, 1976). It is not superimposed upon schistosomal liver disease.

The tumour is very common in Africa (Davies, 1952; Clifford, Linsell, and Timms, 1968; Cook and Burkitt, 1970), Hong Kong, and much of south China (Doll, 1967). There seems no doubt that in Africa at least, it was common before urbanization and industrialization (Davies, Elmes, Mtimavalye, Owor, and Shaper, 1964). In sub-Saharan Africa this is the most common of all tumours, accounting for from 10 to 30 per cent of all malignancies in men (Davies, 1961; Oettlé, 1964; Cook and Burkitt, 1971). In Maputo, Mozambique it accounts for 66 per cent of tumours in men (Prates and Torres, 1965) which is about 1000 times the incidence in most of Europe. A very high rate has also been reported from Senegal (Payet, 1967). In much of east Africa (Davies, Knowelden, and Wilson, 1965) and Nigeria (Edington and MacLean, 1965a), although a common tumour, it does not reach the very high rates seen in Mozambique and Senegal. There is apparently only a five-fold variation within the continent of Africa.

True rates are undoubtedly underestimated in contrast to more easily biopsied tumours such as skin neoplasia (Burkitt, Hutt, and Slavin, 1968).

Cholangiocellular carcinoma is no more common in Africa than in the western world; there is, however, an increased incidence in the Far east (Chapter 14).

9.1. Distribution of HCC

There is no epidemiological evidence, based on geographical distribution, that the disease is related to genetic or ethnic factors, malaria, schistosomiasis, or malnutrition.

The highest incidence rate of all is at Maputo (Prates and Torres, 1965). At Ibadan, 144 cases were seen in a 10-year period (1958–68) (Francis and Smith, 1972); the male, female ratio was 4:1 and death occurred at a mean time of 11 weeks after onset of the first symptom. A high incidence has also been reported from the Sudan (Salih, Satir, Sulieman, and Sabba, 1978). The tumour represented 2 per cent of medical admissions, and 40 per cent of all malignancies. There was a 6:1 male to female ratio. The disease seems to be more common in western Sudan. In Africans in South Africa, 50 per cent of all tumours (Berman, 1951), in Ethiopia, 11 per cent (Pavlica and Samuel, 1970), and in Kenya and Uganda 5 per cent of tumours are hepatomas (Alpert, Hutt, and Davidson, 1968; Clifford, Linsell, and Timms, 1968).

High incidence rates have also been reported from South Africa (Higginson and Oettlé, 1960), western Nigeria (Edington and MacLean, 1965 a and b), Uganda (Davies, Knowelden, and Wilson, 1965), and Chinese living in Singapore (Muir and Shanmugaratnam, 1966). Immigrant Chinese to Singapore are more prone to develop HCC than the Chinese born in Singapore (Shanmugaratnam and Tye, 1970). High rates have also been reported from Senegal (Camain, 1954), Ethiopia (Pavlica and Samuel, 1970), Ghana (Edington, 1956), Zaire (Thijs, 1957), China and Japan (Edington and Gilles, 1976), and Papua New Guinea (McGovern and Kariks, 1966). In Papua New Guinea it is the third most common malignancy in men and the sixth most common in women (*Papua New Guin. med. J.*, 1972; Wagner and Shepherd, 1976). In a prospective analysis at Goroka Base Hospital in the Papua New Guinea highlands, 43 of 141 gastrointestinal malignancies were hepatomas. Hepatoma in Papua New Guinea is usually superimposed on a macronodular cirrhosis (Cooke, 1968), and in all respects the tumour seems very similar to that in Africa. It may be more common in the highlands than the coastal areas. In Egypt (Hashem, Zaki and Hussein, 1961), India (Paymaster, 1964), Brazil (Montenegro, da Silva and Pontes, 1958), Mexico (Lopez-Corrella, Ridaura-Sanz, and Albores-Saavedra, 1968), Columbia (Correa and Llanos, 1966), Jamaica (Bras, Brooks, and Watler, 1961), and the USA (in both blacks and whites) (Dorn and Cutler, 1958), incidence rates tend to be lower. In Indians and Malays in Malaysia the incidence is also low; however the Chinese there have high rates (Marsden, 1958).

9.2. Aetiology of HCC

9.2.1. Relationship to macronodular cirrhosis

Between 55 and 80 per cent of hepatomas in high incidence areas arise in cirrhotic livers. Those figures contrast with ones from temperate countries and South African whites (Becker and Chatgidikas, 1961; Thomson, 1961) where the corresponding figures are 2·5 to 15 per cent; in Mexico a figure of 0·26 per cent has been recorded. Reports from Uganda (Davies, 1952), South Africa (Higginson, 1956), Ghana (Edington, 1957), Uganda (Shaper, 1970), and Ethiopia (Pavlica and Samuel, 1970) all confirm such an association. In Kampala, Uganda, 19 per cent of cirrhotic patients, most with macronodular cirrhosis, were found at post-mortem to have a HCC, while in Boston, USA 4 per cent of cirrhotics have that complication (Hutt, 1972). The association might be due to the fact that a common aetiological agent or agents produces both cirrhosis and hepatoma; it might on the other hand merely mean that abnormal hepatocyte hyperplasia in cirrhosis is a predisposing factor to development of HCC.

In some areas where cirrhosis is common, there is not a high incidence of HCC (Hutt, 1972); the explanation for that is not clear. Although incidence rates of macronodular cirrhosis and HCC are similar in high incidence areas, in certain others HCC occurs in the absence of cirrhosis.

The underlying cirrhosis is usually macronodular; that suggests that liver cell injury, followed by regenerative hyperplasia is important aetiologically; there is a suggestion that the greater the degree of hyperplasia, the greater is the danger of the development of HCC (Anthony, Vogel, and Barker, 1973). Overall it seems very likely that cirrhosis and hepatoma have a similar aetiology.

It is also clear that alcoholic cirrhosis predisposes to a high incidence of HCC (Lee, 1966). A significant time factor is involved there, for when alcoholic cirrhotics give up alcohol, they survive longer than they would otherwise have done, but have a higher risk of developing HCC.

9.2.2. Relationship to hepatitis B virus

Recent work suggests that the hepatitis B virus may be more important than aflatoxin in the pathogenesis of hepatoma in Africa and Asia (*Br. med. J.*, 1978). Reports from African countries show a close correlation between HB_sAg and acute viral hepatitis, post-necrotic cirrhosis, and HCC (Bagshawe, Parker, and Jindani, 1971; Vogel, Anthony, Sadikali, Barker, and Peterson, 1972; Williams, 1972; Samuel, Gebre Selassie, and Bocina, 1974); all of those diseases are common (Teferra and Abdul Kadir, 1968; Pavlica and Samuel, 1970; Boshnakova and Gillum, 1972; Lainovic, 1974). It seems likely therefore that viral hepatitis is a predisposing factor to HCC, and that the intermediate stage is usually cirrhosis (Vogel *et al.*, 1972; Tong, Sun, Schaeffer, Chang, Lo, and Peters, 1971; Hirschman, Vernace, and Schaffner, 1971; *Lancet*, 1971).

Vogel, Anthony, Mody, and Barker (1970), using an insensitive technique found that 40 per cent of patients with HCC in Uganda had HB_sAg in their serum (the positivity rate in a control group was three per cent); the proportion was highest in young patients without underlying cirrhosis: 70 per cent of those under 30 and 17 per cent of those over 50 years. The incidence of HB_sAg in 46 patients with HCC and 106 controls was studied by Tsega, Gold, Shuster, Whittemore, and Lester (1976) in Ethiopia; 30 of the 46 (65 per cent) patients with HCC, and none of the controls had a positive alpha-fetoprotein (AFP) (determined by radioimmunoassay) which is a rather low incidence rate for African patients. Twenty-three of the 46 (50 per cent) of those with HCC had a positive HB_sAg result, whereas four of the 106 (4 per cent) controls had HB_sAg. There was a tendency for the patients with a positive AFP result to be HB_sAg positive but that was not significant. The findings in that study are similar to those reported from Uganda (Vogel and Linsell, 1972). In a study in Dar-es-Salaam, Tanzania, 21 per cent of serum samples from 57 patients with hepatoma gave positive results for HB_sAg (Nantulya, Lindqvist, and Spencer, 1975); in a control group, rates of 5·5 and 1·3 per cent in males and females were reported. An incidence of 31 per cent was reported in patients with HCC in Athens (Hadziyannis, Merikas, and Afroudakis, 1970). In Kenya, HB_sAg was present in 21 per cent of patients with cirrhosis and 14 per cent of those with HCC (Bagshawe, *et al.*, 1971). In Singapore, however, HB_sAg was present in only 2·6 per cent of patients with HCC (Simons, Yap, Yu, Seah, Chew, Fung, Tan, and Shanmugaratnam, 1971). Since then, much higher rates have been reported with the newer and more sensitive techniques (radioimmunoassay and haemagglutination) from Taiwan (Tong, *et al.*, 1971), Africans in South Africa (Kew, Geddes, MacNab, and Bersohn, 1974), Greece (Theodoropoulis, Archimandritis, and Angelopoulos, 1975), Thailand (Chainuvati, Viranuvatti, and Pongpipat, 1975), Senegal (Prince, Szmuness, and Michon, 1975), and south Vietnam (Welsh, Brown, Arnold, Mathews, and Prince, 1976); all of those are areas where at least 7 per cent of the normal population are HB_sAg carriers. HB_sAg is less frequent in hepatomas in France (Prince, Leblanc, Krohn, Masseyeff, and Alpert, 1970) and the USA (Alpert and Isselbacher, 1971), where HB_sAg carriers are less common.

Ninety-five per cent of Africans and Asians with HCC have antibodies to the hepatitis core antigen (anti-HB_c) (Maupas, Werner, and Larouzé, 1975); those authors suggested that some patients may continue to produce core antigen rather than surface antigen. Similarly, Kubo, Okuda, Musha, and Nakashima (1978) found anti-HB_c in 81 per cent of over 200 serum samples from patients with HCC, though only 52 per cent were HB_sAg positive.

Duration of chronic liver disease before hepatoma is detected is significantly shorter in HB_sAg positive, than HB_sAg negative patients (Kubo *et al.*, 1978); however survival after tumour detection was not significantly related to the presence of HB_sAg or duration of the previous liver disease.

If hepatitis B virus causes HCC by initiating the chain of events: acute hepatitis, active chronic hepatitis, cirrhosis, hepatoma, then HB_sAg positivity should be more common when the HCC is secondary to cirrhosis, than when it is unrelated to cirrhosis; that has in fact been found in most series. Thus in California, less than one per cent of non-cirrhotic patients with HCC have markers of hepatitis B infection, but 73 per cent of patients with cirrhosis have HB_sAg positivity (Peters, Afroudakis, and Tatter, 1977). Hepatitis B virus seems to play a role in the aetiology of HCC in Greece (Trichopoulos, Tabor, Gerety, Xirouchaki, Sparros, Munoz, and Linsell, 1978); of 80 patients with HCC the prevalence of HB_sAg was higher if cirrhosis was also present, but without cirrhosis the rate was also higher than in controls. In Uganda, HB_sAg is not found in patients with micronodular cirrhosis, in whom hepatoma is rare. In Greenland however, although the HB_sAg carrier rate is seven to 25 per cent, there is no indication that the incidence rate for HCC is any higher than in northern Europe where hepatitis B is at least ten times less prevalent in the population (Skinhøj, Hart Hansen, Nielsen, Højgaard, and Mikkelsen, 1978).

The possibility of co-carcinogenicity should also be considered. Both hepatitis B virus and aflatoxin may play a joint role (*Br. med. J.*, 1978); there are certainly geographical parallels between high incidence rates of those two factors.

It is difficult to exclude the possibility that the high incidence of HB_sAg in patients with HCC is a result of altered immunological status, rendering infection more likely. Primack, Vogel, and Barker (1973) considered however that that explanation was unlikely to account for the high incidence of HB_sAg

in Ugandan patients with HCC. It is also possible that development of HCC merely activates a latent hepatitis B virus infection with the production of HB_sAg and HB_cAg in infected cells, or alternatively an HB_s antigenaemia might indicate a defective immune response; aflatoxins have immunosuppressive actions (Savel, Forsyth, Schaeffer, and Cardella, 1970). Incidentally, aflatoxin usually produces AFP negative tumours in laboratory animals.

Although therefore there is strong suggestive evidence that hepatitis B virus is aetiologically related to cirrhosis, this is far from proven. No viral particles have been found in ultrastructural studies on hepatoma cells (O'Conor, Tralka, and Hensen, 1972).

Prophylactically, hepatitis B virus vaccine given at an early age might limit the carriage of hepatitis B virus in endemic areas.

9.2.3. Relationship to aflatoxin and other mycotoxins

Throughout the tropics, the possibility of hepatotoxin ingestion in the causation of chronic liver injury should be considered. Certain foodstuffs, herbal remedies, and plant alkaloids are known to be toxic to man (Edington and Gilles, 1976).

The age distribution of HCC, with a peak in young men and a subsequent plateau, contrasts to the rising incidence after 50 years in the western world; that is compatible with the possibility of young men being exposed to an hepatic carcinogen at an early age.

Aflatoxin is a carcinogenic product of *Aspergillus flavus*, a fungus which grows on mouldy groundnuts; it can produce hepatoma in several species of animal (Lancaster, Jenkins, and Philp, 1961; Sargeant, Sheridan, O'Kelly, and Carnaghan, 1961). In Brazil, where groundnuts were first shown to produce hepatoma in turkeys, both macronodular cirrhosis and HCC are uncommon. The fungus penetrates the kernel when the shell is damaged during harvesting or transportation. Young animals seem to be more susceptible than adults; after an initial insult hepatoma may occur some time later, during which time a normal diet is being taken.

In Uganda, the presence of potent hepatotoxins in the environment is well established. Lopez and Crawford (1967) showed that two out of 84 samples of groundnuts sold for human consumption in Uganda contained more than 10 ppm aflatoxin; furthermore there was a seasonal variation in contamination, the highest being at the end of the rainy season. However, those authors concluded that an intake of 16 kg of groundnuts would be required to produce a total concentration which constitutes the LD_{50} in the duckling. In a further survey of the aflatoxin content of common food samples from different parts of Uganda, most were found to be contaminated to some degree, and 3·7 per cent contained more than one μg per kg. The incidence of hepatoma is high throughout Uganda but especially so in Karamoja; in that area a high correlation between the level of aflatoxin in foodstuffs and incidence of HCC was found (Alpert, Hutt, Wogan, and Davidson, 1971). In Nigeria, also, aflatoxin is present at high concentration in most common foods stored for long periods of time (Nwokolo and Okonkwo, 1978). At high concentrations fungal growth would be noted macroscopically.

Aflatoxin has also been incriminated in Papua New Guinea where HCC is also a common disease (Powell and McGovern, 1976); foods from widely divergent parts of the country: the Highlands, the Trobriand Islands, and a market in Port Moresby have been shown, using thin-layer chromatography, to be contaminated (Wookey, 1972). However in another study at Goroka, results of food analyses for hepatotoxins gave uniformly negative results (Cunningham and Le Page, 1972).

It is difficult to evaluate the overall role of mycotoxin in HCC and other forms of chronic liver disease, in the tropics. Whether or not that agent modifies the effect of other factors, e.g., hepatitis virus, malnutrition, or parasitic disease is unknown. A variety of hepatic lesions has been produced in monkeys by aflatoxin administration (Deo, Dayal, and Ramalingaswami, 1970); that report stressed the importance of studying the effect of small doses over a long period of time.

Multinucleate hepatocytes with great variability in their nuclear size are common in the Gambia (Walters and Waterlow, 1954) and Uganda (Hutt, 1971); the latter author has suggested that that is a result of toxic agents to which those populations are exposed at low concentrations.

Although some epidemiological and circumstantial evidence points to their being important, the solution in man is still unresolved. Most aflatoxin-induced hepatomas in laboratory animals are negative for alpha-fetoprotein.

In the Far east, a contaminant of rice, *Penicillium islandicum* produces toxic compounds which can cause liver injury and hepatoma in rats and mice (Miyake, Saito, Enomoto, Shikata, Ishiko, Uraguchi, Sakai, Tatsuno, Tsukioka, and Sakai, 1960); however there is no evidence that that agent is important in man. That mycotoxin has also been isolated from market produce in Addis Ababa (Coady, 1964).

In Ethiopia, hepatoma is associated with cirrhosis in 94·7 per cent of patients (Pavlica and Samuel, 1970); it was felt that mycotoxins and herbal medicines were important. In Jamaica, ingestion of alkaloids of crotalaria give rise to veno-occlusive disease (Bras, Jelliffe, and Stuart, 1954; Hill, 1959) (Chapter 8).

The possibility that aflatoxin, or another mycotoxin, acts synergistically with the hepatitis B virus should be considered.

9.2.4. Other possible aetiological factors

Diet. The role of diet in the production of hepatoma is also not clear. Foy, Kondi, Linsell, Parker, and Sizaret (1970) working in Nairobi detected AFP in the serum of five of 10 baboons who had received a pyridoxine-free diet; furthermore the hepatic lesions histologically resembled hepatomas. Vitamin B_{12} concentrations were elevated. Because low pyridoxine diets are common in the third world, that observation might have a significance but is at present difficult to evaluate.

Alcohol seems to be unimportant; hepatoma is common in Islamic-dominated areas such as northern Nigeria where little alcohol is consumed.

Schistosomiasis. Although hepatoma frequently occurs in areas where schistosomiasis is a great medical problem there is no current evidence of a cause-effect relationship. However there is evidence in experimental animals that schistosomiasis together with a carcinogen results in a greatly increased incidence rate of hepatoma (Domingo, Warren, and Stenger, 1967).

Hydatid disease. On a number of occasions, hydatid disease and hepatoma have been demonstrated in the same liver (Edington and Gilles, 1976); there is no evidence however of a causal relationship.

Hormonal factors. Gynaecomastia is common in many parts of the tropics (Dawson, 1966). Hyperoestrogenism has been suggested as an aetiological factor in HCC in Kampala, Uganda (Davies, 1952; Clifford and Bulbrook, 1966). However, it seems possible that hepatocellular damage is so widespread in those populations that the high circulating oestrogen concentrations are a result, rather than a cause, of the liver changes, and hepatocyte damage. In view of the significantly higher incidence of HCC in men compared with women, that hypothesis makes no obvious sense, although there is a rise in the incidence of HCC in post-menopausal compared with pre-menopausal women.

9.3. Presentation of HCC

The disease involves males much more often than females by a ratio of four or five; average age at presentation is 30 to 40 years (Shaper, 1970). Although cirrhosis is often present, in 15 to 20 per cent the liver is otherwise normal. Excessive alcohol intake is not a consistent feature, and haemosiderosis in liver-biopsy specimens is rare. There does not seem to be any relationship to social class; the tumour is seen in all sections of the community, from labourers to government ministers and even a head of state.

Most patients have pain, anorexia, and weight-loss at presentation and in approximately 95 per cent there is hepatomegaly (Berman, 1940). The liver is usually large and craggy. The majority of patients are aware of the liver enlargement. About 25 per cent are jaundiced at presentation. Signs of cirrhosis (Chapter 8) may dominate the picture clinically.

Acute onset with bleeding into the peritoneal cavity from the growth, occurs in about 10 per cent. In a further 10 per cent presentation is associated with metastases in lungs, bones, or brain. Twelve of one hundred patients with hepatoma studied in Ethiopia presented initially with fever (Tsega, 1977). Unusual presentations have been recorded (Jeshrani and Gatei, 1975).

Examination reveals a grossly enlarged liver; occasionally enlargement is localized and the remainder of the organ is nodular. A bruit is heard over the liver in approximately 40 per cent of hepatomas, although the frequency of that varies in different series (Clain, Wartnaby, and Sherlock, 1966). In a prospective study in Addis Ababa, Ethiopia, 80 per cent of 100 patients with hepatoma had an audible bruit (Tsega, 1977). If that sign is positive there is no reasonable doubt about the diagnosis (Teklu, 1978). The presence of ascites usually denotes portal vein involvement and is often a terminal event. In about one quarter, the ascites is blood-stained. Hypoglycaemic attacks and polycythaemia are common in patients with HCC in both Africa and Hong Kong (MacFadzean and Yeung, 1969). Four cases of hepatoma presenting during pregnancy have been described from Ibadan, Nigeria (Francis, Smith, and Hendrickse, 1974); in three the tumour arose in a non-cirrhotic liver.

Evidence of hepatic decompensation is generally unusual; there is rarely a flapping tremor or foetor hepatis, and although varices are often present haematemeses are not very common. Ankle oedema occurs at a late stage. Growth is at a very great rate, and the downhill course is rapid. On successive ward rounds it is almost possible to visualize the liver edge approaching the umbilicus, without taking measurements. Death, which is usually a result of cachexia often takes place within a few weeks of diagnosis; longer survivals are usually a few months only. Haemoperitoneum resulting from nodules on the liver surface may hasten death. Intercurrent infection and haemorrhage from oesophageal varices also account for death in some patients. A minority become progressively jaundiced and develop hepatic encephalopathy or suffer a terminal haematemesis.

Differential diagnosis. This is nearly always clear-cut and only rarely presents a problem. Over 80 per cent of cases in Africa are correctly diagnosed on clinical assessment (Davies and Owor, 1960; Alpert, Hutt, and Davidson, 1969; Vogel, Anthony, Modi, and Barker, 1970; Tsega, 1977). The most common diagnostic problem is to differentiate the tumour from an amoebic liver abscess (Chapter 12). In that case, there is usually a fever and polymorph leucocytosis, and a bruit is not heard over the liver. If there is any doubt about that diagnosis however, a course of metronidazole should be given. Secondary tumours in the liver are relatively unusual in Africa in comparison with the very high incidence of hepatoma. In Ethiopia and the Middle-east, hydatid cysts should also be considered in the differential diagnosis.

9.4. Pathology of HCC

These tumours arise from the hepatocytes; they are therefore hepatocellular or liver-cell carcinomas. They may be multi- or monocentric in origin and that is usually impossible to be sure about. The incidence of bile-duct carcinomas in Africa and most of the tropics is no different from that in the western world.

Rate of growth is very rapid and tumours may reach an enormous size of up to 4000 g. The tumour may be either single or multinodular and may involve most of the liver (Fig. 9.1). In the nodular type, the liver is hard, scarred, and of abnormal shape; dark green or whitish-grey areas varying from a few mm to several cm in diameter are scattered over the surface. Alternatively there is a massive tumour, usually in the right lobe, and multiple smaller growths are present in the left lobe. Necrosis, haemorrhage, and fatty change may be present. The tumour is superimposed on a macronodular cirrhosis in approximately 80 per cent of cases; the non-tumour liver tissue may be reddish-brown due to siderosis. In a post-mortem study of 144 cases of HCC at Ibadan, 62·5 per cent were associated with cirrhosis which was usually of a macronodular type (Francis and Smith, 1972); however in patients under 10 years and in women over 45 years, cirrhosis was unusual. Metastasis is largely by lymphatic spread to the porta hepatis and head of the pancreas. Spread to hepatic veins with pulmonary metastases is very common (Fig. 9.2). Portal vein thrombosis may be produced by growth into the portal vein. Bone secondaries are occasionally seen. Hilar glands, diaphragm, gall bladder, mesentery, peritoneum, heart, skull, sternum, and brain may also be the sites of metastases. In a study of 144 post-mortem livers at Ibadan, from patients with HCC, metastases had occurred in 53·4 per cent. Cutaneous porphyria is a rare complication (Thompson, Nicholson, Farnan, Whitmore, and Williams, 1970).

There are several histological types, (i) adenoid, (ii) giant-cell, (iii) anaplastic, (iv) pseudoendothelial, and (v) miscellaneous (Edington and Gilles, 1976); there are also mixed types, and the essential histological feature is the resemblance of the cells to hepatocytes. The tumour cells are arranged in nodules of varying size; they are surrounded by sinusoidal spaces containing blood and lined by endothelial-like cells. Kupffer cells and macrophages are not seen. There are usually areas of necrosis.

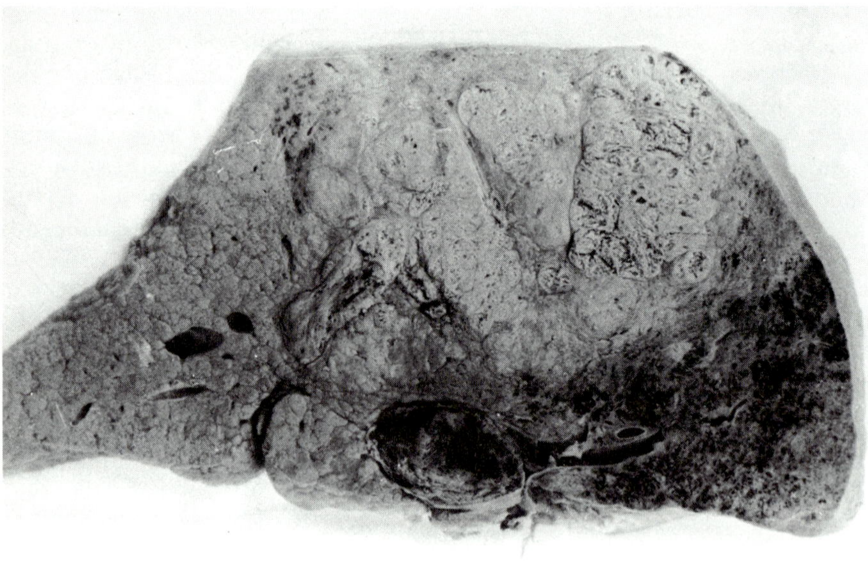

FIG. 9.1. Cut surface of the liver of a Papua New Guinean man from the Central Province. He was admitted with abdominal pain; examination revealed a very large hard liver and ascites, which was bloodstained. He died in hepatic coma a few days later. The section shows macronodular cirrhosis (left); most of the liver tissue has been replaced by a large hepatocellular carcinoma.

The tumour cells are usually large and polyhedral with vesicular nuclei and a well-marked nucleolus; occasionally they are small with dense nuclei. Their cytoplasm is eosinophilic but may show ballooning and feathery degeneration; glycogen may be seen. Mitotic figures and giant cells may also be present. Bile canaliculi with thrombi and bile pigment in the tumour cells may be present. Rarely there may be mucin-secreting cells.

The remaining liver tissue usually shows a macronodular cirrhosis; if there is no cirrhosis (which is the case in approximately 15 to 20 per cent), there may be a fibrous tissue reaction at the periphery of the tumour. There may be regenerative activity in the hepatocytes and focal bile retention.

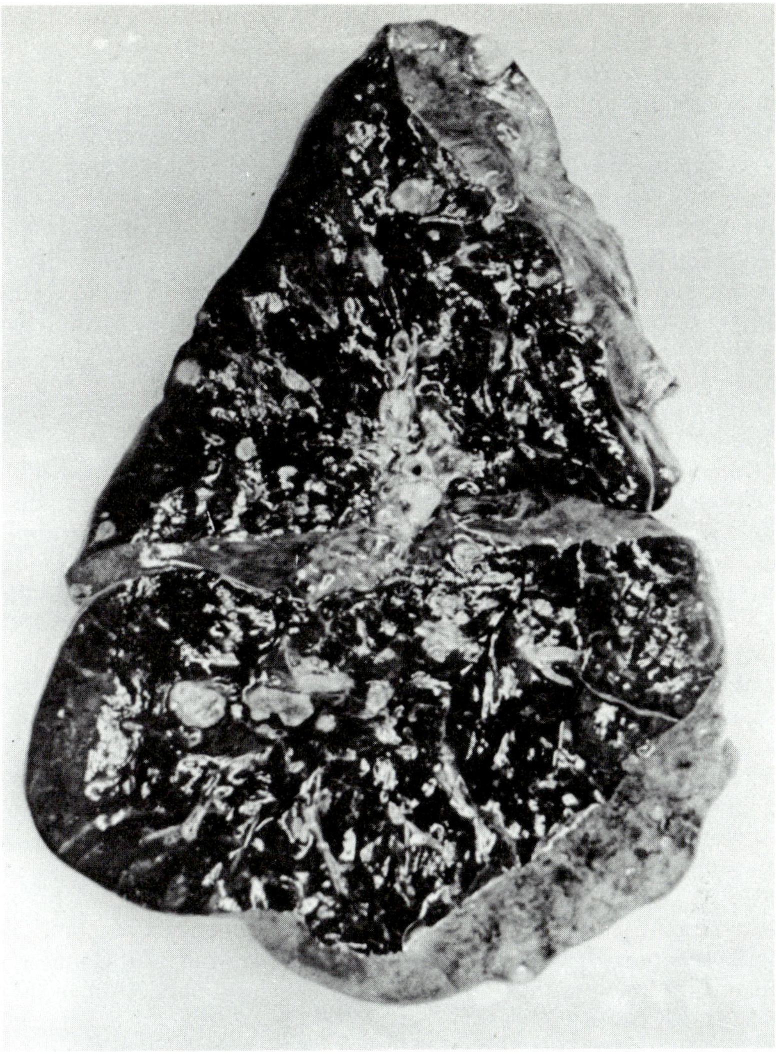

FIG. 9.2. Cut surface of lung from a Zambian woman with a hepatocellular carcinoma. Multiple secondary deposits are clearly demonstrated.

In a histological study of 144 post-mortem livers from patients with HCC at Ibadan, 87 per cent were described as typical trabecular or mixed trabecular, giant cell and adenoid and only eight per cent secreted bile (Francis and Smith, 1972).

9.5. Investigation of HCC

9.5.1. Routine investigations

The condition is usually so obvious clinically that little if any investigation is required. Confirmation of diagnosis has become very much easier since the introduction of serum alpha-fetoprotein (AFP) estimations (see below). Of routine liver-function tests, serum transaminases and alkaline phosphatase are usually elevated. Serum protein electrophoresis usually shows a reduced albumin, and elevated serum gamma-globulin and immunoglobulins IgG, IgA, and IgM; these changes depend however largely on the presence of underlying cirrhosis. Needle liver-biopsy and cytological examination of ascitic fluid are frequently of value in clinching the diagnosis. Ascitic fluid may contain a high concentration of γ-glutamyltransferase, and that is of value in diagnosis (Peters, Seymour, Wells, Fakunle, and Neale, 1977).

An abnormal serum α_1-globulin may be present (Lippi, Villa, Pavan, and Guidi, 1971), serum hydroxylase may be elevated (Keiser, Vogel, and Sadikali, 1972), and the circulating fibrinogen may be abnormal (von Felton, Straub, and Frick, 1969; Vogel and Linsell, 1972).

Serum vitamin B_{12} concentration is often elevated. A further biochemical test of potential value in confirming a diagnosis of hepatoma is serum ferritin; raised concentrations were demonstrated in 58 of 76 Africans with HCC in South Africa (Kew, Torrance, Derman, Simon, MacNab, Charlton, and Bothwell, 1978). There was however no correlation between the ferritin concentration and tumour size, presence or absence of cirrhosis, serum transaminase concentrations, or hepatic iron stores. A significant negative correlation between serum ferritin and AFP was found however. Those authors considered that when an assay utilizing a specific antibody against acidic hepatoma isoferritins can be developed, this test will be a second major biochemical marker in HCC. The chest radiograph shows elevation of the diaphragm on the side of the tumour. Barium-meal examination may show gross displacement of the stomach by a massive hepatoma. Vascular radiology: hepatic angiography and splenic venography, and hepatic scintiscanning, if available, give valuable information on the vasculature and site of the tumour. Peritoneoscopy or laparotomy are the remaining investigations which may lead to a positive diagnosis.

Disorders of carbohydrate metabolism are common and clinical hypoglycaemic reactions are often encountered. In a study in Uganda, blood glucose and insulin responses were delayed and prolonged after oral glucose (Primack and Kajubi, 1974).

9.5.2. Alpha fetoprotein (AFP)

In 1963, Abelev and his colleagues noticed a fetal alphaglobulin in the serum of adult mice with chemically induced hepatomas (Abelev, Perova, Khramkova, Postnikova, and Irlin, 1963). Shortly after that observation, Tatarinov (1964) detected AFP in the serum of patients with HCC. The globulin can be demonstrated within tumour cells by immunofluorescent techniques. Since then AFP has become an extremely valuable immunochemical marker in the diagnosis of hepatoma (Abelev, Assecritova, Kraevsky, Perova, and Perevodchikova, 1967; Uriel, de Nechard, Stanislawski-Birencwajg, Masseyeff, Leblanc, Quénem, Loisillier, and Graber, 1968; Hirai and Miyaji, 1973).

AFP is normally synthesized by the fetal liver and yolk-sac; in the fetus, the highest concentrations occur during the twelfth to fourteenth weeks and begin to decline at about the 32nd week. High values continue however until about five weeks after birth.

In the neonate, AFP is present in the periportal hepatocytes. AFP can also be detected in maternal serum, where concentrations are highest during the second trimester.

In patients with HCC, AFP which is produced by tumour cells, is present at very high concentrations in the serum in from 28 to 87 per cent of individuals; it is found in a focal fashion in the cytoplasm of malignant liver cells (Smith, Francis, Edington, and Williams, 1971). It is also present in cerebrospinal fluid and bile, in patients with HCC in whom the serum concentrations are raised. The highest positivity rates, using fairly crude methods of identification, are in areas where hepatoma is a very common disease:

	per cent positive results
South Africa	78
Senegal	72
Taiwan	73
Indonesia	87
UK	29
USA	28–50

Using an immunodiffusion technique, positive results were obtained in 94 per cent of patients with hepatoma in Papua New Guinea (Woodfield and Oraka, 1972). The reason for the marked geographical variation is not clear. A basic difference in the type of tumour might be important; hepatomas in the UK and USA behave very differently from those in tropical countries. AFP is also most commonly present at high concentration in young people, especially young men with hepatoma, which is the group which is most at risk for hepatomas in tropical countries. Ethnic factors have not been excluded.

Since its introduction many refinements in technique have been made, and *normal* concentrations of AFP in serum can now be measured. However specificity of the test in diagnosing HCC is obviously not nearly so great (Woodfield, Gustaffson, and Oraka, 1973). In Chinese patients with hepatoma, the positivity rate is 93 per cent with an immunoassay and 69 per cent with the immunodiffusion method (Ishii, 1973); in Uganda comparable figures are 93 and 71 per cent (McIntire, Vogel, Princler, and Patel, 1972).

Recent reports using more sensitive techniques, suggest that the percentage of patients with HCC and an elevated AFP is in fact fairly constant throughout the world, but that concentrations merely reach higher levels in tropical countries compared with temperate ones (Johnson, Portman, and Williams, 1978); in that study, using a sensitive radioimmunoassay the incidence of raised AFP in patients with HCC in Britain was in fact 80 per cent. Using the same technique, Kohn and Weaver (1974) also reported a rate of 83 per cent in caucasians with HCC.

With even the most sensitive of modern techniques, however, AFP cannot be detected in a proportion of patients with primary hepatoma. With the sensitive techniques, results from African patients with hepatoma show a very wide range in concentration from just over the normal range of 30 ng per ml to 7 mg per ml (Kew, 1974); the reason for such vast differences in production by different tumours is unknown. A value of 2000 ng per ml in adults makes a diagnosis of hepatoma extremely likely (Nolan, 1978).

Much higher concentrations exist in young compared with old patients with hepatoma; thus a negative result, using an immunodiffusion technique, in a 60-year-old patient would not necessarily rule out hepatoma (Vogel and Linsell, 1972). The elevated concentrations remain very stable in individual patients, until at the point of death a rapid decrease in concentration sometimes occurs; concentrations also fall rapidly after resection of the HCC.

In conclusion, the less sensitive tests are probably of greatest value in routine practice, for diagnosing HCC, while the more sophisticated ones are best used for following the course of the disease, and assessing responses to treatment. Using more sensitive methods for detection, it has been shown that an elevated AFP concentration is not confined to patients with HCC but is present in tumours composed of other tissues, and also in other liver diseases, but at a lower concentration (Kew, 1974).

AFP in other tumours. Most false-positive results have been reported in patients with tumours originating from either the gastrointestinal tract or the primitive foregut; stomach, pancreatic, gall-bladder and pulmonary tumours have all yielded high concentrations. The fetal gastrointestinal tract, as well as the liver, synthesizes AFP. Other tumours associated with a positive AFP are undifferentiated teratocarcinomas. Incidence of positive results is higher in children compared with adults with those tumours (as with hepatomas); the size and degree of malignancy of the tumour seems to correlate with the positivity rate in the presence of those tumours.

AFP in other liver diseases. Liver diseases in which there is extensive necrosis and regeneration of hepatocytes are associated with high concentrations of AFP, using a sensitive technique. In viral hepatitis, maximum concentrations are seen during the recovery phase of the disease. It is very unusual to find elevated titres of AFP in cirrhosis or active chronic hepatitis, although high levels have been demonstrated in Indian childhood cirrhosis; Nayak, Malaviya, Chawla, and Chandra (1972) found AFP in the serum of 45 per cent of patients with that condition. High concentrations have also been reported in congenital biliary atresia and neonatal hepatitis.

Value of AFP in excluding hepatoma. Using a sensitive radioimmunoassay in 30 patients with cirrhosis and hepatoma, and in 100 patients with cirrhosis and no evidence of malignancy, Johnson *et al*. (1978) showed that 29 and one, respectively, had an AFP concentration greater than 10·5 ng per ml. Eleven of 20 in whom hepatoma had arisen in a normal liver had a raised AFP concentration. AFP estimated by that technique is thus of considerable value in excluding hepatocellular carcinoma in cirrhotic patients; however the technique is of less value in distinguishing between primary tumours in patients without cirrhosis and secondary hepatic deposits.

9.6. Treatment of HCC

Single tumours can occasionally be resected (Bremner, 1964; Nugent, 1973), but there are very few surgeons in tropical countries who will undertake that, or in fact have the facilities. Two such operations have been reported from Papua New Guinea (Radford, Nugent, Gray, and Woodfield, 1973); one patient, a 45-year-old woman, was well some 15 months post-operatively. The vast majority of tumours are too advanced, have multiple foci, or have arisen in a cirrhotic liver; they are not therefore amenable to surgery. Hepatic transplantation is clearly not the answer to this problem.

Many chemotherapeutic agents have been tried but without much success. Hepatic arterial infusion of cytotoxic agents has been attempted. Some relief of pain was reported in two patients treated with intrahepatic 5-fluorouracil at Ibadan, Nigeria (Francis, 1972); one of them survived for seven months. Cochrane, Murray-Lyon, Brinkley, and Williams (1977) obtained some improvement in survival using quadruple cytotoxic therapy, but not only was the degree of symptomatic improvement rarely impressive, but side-effects were common. Tormey, Bergevin, Blom, and Petty (1973) demonstrated that doxorubicin ('Adriamycin') had significant antitumour activity in three patients with hepatoma, when combined with bleomycin. Olweny, Toya, Katongole-Mbidde, Mugerwa, Kyalwazi, and Cohen (1975) showed furthermore that all of 11 Ugandan patients treated with doxorubicin showed some improvement. Vogel, Bayley, Brooker, Anthony, and Zeigler (1977) described a partial response in 37 per cent of cases in a series from Africa and the USA. Remission can be induced by doxorubicin in 30–40 per cent of patients (Johnson and Williams, 1978). In a study of 44 patients with hepatoma, Johnson, Williams, Thomas, Sherlock, and Murray-Lyon (1978) have demonstrated a clinical remission in 14 (32 per cent) of them; the dose of doxorubicin given was 60 mg per m^2 at three weekly intervals to a maximum dose of 550 mg per m^2. In three who responded, hepatic arteriography showed clearing of the previously extensive tumour circulation, and in a fourth there was disappearance of the tumour on serial ultrasound examination. Compared with quadruple therapy there were few side-effects of doxorubicin. In those patients who responded, there was a fall in serum AFP which occurred after the first injection, and in those who did not respond the concentration continued to rise. Serial AFP concentrations are of great value in assessing results of treatment (Radford, Nugent, Gray, and Woodfield, 1973).

In assessing the effectiveness of chemotherapy it is often difficult to separate the effect of treatment on the hepatoma from the deterioration in clinical state associated with the cirrhosis.

In an investigation in Greece, oral urea was given in a dose of 2 to 2·5 g at four to six times daily to eight patients with HCC (Danopoulos and Danopoulou, 1974); mean survival was 26·5 months after commencing treatment, and two patients were alive at 36 and 57 months. That form of therapy is very inexpensive and warrants a controlled trial.

Ligation of the hepatic artery has been advocated by some workers (Nugent, 1973); the rationale for that treatment is that hepatomas derive the major part of their blood supply from the hepatic artery rather than the portal vein.

Radiotherapy has also been used in Papua New Guinea, with results which are initially encouraging (J. Niblett, 1980, *unpublished*).

None of those lines of treatment is of much value in treating this tumour, which is extremely malignant; the prognosis overall is appallingly bad.

9.7. Other hepatic malignancies in tropical countries

Benign primary tumours. Adenomata and cavernous haemangiomata are not uncommon; the latter may be accompanied by microangiopathic haemolytic anaemia (Prematilleke, 1972). Cysts and hamartomas are also seen in Africa (Edington and Gilles, 1976).

Hepatoblastoma. This rare childhood tumour has been reported in a Papua New Guinean child (Wilkey and Biddulph, 1970).

Bile-duct (cholangiocellular) carcinoma. This is discussed in Chapter 14; it is important to differentiate this tumour from hepatocellular carcinoma, which can easily be done histologically, because the aetiology is clearly different. In some tumours, cholangiocellular elements as well as liver-cell carcinoma are present giving a combined hepatobiliary picture. Clonorchiasis and opisthorchiasis are usually endemic in areas where it is common.

Mesenchymal tumours. This group includes fibrosarcomas and haemangioendotheliomas which certainly occur in tropical countries; their incidence is unknown (Edington and Gilles, 1976).

Secondary malignant tumours. Secondary tumours are common in tropical countries, as in temperate ones; however their frequency is overshadowed by the very high incidence of HCC (Powell and McGovern, 1976). Burkitt's lymphoma, gastric and chorion carcinoma, malignant melanoma, etc. can all produce secondary deposits in the liver. Burkitt's lymphoma (Chapter 1) may produce single or multiple deposits in the liver; retroperitoneal and paravertebral masses are common. Ascites may be present but is rarely gross. A search for a primary site and needle liver-biopsy from the tumour nodule are important in arriving at a diagnosis.

Direct invasion of metastatic nodules with anaerobic bacteria may occur (Trump, Fahnestock, Cloutier, and Dickman, 1978); that might be an important mechanism in the fever which so often accompanies secondary malignant disease of the liver.

References

Abelev, G. I., Assecritova, I. V., Kraevsky, N. A., Perova, S. D., and Perevodchikova, N. I. (1967). *Int. J. Cancer*, **2**, 551.

——, Perova, S. D., Khramkova, N. I., Postnikova, Z. A., and Irlin, I. S. (1963). *Transplantation,* **1**, 174.

Alpert, M. E., Hutt, M. S. R., and Davidson, C. S. (1968). *Lancet*, **1**, 1265.

——, ——, and —— (1969). *Am. J. Med.,* **46**, 794.

——, ——, Wogan, G. N., and Davidson, C. S. (1971). *Cancer, N.Y.*, **28**, 253.

——, and ISSELBACHER, K. J. (1971). *Lancet*, **2,** 1087.
ANTHONY, P. P., VOGEL, C. L., and BARKER, L. F. (1973). *J. clin. Path.*, **26,** 217.
BAGSHAWE, A. F., PARKER, A. M., and JINDANI, A. (1971). *Br. med. J.,* **1,** 88.
BECKER, B. J. P. and CHATGIDIKAS, C. B. (1961). *Acta Un. int. Cancr.*, **17,** 650.
BERMAN, C. (1940). *S. Afr. med. J.*, **5,** 92.
—— (1951). *Primary carcinoma of the liver.* Lewis, London.
BOSHNAKOVA, T. and GILLUM, R. L. (1972). *Ethiop. med. J.*, **10,** 139.
BRAS, G., JELLIFFE, D. B., and STUART, K. L. (1954). *Archs Path.*, **57,** 285.
——, BROOKS, S. E. H. and WATLER, D. C. (1961). *J. Path. Bact.,* **82,** 503.
BREMNER, C. G. ((1964). *S. Afr. med. J.*, **2,** 71.
Br. med. J. (1978). **2,** 718.
BURKITT, D. P., HUTT, M. S. R., and SLAVIN, G. (1968). *Br. J. Cancer*, **22,** 1.
CAMAIN, R. (1954). *Acta Un. int. Cancr.*, **13,** 617.
CHAINUVATI, T., VIRANUVATTI, V., and PONGPIPAT, D. (1979). *Gastroenterology*, **68,** 1261.
CLAIN, D., WARTNABY, K., and SHERLOCK, S. (1966). *Lancet,* **2,** 516.
CLIFFORD, P., LINSELL, C. A., and TIMMS, G. L. (1968). (eds.) *Cancer in Africa.* East African Medical Journal, East African Publishing House, Nairobi, Kenya.
——, and BULBROOK, R. D. (1966). *Lancet*, **1,** 1228.
COADY, A. (1964). *Br. med. J.*, **1,** 1510.
COCHRANE, A. M., MURRAY-LYON, I. M., BRINKLEY, D. M., and WILLIAMS, R. (1977). *Cancer, N.Y.*, **40,** 609.
COOK, P. and BURKITT, D. (1970). *An epidemiological study of seven malignant tumours in east Africa.* Medical Research Council, London.
COOK, P. J. and BURKITT, D. P. (1971). *Br. med. Bull.*, **27,** 14.
COOKE, R. A. (1968). *Papua New Guin. med. J.*, **11,** 7.
CORREA, P. and LLANOS, C. (1966). *J. natn. Cancer Inst.*, **36,** 717.
CUNNINGHAM, A. and LE PAGE, R. N. (1972). *Papua New Guin. med. J.*, **15,** 102.
DANOPOULOS, E. D. and DANOPOULOU, I. E. (1974). *Lancet*, **1,** 132.
DAVIES, J. N. P. (1952). *W. Afr. med. J.*, **1,** 141.
—— (1961). *Acta Un. int. Cancr.*, **17,** 787.
——, ELMES, S., HUTT, M. S. R., MTIMAVALYE, L. A. R., OWOR, R., and SHAPER, L. (1964). *Br. med. J.*, **1,** 259, 336.
——, KNOWELDEN, J. and WILSON, B. A. (1965). *J. natn. Cancer Inst.*, **35,** 789.
—— and OWOR, R. (1960). *E. Afr. med. J.*, **37,** 249.
DAWSON, J. L. M. (1966). *J. trop. med. Hyg.*, **69,** 175.
DEO, M. G., DAYAL, Y. and RAMALINGASWAMI, V. (1970). *J. Path. Bact.*, **101,** 47.
DOLL, R. (1967). *Prevention of cancer: pointers from epidemiology.* Nuffield Provincial Hospitals Trust. Oxford University Press, London.
DOMINGO, E. O., WARREN, K. S., and STENGER, R. J. (1967). *Am. J. Path.*, **51,** 307.
DORN, H. F. and CUTLER, S. J. (1958). *Publ. Hlth Monogr.*, No. 56.
EDINGTON, G. M. (1956). *Br. J. Cancer*, **10,** 595.
—— (1957). *Trans. R. Soc. trop. Med. Hyg.*, **51,** 48.
—— and GILLES, H. M. (1976). *Pathology in the tropics.* pp. 204, 588. 2nd ed. Edward Arnold, London.
—— and MACLEAN, C. M. U. (1965a). *Br. J. Cancer*, **19,** 471.
—— and —— (1965b). *Br. med. J.*, **1,** 264.
FOY, H., KONDI, A., LINDSELL, C. A., PARKER, A. M., and SIZARET, P. (1970). *Nature, Lond.*, **225,** 952.
FRANCIS, T. I. (1972). *W. Afr. med. J.*, **21,** 18.
—— and SMITH, J. A. (1972). *W. Afr. med. J.*, **21,** 37.
——, ——, and HENDRICKSE, J. P. de V. (1974). *E. Afr. med. J.*, **51,** 789.
HADZIYANNIS, S., MERIKAS, G. E., and AFROUDAKIS (1970). *Lancet*, **2,** 100.
HASHEM, M., ZAKI, S. A., and HUSSEIN, M. (1961). *J. Egypt med. Ass.*, **44,** 579.

HIGGINSON, J. (1956). *Br. J. Cancer*, **10,** 609.
—— and OETTLÉ, A. G. (1960). *J. natn. Cancer Inst.*, **24,** 589.
HILL, K. R. (1959). *Trans. R. Soc. trop. Med. Hyg.*, **53,** 217.
HIRAI, H. and MIYAJI, T. (1973) (eds.) *Alpha-fetoprotein and hepatoma. Gann monograph on cancer research no. 14.* University of Tokyo Press, Japan.
HIRSHMANN, S. Z., VERNACE, S. J. and SCHAFFNER, R. (1971). *Lancet*, **1,** 1099.
HUTT, M. S. R. (1971). *Trans. R. Soc. trop. Med. Hyg.*, **65,** 273.
—— (1972). In *Medicine in a tropical environment* (ed. A. G. Shaper, J. W. Kilbukamusoke and M. S. R. Hutt,), p. 401. BMA, London.
ISHII, M. (1973). In *Alpha-fetoprotein and hepatoma. Gann monograph on cancer research no. 14* (ed. H. Hirai and T. Miyaji) p. 89. University of Tokyo Press, Japan.
JESHRANI, M. K. and GATEI, D. G. (1975). *E. Afr. med. J.*, **52,** 605.
JOHNSON, P. J., PORTMANN, B., and WILLIAMS, R. (1978). *Br. med. J.*, **2,** 661.
—— and WILLIAMS, R. (1978). *Gut*, A451.
——, ——, THOMAS, H., SHERLOCK, S., and MURRAY-LYON, I. M. (1978). *Lancet*, **1,** 1006.
KEISER, H. R., VOGEL, C. L., and SADIKALI, F. (1972). *J. natn. Cancer Inst.*, **49,** 1251.
KEW, M. (1974). *Gut*, **15,** 814.
KEW, M. C., GEDDES, E. W., MACNAB, G. M. and BERSOHN, I. (1974). *Cancer, N.Y.*, **34,** 539.
——, TORRANCE, J. D., DERMAN, D., SIMON, M., MACNAB, G. M., CHARLTON, R. W., and BOTHWELL, T. H. (1978). *Gut.*, **19,** 294.
KOHN, J. and WEAVER, P. C. (1974). *Lancet*, **2,** 334.
KUBO, Y., OKUDA, K., MUSHA, H., and NAKASHIMA, T. (1978). *Gastroenterology*, **74,** 578.
LAINOVIC, D. (1974). *Ethiop. med. J.*, **12,** 13.
LANCASTER, M. C., JENKINS, F. P., and PHILP, J. M. (1961). *Nature, Lond.*, **192,** 1095.
Lancet, (1971). **1,** 1113.
LEE, F. I. (1966). *Gut*, **7,** 77.
LIPPI, U., VILLA, A., PAVAN, R., and GUIDI, G. (1971). *Am. J. clin. Path.*, **56,** 227.
LOPEZ, A. and CRAWFORD, M. A. (1967). *Lancet*, **2,** 1351.
LOPEZ-CORRELLA, E., RIDAURA-SANZ, C., and ALBORES-SAAVEDRA, J. (1968). *Cancer, N.Y.*, **22,** 678.
MACFADZEAN, A. J. S. and YEUNG, R. T. T. (1969). *Am. J. Med.*, **47,** 220.
MCGOVERN, V. J. and KARIKS, J. (1966). *Med. J. Aust.*, **2,** 441.
MCINTIRE, K. R., VOGEL, C. L., PRINCLER, G. L. and PATEL, I. R. (1972). *Cancer Res.*, **32,** 1941.
MARSDEN, A. T. H. (1958). *Br. J. Cancer*, **12,** 161.
MAUPAS, P., WERNER, B., and LAROUZÉ, B. (1975). *Lancet*, **2,** 9.
MIYAKE, M., SAITO, M., ENOMOTO, M., SHIKATA, T., ISHIKO, T., URAGUCHI, K., SAKAI, F., TATSUNO, T., TSUKIOKA, M., and SAKAI, Y. (1960). *Acta path. jap.*, **10,** 75.
MONTENEGRO, M. R., da SILVA, L. C., and PONTES, J. F. (1958). *Gastroenterology*, **34,** 1108.
MUIR, C. S. and SHANMUGARATNAM, K. (1966). In *Cancer incidence in five continents* (ed. R. Doll, P. Payne and J. Waterhouse). p. 124. Springer-Verlag, Berlin, Heidelberg, and New York.
NANTULYA, V. M., LINDQVIST, K. J., and SPENCER, S. (1975). *E. Afr. med. J.*, **52,** 430.
NAYAK, N. C., MALAVIYA, A. N., CHAWLA, V., and CHANDRA, R. K. (1972). *Lancet*, **1,** 68.
NOLAN, J. P. (1978). *Gastroenterology*, **74,** 953.
NUGENT, R. (1973). *Papua New Guin. med. J.*, **16,** 199.
NWOKOLO, C. and OKONKWO, P. (1978). *Trans. R. Soc. trop. Med. Hyg.*, **72,** 329.
OETTLÉ, A. G. (1964). *J. natn. Cancer Inst.*, **33,** 383.
O'CONOR, G. T., TRALKA, T. S., and HENSEN, E. (1972). *J. natn. Cancer Inst.*, **48,** 587.

OLWENY, C. L. M., TOYA, T., KATONGOLE-MBIDDE, E., MUGERWA, J., KYALWAZI, S. K., and COHEN, H. (1975). *Cancer, N.Y.*, **36,** 1250.

Papua New Guin. med. J. (1972). **15,** 65.

PAVILICA, D. and SAMUEL, I. (1970). *Br. J. Cancer*, **24,** 22.

PAYET, M. (1967). *Acta Un. int. Cancr.*, **13,** 712.

PAYMASTER, J. C. (1964). *Cancer, N.Y.*, **17,** 1026.

PETERS, R. L., AFROUDAKIS, A. P., and TATTER, D. (1977). *Am. J. clin. Path.*, **68,** 1.

PETERS, T. J., SEYMOUR, C. A., WELLS, G., FAKUNLE, F., and NEALE, G. (1977). *Br. med. J.*, **1,** 1576.

POWELL, K. C. and MCGOVERN, V. J. (1976). *Papua New Guin. med. J.*, **19,** 140.

PRATES, M. D. and TORRES, F. O. (1965). *J. natn. Cancer Inst.*, **35,** 729.

PREMATILLEKE, M. N. (1972). *Postgrad. Med. J.*, **48,** 111.

PRIMACK, A. and KAJUBI, S. (1974). *E. Afr. med. J.*, **51,** 574.

——, VOGEL, C. L., and BARKER, L. F. (1973). *Br. med. J.*, **1,** 16.

PRINCE, A. M., LEBLANC, L., KROHN, K., MASSEYEFF, R., and ALPERT, M. E. (1970). *Lancet*, **2,** 717.

——, SZMUNESS, W., and MICHON, J. (1975). *Int. J. Cancer*, **16,** 376.

RADFORD. A. J., NUGENT, R., GRAY, F. J., and WOODFIELD, D. G. (1973). *Papua New Guin. med. J.*, **16,** 202.

SALIH, S. Y., SATIR, A. A., SULIEMAN, S. I., and SABBA, H. A. (1978). *J. trop. Med. Hyg.*, **81,** 60.

SAMUEL, I., GEBRE SELASSIE, M., and BOCINA, B. (1974). *Ethiop. med. J.*, **12,** 53.

SARGEANT, K., SHERIDAN, A., O'KELLY, J., and CARNAGHAN, R. B. A. (1961). *Nature, Lond.*, **192,** 1096.

SAVEL, H., FORSYTH, B., SCHAEFFER, W., and CARDELLA, T. (1970). *Proc. Soc. exp. Biol. Med.*, **134,** 1112.

SHANMUGARATNAM, K. and TYE, C. Y. (1970). *J. chron. Dis.*, **23,** 443.

SHAPER, A. G. (1970). *Trop. geogr. Med.*, **22,** 161.

SIMONS, M. J., YAP, E. H., YU, M., SEAH, C. S., CHEW, B. K., FUNG, W. P., TAN, A. Y. O., and SHANMUGARATNAM, K. (1971). *Lancet*, **1,** 1149.

SKINHØJ, P., HART HANSEN, J. P., NIELSEN, N., HØJGAARD, and MIKKELSEN, F. (1978). *Dan. med. Bull.*, **25,** 223.

SMITH, J. A., FRANCIS, T. I., EDINGTON, G. M., and WILLIAMS, A. O. (1971). *Br. J. Cancer*, **25,** 343.

TATARINOV, Y. S. (1964). *Vop. med. Khim.*, **10,** 90.

TEFERRA, A. and ABDUL KADIR, J. (1968). *Ethiop. med. J.*, **6,** 95.

TEKLU, B. (1978). *Lancet*, **2,** 259.

THEODOROPOULIS, G., ARCHIMANDRITIS, A., and ANGELOPOULOS, B. (1975). *Ann. intern. Med.*, **82,** 809.

THIJS, A. (1957). *Annls Soc. belge Méd. trop.*, **37,** 483.

THOMSON, J. G. (1961). *Acta Un. int. Cancr.*, **17,** 623.

THOMPSON, R. P. H., NICHOLSON, D. C., FARNAN, T., WHITMORE, D. N., and WILLIAMS, R. (1970). *Gastroenterology*, **59,** 779.

TONG, M. J., SUN, S. C., SCHAEFFER, B. T., CHANG, N. K., LO, K. J., and PETERS, R. L. (1971). *Ann. intern. Med.*, **75,** 687.

TORMEY, D. C., BERGEVIN, P., BLOM, J., and PETTY, W. (1973). *Cancer Chemother, Rep. part 1*. **57,** 413.

TRICHOPOULOS, D., TABOR, E., GERETY, R. J., XIROUCHAKI, E., SPARROS, L., MUNOZ, N., and LINSELL, C. A. (1978). *Lancet*, **2,** 1217.

TRUMP, D. L., FAHNESTOCK, R., CLOUTIER, C. T., and DICKMAN, M. D. (1978). *Cancer, N.Y.*, **41,** 682.

TSEGA, E. (1977). *E. Afr. med. J.*, **54,** 281.

——, GOLD, P., SHUSTER, J., WHITTEMORE, B., and LESTER, F. T. (1976). *J. trop. Med. Hyg.*, **79,** 230.

URIEL, J., de NECHAUD, B., STANISLAWSKI-BIRENCWAJG, M., MASSEYEFF, R., LEBLANC, L., QUÉNEM, C., LOISILLIER, F., and GRABER, P. (1968). *Presse méd.*, **76,** 1415.

VOGEL, C. L., ANTHONY, P. P., MODY, N., and BARKER, L. F. (1970). *Lancet,* **2,** 621.

——, ——, SADIKALI, F., BARKER, L. F., and PETERSON, M. R. (1972). *J. natn. Cancer Inst.*, **48,** 1583.

——, BAYLEY, A. C., BROOKER, R. J., ANTHONY, P. P., and ZIEGLER, J. L. (1977). *Cancer, N.Y.*, **39,** 1923.

—— and LINSELL, C. A. (1972). *J. natn. Cancer Inst.*, **48,** 567.

VON FELTON, A., STRAUB, P. W., and FRICK, P. G. (1969). *New Engl. J. Med.*, **280,** 405.

WAGNER, F. B. and SHEPHERD, A. (1976). *Papua New Guin. med. J.*, **19,** 156.

WALTERS, J. H. and WATERLOW, J. C. (1954). *Spec. Rep. Ser. med. Res. Coun.*, no. 285.

WELSH, J. D., BROWN, J. D., ARNOLD, K., MATHEWS, H. M., and PRINCE, A. M. (1976). *Gastroenterology*, **70,** 392.

WILKEY, I. S. and BIDDULPH, J. (1970). *Papua New Guin. med. J.*, **13,** 95.

WILLIAMS, A. O. (1972). *Scientific groups on viral B hepatitis*, W.H.O. Geneva.

WOODFIELD, D. G., GUSTAFFSON, A., and ORAKA, R. (1973). *Papua New Guin. med. J.*, **16,** 206.

—— and ORAKA, R. (1972). *Papua New Guin. med. J.*, **15,** 98.

WOOKEY, S. J. (1972). *Papua New Guin. med. J.*, **15,** 113.

10

Schistosomal involvement of the liver

HEPATIC schistosomiasis has been termed 'one of the great neglected diseases of mankind' (Warren, 1978a); it affects something of the order of 100 million of the world's population. Thirty per cent of infected populations have significant hepatomegaly; however that is a result of heavy infections, and is unusual in mild cases (Siongok, Mahmoud, Ouma, Warren, Muller, Handa, and Houser, 1976), and that observation applies particularly to children (Lehman, Mott, Morrow, Muniz, and Boyer, 1976).

The parasites *Schistosoma mansoni, S. japonicum*, and *S. haematobium* (Carter and Shaldon, 1959) produce scattered granulomata throughout the liver (Chapter 5); ova which have been released from the intestine, into the portal venous system, stimulate granuloma formation. Progression to extensive fibrosis is relatively unusual. However, with very heavy and repeated infections with *S. mansoni* and *S. japonicum*, broad bands of fibrous tissue are laid down; they intersect the liver and give rise to a condition known as 'pipe-stem' fibrosis (Hashem, 1947), the mechanism of production of which is not clear. Advanced schistosomal liver disease is very common in Egypt and the Nile Delta; although it occasionally occurs, it is uncommon in most other parts of Africa, and that is probably due to the lower concentrations of infection. Diffuse destruction of hepatocytes, accompanied by regenerative nodule formation does not occur so that, by definition, that is not a true cirrhosis; in Japan, there is limited evidence which suggests that *S. japonicum* might be causally associated with cirrhosis (Miyake, 1967). When chronic liver disease is fully established it may be very difficult to find typical ova and granulomata of schistosomiasis. A presinusoidal obstruction to hepatic blood flow in association with normal overall blood flow, due to pronounced arterialization, has been demonstrated (Andrade and Cheever, 1971) (Chapter 11).

10.1. Hepatic schistosomiasis (HS)

10.1.1. History of HS

A classical description of hepatic schistosomiasis was made by the English pathologist William Saint Clair Symmers, working in Egypt, in 1904. The pathology was, he believed, dependent on the presence of schistosomal ova. At about the same time as that report, another major form of the disease, i.e. that due to *S. japonicum*, was discovered in the Far east. Most early workers considered that the chronic liver disease resulting from schistosomiasis was a true cirrhosis. It was later appreciated, however, that the histological abnormalities were limited to periportal fibrosis and that there was only minimal involvement of the hepatocytes (Hashem, 1947; Bogliolo, 1957). Those early descriptions cannot be substantially improved today; however, they contribute very little to the pathogenesis of hepatic schistosomiasis (Warren, 1978b).

10.1.2. Distribution of HS

Schistosomiasis affects more than 200 million people in approximately 70 countries of Asia, Africa, South America, and the Caribbean (Van den Bossche, 1978) (Chapter 26); many of those are children. Advanced disease is extremely common in Egypt (El-gholmy, Nabawy, Gabr, Aidaros, and Omar, 1955; Aidaros and Soliman, 1961), the Sudan (Malik, Satir, Veress, and El Hassan, 1975), Brazil (Bogliolo, 1957) and the Middle east. Irrigation has accounted for most of that increase; a rise from a five to an 80 per cent prevalence rate has, for example, been recorded in lower Egypt following the introduction of perennial irrigation. Populations of tropical countries without this disease, e.g. Papua New Guinea, should realize how extremely fortunate they are.

10.1.3. Parasitology and immunology of HS

'Swimmers' itch' follows the entry of cercariae into the body (Chapter 26) and their subsequent death in the skin; a relatively specific sensitization occurs, and biopsies show hypersensitivity reactions of immediate and delayed types. An acute illness develops in a minority of individuals when the worms start egg-laying. Both that event and the glomerulonephritis which occasionally occurs in *S. mansoni* infections are immune-complex diseases (Da Silva, De Brito, Camargo, De Boni, Lopes, and Gunji, 1970; Andrade, Andrade, and Sadigursky, 1971); IgG and IgM complexes can be demonstrated in renal biopsies.

In the definitive host (man), schistosomes do not replicate. The large number of ova produced daily for many years, approximately half of which are retained in the host's tissues (Warren, 1978a), are the cause of many of the major features of chronic schistosomiasis. The degree of involvement depends on the intensity of infection; the greater oviposition in *S. japonicum* infections is associated with earlier and more severe liver involvement than in *S. mansoni* infections. Quantitative relationships between the severity of the pathological changes, number of ova in the tissues, number of worms in the blood vessels, and intensity of excretion of ova in the faeces have been demonstrated (Cheever, 1968; Cheever, Kamel, Elwi, Mosimann, and Danner, 1977). The number of ova entering the tissues is directly related to the number of worm pairs; thus a 60 per cent retention of *S. mansoni* ova would mean approximately 180 ova daily for one worm pair, and in an individual harbouring 1000 worm pairs that would mean 180 000 ova. Most infected individuals carry only a small number of parasites; in many endemic areas less than 10 per cent of the population has a heavy infection, and even in areas of maximum prevalence only about 30 per cent of the population has such an infection. Hepatomegaly and splenomegaly have been shown to have a direct relationship to intensity of infection in Uganda (Ongom and Bradley, 1972), Kenya (Siongok, *et al.*,

1976), St. Lucia (Cook, Baker, Warren, and Jordan, 1974), and Brazil (Lehman, *et al.*, 1976). The granulomatous reaction around the ova (Fig. 10.1), and subsequent fibrosis have been shown to be essential for the development of the chronic disease (Bloch, Wahab, and Warren, 1972); the host response is an immunological reaction of the delayed, cell-mediated type (Warren, 1978a) (see below). Various antigens have now been isolated from the ova (Pelley and Pelley, 1976; Warren, 1978b).

Hepatosplenomegaly is therefore the result of hypersensitivity reactions of the host to schistosome ova trapped in the tissues; only when ova production is occurring do hepatomegaly and splenomegaly, portal hypertension, and oesophageal varices develop (Warren, 1972). As the large avascular granulomas form around the ova—often 100 times the volume of the ova themselves—the local blood flow is obstructed, and the surrounding area destroyed; that is a cell-mediated immunological reaction. Later, fibrous tissue is deposited and new arterial vessels develop; this arterialization ensures a good hepatic blood-flow, and hepatocyte function is maintained despite the development of portal hypertension. Thus it is the granulomatous reaction of the host (man) to the ova, which forms the basis for the chronic disease.

10.1.4. Presentation of HS

The clinical features of this disease have been described by Mahmoud (1977). All ages and both sexes are involved; many patients are less than 30 years of age. Cutaneous evidence of liver disease (Chapter 8) is usually absent. Jaundice and hepatocellular failure are also unusual. Evidence of portal hypertension is, however, frequently very obvious; a collateral circulation, ascites and hypoproteinaemia are often present. Gross abdominal distension, due to ascites, often with dilated veins over the anterior abdominal wall and marked hepatosplenomegaly, are prominent features of the disease. In Egypt the gross splenic enlargement has for long been termed Egyptian splenomegaly. Ultimately, oesophageal and gastric varices are formed, and haemorrhage is a common cause of death. Haemorrhage can also cause hepatic anoxia with acute liver failure and coma; however that is an unusual event (Warren and Rebouças, 1964; Sulit, Domingo, Dalmacio-Cruz, De Peralta, and Imperial, 1964). Loss of muscle bulk is a common sequel. Ankle oedema occurs. Blood ammonia concentrations are normal or only mildly elevated. If there is cardiac failure or portal vein thrombosis, liver failure may be a sequel. Splenic vein thrombosis is a further possibility.

There may be evidence of hypersplenism (Chapter 16).

10.1.5. Pathology of HS

Hepatomegaly and splenomegaly often occur during the invasive stage of schistosomiasis; inflammatory changes and often an eosinophilia can be demonstrated in liver-biopsy specimens. Ova and pseudotubercles may be seen adjacent to the portal tracts; they result in small focal scars. Lobular architecture is however intact. The specific lesion is the schistosomal granuloma in its various evolutionary stages (Fig. 10.1). Ova are present in portal and periportal areas, and reactions from an acute eosinophilia to a dense collagenous

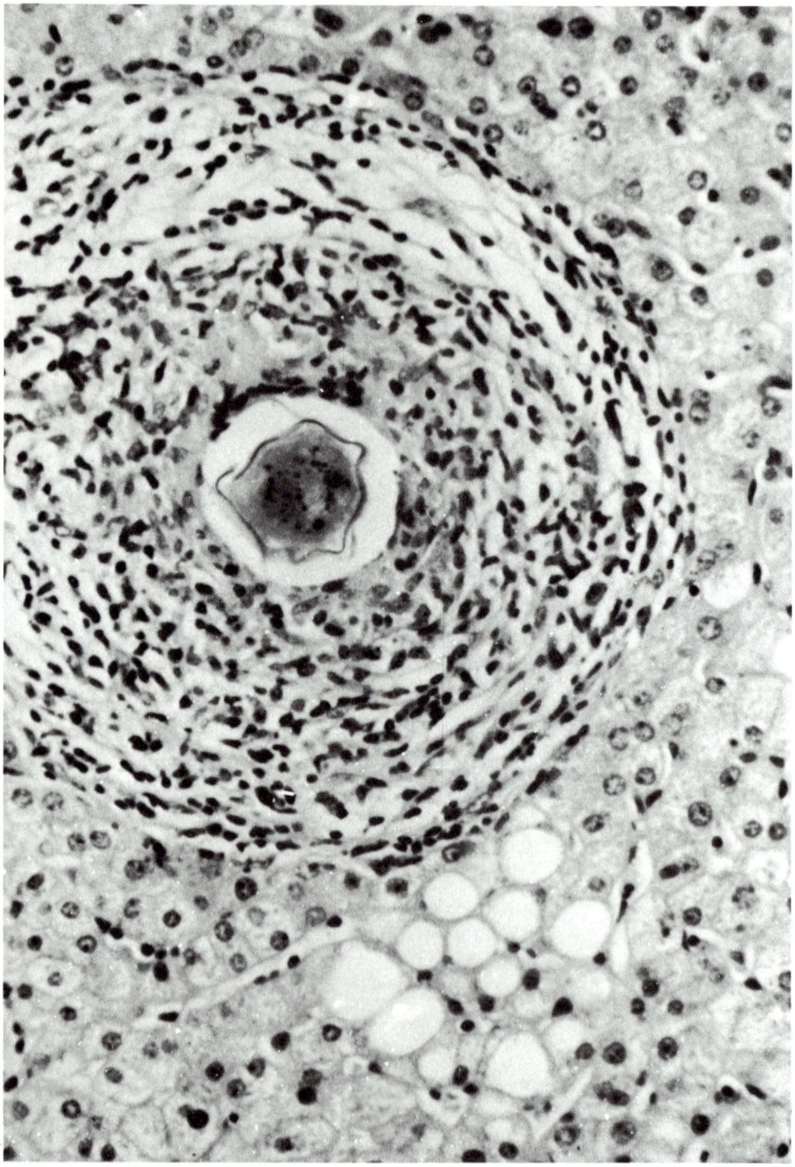

FIG. 10.1. Needle liver-biopsy section (haematoxylin and eosin) from a 30-year-old Zambian woman who was admitted with weight loss and fever; she was subsequently shown to have abdominal tuberculosis. The section shows a typical schistosomal granuloma surrounding an ovum of *Schistosoma mansoni*.

reaction may be present. In liver-biopsy sections, even where serial sections are made, the ovum may be missed and only a non-specific granuloma is seen. The presence of laminated fibrous tissue or eosinophils in a liver granuloma is however very suggestive of schistosomiasis (Hutt, 1971).

In *S. japonicum* infections, ova may adhere to each other by a transparent substance of parasitic origin; large abscesses may form with a subsequent delay in pseudotubercle and fibrous tissue formation (Areán, 1964). Although granuloma formation is very common in *S. haematobium* infections, the parasite very rarely produces advanced hepatic disease.

Schistosomal pigment, which is brownish-yellow and consists of a complex porphyrin composed of haematin and a nitrogenous moiety, may be present in the Kupffer cells (Koppisch, 1941), histiocytes, and portal tracts. That is evidence of the presence of adult worms and is a residue of the host's red blood-cells after they have been metabolized by the parasite; it can be differentiated by chemical and electron microscopical techniques from malarial pigment. A suggestion that pylephlebitis may result from death of adult worms in portal veins has not been substantiated.

In the established chronic disease, the liver may be normal, small, or enlarged in size; the left lobe is sometimes disproportionately enlarged (Cheever and Andrade, 1967). The surface shows a fine or coarse nodularity. The organ is firm, and there are white clay 'pipe-stems' throughout the parenchyma which may be round, oval, or 'stellate' and are a result of the fibrotic reaction caused by ova in and around the portal venous radicles; that is set against a background of relatively normal pink-brown liver tissue. There may be focal nodular hyperplasia in the subcapsular region, or a fine periportal fibrosis (Hashem, 1947). Dilated portal veins can be seen in some of the scars, and in others they are obliterated.

In fully developed cases, the classical 'pipe-stem' fibrosis can be demonstrated histologically. The disease involves mesenchymal, vascular, and reticuloendothelial components.

The hepatocytes are usually unaffected, unless there is widespread vascular damage and anoxia. Fatty change, and focal atrophy and haemorrhage, accounting for the nodular hypertrophy in the subcapsular region, are occasionally seen. Following massive haematemeses from oesophageal varices, or after portal vein thrombosis or cardiac failure, acute massive necrosis may be seen (Andrade, 1965). Inflammation and severe fibrosis is present in presinusoidal portal areas. When the disease is fully developed, schistosomal granulomas and ova are often very difficult to find in liver-biopsy specimens. There is periportal fibrosis and gross intimal and medial thickening of the portal triads (Areán, 1964). As portal hypertension develops, thrombotic changes occur, and there may be portal venous thrombosis as a complication of the 'pipe-stem' fibrosis. Ova are trapped in intrahepatic portal venules and sometimes reach the sinusoids; occasionally adult worms can be demonstrated in the vessels. Portal vein branches in the portal triads are severely damaged due to the reaction caused by the presence of ova, and may be completely destroyed; sclerosis of the portal vein branches occurs. Portal tracts may also contain hypertrophied bile ducts and nerves. There is an increase in the number and size of the intrahepatic arterial branches, which explains the normal hepatic blood flow (Coutinho, 1968; Andrade and Cheever, 1971).

10.1.6. Investigation of HS

Liver function tests are frequently non-contributory and show only a raised serum gamma-globulin concentration. Concentrations of serum transaminases are however sometimes elevated (Salah, Kheireldin, Mansour, and Hussein, 1976); glutamic pyruvic and glutamic oxaloacetic (Higazi, Fahmy, and Kaddah, 1960; Wroblewski and Le Due, 1956) transaminases may be raised. In addition, ornithine carbamyl transferase, sorbitol dehydrogenase, 5-nucleotidase and LDH_4 may be increased (Salah, *et al.*, 1976); in that study β-glucuronidase was unchanged. Alkaline phosphatase may be elevated (Barreto, 1971). Serum α_2 and γ-globulin concentrations may be elevated. Bromsulphthalein retention may be abnormal, especially in *S. japonicum* infections. A fall in serum cholinesterase activity has been reported from Egypt. Liver-biopsy may give diagnostic information; a Vim-Silverman needle should be used because the liver is usually firm or hard.

Numerous ova in the periportal fibrous tissue are often present. Rectal biopsy is usually positive for *S. mansoni* or *S. japonicum* ova. Splenovenography and hepatic vein catheterization (if facilities are available) provide valuable information on haemodynamics; portal vein pressure is high, and occluded suprahepatic vein pressure is normal, which differentiates the condition from macronodular cirrhosis. It is important to recognize that a splenovenogram showing a thrombosed portal vein in a patient indigenous to a tropical country, must not be assumed to indicate a normal liver as would usually be the case in a temperate area (Hutt, 1971) (Chapter 11). Laparoscopy and wedge-biopsy at a limited laparotomy may also clinch the diagnosis; laparoscopy is an effective diagnostic procedure which is relatively free of postoperative complications (Barry, Brown, and Read, 1978). Intradermal and serological methods of diagnosis for schistosomiasis are dealt with in Chapter 26.

In a fully developed case there is presinusoidal portal hypertension (Chapter 11). Portal haemodynamic studies have been carried out in Egypt (Bibawi, 1961; Mousa and El-Garem, 1959). In Nairobi, Kenya, bleeding from oesophageal varices accounted for 20 per cent of admissions to hospital with acute upper gastrointestinal haemorrhage in a series of 66 African patients (mean age 28 years); there was a close correlation between splenomegaly and presence of schistosomiasis in the areas from which the patients came (Hansen and Daly 1978). HB_sAg is evenly distributed amongst those areas. Another report from Kenya indicated that bleeding from oesophageal varices resulting from schistosomal liver disease was the commonest cause of upper gastrointestinal bleeding in Nairobi (Miller, 1967). Bleeding varices caused by schistosomal disease are also commonly encountered in the Sudan (Malik, *et al.*, 1975). Other reports from Africa support those conclusions (Carvalho and Ojiambo, 1974; Wicks, Thomas, and Clain, 1975).

10.1.7. Treatment of HS

The therapeutic agents effective in schistosomiasis are discussed in Chapter 26.

All cases must be treated when hepatic involvement is present; not only is further progression of disease arrested if treatment is satisfactory, but regression of hepatosplenomegaly often takes place. Drug metabolism in patients with clinically compensated hepatic schistosomiasis seems to be normal (Homeida, Salih, and Branch, 1978). Niridazole ('Ambilhar') must however be used with caution if portal-systemic anastomoses are present, because neuropsychiatric side-effects are common. The agent of choice in advanced cases of *S. mansoni* infection is probably oxamniquine (Omer, 1978) (Chapter 26). Hycanthone ('Etrenol'), the 4-hydroxy-methyl derivative of lucanthone, has clear hepatotoxic properties; it is contraindicated if there is a history of jaundice or liver disease. A rise in transaminases after a single intramuscular injection is well established (Cook and Jordan, 1971; Cook, Jordan, Woodstock, and Pilgrim, 1977; Farid, Bassily, Young, El Masry, and Hassan, 1973; Oostburg, 1972), but that might be partly due to muscle injury during the injection (Cook *et al.*, 1977). Overt hepatitis (Farid, Smith, Bassily, and Sparks, 1972; Kallmeyer, MacSearraigh, and Godlonton, 1977), and several deaths due to acute hepatic necrosis (Gane, 1971; Hatchuel, 1978) seem however to have been caused by that compound. Hepatic histology shows features of toxic hepatitis (Farid *et al.*, 1972; Cohen, 1978), and in those who die there may be massive hepatic necrosis. After recovery, chronic persistent hepatitis has been described one year later (Cohen, 1978). The risk of such complications is however low and has been estimated at 1 in 20 000 injections of hycanthone (WHO Report, 1972). With pre-existing liver disease, overdosage with hycanthone, and polypharmacy should be avoided; when care is taken, liver complications are rare, and in one study no toxicity was noted in 2723 patients who were treated with that agent (Cook and Jordan, 1976).

Davey (1968) has summarized the indications for surgery in patients with hepatic schistosomiasis as follows: (i) portal hypertension requiring portal-systemic anastomosis, (ii) hypersplenism (which requires splenectomy), and (iii) operations for rectal prolapse, intestinal obstruction, and intussusception (Chapter 26).

Few patients qualify for portacaval anastomosis, due to the advanced nature of the disease; it is exceedingly difficult to lay down hard and fast indications for that operation in this disease. Although hepatocyte function is good, there is undoubtedly a high incidence of chronic portal-systemic encephalopathy after portacaval anastomosis (Warren, Rebouças, and Baptista, 1965); the explanation for that is by no means clear. If portacaval anastomosis is carried out there is a danger of the development of cor pulmonale because living worms may be carried to the lungs.

10.2. Other diseases related to hepatic schistosomiasis

10.2.1. Predisposing factors

Only some patients with heavy *S. mansoni* infections develop hepatic disease, although the intensity and chronicity of the infection are important. There are clearly other factors to consider, one of which is the possibility of a genetic predisposition. The possible role of $alpha_1$ antitrypsin deficiency (Chapter 8) being relevant has been investigated (Goodgame and Bartholomew, 1978); in that study, all 90 patients with hepatosplenic schistosomiasis had normal $alpha_1$ antitrypsin concentrations.

There is experimental evidence which indicates that malnutrition has a protective effect from schistosomiasis of the liver; ova output by the adult worm is decreased in that condition (Chapter 13).

10.2.2. Sequelae of HS

In experimental animals, schistosomiasis in the presence of an hepatic carcinogen results in an increased incidence of hepatoma (Chapter 9).

In *S. mansoni* infections, salmonellosis with a prolonged fever has been described (Chapter 26); that might be due to defective sequestration by liver Kupffer cells as occurs in cirrhosis (Chapter 8).

A high carrier rate for HB_sAg has been noted in the presence of hepatic schistosomiasis (Chapter 8); in such carriers there is not only more chronic inflammation in the liver but also more clinical evidence of chronic liver disease.

References

AIDAROS, S. M. and SOLIMAN, L. A. M. (1961). *J. Path. Bact.*, **82,** 19.

ANDRADE, Z. A. (1965). In *Progress in Liver Disease* (ed. H. Popper and F. Schaffner). **2,** 228. Grune and Stratton, New York and London.

——, ANDRADE, S. G., and SADIGURSKY, M. (1971). *Am. J. trop. Med. Hyg.*, **20,** 77.

—— and CHEEVER, A. W. (1971). *Am. J. trop. Med. Hyg.*, **20,** 425.

AREÁN, V. M. (1964). *Revta clín. esp.*, **94,** 1.

BARRETO, V. S. (1971). *Ann. intern. Med.*, **74,** 450.

BARRY, R. E., BROWN, P., and READ, A. E. (1978). *Br. med. J.*, **2,** 1276.

BIBAWI, E. (1961). *Am. J. trop. Med. Hyg.*, **10,** 716.

BLOCH, E. H., WAHAB, M. F. A., and WARREN, K. S. (1972). *Am. J. trop. Med. Hyg.*, **21,** 546.

BOGLIOLO, L. (1957). *Ann. trop. Med. Parasitol.*, **51,** 1.

CARTER, R. A. and SHALDON, S. (1959). *Lancet*, **2,** 1003.

CARVALHO, G. R. and OJIAMBO, H. P. (1974). *E. Afr. med. J.*, **51,** 63.

CHEEVER, A. W. (1968). *Am. J. trop. Med. Hyg.*, **17,** 38.

—— and ANDRADE, Z. A. (1967). *Trans. R. Soc. trop. Med. Hyg.*, **61,** 626.

——, KAMEL, I. A., ELWI, A. M., MOSIMANN, J. E. and DANNER, R. (1977). *Am. J. trop. Med. Hyg.*, **26,** 702.

COHEN, C. (1978). *Gastroenterology*, **75,** 103.

COOK, J. A., BAKER, S. T., WARREN, K. S. and JORDAN, P. (1974). *Am. J. trop. Med. Hyg.*, **23,** 625.

—— and JORDAN, P. (1971). *Am. J. trop. Med. Hyg.*, **20,** 84.

—— and —— (1976). *Am. trop. Med. Parasit.*, **70,** 109.

——, ——, WOODSTOCK, L., and PILGRIM, V. (1977). *Ann. Trop. Med. Parasit.*, **71,** 197.

COUTINHO, A. (1968). *Am. J. Med.*, **44,** 547.

DA SILVA, L. C., DE BRITO, T., CAMARGO, M. E., DE BONI, D. R., LOPES, J. D., and GUNJI, J. (1970). *Bull. Wld Hlth Org.*, **42,** 907.

DAVEY, W. W. (1968). *Companion to Surgery in Africa*. pp. 74 and 195. Churchill Livingstone; Edinburgh, London and New York.

EL-GHOLMY, A., NABAWY, M., GABR, M., AIDAROS, S., and OMAR, A. (1955). *J. trop. Med. Hyg.*, **58,** 25.

FARID, Z., BASSILY, S., YOUNG, S., EL MASRY, N. A., and HASSAN, A. (1973). *Ann. trop. Med. Parasit.*, **67,** 233.

——, Smith, J. H., Bassily, S., and Sparks, H. A. (1972). *Br. med. J.*, **2,** 88.
Gane, N. F. C. (1971). *Cent. Afr. med. J.*, **17,** 108.
Goodgame, R. W. and Bartholomew, R. K. (1978). *Am. J. trop. Med. Hyg.*, **27,** 779.
Hansen, D. P. and Daly, D. S. (1978). *Am. J. trop. Med. Hyg.*, **27,** 197.
Hashem, M. (1947). *J. Egypt med. Ass.*, **30,** 48.
Hatchuel, W. (1978). *S. Afr. med. J.* **54,** 808.
Higazi, A. M., Fahmy, A. R., and Kaddah, S. (1960). *J. Egypt Med. Ass.*, **43,** 923.
Homeida, M., Salih, S. Y., and Branch, R. A. (1978). *Gut*, **19,** 808.
Hutt, M. S. R. (1971). *Trans. R. Soc. trop. Med. Hyg.*, **65,** 273.
Kallmeyer, J. C., Macsearraigh, E. T. M., and Godlonton, J. D. (1977). *S. Afr. med. J.*, **51,** 109.
Koppisch, E. (1941). *Puerto Rico J. publ. Hlth trop. Med.*, **16,** 395.
Lehman, J. S., Mott, K. E., Morrow, R. H., Muniz, T. M. and Boyer, M. H. (1976). *Am. J. trop. Med. Hyg.*, **25,** 285.
Mahmoud, A. A. (1977). *New Engl. J. Med.*, **297,** 1329.
Malik, M. O. A., Satir, A. A., Veress, B., and El Hassan, A. M. (1975). *E. Afr. med. J.*, **52,** 183.
Miller, J. R. M. (1967). *E. Afr. med. J.*, **44,** 376.
Miyake, M. (1967). In *Bilharziasis* (ed. F. K. Mostofi). p. 140. Springer-Verlag, New York.
Mousa, A. H. and El-Garem, A. (1959). *J. Egypt med. Ass.*, **42,** 444.
Omer, A. H. S. (1978). *Tropical Doctor*, **8,** 3.
Ongom, V. L. and Bradley, D. J. (1972). *Trans. R. Soc. trop. Med. Hyg.*, **66,** 835.
Oostburg, B. F. J. (1972). *Trop. geogr. Med.*, **24,** 148.
Pelley, R. P. and Pelley, R. J. (1976). In *Biochemistry of parasites and host parasite relationships* (ed. H. Van den Bosshe). p. 283. Elsevier (North Holland Biomedical Press): Amsterdam.
Salah, L. A., Kheireldin, A. A., Mansour, M. M., and Hussein, F. (1976). *J. trop. Med. Hyg.*, **79,** 270.
Siongok, T. K. A., Mahmoud, A. A. F., Ouma, J. H., Warren, K. S., Muller, A. S., Handa, A. K., and Houser, H. B. (1976). *Am. J. trop. Med. Hyg.*, **25,** 273.
Sulit, Y. S. M., Domingo, E. O., Dalmacio-Cruz, A. E., De Peralta, D. S., and Imperial, E. S. (1964). *J. Philipp. Med. Ass.*, **40,** 1021.
Symmers, W. St. C. (1904). *J. Path. Bact.*, **9,** 237.
Van den Bossche, H. (1978). *Nature, Lond.*, **273,** 626.
Warren, K. S. (1972). *Trans. R. Soc. trop. Med. Hyg.*, **66,** 417.
—— (1978a). *Gut*, **19,** 572.
—— (1978b). *Nature, Lond.*, **273,** 609.
—— and Rebouças, G. (1964). *New Engl. J. Med.*, **271,** 921.
——, ——, and Baptista, A. G. (1965). *Ann. intern. Med.*, **62,** 1113.
WHO Reports on Schistosomal drugs (1972). *Boln Of. sanit. pan-am*, **6,** 82.
Wicks, A. C. B., Thomas, G. E., and Clain, D. J. (1975). *Br. med. J.*, **4,** 259.
Wroblewski, F. and La Due, J. S. (1956). *Ann. intern. Med.*, **45,** 801.

11

The portal venous system and portal hypertension (PH) in the tropics

TABLE 11.1 summarizes the main diseases responsible for portal hypertension (Miller, 1972; Sherlock, 1975; 1978). All causes may be encountered in tropical countries, but by far the commonest are macronodular cirrhosis (Chapter 8), schistosomal hepatic fibrosis (caused by *Schistosoma mansoni* and *S. japonicum*, and less commonly *S. intercalatum*) (Chapter 10) and the tropical splenomegaly syndrome (TSS) (Chapter 16); in the latter condition there is a greatly increased portal blood-flow.

TABLE 11.1. *Classification of portal hypertension.*

Site of pathology	*Cause*
Prehepatic	*† Tropical splenomegaly syndrome (TSS) (increased portal blood flow)
	*† Portal vein occlusion
	† Splenic vein occlusion
Intrahepatic	*† Schistosomal ('pipe-stem') fibrosis
	* Cirrhosis (usually macronodular)
	* Veno-occlusive disease (VOD)
	† Congenital hepatic fibrosis
Posthepatic	Cardiac failure (usually due to chronic rheumatic cardiac disease)
	* Endomyocardial fibrosis (right-sided)
	* Constrictive pericarditis
	Inferior venacaval obstruction
	Hepatic vein thrombosis (Budd–Chiari syndrome)

* causes which are commonly encountered in tropical countries.
† portal hypertension is predominantly presinusoidal.

The livers of many indigenous people in the tropics contain evidence of portal inflammation with mild fibrosis (Chapter 5); occasionally the degree of fibrosis may be severe and portal hypertension may ensue (McGovern and Kariks, 1966; Powell and McGovern, 1976). In a small proportion of patients, portal hypertension has been reported in the presence of normal liver structure and function (Polish, Christie, Cohen, and Sullivan, 1962; Siderys and Vellios, 1964); splenic pulp pressure is increased but hepatic wedge pressure is normal. The cause is probably similar to that in TSS and is related to increased portal blood-flow due to splenic and possibly other factors.

Ramalingaswami, Wig, and Sama (1962) described a group of patients with portal hypertension in India, in whom there was no clinical or histological evidence of cirrhosis. In India also, Boyer, Sen Gupta, Biswas, Pal, Mallick, Iber, and Basu (1967) have described 21 cases of idiopathic portal hypertension (noncirrhotic portal fibrosis) in which there was portal fibrosis associated with intra- and extra-hepatic portal vein sclerosis; splenovenograms showed changes similar to those in schistosomal pipe-stem fibrosis and TSS. However there was no hepatic sinusoidal lymphocytosis. Hypersplenism is not a feature of this condition. Nayak and Ramalingaswami (1969) have described an obliterative occlusion of the portal veins unassociated with cirrhosis or extrahepatic portal vein obstruction in India. There is marked subendothelial thickening of the larger intrahepatic branches of the portal vein. A patchy segmental distribution leads to portal hypertension. The aetiology is unknown, but the disease seems to be relatively common in India. Thrombosis and sclerosis of the portal system take place in Hong Kong in both patients with gross splenomegaly and also cirrhosis (Hou and McFadzean, 1965). The cause (or causes) of the noncirrhotic liver disease in India which gives rise to portal hypertension is unknown; 'local' medicines, opium obtained illegally, and arsenic in drinking water have all been incriminated (Datta, 1976; 1977; Datta and Kaul, 1976).

Recently, reversible portal hypertension in association with an amoebic liver abscess has been reported from India (Naik, Achar, and Mehta, 1978) (Chapter 12).

11.1. Aetiology of PH

11.1.1. Prehepatic PH

In the tropical splenomegaly syndrome (Chapter 16), the degree of elevation of portal pressure varies greatly from case to case, and is largely the result of a greatly increased splenic blood-flow (Leather, 1961; Marsden, Hutt, Wilks, Voller, Blackman, Shah, O'Connor, Hamilton, Banwell, and Lunn, 1965). There is also sometimes an increase in presinusoidal resistance (Williams, Parsonson, Somers, and Hamilton, 1966). That condition is probably malarial in origin. Liver-biopsy histology shows a sinusoidal lymphocytosis (with mature lymphocytes) which might be partly responsible for the portal hypertension (Butler, Boyer, Farrell, Goldstein, Schaeffer, and Loan, 1973); portal hypertension cannot however be correlated with the intensity of the sinusoidal lymphocytosis (Leather, 1961; Williams, *et al.*, 1966). Other causes of splenomegaly such as cirrhosis, schistosomiasis, blood dyscrasias, etc, must be excluded. In TSS, haemolytic jaundice, anaemia, and hypoalbuminaemia, which results from the plasma volume expansion, may be present (Pryor, 1967).

In many parts of the tropics, portal vein thrombosis with normal liver histology is common (Miller, 1967); in both India (Basu and Aikat, 1963) and Nairobi, Kenya (Bagshawe and Miller, 1972) high incidence rates have been recorded. Working in Nairobi, Kenya, Bagshawe and Miller (1970) demonstrated that oesophageal varices were associated with portal vein thrombosis in approximately 50 per cent of patients studied; percutaneous splenic venography was used for diagnosis. Although no clear cause has been found it seems probable that umbilical sepsis which is extremely common in some parts of Africa (especially west Africa) is a common predisposing factor. In some parts of west Africa, cow dung is rubbed into the umbilicus after detachment of the umbilical cord; pyogenic liver infections, tetanus, and umbilical hernia are other sequelae. Severe dehydrating diseases such as dysentery, cholera, and typhoid have also been implicated. Portal venous obstruction is also not uncommonly a result of compression of the vein by an hepatocellular carcinoma (Chapter 9). The condition may be diagnosed at any age and may be associated with bleeding from oesophageal varices (Fig. 11.1).

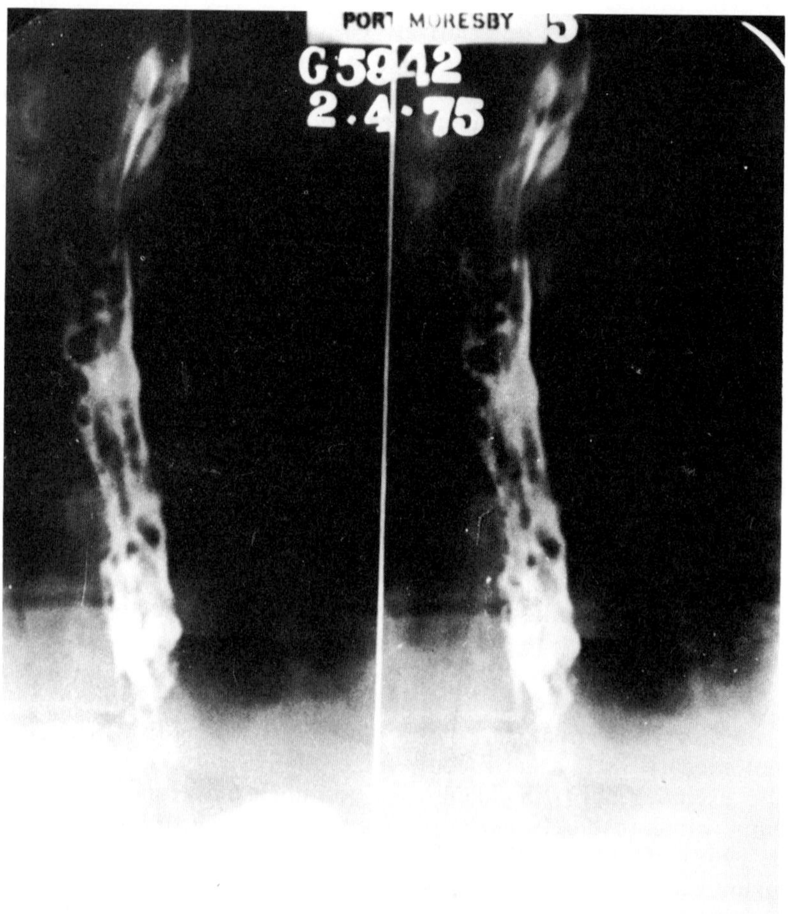

FIG. 11.1. Barium-swallow in a 21-year-old Papua New Guinean man who was admitted with a massive haematemesis; gross oesophageal varices are shown. A splenovenogram showed numerous anastomoses but the portal vein could not be demonstrated. The diagnosis was hepatic vein thrombosis.

11.1.2. Intrahepatic PH

In this form of portal hypertension, liver failure sometimes follows a haematemesis, which is not the case with the prehepatic type. In Africa and Asia, cirrhosis and schistosomal fibrosis, and in the Caribbean, veno-occlusive disease, are the most common causes of intrahepatic PH.

In cirrhosis, regenerating nodules of liver tissue distort the portal vascular bed; venous outflow from the hepatic sinusoids is therefore obstructed giving rise to postsinusoidal hypertension. Shunting between the tributaries of the hepatic artery and portal vein, and the portal vein and hepatic vein occurs.

The extent of the 'pipe-stem' fibrosis in schistosomiasis depends on many factors (Chapter 10) but especially parasite load and duration of infection. Ova are present in the terminal radicles of the portal vein and are initially surrounded by a granulomatous reaction; hepatic fibrosis is a direct sequel. A fibrous tree, not unlike the baobab tree (Davey, 1968) is then formed. Because the process develops very slowly there is time for large collateral portal-systemic anastomoses to develop; that possibly accounts for the low incidence of haematemeses in that condition. Nevertheless blood flow is impeded and that gives rise to presinusoidal hypertension. Hepatocellular dysfunction is very much less severe than in cirrhosis, with comparable levels of portal hypertension.

Intrahepatic portal hypertension is usually accompanied by features of chronic liver disease, e.g. hepatic encephalopathy, gynaecomastia, jaundice, oedema, and ascites. Transient ascites and oedema can occur after haemorrhage in the absence of chronic liver disease. Dilated anterior abdominal veins, in which blood flows away from the umbilicus, are indicative of intrahepatic portal hypertension, but that sign is rarely diagnostic.

11.1.3. Posthepatic PH

Posthepatic portal hypertension is associated with hepatomegaly, which is often tender. Rightsided endomyocardial fibrosis and constrictive pericarditis (Basu, 1965) are relatively common causes in tropical countries (Chapter 8). If the underlying cause is cardiac disease, the jugular venous pressure is raised and electrocardiographic and radiological abnormalities are present. Inferior venacaval obstruction causes gross oedema of the lower limbs and anterior abdominal wall.

11.2. Presentation of PH

Splenomegaly, which may be gross, results from portal hypertension; the degree of splenic enlargement is not directly related however to the level of hypertension. Consequences of hypersplenism—anaemia, leucopenia, and thrombocytopenia—develop *pari passu* with the splenic hypertrophy. Three major complications are attributable to portal hypertension: (i) haemorrhage from oesophageal varices, (ii) hepatic encephalopathy, and (iii) in the presence of hypoalbuminaemia, which occurs in cirrhosis, ascites develops.

In areas of Africa and Asia where other causes of splenomegaly, such as visceral leishmaniasis, are common, mere palpation of the spleen (which is of value in arriving at a clinical diagnosis of portal hypertension in a temperate area) will not help in deciding whether the haematemesis is the result of portal hypertension (Shaper, 1969).

Whereas liver size in primary portal vein thrombosis is normal, in cirrhosis it is small. Schistosomiasis is usually associated with a large liver. In TSS a smooth hepatomegaly, which usually involves the left lobe more than the right, is present.

Development of collateral vessels is less common in TSS than when other causes of portal hypertension exist.

Other causes of haematemesis must be considered in the differential diagnosis; the incidence of peptic ulcer with subsequent haemorrhage varies in different parts of the tropics (Chapter 4).

11.3. Investigation of PH

A barium-swallow outlines oesophageal varices, which show up as space-filling defects in the oesophagus (Fig. 11.1). These are common in both cirrhosis, and portal vein obstruction. Oesophagoscopy gives a similar positivity rate compared with barium-swallow. Portal hypertension is confirmed by demonstrating a raised intrasplenic pressure, or the demonstration of an abnormal portal venogram, usually with abdominal collaterals.

Measurement of intrasplenic pressure closely correlates with portal vein pressure. Basic precautions, i.e. measurement of prothrombin time and platelet count, must however be taken before the procedure is carried out. Deep jaundice is also a contraindication. After measurement of the splenic pressure, splenic venography can be performed. Bagshawe and Miller (1972) have stressed that highly sophisticated apparatus is not essential for splenic manometry and venography; they have given details of simple equipment which they have found to be of value. However, sterile precautions must be strictly adhered to. Normal values for portal venous pressure have been given for Indians in Calcutta (Boyer, Sen Gupta, Biswas, Pal, Mallick, Iber, and Basu, 1967) and Africans in Nairobi (Miller, 1967). More sophisticated procedures, such as selective visceral angiography, umbilical vein catheterization, transhepatic catheterization, and recently developed ultrasound procedures are very rarely available in the third world.

Having established the presence of portal hypertension, the cause must be determined. Biochemical tests of liver function assist in the differentiation between intra- and posthepatic portal hypertension, and portal vein obstruction. Liver-biopsy with the Menghini needle often gives valuable information. Both schistosomiasis and cirrhosis can usually be diagnosed by that technique, although sampling-error is important, especially in hepatic schistosomiasis. Sinusoidal lymphocytosis with Kupffer cell hypertrophy and hyperplasia strongly suggests the tropical splenomegaly syndrome (Chapter 16). Normal liver-biopsy histology in the presence of portal hypertension strongly suggests portal-vein obstruction.

11.4. Treatment of PH

Management of PH has been summarized by Sherlock (1978). If it is available, fibre-optic oesophagogastroduodenoscopy will usually visualize the site of bleeding; although varices are the most frequent cause, acute mucosal ulcers may be responsible. Acute haemorrhage is managed by blood replacement; transfusion is lifesaving and must be rapid and adequate. Blood pressure and pulse rate are used to estimate the quantity required. Sedation with chlorpromazine or phenobarbitone should usually be avoided if possible; both are moderately safe in the presence of compensated liver disease, but not following haemorrhage. Intramuscular vitamin K and oral cimetidine should be given if available to attempt correction of the bleeding diathesis and to reduce gastric bleeding, respectively. Although haemorrhage from oesophageal varices may stop spontaneously, other measures are frequently required. 20 units of vasopressin ('Pitressin') (posterior pituitary extract) in 100 ml glucose given intravenously over 10 minutes causes constriction of the mesenteric arterial bed; unfortunately its efficacy declines with repeated administration. A continuous infusion of 40 units over 60 min may also be used. Because it causes coronary artery constriction, vasopressin is potentially dangerous in elderly people; in any case its vasoconstrictive effect often gives rise to faintness and defaecation, or vomiting. Alternatively, the Sengstaken tube (gastro-oesophageal tamponade), by producing pressure on the bleeding varices, may be used. Again it is unpleasant for the patient, but is usually effective, and is of particular value while transporting a patient over a considerable distance.

Occasionally surgery is necessary to reduce portal venous pressure. In cirrhosis, the patient's condition is usually poor and his liver function abnormal; there is therefore a high postoperative mortality rate. Hepatocellular function deteriorates after portacaval anastomosis. Subsequent hepatic encephalopathy is more severe after the side-to-side than the end-to-side shunt (Iwatsuki, Mikkelsen, Redeker, Reynolds, and Turrill, 1971). Portal blood may be important in preserving normal hepatocyte function; it is possible that insulin and glucagon are the responsible hormones (Bucher and Swaffield, 1975; Starzl, Watanabe, Porter, and Putnam, 1976). However, if they are in fact important, their mode of action is unclear. Emergency and prophylactic portacaval shunt operations are not currently in favour. Emergency ligation, or injection, of oesophageal varices, or oesophageal transection may be necessary, if other measures have failed. Splenectomy should not be carried out. In hepatic schistosomiasis, hepatocellular function should theoretically be preserved, and surgery would be expected to be tolerated much better than in cirrhosis; in practice severe encephalopathy is not uncommon, however (Chapter 10). In portal vein thrombosis no surgical procedure is of proven value; bleeding is however sometimes self-limiting; the only possible operations are splenorenal or mesocaval shunts, thrombosis of which is common. Elective surgery is best undertaken at a later date if a surgeon accomplished at the procedure, and suitable operating and postoperative conditions are available. Portacaval shunting is indicated in patients with intrahepatic portal hypertension who have already bled from proven varices, after a patent portal vein has been demonstrated. Age and profession of the patient, liver function ('active' liver-cell disease is a contraindication), and the type of cirrhosis must be taken into account; alcoholic has a better prognosis than postviral cirrhosis, if alcohol intake is stopped. Distance of the patient from a centre where emergency treatment can be carried out is also an important factor. The ideal candidate for a shunt is under 40 years old, has had at least one major bleed, has no evidence of jaundice, encephalopathy or ascites, and good biochemical evidence of liver function with minimal evidence of 'activity'.

Hepatic encephalopathy should be treated with a low protein, or protein-free diet, aspiration of blood from the stomach, and oral neomycin, one gram four hourly. Purgation is of value. Oral lactulose has been successfully used (Zeegen, Drinkwater, Fenton, Vince, and Dawson, 1970), although the mode of action is not yet understood (Conn, 1978). Lactulose ('Duphalac'), 30 to 50 ml (20·1 to 33·5 g) thrice daily should be tried; the size of the dose may be limited by diarrhoea. Morphine and other drugs metabolized by the liver must obviously be avoided.

References

Bagshawe, A. and Miller, J. R. M. (1970). *E. Afr. med. J.*, **47,** 185.

—— and —— (1972). In *Medicine in a Tropical environment* (ed. A. G. Shaper, J. W. Kibukamusoke, and M. S. R. Hutt). p. 409. B.M.A., London.

Basu, A. K. (1965). (ed.) In *Tropical Surgery.* p. 172. Butterworths, London.

—— and Aikat, B. K. (1963). *Tropical splenomegaly.* p. 107. Butterworths, London.

Boyer, J. L., Sen Gupta, K. P., Biswas, S. K., Pal, N. C., Mallick, K. C. B., Iber, F. L., and Basu, A. K. (1967). *Ann. intern. Med.*, **66,** 41.

Bucher, N. L. R. and Swaffield, M. N. (1975). *Proc. natn. Acad. Sci. U.S.A.*, **72,** 1157.

Butler, T., Boyer, J. L., Farrell, R. L., Goldstein, H. M., Schaeffer, B. T. and Loan, N. T. (1973). *Am. J. trop. Med. Hyg.*, **22,** 6.

Conn, H. O. (1978). *Gastroenterology*, **74,** 624.

Datta, D. V. (1976). *Lancet*, **1,** 433.

—— (1977). *Lancet*, **1,** 484.

—— and Kaul, M. K. (1976). *Jl. Ass. Physns India*, **24,** 599.

Davey, W. W. (1968). *Companion to Surgery in Africa.* p. 201. E. and S. Livingstone. Edinburgh and London.

Hou, P. C. and McFadzean, A. J. S. (1965). *J. Path. Bact.*, **89,** 473.

Iwatsuki, S., Mikkelsen, W. P., Redeker, A. G., Reynolds, J. B., and Turrill, F. L. (1971). *Ann. Surg.*, **178,** 65.

Leather, H. M. (1961). *Br. med. J.*, **1,** 15.

McGovern, V. J. and Kariks, J. (1966). *Med. J. Aust.*, **2,** 441.

Marsden, P. D., Hutt, M. S. R., Wilks, N. E., Voller, A., Blackman, V., Shah, K. K. O'Conner, D. H., Hamilton, P. J. S., Banwell, J. G., and Lunn, H. F. (1965). *Br. med. J.*, **1,** 89.

Miller, J. R. M. (1967). *E. Afr. med. J.*, **44,** 376.

—— (1972). *E. Afr. med. J.*, **49,** 243.

Naik, S. R., Achar, B. G., and Mehta, S. K. (1978). *J. trop. Med. Hyg.*, **81,** 116.

Nayak, N. C. and Ramalingaswami, V. (1969). *Archs Path.*, **87,** 359.

Polish, E., Christie, J., Cohen, A., and Sullivan, B. (1962). *Ann. intern. Med.*, **56,** 624.

Powell, K. C. and McGovern, V. J. (1976). *Papua New Guin. med. J.*, **19,** 140.

Pryor, D. S. (1967). *Q. Jl. Med.*, **36,** 337.

Ramalingaswami, V., Wig, K. L., and Sama, S. K. (1962). *Archs intern. Med.*, **110,** 350.

Shaper, A. G. (1969). *Trans. R. Soc. trop. Med. Hyg.*, **63,** 206.

Sherlock, S. (1975). *Diseases of the liver and biliary system.* 5th ed. p. 150. Blackwell, Oxford, London, Edinburgh, and Melbourne.

—— (1978). *Gut,* **19,** 70.

Siderys, H. and Vellios, F. (1964). *Am. J. Surg.*, **108,** 785.

Starzl, T. E., Watanabe, K., Porter, K. A., and Putnam, C. W. (1976). *Lancet*, **1**, 821.
Williams, R., Parsonson, A., Somers K., and Hamilton P. J. S. (1966). *Lancet*, **1**, 329.
Zeegen, R., Drinkwater, J. E., Fenton, J. C. B., Vince, A., and Dawson, A. M. (1970). *Q. Jl. Med.*, **39**, 245.

12

Space-occupying hepatic lesions: amoebic and pyogenic abscess, and hydatid disease

12.1. Amoebic abscess of the liver (AAL)

HEPATIC amoebiasis is the most common systemic complication of the intestinal form of the disease (Chapter 25) (Ochsner and De Bakey, 1943; Wilmot, 1962; Reynolds, 1971). Reports have been made from most tropical countries including Sierra Leone (Rowland, 1963), Kenya (Whitaker, 1963), Zimbabwe Rhodesia (Gelfand, 1966), Papua New Guinea (Rhodes, 1972), and the Caribbean (Grell and Watty, 1978). In most cases intestinal symptoms are absent and presentation is with a sick patient with a large tender liver. Only acute awareness of the condition in all patients with right hypochondrial tenderness and tender hepatomegaly, especially if there is a history of tropical exposure, will lead to early diagnosis and the forestalling of complications and a subsequent high mortality rate (Archampong, 1977). The condition can present several decades after a tropical exposure.

12.1.1. Presentation of AAL

The clinical signs of this disease have been summarized by Paul (1960) and Adi (1965). Throughout the world there is a highly significant male sex predominance, often as great as 8:1. About two-thirds to three-quarters of abscesses are single, and the remainder multiple. The right lobe is affected approximately four times as often as the left. Approximately 50 per cent of patients have had amoebic dysentery in the previous month (Davey, 1968), but far fewer have dysentery at the time of presentation. Severe trauma over the liver may occasionally be followed by an amoebic abscess of the right lobe (Ramachandran and Edwards, 1978).

The patient is usually obviously ill, and there is a high fever, although in chronic cases this may be low-grade. Jaundice is overall uncommon; however, two studies have shown incidence rates as high as 29 (Salako, 1967) and 15 per cent (Vakil, Mehta and Desai, 1970), respectively. In Swaziland, two of 23 cases seen over a 12-month period were jaundiced (Mokhobo, 1971). In long-standing cases, anaemia is common. Local signs are absent until the abscess reaches the surface of the liver; when that occurs, pain associated with tender hepatomegaly is usually present. Signs in the right lower chest, consisting of elevation of the diaphragm, frequently with pleural effusion and atelectasis, are common. Abnormal physical signs in the right lower chest in anyone who has had exposure to the tropics or subtropics should strongly suggest amoebic liver abscess.

Although the majority of cases behave in this classical way, atypical manifestations are not uncommon (Vakil, *et al.*, 1970); hepatocellular and cholestatic jaundice, and hepatic coma and precoma may confuse the clinical presentation.

Corticosteroids have a deleterious effect in patients with hepatic amoebiasis (Stuiver and Goud, 1978); in that study, three patients had progressive fulminating hepatic disease after prednisone had been mistakenly given for liver disease which was ultimately shown to be amoebic. A similar problem has been reported from Egypt (El-Hennawy and Abd-Rabbo, 1978); in that study eight of 12 cases of hepatic amoebiasis had received corticosteroids within the previous three months.

Differentiation on clinical grounds from hepatoma may be extremely difficult. Both lesions occur commonly in similar geographical settings and physical findings can be astonishingly similar. If there is doubt about the diagnosis, there is nothing to be lost, and everything to be gained by giving a course of metronidazole (see below).

Amoebic hepatitis. This is a clinical entity, and there is little concrete evidence of a genuine hepatitis caused by *Entamoeba histolytica*; it seems, however, reasonable to assume that that does occur before the formation of an abscess. Most physicians who have worked in tropical countries are aware of a clinical situation where there is a large tender liver, fever, and leucocytosis; there is no evidence of abscess formation, and that responds dramatically to anti-amoebic agents.

Doxiades, Candreviotis, Tiliakos, and Polymeropoulos (1961) have demonstrated amoebae in liver-biopsy sections from patients with 'chronic diffuse non-suppurative amoebic hepatitis', without a well developed abscess; however other investigators have failed to provide convincing evidence of the presence of amoebae, and have found only Kupffer cell hypertrophy and hyperplasia, and portal infiltration with chronic inflammatory cells.

12.1.2. Aetiology and pathology of AAL

Entry of *E. histolytica* trophozoites into the portal venous radicles gives rise to hepatic metastases; they also enter the lymphatics but are presumably destroyed in the lymph glands, for they cannot be demonstrated entering the blood stream via the thoracic duct. There are however no records of amoebae being detected in the abdominal lymph glands (Edington and Gilles, 1976). Using isoenzyme electrophoresis, Sargeaunt, Williams, and Grene (1978) have demonstrated that virulent (invasive) strains of *E. histolytica* can be distinguished from avirulent strains by a constant positioning of the phosphoglucomutase band (*Lancet*, 1979). A spherical liver abscess, usually in the right lobe, is formed (Fig. 12.1) which may contain many litres of 'anchovy sauce' pus. Multiple abscesses are not uncommon. It is unusual to find an amoebic abscess in a cirrhotic liver.

Histologically, there is lysis of hepatocytes, mainly in the periportal region and necrosis follows. The pus is chocolate-coloured, due to a mixing of portal

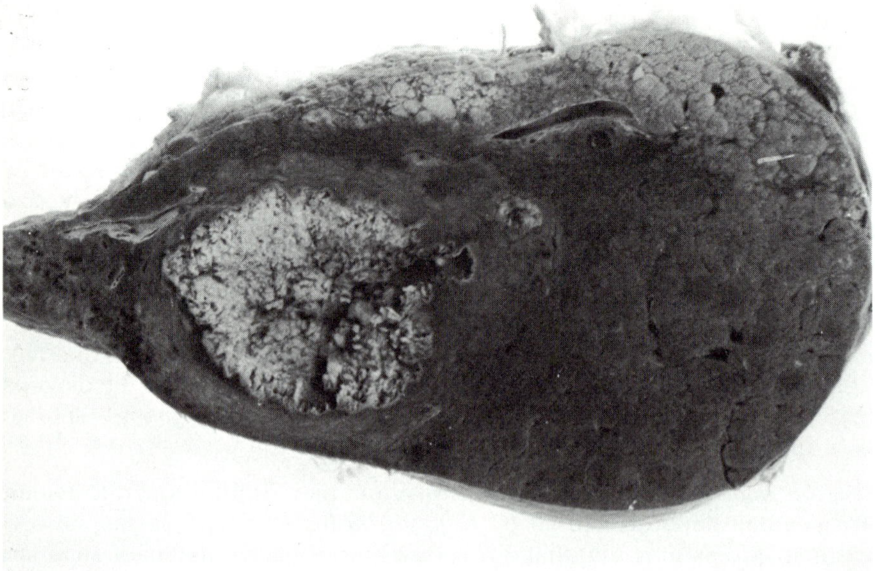

FIG. 12.1. Liver-section from a Papua New Guinean man. An amoebic abscess, approximately 10 cm in diameter is shown; the remainder of the liver shows a coarse macronodular cirrhosis. Death was caused by rupture of the abscess into the peritoneal cavity.

blood with bile and a few pus cells, and is sterile. The periphery of the abscess is irregular and shaggy and consists of stroma and layers of compressed liver parenchyma; there is little fibrous tissue formation, but monocytes, plasma cells, lymphocytes, and fibroblasts are present. *E. histolytica* are often found in large numbers in the tissue at the periphery of the lesion. Trophozoites, usually containing ingested red blood-cells, may also be found in the pus if it is examined immediately after aspiration. Secondary infection may occur, especially after surgical intervention; the pus then becomes yellow, creamy, or green and amoebae are usually very difficult to identify; *Escherichia coli, Bacillus pyocyaneus*, and *Salmonella typhi* have all been identified as secondary invaders. It has been suggested, but not proved, that both alcohol and malnutrition may predispose to invasion of the tissues by *E. histolytica.*

12.1.3. Complications of AAL

Complications of hepatic amoebiasis have been summarized by Wilmot (1962) and Adi (1966). Direct extension to the right pleural cavity or base of the right lung is common; the diaphragm is raised and its movements restricted. The major complications are however the results of rupture of an abscess. Rupture to the right lower chest, with pleural effusion and atelectasis, is not uncommon; 'anchovy sauce' may be coughed up if a bronchus is eroded; rupture to the left base is relatively uncommon. Formation of a subphrenic abscess is a possibility, but is unusual.

A serous pericardial effusion may be present (McLeod, Wilmot, and Powell, 1966); however, if rupture to the pericardial sac from a left-lobe abscess occurs, an amoebic pericarditis which has a bad prognosis may result (McLeod *et al.*, 1966). There is usually thickening of the parietal pericardium, and thick greenish-yellow material is present between the layers, the surfaces of which are yellowish-grey and granular. Amorphous necrotic tissue, containing amoebae and monocytes and lymphocytes, may be present. The pericardium subsequently undergoes coagulative necrosis, and granulation and fibrous tissue are formed. Pericarditis has been reported in 7·5 per cent of patients with hepatic abscess in one series (Paulley, 1965). Acute tamponade may be immediately fatal. Constrictive pericarditis may occur as a chronic complication.

Rupture into the peritoneal cavity is often followed by severe shock, hypotension, and death (Singha, 1959); however 'silent' perforations with little reaction may also occur. Occasionally a tender localized abscess may form within the peritoneal cavity.

Any viscus may in fact be involved, including the stomach, intestine, and hepatic vein; venacaval thrombosis is rare. Rupture through the skin is a further possibility. Distant spread to the brain is a rare complication. Other complications consist of massive haemorrhage and secondary infection, frequently by bacteria introduced during aspiration.

Rarely, portal hypertension (Chapter 11) which is reversible after treatment, may occur (Naik, Achar, and Mehta, 1978); in that study a 58-year-old man had radiological and endoscopic evidence of oesophageal varices associated with an amoebic liver abscess, which resolved after treatment with metronidazole.

12.1.4. Investigation of AAL

Aspiration of 'pus' in which amoebae can be identified is the only sure way of diagnosis (Krogstad, Spencer, Healy, Gleason, Sexton, and Herron, 1978). An indirect immunofluorescent technique has been applied to the demonstration of *E. histolytica* in tissue (Parelkar, Stamm, and Hill, 1971). Stools show amoebae in only about 10 per cent of cases. A polymorphonuclear leucocytosis is usual. A mild anaemia is common. Liver-function tests give variable results; serum bilirubin is rarely more than 34 μmol per l (Salako, 1967); serum alkaline phosphatase and transaminases may be mildly increased. Rarely, the alkaline phosphatase concentration is markedly elevated. In a study of liver function tests in 11 patients with hepatic amoebiasis (El-Zayadi, Hartmann, and Mohr, 1976), serum bilirubin was raised in one, alkaline phosphatase in seven, transaminases in two, and lactic dehydrogenase (LDH) in seven; all of those with an abscess had raised LDH concentrations. All had hypoalbuminaemia, and elevated serum α_2 globulin concentrations. Defective B_{12} absorption has been reported (Devakul, Areekul, and Viravan, 1967).

Radiology is often of value. The right diaphragm may be raised with restricted movement; localized bulging is occasionally apparent. A small pleural effusion or basal atelectasis may be present. There may be pulmonary consolidation, with or without abscess formation. Amoebic lung abscesses are usually thick-walled, and in the anterior basal segment of the right lower lobe.

Aspiration of the abscess, with air or lipiodol replacement, splenic venography, and induction of a pneumoperitoneum (Ellman, McLeod, and Powell, 1965) are also of value.

Isotope scanning of the liver (de Dominicis, Balastrieri, and Assumma, 1966) and ultrasonic sounding (Vicary, 1977) are of value in localizing an abscess, if those procedures are available.

Serological tests. Serology is of great value in the diagnosis of hepatic amoebiasis, as it is in all other forms of *invasive* amoebic disease (Wéry-Paskoff, Renoirte, and Wéry, 1974; *Br. med. J.*, 1978). The complement-fixation test is positive in 100 per cent of cases of hepatic amoebic abscess (Robinson, 1972); all controls give negative results and titres fall more rapidly after treatment of the disease than do haemagglutination titres. The indirect haemagglutination test (Kessel, Lewis, Pasquel, and Turner, 1965) is positive in 100 per cent of patients with amoebic liver abscess; unfortunately however, titres are positive many years after treatment. The amoebic gel-diffusion test (Powell, Maddison, Wilmot, and Elsdon-Dew, 1965) is positive in 96 per cent of patients with amoebic liver abscess; unfortunately it is also positive in 15 per cent of Africans with other diseases. A fluorescent-antibody test (FAT) (Parelkar and Stamm, 1973) in which there is fluorescence of cultured *E. histolytica* when they are exposed to serum from a patient with invasive amoebic disease is of value in acute and chronic cases; however there seem to be some false positive results. A simple latex test (Morris, Powell, and Elsdon-Dew, 1970) presented as a commercial kit ('Serameba') is also of value (Stamm, Ashley, and Parelkar, 1973). Thus, several serological tests remain positive long after successful treatment, and are of limited value in assessing cure (Krupp and Powell, 1971); the gel-diffusion test is a better guide than the FAT. It seems likely that within the next few years the enzyme-linked immunosorbent assay (ELISA) technique will add to greater sensitivity in detection of serum *E. histolytica* antibody (Krogstad, Spencer, and Healy, 1978).

Rarely the abscess is surrounded by a thick fibrous wall (Abioye, 1976); in that case not only are all immunodiagnostic tests negative, but there is a lack of response to antiamoebic agents. The explanation presumably lies in the impenetrability of blood through the fibrous tissue.

12.1.5. Treatment of AAL

Treatment has become fairly straightforward since the discovery that metronidazole ('Flagyl') is an effective and safe antiamoebic agent; however, in patients who have contracted their disease in India a high failure rate, using that agent, has been reported (Chapter 25). Metronidazole should be given as an oral dose of 800 mg three times daily for 10 days. However, response to a course of metronidazole should not be accepted as proof of amoebic disease because that agent is effective against enterococci as well as *E. histolytica* (Archampong, 1977). Mild side-effects, such as nausea and lethargy, are common. The drug has an antabuse action and the patient should be warned not to take alcohol while the treatment is taking place. Powell, Wilmot, and Elsdon-Dew (1969) reported a 100 per cent cure rate with metronidazole in amoebic liver disease; however Vigg, Shay, and Lingam (1971) gave a rate of only 70 per cent. A recently used alternative to metronidazole, tinidazole (Miller, Howes, and English, 1969) has also given promising results (Islam and Hasan, 1978); 94 per cent of a tinidazole treated group and 80 per cent of a metronidazole treated group were cured of the disease. A 100 per cent cure rate using 2g daily for two to three days in 35 patients has also been reported (Quaderi, Rahman, Rahman, and Islam, 1978). In children with amoebic liver abscesses tinidazole seems to be an effective agent (Scragg and Proctor, 1977); 23 of 25 children were cured with a daily dose of 50 mg per kg bodyweight for three or five days. However, two required surgical drainage followed by other amoebicides and one of them died from bronchopneumonia. Tinidazole has the advantage of being given as a single oral dose daily. Alternatively one of the older regimes which include emetine, chloroquine, and tetracycline may be given; the role of the latter agent has never been established in an uninfected abscess. If emetine (which is cardiotoxic) is used, electrocardiographic monitoring before and during treatment is an advantage; blood pressure recordings should also be made.

If the abscess is large and the patient severely ill, needle aspiration is indicated; however even with large abscesses, resolution usually occurs after a course of metronidazole (Krogstad, Spencer, and Healy, 1978). Davey (1968) has summarized the indications for *aspiration* as follows: (i) a large tender liver with lack of response to anti-amoebic agents, (ii) localized signs of surface inflammation—swelling, oedema, tenderness, shiny skin, and fluctuation, and (iii) changes at the right lung base, especially elevation of the diaphragm. Small abscesses do not as a rule require evacuation, and resolve with metronidazole; however, if there is a clinical indication of impending rupture, aspiration should be undertaken. Complications of aspiration are secondary infection and haemorrhage. A space-occupying defect on liver 'scan' often persists for many months. Using such a technique, Sheehy, Parmley, Johnston, and Boyce (1968) reported that up to one year was required for complete resolution. Bhasin, Mittal, Shrivastava, Bhardwaj, Sachdev, and Gupta (1978), using a micro-opaque barium sulphate technique for outlining the abscess cavity, found a mean resolution time of 75 (24–184) days in 20 patients with amoebic liver abscess; there was no relationship between resolution time and size of the abscess.

Davey (1968) has summarized the indications for *open drainage* as follows: (i) the pus is too thick to be aspirated, and may contain a slough, (ii) a very large amount of pus is present, i.e. up to 500–1000 ml is being aspirated daily, (iii) the pus is secondarily infected, (iv) rupture has already occurred, and (v) there is evidence of impending rupture, especially from a left lobe abscess. A drain should always be inserted, and connected to an underwater seal; that must however be removed as soon as possible due to the risk of haemorrhage into the liver, or biliary fistula formation. Furthermore, it is very important that the tube does not have a flange, or cup, which might tear the liver substance during removal. When there is doubt about diagnosis of perforation to the peritoneal cavity, laparotomy should be performed; a localized swelling can be aspirated while a generalized perforation should be treated by peritoneal toilet, and the abscess cavity sucked out. A soft tube may then be placed at the entrance to the cavity and omentum drawn round it; the tube is connected to an underwater seal. An antibiotic, as well as an antiamoebicide cover is required. Because the serum pseudocholine esterase concentration may be low, anaesthesia can be a hazardous undertaking (Mullan and Williams, 1965).

12.2. Pyogenic abscess of the liver (PAL)

Compared with amoebic liver abscess, pyogenic liver abscess is a rarity in tropical countries. The liver is a vast filtration system which sieves all intestinal bacteria which pass into the portal system; that this condition is unusual is therefore surprising. However a pyogenic liver abscess is occasionally encountered and early diagnosis is important. Because of the lateness of diagnosis in the majority of cases, pyogenic abscess has a high mortality rate; in one series of 20 cases, 11 multiple and 9 solitary, there was an 81 per cent mortality rate in the former and 33 per cent in the latter subgroup (Warren and Hardy, 1968). Any organism, including *Streptothrix actinomyces* may be involved. The role of *Ascaris lumbricoides* in the production of liver abscess is difficult to assess; it has been thought by some investigators to be important (Reay, Dignan, and Maunder, 1964), but the majority of physicians in tropical areas consider it to be of minor importance (Chapter 5).

McFadzean, Chang, and Wong, (1953) reported 14 cases of solitary hepatic pyogenic abscess, from Hong Kong; they were seen over a two-year period in which 2868 admissions were made to the University Department of Medicine. Those authors considered that that was an unusually high incidence. There was a male predominance which agrees with most other series; it was a disease of the younger age groups. Stokes (1960) described four cases of the disease in London; Butler and McCarthy (1969) recorded 48 cases of pyogenic liver abscess from Bristol, England, of whom 17 died. In a three-year prospective analysis of hospital admissions at the Goroka Base Hospital, Papua New Guinea, Wagner and Shepherd (1976) reported four cases of staphylococcal liver abscess; during the same period there were 12 cases of amoebic liver abscess amongst 124 patients with disease of the liver and biliary tract.

12.2.1. Presentation of PAL

In the series reported by McFadzean, *et al.* (1953), mean duration of symptoms was 18 (8–30) days prior to admission; the onset was acute in only one case. Fever, malaise, and pain were the most frequent symptoms. Pain, which was usually dull in character, was by no means constant and was a dominant complaint in 12 cases. Anorexia, nausea, and vomiting were common. Eight cases had respiratory symptoms. Butler and McCarthy (1969) also commented on the insidious onset in their cases; most patients were uncertain at the beginning of their illness, and in some that was probably as long as three years before.

On examination, all of the cases described by McFadzean, *et al.* (1953) had a 'dusky' skin-pigmentation. Although not jaundiced, four had mildly elevated bilirubin concentrations. All had a fever. Acute onset of clubbing was noted in three cases. A visible mass over the liver was seen in two, and localized oedema of the right lateral thoracic wall and abdomen was present in three. Mild involuntary rigidity was usual. Thirteen had hepatomegaly, and a fluctuant swelling, with acute tenderness, could sometimes be palpated; general liver tenderness was usual. Ascites and splenomegaly were not encountered. Pulmonary signs, in the right lower chest, were present in 11 cases. Nearly half of the cases described by Butler and McCarthy (1969) were jaundiced. Anaemia, and occasionally oedema, caused by hypoalbuminaemia, were also seen in a minority of that series; the latter sign had a bad prognostic significance.

Amoebic liver abscess and hepatoma are the two conditions which must be borne in mind in the differential diagnosis. Usually, however, the diagnosis is straightforward (McFadzean, *et al.*, 1953).

Signs of bad prognostic significance have been summarized by Butler and McCarthy (1969). They are features of gross liver destruction and poor 'defence mechanisms', severe jaundice, coma, hypotension, associated diabetes mellitus, a serum albumin concentration below 20g per l, absence of a leucocytosis, and a blood urea concentration of less than 2·0 mmol per l. Positive blood cultures, multiple abscesses, an age of more than 50 years, anaemia, and an elevated serum bilirubin concentration were considered to be factors of grave significance in a recent series of 33 cases described by Satiani and Davidson (1978).

12.2.2. Aetiology and pathology of PAL

Most cases of pyogenic, as well as amoebic, liver abscess involve the right lobe (Butler and McCarthy, 1969). Routes of infection are: (i) the portal vein, (ii) the biliary tree, (iii) the hepatic artery, (iv) direct extension from an adjacent infective process, and (v) penetrating injuries of the liver. Contamination of a primary hepatic lesion, such as a neoplasm, may also occur. In addition, in infants umbilical sepsis is occasionally a cause; portal vein thrombosis and tetanus are other consequences of such an infection. It is possible that *Ascaris lumbricoides* infections may be causally related, but that is not proven (see above). Pyogenic liver abscess is common in people with sickle-cell (SS) disease (Schulman and Beem, 1971).

Appendicitis, bacillary dysentery, infected haemorrhoids, diverticulitis, and ulcerative colitis are possible foci for portal vein spread; the three latter conditions are uncommon in many indigenous tropical populations (Chapter 29). Suppurative cholangitis, which is common in Hong Kong (McFadzean, *et al.*, 1953), may be associated with *Clonorchis sinensis* infection. Multiple liver abscesses in the Far east—Japan, Korea, China, Taiwan, and Vietnam—are usually a result of a secondary infection of disease caused by liver flukes (Chapter 14). Abscesses associated with the presence of adult worms of *Paragonimus westermani* (the lung fluke) have been reported; that parasite occurs focally in the Far east, south-east Asia, the Pacific islands, west Africa, and parts of south America. If *A. lumbricoides* is a contributory factor, secondary infection may follow its invasion of the biliary tree. Any condition which produces bacteraemia, septicaemia, or pyaemia can produce an abscess via the hepatic artery. There is a group in which no obvious route can be found; that was the case in all of the patients described by Stokes (1960), and in many of those described by Butler and McCarthy (1969).

Escherichia coli, anaerobic streptococcus, and *Staphycoccus aureus* were causative in the cases described by McFadzean, *et al.* (1953); in two of those cases the pus was sterile. The bulk of the series described by Butler and McCarthy (1969) contained *E. coli* either alone, or in association with *Streptococcus faecalis.* In the cases described by Stokes (1960) anaerobic cocci were recovered from the pus in every case. *Salmonella typhi* has also been implicated (Hirschowitz, 1952).

12.2.3. Investigation of PAL

A marked polymorphonuclear leucocytosis is usual; this is usually higher than in amoebic liver abscess. Serum bilirubin was mildly elevated in four, and alkaline phosphatase in all of the cases, in whom they were determined, described by McFadzean, *et al.* (1953). Most of those described by Butler and McCarthy (1969) had a raised serum alkaline phosphatase; those who died had very high phosphatase concentrations, and serum albumin concentrations were less than 20 g per l. Serum B_{12} concentrations are frequently elevated (Butler and McCarthy, 1969). Chest radiography frequently shows no abnormality; however the right diaphragm usually moves poorly. If available, a liver 'scan' is of great value in establishing the diagnosis and in localization (Butler and McCarthy, 1969). Technetium and gallium scans and sonography, if available, are of great help in making an early diagnosis, and in differentiating collections of pus from other intrahepatic lesions (Taylor, Wasson, DeGraaff, Rosenfield, and Andriole, 1978). Lipiodol instillation into the cavity is also of value in localization (McFadzean, *et al.*, 1953).

12.2.4. Treatment of PAL

Early recognition, aggressive surgical drainage, and appropriate long-term antibiotic therapy are vital, for this is potentially a fatal disease. Butler and McCarthy (1969) stressed the importance of accurate localization of the abscess before drainage, i.e. if the necessary apparatus is available.

Antibiotics and drainage of the abscess through a needle have been used, but surgical drainage is superior. All of the cases described by Stokes (1960) were infected with organisms sensitive to penicillin and streptomycin. Those reported by Butler and McCarthy (1969) all received either tetracycline, or penicillin and streptomycin therapy. Similar treatment was followed by immediate improvement in 13 of the cases described by McFadzean, *et al.* (1953); in the other patient a second aspiration was necessary to produce a cure. In a recent series of 33 pyogenic liver abscesses, the six patients who were not explored surgically died (Satiani and Davidson, 1978); in the remainder, who were explored, the mortality rate was 13 per cent.

12.3 Hydatid disease of the liver (HDL)

Hydatid disease is usually the result of infection with the larvae of *Echinococcus granulosus*; the related species *E. multilocularis,* and *E. oligaettas* are responsible for some cases.

References to hydatid cysts appear in the Talmud, the writings of Hippocrates, and those of Al-Rhazi; there are also other early writings (Naji, 1976).

Although often looked upon as a 'tropical disease', that is really not the case. Hydatid disease occurs wherever sheep and cattle raising takes place, for instance in such non-tropical countries as Wales and New Zealand. It is common in the nomadic tribes of east Africa (Rottcher, 1973). It is a major problem in Chile, the Middle-east (Naji, 1976; Nourmand, 1976), Bangladesh (Islam, 1977), Libya (Taguri and Dar, 1978), Ethiopia, Kenya (O'Leary, 1976), and northern Uganda (Owor and Bitakaramire, 1975).

12.3.1. Presentation of HDL

There may be a mild febrile reaction with urticarial skin eruptions during the migratory stage. Frequently a hydatid cyst of the liver starts its life in childhood and there are no symptoms until sometime in adult life; there may be an interval of at least 30 years between infection and presentation. At presentation there is usually hepatomegaly, and a cyst of 5 to 10 cm is present in the right lobe of the liver; it is surrounded by greyish-white fibrous tissue and compressed liver tissue. An 'hydatid thrill' may be present, but is usually difficult to elicit (Taguri and Dar, 1978). Secondary infection may occur; pyogenic organisms and salmonellae have been found. Secondary infection, trauma, needle liver-biopsy, or operative intervention may produce rupture; allergic manifestations with shock, sometimes leading to death, may then occur. Escape of cyst fluid and 'hydatid sand' may cause a severe allergic reaction with urticaria, pruritis, fever, abdominal pain, dyspnoea, delirium, and syncope. Alternatively secondary abdominal spread, with multiple cysts within the peritoneal cavity may occur. Ruptures to the gall bladder, biliary tree, pleural cavity, hepatic vein, or lungs are also recorded.

Presentation may be with jaundice, fever, pain in the right upper abdomen, and an enlarged tender liver (Zielinski and Elmslie, 1969); that syndrome is caused by rupture of the cyst, producing biliary obstruction. If the hydatid cyst is present in another organ, presentation consists of symptoms related to that organ. The disease is so common in Iraq, that if all lumps in the body are diagnosed as being due to hydatid disease, there is a 50 per cent chance of being correct (Naji, 1976).

12.3.2. Parasitology and pathology of HDL

The definitive host, usually the dog or wolf, is infected with the adult echinococcus which is about 5 mm in length, and inhabits the upper small intestine. Ova passed in the faeces are ingested by an intermediate host; men, sheep, cattle, and horses may be involved. Ova are rapidly destroyed by sunlight and high temperatures. Man acquires infection by not washing his hands after close contact with his dogs, often in childhood; dog faeces contaminating sheep fleeces are also a source of infection. In Libya, infection is apparently occasionally caused by the hot wind from the desert which brings dust, containing hydatid ova from the faeces of dogs and jackals (Fossati, 1970). Following ingestion, an embryo is liberated in the duodenum which, after penetrating the intestinal mucosa, is transferred to the liver by the portal circulation. There it is either trapped by the hepatic filtration mechanism or passes into the lungs, and in a minority of cases on to the systemic circulation. Wherever its progress is arrested, it may develop into a hydatid cyst. The right lobe of the liver is obviously therefore the most common site for a hydatid cyst; when other organs are involved the order of frequency is: lungs 71, brain 5, muscle and cellular tissues 5, spleen 2·5, kidneys 2, other abdominal organs 5 and bone 0·5 per cent; other organs including the heart and thyroid are only very unusually involved. The cyst is sometimes unilocular and develops a two-layered wall. The inner, or germinal layer produces brood-capsules, from which scolices (or heads) are produced; some break loose within the cyst and form 'hydatid sand'. As the cyst enlarges 'daughter cysts' are produced. If there is no effective encapsulation, and that occurs with *E. multilocularis*, the daughter cysts produce a multilocular hydatid cyst. The definitive host is infected by eating the hydatid cyst, usually in the infected viscera of sheep or cattle, and the larvae develop into sexually mature worms within a few weeks, thus completing the life-cycle.

At operation or post-mortem the cyst may be (i) unilocular, or (ii) alveolar. The unilocular type is usually sterile and fertile, and surrounded by fibrous tissue and a granulomatous reaction. Initially there is an eosinophilic reaction to the larva, but that subsides as the cyst becomes walled off by thick fibrous tissue. If rupture occurs dissemination of daughter cysts and scolices may give rise to secondary metastatic hydatids. The alveolar type is multiloculated and the liver is its usual site; microscopically it is sponge-like. Small cysts are usually sterile and are separated from each other by connective and fibrous tissue of the host, in which may be areas of necrosis and calcification; however a minority of the cysts are fertile and metastasise.

12.3.3. Investigation of HDL

In the invasive stage and following leakage or rupture there is an eosinophilia. Contents of the cysts may be found in the stool, sputum, or urine samples, after rupture.

Liver biopsy must on no account be performed if there is any possibility of an hydatid cyst being present; that is because of the possibility of rupturing a cyst, with disastrous results.

Radiology, radioisotope scanning, and ultrasound are of value in the localization of cysts (Vicary, 1977). Selective angiography has also proved of value (McNulty, 1968).

Intradermal and serological tests. Much of the difficulty with these tests is that once the cyst is sealed off by fibrous tissue, very little or no antigen escapes from it; antibody production cannot therefore take place. Also, when once positive these tests remain so for long periods of time and are of no value in the immediate assessment of a cure.

The intradermal Casoni test, which utilizes crude, sterile hydatid fluid, is unreliable in most hands but depends upon the source of the antigen; it is positive in from 50 to 100 per cent of cases. In a recent report from Iran, the Casoni test gave positive results in 84 per cent of 58 patients with proven hydatid disease (Nourmand, 1976). The test is of no value in assessing a cure because it remains positive for five years or more after the excision or death of a cyst. An extract of lyophilized cyst material from *E. multilocularis* seems to give more reliable results (Kagan, Osimani, Varela, and Allain, 1966). The complement-fixation test is positive in 70 per cent of cases, and persists for up to two years after excision of the cyst (Nobili, Cascio, and Cosentino, 1966). An indirect haemagglutination test (Arabatzis and Papapanagiotou, 1963) is positive in 90 per cent of cases, and rarely gives false positive results; it has been shown to be of value as a screening technique in field studies (Varela-Díaz, Coltorti, Ricardes, Prezioso, Schantz, and Garcia, 1976). Various flocculation tests have also been used. An indirect immunofluorescence test seems to be of value (Moroni and Sorice, 1966; Gore, Sadun, and Hoff, 1970); a scolex antigen gave the best results (Beggs and Fischman, 1970). A commercially available slide-latex agglutination test (Italdiagnostico, Italy) seems to be as satisfactory as the Casoni test (Hoghooghi, Sabbaghian, Ghadirian, Kagan, and Schiller, 1976); a positivity rate of 80 per cent, compared with one of 82 per cent with the Casoni test, with false positive rates of 6·7 and 4·8 per cent respectively in patients who were free of hydatid disease, has been recorded.

12.3.4. Treatment of HDL

This consists of surgical removal of the cyst by an experienced surgeon, after 5 per cent formalin has been injected into it, to sterilize it (Naji, 1976). When properly carried out, the mortality rate is extremely low (Nourmond, 1976).

Mebendazole ('Vermox') (Chapter 19) has given encouraging results in experimental conditions. Given to mice with long-standing, heavy infections with *E. granulosus* a significant decrease in the number of cysts has been reported (Heath, Christie, and Chevis, 1975; Kammerer and Judge, 1976). In *E. multilocularis* infections also, mebendazole gave encouraging results in both mice and rats (Campbell, McCracken, and Blair, 1975). In man, favourable results have also been reported, although it is difficult to understand how mebendazole can penetrate the fibrous tissue surrounding the cyst. Mebendazole was given to four patients with hepatic hydatid cysts, in an oral dose of 400–600 mg three times daily for 21–30 days (Bekhti, Schaaps, Capron, Dessaint, Santoro, and Capron, 1977); after 4–13 months, ultrasonic echotomography showed complete regression of the cysts in all four patients. However, the treatment had subsequently to be repeated in three of them. After similar treatment, complete degeneration of the germinal layer and absence of protoscolices and brood-capsules has been demonstrated in three hydatid cysts removed from a 20-year-old woman (Al-Moslih, Al-Janabi, Al-Rawas, Shafik, Rassam, Al-Ani, and Al-Dabagh, 1978).

12.4. Other space-occupying lesions of the liver

12.4.1. Acute bacterial infections

Clostridium welchii infections. Production of gas-filled cysts in the liver, and also spleen, may occur in debilitated patients infected with *Cl. welchii* (Ashley, 1965); that is however an unusual event. The exotoxin may also produce massive haemolysis and jaundice.

Pasteurella pseudotuberculosis. This disease causes acute mesenteric lymphadenitis. The liver may be affected and if death occurs the causative organism can be cultured from numerous abscesses in the liver and spleen.

Melioidosis. In the Far east and Papua New Guinea, multiple hepatic abscesses are occasionally caused by this disease which results from infection with *Pseudomonas pseudomallei.*

12.4.2. Tuberculoma

This is a rare space-occupying lesion of the liver. Involvement of the liver by tuberculosis usually results in no more than scattered granulomatous lesions (Chapters 5 and 8). However it is important in that it can occasionally closely mimic hepatoma (Campbell, 1966).

12.4.3. Hepatic infarction

Massive hepatic infarction with necrosis, is a rare event (Chen, Hamilton, and Qizilbash, 1976) and has been associated with the sickle-cell trait (AS) (Mengel, Schauble, and Hammond, 1963).

References

Abioye, A. A. (1976). *J. trop. Med. Hyg.*, **79,** 252.

Adi, F. C. (1965). *W. Afr. med. J.*, **14,** 181.

—— (1966). *W. Afr. med. J.*, **15,** 43.

Al-Moslih, M. I., Al-Janabi, T. A., Al-Rawas, A. Y., Shafik, M. A., Rassam, S., Al-Ani, M. S., and Al-Dabagh, M. A. (1978). *Br. med. J.*, **2,** 1435.

Arabatzis, G. and Papapanagiotou, J. (1963). *Bull. Wld Hlth Org.*, **28,** 266.

Archampong, E. Q. (1977). *Tropical Doctor*, **7,** 161.

Ashley, D. J. B. (1965). *J. clin. Path.*, **18,** 170.

Beggs, W. A. and Fischman, A. (1970). *Bull. Wld Hlth Org.*, **42,** 331.

Bekhti, A., Schaaps, J-P, Capron, M., Dessaint, J-P., Santoro, F., and Capron, A. (1977). *Br. med. J.*, **2,** 1047.

Bhasin, A. S., Mittal, K. P., Shrivastava, P. N., Bhardwaj, O. P., Sachdev, S., and Gupta, P. S. (1978). *J. trop. Med. Hyg.*, **80,** 169.

Br. med. J. (1978). **2,** 379.

Butler, T. J. and McCarthy, C. F. (1969). *Gut*, **10,** 389.

Campbell, C. H. (1966). *Papua New Guin. med. J.*, **9,** 152.

Campbell, W. C., McCracken, R. O., and Blair, L. S. (1975). *J. Parasit.*, **61,** 844.

Chen, V., Hamilton, J., and Qizilbash, A. (1976). *Archs Path.*, **100,** 32.

Davey, W. W. (1968). *Companion to Surgery in Africa*. p. 251. E. and S. Livingstone, Edinburgh and London.

De Dominicis, A., Balestrieri, A., and Assumma, M. (1966). *Archo ital. Sci. med. trop. Parassit.*, **47,** 215.

Devakul, K., Areekul, S., and Viravan, C. (1967). *Ann. trop. Med. Parasit.*, **61,** 29.

Doxiades, T., Candreviotis, N., Tiliakos, M., and Polymeropoulos, I. (1961). *Brit. med. J.*, **1,** 460.

Edington, G. M. and Gilles, H. M. (1976). *Pathology in the tropics*. 2nd ed. pp. 71 and 201. Edward Arnold, London.

El-Hennawy, M. and Abd-Rabbo, H. (1978). *J. trop. Med. Hyg.*, **81,** 71.

Ellman, B., McLeod, I. N., and Powell, S. J. (1965). *Br. med. J.*, **2,** 1406.

El-Zayidi, A. M., Hartmann, M. G., and Mohr, W. (1976). *J. trop. Med. Hyg.*, **79,** 120.

Fossati, C. J. (1970). *Revta ibér. Parasit.*, **30,** 587.

GELFAND, M. (1966). *Cent. Afr. med. J.*, **12,** 211.
GORE, R. W., SADUN, E. H., and HOFF, R. (1970). *Expl Parasit.*, **28,** 272.
GRELL, G. A. C. and WATTY, E. I. (1978). *W. Indian med. J.*, **27,** 40.
HEATH, D. D., CHRISTIE, M. J., and CHEVIS, R. A. F. (1975). *Parasitology*, **70,** 273.
HIRSCHOWITZ, B. I. (1952). *Gastroenterology*, **21,** 291.
HOGHOOGHI, N., SABBAGHIAN, H., GHADIRIAN, E., KAGAN, I. G., and SCHILLER, E. L. (1976). *Am. J. trop. Med. Hyg.*, **25,** 660.
ISLAM, N. (1977). *Lancet*, **2,** 33.
—— and HASAN, M. (1975). *Curr. ther. Res.*, **17,** 161.
—— and —— (1978). *J. trop. Med. Hyg.*, **81,** 20.
KAGAN, I. G., OSIMANI, J. J., VARELA, J. C., and ALLAIN, D. S. (1966). *Am. J. trop. Med. Hyg.*, **15,** 172.
KAMMERER, W. S. and JUDGE, D. M. (1976). *Am. J. trop. Med. Hyg.*, **25,** 714.
KESSEL, J. F., LEWIS, W. P., PASQUEL, C. M., and TURNER, J. A. (1965). *Am J. trop. Med. Hyg.*, **14,** 540.
KROGSTAD, D. J., SPENCER, H. C., HEALY, G. R. (1978). *New Engl. J. Med.*, **298,** 262.
——, ——, ——, GLEASON, N. N., SEXTON, D. J., and HERRON, C. A. (1978). *Ann. intern. Med.*, **88,** 89.
KRUPP, I. M. and POWELL, S. J. (1971). *Am. J. trop. Med. Hyg.*, **20,** 421.
Lancet (1979). **1,** 303.
MCFADZEAN, A. J. S., CHANG, K. P. S., and WONG, C. C. (1953). *Br. J. Surg.*, **41,** 141.
MCLEOD, I. N., WILMOT, A. J., and POWELL, S. J. (1966). *Q. Jl. Med.*, **35,** 293.
MCNULTY, J. G. (1968). *Am. J. Roentg.*, **102,** 380.
MENGEL, C. E., SCHAUBLE, J. F., and HAMMOND, C. B. (1963). *Archs intern. Med.*, **111,** 93.
MILLER, M. W., HOWES, H. L., and ENGLISH, A. R. (1969). *Antimicrob. Agents Chemother.*, **9,** 257.
MOKHOBO, K. P. (1971). *W. Afr. med. J.*, **20,** 365.
MORONI, M. and SORICE, F. (1966). *G. Mal. infett. parassit.*, **18,** 471.
MORRIS, M. N., POWELL, S. J., and ELSDON-DEW, R. (1970). *Lancet*, **1,** 1362.
MULLAN, D. P. and WILLIAMS, N. E. (1965). *Br. med. J.*, **1,** 235.
NAIK, S. R., ACHAR, B. G., and MEHTA, S. K. (1978). *J. trop. Med. Hyg.*, **81,** 116.
NAJI, K. (1976). *Tropical Doctor*, **6,** 70.
NOBILI, I., CASCIO, G., and COSENTINO, G. (1966). *Riv. 1st. sieroter. ital.*, **41,** 237.
NOURMAND, A. (1976). *Am. J. trop. Med. Hyg.*, **25,** 845.
OCHSNER, A. and DE BAKEY, M. (1943). *Surgery, St Louis,* **13,** 460 and 612.
O'LEARY, P. (1976). *E. Afr. med. J.*, **53,** 540.
OWOR, R. and BITAKARAMIRE, P. K. (1975). *E. Afr. med. J.*, **52,** 700.
PARELKAR, S. N. and STAMM, W. P. (1973). *Trans. R. Soc. trop. Med. Hyg.*, **67,** 659.
——, ——, and HILL, K. R. (1971). *Lancet*, **1,** 212.
PAUL, M. (1960). *Br. J. Surg.*, **47,** 502.
PAULLEY, J. W. (1965). *Postgrad. med. J.*, **41,** 575.
POWELL, S. J., MADDISON, S. E., WILMOT, A. J., and ELSDON-DEW, R. (1965). *Lancet*, **2,** 602.
——, WILMOT, A. J. and ELSDON-DEW, R. (1969). *Ann. trop. Med. Parasit.*, **63,** 139.
QUADERI, M. A., RAHMAN, M. S., RAHMAN, A., and ISLAM, N. (1978). *J. trop. Med. Hyg.*, **81,** 16.
RAMACHANDRAN, S. and EDWARDS, R. (1978). *J. trop. Med. Hyg.*, **81,** 40.
REAY, H. A. J., DIGNAN, A. P., and MAUNDER, C. (1964). *Br. med. J.*, **2,** 553.
REYNOLDS, T. B. (1971). *Gastroenterology*, **60,** 952.
RHODES, F. A. (1972). *Papua New Guin. med. J.*, **15,** 160.
ROBINSON, G. L. (1972). *Trans. R. Soc. trop. Med. Hyg.*, **66,** 435.
ROTTCHER, K. H. (1973). *E. Afr. med. J.*, **50,** 466.
ROWLAND, H. A. K. (1973). *J. trop. Med. Hyg.*, **66,** 113.

SALAKO, L. A. (1967). *J. trop. Med. Hyg.*, **70,** 19.
SARGEAUNT, P. G., WILLIAMS, J. E., and GRENE, J. D. (1978). *Trans. R. Soc. trop. Med. Hyg.*, **72,** 519.
SATIANI, B. and DAVIDSON, E. D. (1978). *Am. J. Surg.*, **135,** 647.
SCHULMAN, S. T. and BEEM, M. O. (1971). *Pediatrics*, **47,** 1019.
SCRAGG, J. N. and PROCTOR, E. M. (1977). *Archs Dis. Childh.*, **52,** 408.
SHEEHY, T. W., PARMLEY, L. F., JOHNSTON, G. S., and BOYCE, H. W. (1968). *Gastroenterology*, **55,** 26.
SINGHA, H. S. K. (1959). *Br. J. Surg.*, **47,** 198.
STAMM, W. P., ASHLEY, M. J., and PARELKAR, S. N. (1973). *Trans. R. Soc. trop. Med. Hyg.*, **67,** 211.
STOKES, J. F. (1960). *Lancet*, **1,** 355.
STUIVER, P. C. and GOUD, T. J. L. M. (1978). *Br. med. J.*, **2,** 394.
TAGURI, S. and DAR, F. K. (1978). *Trans. R. Soc. trop. Med. Hyg.*, **72,** 338.
TAYLOR, K. J. W., WASSON, J. F. M., DE GRAAFF, C., ROSENFIELD, A. T., and ANDRIOLE, V. T. (1978). *Lancet*, **1,** 83.
VAKIL, B. J., MEHTA, A. J., and DESAI, H. N. (1970). *J. trop. Med. Hyg.*, **73,** 63.
VARELA-DÍAZ, V. M., COLTORTI, E. A., RICARDES, M. I., PREZIOSO, U., SHANTZ, P. M., and GARCIA, R. (1976). *Am. J. trop. Med. Hyg.*, **25,** 617.
VICARY, F. R. (1977). *Gut*, **18,** 386.
VIGG, B. L., SHAY, B. K., and LINGAM, K. P. (1971). *J. Ass. Physns India*, **19,** 515.
WAGNER, F. B. and SHEPHERD, A. (1976). *Papua New Guin. med. J.*, **19,** 156.
WARREN, K. W. and HARDY, K. J. (1968). *Archs Surg., Chicago*, **97,** 40.
WÉRY-PASKOFF, S., RENOIRTE, R., and WÉRY, M. (1974). *Annls Soc. belge Méd. trop.*, **54,** 65.
WHITTAKER, L. R. (1963). *E. Afr. med. J.*, **40,** 95.
WILMOT, A. J. (1962). *Clinical Amoebiasis*. p. 75. Blackwell, Oxford.
ZIELINSKI, V. E. and ELMSLIE, R. G. (1969). *Med. J. Aust.*, **1,** 839.

13

Effect of undernutrition and alcohol on the liver

13.1. Undernutrition and the liver

SEVERE protein deficiency (kwashiorkor) in childhood has been suggested as a possible precursor of cirrhosis in later life in tropical countries (Himsworth, 1950). Marasmus (starvation) leads to liver atrophy rather than fatty infiltration; that probably accounts for the descriptions of the small shrunken liver in old reports of tropical malabsorption (Cook, 1978). There is no evidence to support the idea that cirrhosis is a result of a *specific* nutritional deficiency.

13.1.1. The liver in kwashiorkor

Kwashiorkor is a word used by the Ga tribe of Ghana to describe a clinical syndrome which was first recorded by Cicely Williams (1933). The disease is widespread throughout the tropics, and is especially common in populations living on maize, rice, yams, cassava, and plantains. It usually occurs between one and four years of age, often during the weaning period, and is related to a protein deficiency in the diet; the aetiology is however by no means clear. Kwashiorkor also rarely occurs in adults; in them it is usually secondary to another condition, not infrequently severe malabsorption caused by intestinal tuberculosis (Chapter 23).

Associated infections, such as measles, tuberculosis and salmonellosis, and other forms of diarrhoeal disease, are common (Phillips and Wharton, 1968). They are partly due to an impaired immune response associated with the disease. In severe kwashiorkor, cellular immunity is impaired, partially as a result of thymic atrophy (Watts, 1969). An immune-deficiency state predisposes to some viral infections, including disseminated herpes simplex, in which characteristic focal necrosis of hepatocytes is seen (Templeton, 1970) (Chapter 7).

Kwashiorkor is easily diagnosed clinically. The affected child is irritable and apathetic. There is discolouration of the hair, a characteristic dusky red dermatosis with desquamation, and oedema. Evidence of at least one infection is usually present. The liver is frequently enlarged on clinical examination. There is hypoproteinaemia. Evidence of hepatic failure is extremely unusual.

Treatment consists of dealing with the infections and improving nutritional status with aminoacids and vitamin supplements; numerous therapeutic regimes have been used. In kwashiorkor, the liver is frequently densely infiltrated with fat within the hepatocytes (Trowell, Davies, and Dean, 1954;

Kariks, 1960; Waterlow, Cravioto, and Stephen, 1960) (Fig. 13.1); that is due to the failure of the hepatocyte to handle fat in the presence of a severe amino-acid deficiency. The role of the pancreatic deficiency, which is a major feature of kwashiorkor, in the fat deposition is unclear (Trowell, *et al.*, 1954).

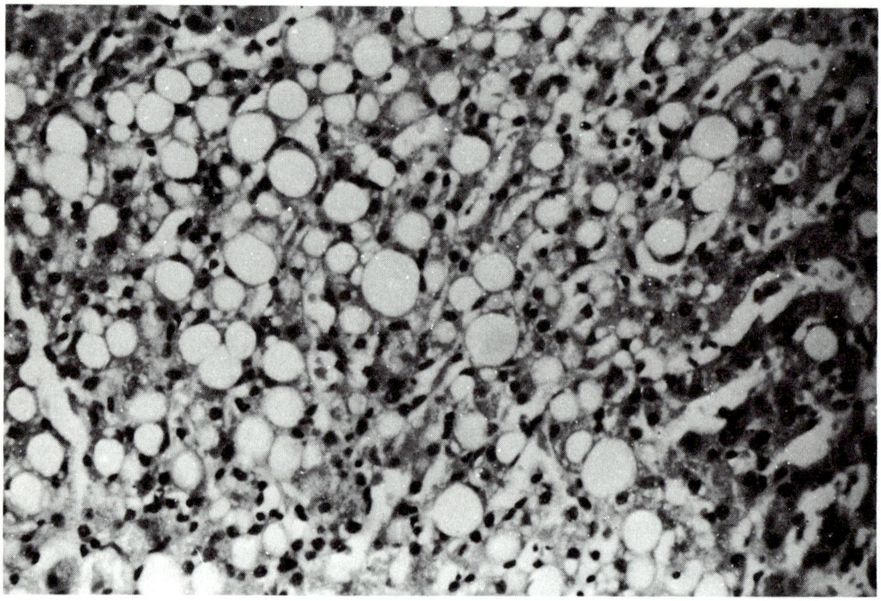

FIG. 13.1. Liver-biopsy section (haematoxylin and eosin) from a 23-year-old Zambian woman from the Chewa tribe, with 'adult kwashiorkor'; the primary pathology was shown to be abdominal tuberculosis. Haemoglobin concentration was 8·3 g per dl. Serum albumin concentration was 14, and gamma-globulin 24 g per l. The section shows marked fatty infiltration of the hepatocytes; there is no disturbance of architecture.

13.1.1. Liver morphology in kwashiorkor

Macroscopically, the liver is yellow, firm, and greasy. There is massive fatty change in the hepatocytes which begins in the periportal regions; the hepatocyte often consists in fact of a fat globule with the nucleus flattened against the cell membrane. Rarely, focal areas of necrosis may occur. Electron microscopy shows a thickened cell membrane, swollen mitochondria, and a decrease in endoplasmic reticulum (Camain, Rouiller, and Dupin, 1959). Hepatic pathology seems to differ in different areas; in Papua New Guinea, atrophy and vacuolization of hepatocytes is apparently more common than the fatty infiltration which is the dominant feature in Africa and the West Indies (Bailey, 1966). Portal tracts are widened and fibrous tissue may radiate into the lobule ('stellate fibrosis'). Malarial pigment may be seen in the Kupffer cells, and a cellular infiltrate consisting of lymphocytes and monocytes may be present; those changes are the result of other environmental stimuli (Chapter 5) and not malnutrition.

13.1.2. Hepatic function in kwashiorkor

Liver function is usually well preserved in kwashiorkor; jaundice is unusual. However, in Jamaica hepatic failure has been reported (McLean, 1962). Also, using intravenous galactose to test liver function, a significant impairment in clearance rate has been demonstrated in seven malnourished adults (Royle, Kettlewell, Ilic, and Williamson, 1978); this was considered to be related to changes in hepatic blood flow. The rise in blood glucose and lactate after galactose, was also impaired in that study.

13.1.3. Possible long-term sequelae of kwashiorkor on the liver

The suggestion has been made, largely as a result of extensive animal experimentation (Himsworth and Glynn, 1944; Himsworth, 1950), that those changes may be a precursor of chronic liver disease, including cirrhosis, in adult life. The fact that cirrhosis is common in many areas where malnutrition is common also fostered such conclusions, i.e., that there was a cause-effect relationship between the two. Alternatively, it has been suggested that the liver in a malnourished individual is more susceptible to damage by other agents, including viral hepatitis.

There are now no grounds for considering in man that malnutrition predisposes to chronic hepatic disease. In a liver-biopsy follow-up investigation of 20 children with kwashiorkor in South Africa (Suckling and Campbell, 1957), there was no evidence of progressive disease. Studies in India (Srikantia, Sriramachari, and Gopalan, 1958) and Jamaica (Bras, Brooks, and Watler, 1961) have also failed to demonstrate an association between kwashiorkor and cirrhosis. Similarly in Uganda liver-biopsy histology has been shown to return to normal after disappearance of the fatty infiltration (Cook and Hutt, 1967); in that study liver-biopsies and liver function tests were performed in 50 children, 7·0 (4·0–11·3) years after recovery from kwashiorkor. Only one biopsy showed evidence of fatty change while five showed 'stellate fibrosis' radiating from the portal triads, which is normal for Africans' livers (Chapter 5). It is difficult however to rule out the possibility that prolonged untreated kwashiorkor gives rise to chronic liver disease (Ramalingaswami, 1964), but that seems very unlikely.

In African adults, fatty change is frequently associated with chronic alcoholism; such patients are not usually wasted, and fatty change is rarely severe. In chronic calcific pancreatic disease in adults, fatty change in liver-biopsy specimens is also common and often severe (Kajubi, Shaper, and Owor 1972); in that study the change seemed to be predominantly the result of secondary malnutrition caused by malabsorption and steatorrhoea. There was not a higher incidence of cirrhosis.

13.1.4. Effect of other diseases on the kwashiorkor liver

Schistosomiasis. Work in this field is limited. However, in experimental animals malnutrition seems to have a protective effect, as shown by diminished ova output by the adult worms and a lower rate of granuloma formation (Kanuft and Warren, 1969; Akpom and Warren, 1975).

Viral hepatitis. It seems probable that a fatal outcome in viral hepatitis is more common in undernourished individuals; acute hepatic necrosis is certainly more common in tropical than in temperate countries and that might be associated with poor nutrition (Chapter 7).

The possibility that malnutrition predisposes to hepatic injury from another unknown agent is difficult to eliminate. However the geographical distribution of malnutrition and cirrhosis does not support that hypothesis (Edington and Gilles, 1976).

13.2. Alcoholic liver disease (ALD)

Alcoholism is a very important problem in many parts of Africa as well as the western world. In the eighteenth and nineteenth centuries, excessive alcohol consumption was a much greater problem in Britain than it is today (Spring and Buss, 1977); that was due to several factors, not least the existing social pressures. Such pressures are present in most newly independent countries, especially in the upper classes. In some instances also, increased availability of alcohol and the wherewithal to purchase it suddenly appeared as colonial rule gave way to independence. In expatriates living in tropical countries, boredom is not infrequently an initiating factor on the path to alcoholism.

In many third-world countries alcohol is now a very great menace; a high proportion of traffic accidents, which are exceedingly common, are associated with alcoholism.

13.2.1. Aetiology of ALD

Excess alcohol intake superimposed on a poor nutritional background seems to be associated with a high incidence of liver disease. Fatty liver, alcoholic hepatitis, and cirrhosis is the usual course of events (Lieber, Carli, and Rubin, 1975; *Br. med. J.*, 1978). Regular drinkers seem much more prone to cirrhosis than those with an intermittent pattern of consumption (Brunt, Kew, Scheuer, and Sherlock, 1974). In an investigation of 319 men with both a reliable history of alcohol intake and available liver-biopsies, mean daily alcohol intake in those with normal histology was 139g; those with fatty livers, chronic hepatitis, and cirrhosis had intakes of 172, 203, and 245g daily (Lelbach, 1974). A study in France however suggests that 60g in men and 20g in women is enough to produce liver damage (Pequignot, Chabert, Eydoux, and Courcoul, 1974). That evidence suggests a direct hepatotoxic effect of alcohol on the liver. The possibility of genetic or immunological factors has to be considered, especially because the intake of alcohol required to produce chronic liver disease in women seems to be significantly less than that in men (Pequignot, *et al.*, 1974). Existence of a sex difference seems to have been confirmed in a study in which women had more severe liver damage, and also an increased incidence of smooth muscle and antinuclear antibodies and higher serum IgG and IgM concentrations, compared with men consuming similar amounts of alcohol (Krasner, Davis, Portmann, and Williams, 1977). Alcoholics with cirrhosis have a higher incidence of histocompatibility antigen HLA-B8 than those who have only fatty change (Bailey, Krasner, Eddleston, Williams, Tee, Doniach, Kennedy, and Batchelor, 1976).

The development of alcoholic hepatitis and its progression to cirrhosis might be mediated by immune mechanisms; both humoral and cell-mediated factors have been implicated. Alcoholic hyaline may be detected in the serum of patients soon after the development of alcoholic hepatitis, and that might evoke an immune response with the production of antibodies (Leevy, Chen, and Zetterman, 1975; Kakumu and Leevy, 1977). Titres of antibodies increase with repeated attacks of hepatitis. To date there is no evidence however that that antibody is responsible for hepatocyte damage. It is possible that cytotoxic lymphokines elaborated by T-lymphocytes are important in the perpetuation of liver-cell injury and the initiation and perpetuation of fibrosis.

Mechanism of the fat deposition. Despite intensive study the pathogenesis of alcoholic-induced fatty liver is still uncertain. Much work was initiated by the possibility that the fatty liver might predispose to the development of cirrhosis. However the presence of fat is not directly related to the histological changes leading to cirrhosis; that is related to hepatocellular necrosis and regeneration, and is independent of fat accumulation. Current evidence suggests that a major factor in the development of fatty liver is the increased esterification of fatty acids to triglycerides—possibly stimulated by a massive influx of free fatty acids mobilised from adipose tissue. The accumulation of fat may reflect an imbalance between massive triglyceride synthesis and the ability of the liver to assemble and secrete triglycerides in the form of very low density lipoproteins. Some degree of hypertriglyceridaemia is often present, and evidence of hyperlipidaemia is a constant finding in patients with alcoholic hepatitis.

In baboons, if sclerosis has developed around the central vein, in addition to the fatty change, progression to cirrhosis is inevitable (Waes and Lieber, 1977; *Lancet*, 1978).

Alcoholic hepatitis. Acute hepatocellular injury brought about by an alcohol excess results in a wide spectrum of clinical manifestations, from asymptomatic hepatomegaly to massive steatonecrosis, and fulminant hepatic failure (Sabesin, Hawkins, Bertram, Mann, and Peace, 1978).

It has been suggested that mitochondrial damage is a significant factor in the pathogenesis of alcoholic liver disease (Rubin, Beattie, and Lieber, 1970; Svoboda and Manning, 1964; Konttinen, Härtel, and Louhija, 1970). However mitochondrial enzymes (glutamate dehydrogenase, malate dehydrogenase, and aspartate aminotransferase) are significantly raised in chronic alcoholics with steatosis (Jenkins and Peters, 1978); that suggests that there is not significant mitochondrial damage in alcoholic liver disease, and that the raised concentrations are an adaptive response to alcohol.

13.2.2. Presentation of ALD

The alcohol intake is frequently of the order of 160g alcohol (equivalent to about two-thirds of a bottle of whisky) daily. Alcoholic hepatitis (Beckett, Livingstone, and Hill, 1961; 1962) is by no means uncommon in both indigenous and expatriate populations in tropical countries, and is undoubtedly underdiagnosed. In alcoholic hepatitis there is loss of appetite, weakness, right upper-abdominal discomfort, and weight-loss. Jaundice is apparent on clinical examination. There is often a pyrexia which may be as high as 40°C at times. Hepatomegaly, and sometimes splenomegaly are present. There is usually some muscle wasting. If cirrhosis has developed, the clinical signs of that disease may be present (Chapter 8). There may also be parotid hypertrophy. Associated pancreatitis and peripheral neuropathy may be present.

Death is frequently associated with haemorrhage or hepatic coma; sepsis and disseminated intravascular coagulation may dominate the picture. There is a high mortality rate in the acute attack of alcoholic hepatitis; the disease sometimes takes a fulminant course. In that event, in addition to massive fat deposition and polymorphonuclear infiltration, there is extensive hepatocellular necrosis. There may be associated underlying chronic liver disease but that is certainly not always the case.

Untreated, recovery is slow with a gradual decrease in hepatic size, appetite recovery, and return of liver-function tests to normal, over several weeks. This course of events usually recurs at varying periods of time depending on the alcohol consumption, which is usually erratic. After several years, cirrhosis develops, and ascites and signs of liver cell failure (Chapter 8) become apparent.

13.2.3. Pathology of ALD

Most cases of cirrhosis in tropical countries are of the macronodular type (Chapter 8), which is usually a result of viral hepatitis; that end result can also result from an alcohol excess. A minority are cases of micronodular cirrhosis, the bulk of which seem to be an end result of a high alcohol intake over many years. Serial liver-biopsy sections show progressive changes. The fatty infiltration gives way to increasing hepatocellular necrosis and eventually micronodular cirrhosis (Fig. 13.2.). Macroscopically, the liver is usually of normal shape but reduced in size, and varies from pale yellow (due to an excess of fat) to brownish-green; on section it shows a fine uniform nodularity, the nodules being usually less than 4 mm in diameter. Although hepatoma was formerly thought to be an unusual complication of micronodular cirrhosis that is now known not to be the case (Lee, 1966).

Nodules, roughly the size of lobules are cut out by fine bands of fibrous tissue, joining portal tracts with central veins; that fibrous tissue contains bile ducts, blood vessels, pseudoductules, together with lymphocytes, histiocytes, and polymorphonuclear leucocytes. The nodules do not show the usual lobular structure and hepatic-vein radicles. Fatty vacuoles, without a surrounding inflammatory reaction, may be present. There are no normal portal tracts. The hepatocytes are swollen and the nucleus is compressed to one side by fatty vacuoles. A coarse irregular hyaline network which stains deeply with eosin and phosphotungstic-acid haematoxylin sometimes appears in the cytoplasm (Mallory's alcoholic hyaline) (Mallory, 1911); that is followed by leucocyte infiltration and destruction of affected cells. The combination of Mallory's hyaline with fatty infiltration strongly suggests that a case of micronodular cirrhosis is a result of alcohol excess. Haemosiderin may be present in excess in both hepatocytes and Kupffer cells. In post-mortem specimens, when death has occurred after a large haematemesis, areas of necrosis may be seen. Intralobu-

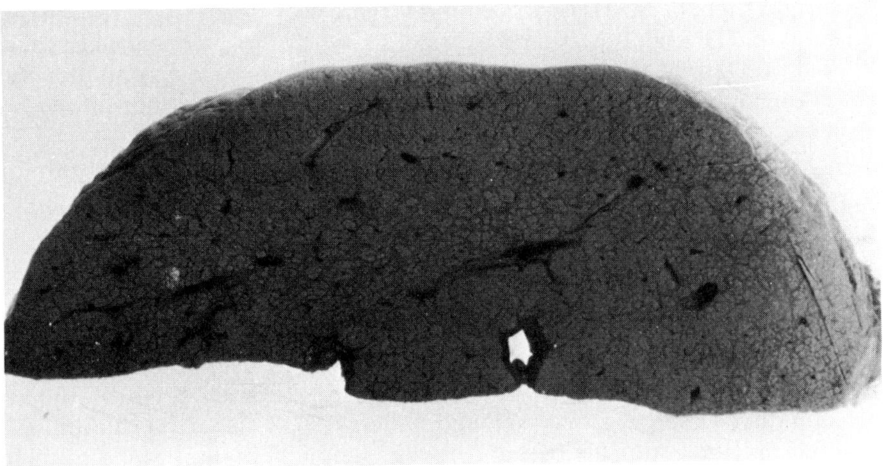

FIG. 13.2. Liver-section from a Papua New Guinean man, showing a fine micronodular cirrhosis. There was a history of heavy alcohol consumption over several years.

lar cholestasis with bile plugging is variable, but may be very marked; approximately 50 per cent of biopsies show evidence of cholestasis. Differentiation from large duct obstruction may be difficult and other measures such as percutaneous transhepatic cholangiography, or endoscopic retrograde cholangiopancreatography are sometimes required for diagnosis.

The early hepatic lesions of acute alcoholic hepatitis have been described by Edmondson, Peters, Frankel, and Borowsky (1967) and Rubin and Lieber (1967).

13.2.4. *Investigation of ALD*

Laboratory investigations show a raised white-blood-cell count, occasionally up to 30–40 000 per mm^3; the reason for that is unknown, but is probably associated with liver-cell necrosis. Serum albumin is usually low, and serum bilirubin, transaminases, and alkaline phosphatase concentrations elevated, all to very high levels in a severe case. Marked prolongation of the prothrombin time indicates a poor prognosis in severe cases (Porter, Simon, Pope, Volwiler, and Fenster, 1971; Maddrey, Boitnott, Bedine, Weber, and Mezey, 1977) as in acute viral hepatitis. Cholestasis may be severe. Needle liver-biopsy histology usually clinches the diagnosis.

13.2.5. *Treatment of ALD*

Most patients with pure fatty infiltration of the liver improve markedly during the 10 days after they stop taking alcohol. If however drinking continues, and clinical and pathological evidence of alcoholic hepatitis occurs there is an 80 per cent chance that cirrhosis will develop in five years (Hawkins, 1978).

Nutrition. It is now considered that alcohol is a direct hepatotoxin, and that the development of liver disease is not closely related to the nutritional status of the subject; thus baboons given a good diet still develop alcoholic liver injury

(Rubin and Lieber, 1974). However in rats there is evidence of protection on a nutritious diet (Patek, Bowry, and Sabesin, 1976). There might even be species differences. Despite the controversies, it seems wise to give a good diet with added folic acid, vitamin B_6, thiamine and niacin, and zinc.

Role of corticosteroids in alcoholic hepatitis. There is renewed interest in this in view of the recent suggestion that alcoholic hepatitis might have an immunological basis (Reynolds and Edmondson, 1971). In one investigation (Helman, Temko, Nye, and Fallon, 1971), three groups of patients with proven alcoholic hepatitis, of varying severity, were given high protein and calorie diets with vitamin supplements. They were randomly divided into groups who were given either 40 mg prednisolone daily, or a placebo for four weeks. In the severe group (with hepatic coma), prednisolone seemed to decrease the mortality rate. Results of a further study in patients with alcoholic hepatitis and encephalopathy (Lesesne, Bozymski, and Fallon, 1978) also support the use of prednisolone; of seven patients on calorie supplementation alone all died, whereas only two of seven treated with prednisolone died ($P<0{\cdot}01$). Porter, *et al.* (1971) found no difference between groups of patients treated with corticosteroids and those with a placebo. In a further study also (Campra, Hamlin, Kirshbaum, Olivier, Redeker, and Reynolds, 1973) there was no significant difference in clinical status, appetite, rate of recovery, progression of disease, or mortality, in groups treated with prednisone and a placebo. These findings were confirmed by Maddrey, Boitnott, Bedine, Weber, and Mezey (1977); however, Maddrey, Boitnott, Bedine, Weber, Mezey, and White (1978) reported a significant reduction in mortality in a group treated with prednisolone ($P < 0{\cdot}05$).

With the available evidence it seems reasonable therefore to give corticosteroids to patients with severe alcoholic hepatitis, and encephalopathy; however the beneficial effect is at present inconclusive (Conn, 1978).

References

Akpom, C. A. and Warren, K. S. (1975). *J. infect. Dis.*, **132,** 6.

Bailey, K. V. (1966). *Med. J. Aust.*, **1,** 572.

Bailey, R. J., Kransner, N., Eddleston, A. L. W. F., Williams, R., Tee, D. E. H., Doniach, D., Kennedy, L. A., and Batchelor, J. R. (1976). *Br. med. J.*, **2,** 727.

Beckett, A. G., Livingstone, A. V., and Hill, K. R. (1961). *Br. med. J.*, **2,** 1113.

——, ——, and —— (1962). *Br. med. J.*, **2,** 580.

Bras, G., Brooks, S. E. H., and Watler, D. C. (1961). *J. Path. Bact.*, **82,** 503.

Br. med. J. (1978). **2,** 381.

Brunt, P. W., Kew, M. C., Scheuer, P. J., and Sherlock, S. (1974). *Gut*, **15,** 52.

Camain, R., Rouiller, C., and Dupin, H. (1959). *Annls Anat. path.*, **4,** 220.

Campra, J. L., Hamlin, E. M., Kirshbaum, R. J., Olivier, M., Redeker, A. G., and Reynolds, T. B.(1973). *Ann. intern. Med.*, **79,** 625

Conn, H. O. (1978). *Gastroenterology*, **74,** 319.

Cook, G. C. (1978). *Jl. R. Coll. Phycns.*, **12,** 329.

—— and Hutt, M. S. R. (1967). *Br. med. J.*, **3,** 454.

Edington, G. M. and Gilles, H. M. (1976). *Pathology in the tropics.* 2nd ed. p. 676. Edward Arnold, London.

Edmondson, H. A., Peters, R. L., Frankel, H. H., and Borowsky, S. (1967). *Medicine, Baltimore*, **46,** 119.

HAWKINS, H. L. (1978). *Gastroenterology*, **74**, 285.
HELMAN, R. A., TEMKO, M. H., NYE, S. W., and FALLON, H. J. (1971). *Ann. intern. Med.*, **74**, 311.
HIMSWORTH, H. P. (1950). 2nd ed. p. 48. *The liver and its diseases.* Blackwell, Oxford.
—— and GLYNN, L. E. (1944). *Lancet*, **1**, 457.
JENKINS, W. J. and PETERS, T. J. (1978). *Gut*, **19**, 341.
KAJUBI, S. K., SHAPER, A. G., and OWOR, R. (1972). in *Medicine in a tropical environment* (ed. A. G. Shaper, J. W. Kibukamusoke, and M. S. R. Hutt) p. 380. BMA, London.
KAKUMU, S. and LEEVY, C. M. (1977). *Gastroenterology*, **72**, 594.
KARIKS, J. (1960). *Papua New Guin. med. J.*, **4**, 5.
KANUFT, R. F. and WARREN, K. S. (1969). *J. infect. Dis.*, **120**, 560.
KONTTINEN, A., HÄRTEL, G. and LOUHIJA, A. (1970). *Acta med. scand.*, **188**, 257.
KRASNER, N., DAVIS, M., PORTMANN, B., and WILLIAMS, R. (1977). *Br. med. J.*, **1**, 1497.
Lancet, (1978). **2**, 353.
LEE, F. I. (1966). *Gut*, **7**, 77.
LEEVY, C. M., CHEN, T., and ZETTERMAN, R. K. (1975). *Ann. N.Y. Acad. Sci.*, **252**, 106.
LELBACH, W. K. (1974). In *Research Advances in Alcohol and Drug problems* (ed. R. J. Gibbins *et al.*) 1. p. 214. John Wiley, New York.
LESESNE, BOZYMSKI, E. M., and FALLON, H. J. (1978). *Gastroenterology*. **74**, 169.
LIEBER, C. S., DE CARLI, L. M. and RUBIN, E. (1975). *Proc. natn. Acad. Sci. U.S.A.*, **72**, 2.
MCLEAN, A. E. M. (1962). *Lancet*, **2**, 1292.
MADDREY, W. C., BOITNOTT, J. K., BEDINE, M. S., WEBER, F. L. and MEZEY, E. (1977). *Gastroenterology*, **72**, 1171.
——, ——, ——, ——, ——, and WHITE, R. I. (1978). *Gastroenterology*, **75**, 193.
MALLORY, F. B. (1911). *Bull. Johns Hopkins Hosp.*, **22**, 69.
PATEK, A. J., BOWRY, S. C., and SABESIN, S. M. (1976). *Archs Path.*, **100**, 19.
PEQUIGNOT, G., CHABERT, C., EYDOUX, H., and COURCOUL, M. A. (1974). *Revue de L'alcoolisme*, **20**, 191.
PHILLIPS, I. and WHARTON, B. (1968). *Br. med. J.*, **1**, 407.
PORTER, H. P., SIMON, F. R., POPE, C. E., VOLWILER, W., and FENSTER, L. F. (1971). *New Engl. J. Med.*, **284**, 1350.
RAMALINGASWAMI, V. (1964). *Nature, Lond.*, **201**, 546.
REYNOLDS, T. B. and EDMONDSON, H. A. (1971). *Ann. intern. Med.*, **74**, 440.
ROYLE, G., KETTLEWELL, M. G. W., ILIC, V., and WILLIAMSON, D. H. (1978). *Clin. Sci. molec. Med.*, **55**, 199.
RUBIN, E., BEATTIE, D. S., and LIEBER, C. S. (1970). *Lab. Invest.*, **23**, 620.
—— and LIEBER, C. S. (1967). *Gastroenterology*, **52**, 1.
—— and —— (1974). *New Engl. J. Med.*, **290**, 128.
SABESIN, S. M., HAWKINS, H. L., BERTRAM, P. D., MANN, J. A., and PEACE, R. J. (1978). *Gastroenterology*, **74**, 276.
SPRING, J. A. and BUSS, D. H. (1977). *Nature, Lond.*, **270**, 567.
SRIKANTIA, S. G., SRIRAMACHARI, S., and GOPALAN, C. (1958). *Indian J. med. Res.*, **46**, 121.
SUCKLING, P. V. and CAMPBELL, J. A. H. (1957). *J. trop. Pediat.*, **2**, 173.
SVOBODA, D. J. and MANNING, R. T. (1964). *Am. J. Path.*, **44**, 645.
TEMPLETON, A. C. (1970). *J. clin. Path.*, **23**, 24.
TROWELL, H. C., DAVIES, J. N. P., and DEAN, R. F. A. (1954). *Kwashiorkor*, p. 128. Edward Arnold, London.
WAES, L. V. and LIEBER, C. S. (1977). *Gastroenterology,* **73**, 646.
WATERLOW, J. C., CRAVIOTO, J., and STEPHEN, J. M. L. (1960). *Adv. Protein Chem.*, **15**, 131.
WATTS, T. (1969). *J. trop. Pediat.*, **15**, 155.
WILLIAMS, C. D. (1933). *Archs Dis. Childh.*, **8**, 423.

14

Diseases of the gall-bladder and biliary system

14.1. The gall-bladder in the tropics

In general the gall-bladder in the tropics is a far more healthy organ than it is in western countries. However all of the diseases of the western world, including cholelithiasis, do occur albeit less commonly. In rural Africa, gall-bladder disease is something of a rarity. As the standards of living improve, however, and life becomes more sophisticated and more similar to that in the western world, disease of the gall-bladder seems to become more common.

14.1.1. Cholecystitis and gall-stones

In Uganda, only 22 cases of gall-bladder disease were seen in seven years (Shaper and Patel, 1964). In a post-mortem study at the Mulago Hospital, Kampala (1950–62) the incidence of gall-stones was 0·87 per cent (Owor, 1964); pure pigment stones were the most common, mixed-facetted stones uncommon, and solitary cholesterol stones rare. A report from Nairobi, Kenya, also emphasized the rarity of gall-bladder and extrahepatic biliary disease in Africans in Kenya (Amollo-Odhiambo and Kamidigo, 1976); however those authors were able to assemble data on 35 patients who had had gall-bladder and biliary pathology during a seven-year period 1968–74.

In Nigeria during a five-year period (1957–62, 35 patients were treated at the University Hospital, Ibadan, for gall-bladder disease (Parnis, 1964). In Senegal, 10 female patients with disease of that organ were described; three had calculi, and seven biliary dyskinesia which was possibly secondary to schistosomiasis (Conté, Doumbia, and Sérafino, 1959). Reports from other African countries also give low incidence rates. Five cases of gall-bladder disease with gall-stones and three of gall-bladder carcinoma were reported by Wagner and Shepherd (1976) in a three-year survey of hospital admissions to Goroka Base Hospital, Papua New Guinea.

The low incidence of cholesterol gall-stones is undoubtedly related to the low concentrations of serum cholesterol and other lipids in Africans (Bronte-Stewart, Keys, and Brock, 1955; Shaper, 1974). Although most are pigment-stones, they too are surprisingly unusual in Africa (Weens, 1945; Lorentz, 1966); there is a very high incidence of haemolysis, much of it associated with sickle-cell disease, in some areas (Davey, 1968). Cholelithiasis is common in patients with sickle-cell (SS) disease in America (Margolies, 1951; Cameron, Maddrey, and Zuidema, 1971); however for an unexplained reason it seems to be uncommon in west Africa.

14.1.2. Salmonellosis (the typhoid carrier state)

The typhoid carrier state (Chapter 22) is a cause of gall-bladder disease; *Salmonella typhi* readily multiplies in bile. Although that is usually a chronic state, the cholecystitis may be acute. In chronic cholecystitis there is a superficial infiltrate of mononuclear cells with secondary lymphoid follicles in the mucosa and submucosa. Although typhoid is a very common disease in most tropical countries, the gall-bladder carrier is not a great practical problem (McFadzean and Ong, 1966). Gall-stones may form on a nucleus of *S. typhi*, but that is a very unusual complication in Africa. In both Ibadan, Nigeria (Davey, 1968), and Hong Kong (McFadzean and Ong, 1966), removal of an infected gall-bladder usually fails to relieve the carrier state; the source of infection seems in most cases to be intrahepatic (Erlik and Reitler, 1960). High dose amoxycillin should be given orally (Chapter 22) (Nolan and White, 1978); that compound is absorbed rapidly from the jejunum, and reaches very high blood concentrations.

14.1.3. Schistosomiasis of the gall-bladder

Schistosomal cholecystitis, with formation of stones in the biliary tract has been reported from South Africa (Botha, 1963). Pseudotubercles and ova have been observed in the gall-bladder wall, where they are associated with cholecystitis.

14.1.4. Other causes of cholecystitis

In Malaysia, biliary tract disease is more common in Indians and Malays than in Chinese (King, 1971). As well as the 'western type' of cholelithiasis, there is a condition known as oriental cholangitis, which is similar to that seen in Hong Kong, Singapore, Korea, China, and Japan. That disease has been called 'recurrent pyogenic cholangitis', 'cholangiohepatitis', 'Chinese biliary obstruction syndrome', and 'Japanese cholelithiasis'. The sex incidence is approximately equal. It is usually a disease of middle age. An enlarged gall-bladder, jaundice, fever, and infected bile are usual; soft pigment stones are found in dilated intra- and extrahepatic ducts. In only one of 44 patients was *Clonorchis sinensis* detected. It is considered possible that intestinal parasites, e.g. *Ascaris lumbricoides* (see below) and acute gastroenteritis are responsible. Death may occur from renal failure or septicaemia.

In adult male Chinese in Singapore, a close association between opium addiction and cholelithiasis has been noted (Edington and Gilles, 1976).

The gall-bladder is never affected in amoebic liver disease. That is presumably because amoebae cannot survive in bile. Although a great problem in the biliary tree, *Clonorchis sinensis* cannot exist in the gall-bladder; in heavy infections hard, friable dark bodies may be found. Cholecystitis and cholelithiasis have been reported in fascioliasis (see below). Empyema of the gall-bladder has been reported in opisthorchiasis.

14.1.5. Carcinoma of the gall-bladder

This tumour seems to be rare throughout Africa; when it does occur, it is an adenocarcinoma. At 4500 post-mortems in Johannesburg, there were four gall-bladder carcinomas (Becker and Chatgidakis, 1952). In Kampala, Uganda, six gall-bladder carcinomas were encountered in seven years (Owor, 1964).

14.2. Bile duct disease

14.2.1. Causes of biliary obstruction in the tropics

Extrahepatic causes of cholestasis differ in tropical countries from those in the western world (Sherlock, 1975), and there is furthermore a marked difference within the tropics. Although pancreatic carcinoma is seen throughout the world, it does not assume the place it has in Europe and the USA. In Africa, gall-stones are very unusual.

Throughout the tropics chronic calcific pancreatitis (Chapter 15) and ascariasis (Chapter 19) are relatively common causes of large duct obstruction. Although chronic pancreatitis is a rare cause of obstructive jaundice in the western world, it not infrequently gives rise to that complication in Africa (Owor, 1972). In addition, in much of the Far east, clonorchis and other liver-flukes are important (see below).

Intrahepatic cholestasis is usually associated with viral hepatitis, systemic bacterial infections (Chapter 6), and occasionally acute alcoholic hepatitis. In addition, patients with macronodular cirrhosis and hepatoma occasionally have this complication. The Dubin-Johnson syndrome seems unusually common in Papua New Guinea (Chapter 6). Primary biliary cirrhosis, biliary atresia, therapeutic agents, reticuloses, and sclerosing cholangitis fade into insignificance in the tropics.

14.2.2. Ascariasis involving the biliary tract

In parts of the tropics where gall-stones are uncommon, and that applies to most developing countries, any young person presenting with symptoms and signs of biliary tract disease should be suspected of having ascariasis (Louw, 1966). Usually the adult worm blocks the sphincter of Oddi and that gives rise to obstruction of both biliary and pancreatic ducts (Yang and Loube, 1946). Ascending pyogenic cholangitis, cholecystitis, granulomatous strictures, abscesses, and even perforation of the bile ducts may ensue (Muazzam, Khaleque, and Ibrahim, 1960; Hsu, 1962; Yue, 1974). There may be formation of biliary calculi, which contain ova and fragments of adult worms. In Japan, pigmented calcium stones are often found in the bile-ducts and gall-bladder and are also considered to be due to the ova of *Ascaris lumbricoides* (Maki, 1961).

Ascariasis of the bile ducts should be suspected on clinical grounds in areas where ascariasis is common. Adult roundworms may or may not have been passed in the stools (Louw, 1974). There is often right upper quadrant pain, which is associated with tenderness and occasional vomiting. Obstructive jaundice may be present. There is tenderness in the right hypochondrium, with hepatomegaly and sometimes a palpable gall-bladder. I have seen this condition diagnosed, tragically, at post-mortem in an elderly Ugandan who was considered on clinical grounds to have a pancreatic carcinoma; laparotomy was not carried out.

Radiology and laparotomy are the only procedures which help with the diagnosis. Intravenous cholangiography frequently outlines the adult ascaris in the common bile-duct (Cywes and Krige, 1960); in 73 per cent of cases, the worms show up using that technique (Cremin, 1969). Where doubt exists, endoscopy and retrograde-cholangiography are of value (van der Spuy, 1978).

In that study three of four children suspected of having the disease, were found to have at least one adult ascaris in the biliary tree; the procedure was also of value in deciding whether the ducts were clear after medical treatment (Chapter 19).

Treatment with antibiotics and antispasmodics, to relax the sphincter of Oddi, together with gastric suction and intravenous fluids should be instituted. Piperazine should be given after the acute attack has subsided (Chapter 19). Surgery is indicated (Davey, 1968): (i) when medical treatment fails, (ii) when gross hepatomegaly is present, and there is evidence of peritonitis, (iii) in the presence of deep jaundice, and (iv) if there is persistence of a worm-outline on the intravenous cholangiogram at a second examination. At operation the dead worm(s) should be removed from the common bile-duct and that should be followed by temporary T-tube drainage.

14.2.3. Clonorchiasis (oriental liver-fluke)

Disease due to liver-flukes is usually caused by organisms from the orient, *Clonorchis sinensis* and *Opisthorchis* spp. (Komiya, 1966). It is confined to south-east Asia, but Chinese immigrants to many parts of the world, including the United Kingdom, may harbour the infection (*Br. med. J.*, 1978). In Montreal, Canada, 62 (15 per cent) of 400 Chinese immigrants examined were infected with *Clonorchis sinensis* (Seah, 1973). Infection is acquired by eating raw freshwater fish. Presentation is usually with obstructive jaundice. Obstructive jaundice in an immigrant Chinese in a western country is an indication for a thorough search for evidence of liver flukes. In Hong Kong, and other areas where liver flukes are endemic, cholangiohepatitis is a common surgical emergency. Presentation is with acute abdominal pain, pyrexia, and jaundice; remission with further exacerbations may occur. The disease may be complicated by perforation of the gall-bladder; strictures may form in the intrahepatic bile-duct system, resulting in abscess formation. Cholangiocarcinoma may also complicate such infections.

Clonorchis sinensis. Otherwise known as the oriental liver-fluke, this organism causes disease in the Far east, Japan, Korea, China, Taiwan, and Vietnam. Approximately 36 per cent of the population of Hong Kong is affected (Huang, Wong, Ma, and Sun, 1969). Incidence of infection rises steeply between two and 21 years, and flattens thereafter (Hou and Pang, 1964); all social groups eat raw fish and all are therefore affected.

It is a flat fluke, 10–25 mm in length and 3–5 mm broad, which lives in the bile and pancreatic ducts of man and other mammals who eat freshwater fish. Fish ponds fertilized with human faeces are responsible for many infections. Ova pass down the common bile-duct to be excreted in the faeces. When they reach water they hatch in the digestive tract of a suitable snail and eventually escape as cercariae. They in turn penetrate the skin of certain freshwater fish and encyst in their flesh, skin, and gills; there they develop into the infective form, encysted metacercariae. After ingestion the metacercariae are liberated by intestinal digestive juices and, after migration to the common bile-duct, the larvae develop into adults in the biliary tree; the worms can live for 25 to 30 years.

Most infections are asymptomatic. There may however be mild abdominal and digestive disturbances, fever, anorexia, and epigastric pain. Jaundice and pyogenic cholangitis may occur (Strauss, 1962). Suppurative pancholangitis with coma, jaundice, fever, rigors, and hypoglycaemia have been described (McFadzean and Yeung, 1965). In infected individuals, the typhoid carrier state seems to be abnormally high (McFadzean and Ong, 1966).

The left lobe of the liver is involved more often than the right. The bile-ducts are dilated with reddish transparent parasites; with heavy infections, localized dilatations of intrahepatic bile ducts appear as pale-blue cystic structures on the serous surface (Hou, 1955). The surrounding liver is normal. Generalized duct dilatation is unusual unless the common bile-duct is obstructed by a stone, tumour, or an inflammatory stricture (Hou, 1955). If there is secondary infection, usually caused by *Escherichia coli* cholangitis, cholangiohepatitis, pylephlebitis, and multiple abscesses may occur. Although both micronodular and biliary cirrhosis have been described, the role of the liver-fluke in their production is not clear. There seems no doubt that *Clonorchis sinensis* infection is associated with bile-duct carcinoma, which is distinct from the hepatocellular cancer seen so commonly in tropical countries (Chapter 9). Desquamation and proliferation of epithelial-lining cells, and excessive mucin formation are found in the bile-ducts. Adenomatous changes occur in the epithelium due to the mechanical irritation of the worm and its metabolic and degradation products. The bile-duct walls become infiltrated with leucocytes, most of which are eosinophils, and their vascularity is increased; smaller portal vein branches become fibrosed with increased portal pressure (Hoeppli, 1932). Blockage of bile-ducts with cystic dilatation may occur. Pigment-stones, ova, and inflammatory products may give rise to 'biliary mud'.

Opisthorchis felineus and *O. viverrini.* Opisthorchiasis is a major problem in Thailand and the Ukraine. In Thailand up to 90 per cent of people over 10 years old are infected with *O. viverrini*, i.e. approximately 3·5 million people (Harinasuta, 1969). The disease is most common in the late rainy season and early dry season (Sadun, 1955). Those residents who do not eat raw fish are not infected (Harinasuta and Vajasthira, 1960). *O. felineus* is common in India, Vietnam, Japan, and the Philippines; *O. viverrini* has been reported from Thailand and Laos.

The adult flukes are approximately 10 mm in length and 2 mm in breadth. The life cycle is similar to that of *Clonorchis sinensis.* Infection in man and other animals, including the cat (*O. felineus*), occurs from eating freshwater fish which has been infected by water contaminated with faeces.

The pathology is similar to that in *Clonorchis sinensis* infection; there is a high incidence of cholangiocellular carcinoma.

Diagnosis of oriental liver-fluke infection is made by finding characteristic ova in the stool or duodenal fluid, in a direct smear. A leucocytosis with an eosinophilia is usual. There may be evidence of biliary obstruction with a raised serum conjugated bilirubin and alkaline phosphatase. Hypoglycaemia is common. Intradermal and serological tests are at present of limited value; an indirect haemagglutination test is however useful (Pacheco, Wykoff, and Jung,

1960). In *Opisthorchis* infections, percutaneous cholangiography may show: (i) a single cyst cavity, (ii) mulberry-like dilatations of the intrahepatic bile-ducts, (iii) a combination of (i) and (ii), or (iv) dilatation of intrahepatic bile-ducts (Viranuvatti, 1968).

Treatment is difficult, and there is at present no satisfactory therapeutic agent. Chloroquine phosphate diminishes ova production but does not kill the flukes. Six hundred mg (base) should be given daily for six weeks; the possibility of retinal complications should be borne in mind. Bithional, 40 mg per kg bodyweight on alternate days for 20–30 days may also be tried. When it is available, hexachloroparaxylol is effective. That agent has been used successfully in China (Chung, Hsu, Ts'ao, K'o, Kuo, Hsu, Li, Cheng, Chang, Yuan, and Chang, 1965; Wang, Chang, Shen, Huei, Chou, Hsu, Chao, Wu, Lan, Ts'ao, Cheng, Li, Cheng, and Sung, 1965), but is difficult to obtain in the western world. In heavy infections, 250 mg per kg bodyweight should be given orally, twice daily on alternate days over a 20 day period; in light infections, half of that dose should be given. Side effects are usually mild and consist of gastro-intestinal disturbances, dizziness, sweating, and fatigue.

14.2.4. Fascioliasis (sheep liver-fluke)

Another trematode, *Fasciola hepatica* (sheep liver-fluke) has a worldwide distribution but is most common in sheep-producing areas. It is of considerable importance in the Middle east; it is also a problem in some non-tropical countries, e.g. Wales. A further species, which is common in domestic ruminants throughout the tropics, *F. gigantica* (Hammond, 1974), frequently affects man in Hawaii (Alicata, 1953; Stemmermann, 1953) and parts of central Africa.

The adult worm is flat and leaf-shaped, 30 mm in length and 13 mm in breadth; it lives in the bile-ducts and liver parenchyma of sheep, cattle, goats, and man. After passage in the stool to moist and swampy terrain, the ova hatch and release miracidia which, after entering certain species of snail, develop with the ultimate production of cercariae. The cercariae encyst on grasses and water plants, especially water-cress and lettuce, which is eaten by the appropriate host, usually in raw salad; larvae are liberated, penetrate the mucosa, enter the portal circulation, and undergo a period of about three months maturing in the bile-ducts by ingesting biliary secretions.

There may be pain in the right upper abdomen with mild fever during the migratory phase. The illness may be clinically similar to viral hepatitis, with jaundice and tender hepatomegaly, or may even be asymptomatic (D'Sa, 1970). Biliary obstruction is possible. Later, portal hypertension and its various manifestations may occur. Adult worms occasionally reach ectopic sites and may produce subcutaneous abscesses in the thorax; epileptic attacks have been recorded following cerebral involvement. These flukes may invade the pharynx and are one of the agents responsible for the condition known as 'halzoun' in parts of the Middle east (Chapter 2).

Desquamation and adenomatous hyperplasia of the bile-duct epithelium occur. There is a pericholangitis and cystic dilatation of the ducts; eosinophils dominate the infiltrate. There may be small necrotic foci or microabscesses infiltrated with eosinophils and leucocytes (Belding, 1965). Fibrosis of the portal tracts occurs, and the adjacent liver tissue is compressed. Portal hypertension, splenomegaly, and ascites follow; malignant change has not been recorded. A focal inflammatory reaction with subsequent fibrosis around ova may occur in various other tissues.

There is usually a leucocytosis and eosinophilia, which is often gross, during the migratory stage. In the early stages, liver-biopsy shows marked infiltration with eosinophils (Facey and Marsden, 1960).

Ova are found in the stool, but not until three months after infection; duodenal juice often contains ova at an earlier stage (Lavier and Deschiens, 1956). Serological diagnosis is of use (Taillez and Korach, 1970); intradermal and haemagglutination tests are of limited value.

The therapeutic agent of choice is bithionol (Knodell, Kirsch and, Rygg, 1972); 40 mg per kg bodyweight should be given on alternate days over a period of 20–30 days. Side-effects consist of nausea and diarrhoea and are mild. Hexachloroparaxylol has been found effective in the USSR (Plotnikov, Karnaukhov, Zalnova, Alekseeva, Borisov, and Stromskaya, 1965); the dosage is the same as for clonorchiasis, but of shorter duration. Emetine hydrochloride, 1 mg per kg bodyweight (maximum 65 mg daily) may be given intramuscularly for 10 days, as an alternative.

14.2.5. Other infections which may involve the biliary tree

Salmonellosis (typhoid fever). Although chronic gall-bladder disease is common, cholangitis is rare in typhoid fever (Edington and Gilles, 1976).

Hydatid disease. Occasionally a hydatid cyst within the liver ruptures into the gall-bladder or biliary tree. The outcome is usually satisfactory; the contents of the cyst pass down the biliary tree and an allergic reaction and shock do not occur.

Tapeworms. Rarely tapeworms (Chapter 19) ascend the biliary system; a blocked cystic duct and cholecystitis have been reported.

Dicrocoeliasis. A small trematode, *Dicrocoelium dendriticum*, may invade the intrahepatic bile-ducts, with the production of fibrous thickening of the portal tracts (Roche, 1948) and progressive obstructive jaundice (Mandoul, Demartial, Pestre, and Moulinier, 1966); it is not uncommon in Nigeria. The adult worm is approximately 10 mm in length. The ova are ingested by various species of land snail; they develop into cercariae which are eaten by ants in which they develop into metacercariae. Man is usually infected accidentally by eating live ants.

14.2.6. Bile-duct (cholangiocellular) carcinoma

This tumour is usually found in areas where liver-flukes are common (see above). It is unusual in areas where hepatocellular carcinoma (hepatoma) is a problem (Chapter 9); the disease is not associated with cirrhosis. The tumours are usually white or grey in colour and may be difficult to distinguish histologically from a liver-cell carcinoma. Some tumours are mixed with liver-cell carcinomas, both elements being present in the same tumour. They are usually in close proximity to the bile-ducts.

There is often evidence of cholangitis and of parasitic, usually clonorchis, infection. In *Clonorchis sinensis* infections, multifocal adenocarcinomas arise from adenomatous hyperplasia of the bile-duct epithelium (Hou, 1956). They do not show a uniform pattern, and can be classified as: (i) polypoid adenocarcinomas (Yamagata, Takanaka, Yaegashi, Watanabe, Abe, and Kanno, 1964), and anaplastic carcinomas arising from the lining epithelial cells of the bile-ducts, (ii) carcinomas arising from adenomas of the bile ducts, and (iii) a mixture of types (i) and (ii). The anaplastic variety, which is uncommon, resembles primary liver-cell carcinoma. Areas of necrosis are common; squamous metaplasia occasionally occurs. Mucin may be present; there is no glycogen or bile pigment. The tumours metastasize to regional lymph glands, and to most organs of the body.

Cholangiolocellular carcinoma. These tumours consist of small cells with an eosinophilic cytoplasm and dense hyperchromatic nuclei. They arise from the cholangioles (the canals of Hering). The cells lie in small simple cords which often contain a small canaliculus and are separated by dense connective tissue; areas of liver-cell or cholangiocellular carcinoma may also be present.

14.3. Biliary cirrhosis

Biliary cirrhosis seems to be uncommon in tropical countries. Although biliary parasites enter the bile-ducts, and may even cause large-duct obstruction (see above), they rarely produce longstanding stasis and cirrhosis. Gall-stones, an important cause of biliary cirrhosis in temperate areas, are generally not common in most tropical countries (see above). Rare forms of cirrhosis, due to congenital absence of bile ducts, and primary biliary cirrhosis, apparently occur in tropical as well as temperate countries, but are universally rare.

References

Alicata, J. E. (1953). *Hawaii med. J. inter-Isl. Nurs. Bull.*, **12,** 196.

Amollo-Odhiambo, P. B. and Kamidigo, N. O. (1976). *E. Afr. med. J.*, **53,** 74.

Becker, B. J. P. and Chatgidakis, C. B. (1952). *S. Afr. J. clin. Sci.*, **3,** 13.

Belding, D. L. (1965). *Textbook of Clinical Parasitology*. 3rd ed. Appleton-Century-Crofts, New York.

Botha, D. J. (1963). *Br. J. Surg.*, **50,** 543.

Br. med. J. (1978). **1,** 1091.

Bronte-Stewart, B., Keys, A., and Brock, J. F. (1955). *Lancet*, **2,** 1103.

Cameron, J. L., Maddrey, W. C., and Zuidema, G. D. (1971). *Ann. Surg.*, **174,** 702.

Chung, H-L., Hsu, C-P., T'sao, W-C., K'o, H-Y., Kuo, C-H., Hsu, H-C., Li, P-H., Cheng, S., Chang, H-Y., Yuan, C-T., and Chang, Y-C. (1965). *China med. J.*, **84,** 232.

Conté, S., Doumbia, F., and Sérafino, X. (1959). *Bull. Mém. Éc. prép. Méd. Pharm. Dakar.*, **7,** 43.

Cremin, B. J. (1969). *Br. J. Radiol.*, **42,** 506.

Cywes, S. and Krige, H. (1960). *S. Afr. med. J.*, **34,** 478.

Davey, W. W. (1968). *Companion to Surgery in Africa*. p. 195, 219. E. and S. Churchill, Edinburgh and London.

D'sa, C. J. (1970). *Proc. R. Soc. Med.*, **63,** 285.

Edington, G. M. and Gilles, H. M. (1976). *Pathology in the tropics*. 2nd ed. p. 324, 598. Edward Arnold, London.

Erlik, D. and Reitler, R. (1960). *Lancet*, **1,** 1216.

Facey, R. V. and Marsden, P. D. (1960). *Br. med. J.*, **2,** 619.

HAMMOND, J. A. (1974). *Trans. R. Soc. trop. Med. Hyg.*, **68,** 253.
HARINASUTA, C. (1969). *In Proceedings of the fourth S. E. Asian Seminar on Parasitology and Tropical Medicine*, p. 253.
—— and VAJRASTHIRA, S. (1960). *Ann. trop. Med. Parasit.*, **54,** 100.
HOEPPLI, R. (1932). *China med. J.*, **46,** 1179.
HOU, P. C. (1955). *J. Path. Bact.*, **70,** 53.
—— (1956). *J. Path. Bact.*, **72,** 239.
—— and PANG, L. S. C. (1964). *J. Path. Bact.*, **87,** 245.
HSU, H. F. (1962). *Nagoya J. med. Sci.*, **24,** 215.
HUANG, C. T., WONG, M. M., MA, S. L., and SUN, T. (1969). *Trop. Med.*, **11,** 136.
KING, M. S. (1971). *Br. J. Surg.*, **58,** 829.
KNODELL, R. G., KIRSCH, E., and RYGG, G. C. (1972). *Calif. Med.*, **117,** 72.
KOMIYA, Y. (1966). *Adv. Parasitol.*, **4,** 53.
LAVIER, G. and DESCHIENS, R. (1956). *Bull. Soc. Path. exot.*, **49,** 541.
LORENTZ, T. G. (1966). *Br. J. Surg.*, **53,** 503.
LOUW, J. H. (1966). *Br. J. Surg.*, **53,** 510.
—— (1974). *S. Afr. J. Surg.*, **12,** 219.
MCFADZEAN, A. J. S. and ONG, G. B. (1966). *Br. med. J.*, **1,** 1567.
—— and YEUNG, R. T. T. (1965). *Trans. R. Soc. trop. Med. Hyg.*, **59,** 179.
MAKI, T. (1961). *Archs Surg., Chicago*, **82,** 599.
MANDOUL, R., DEMARTIAL, L., PESTRE, M. and MOULINIER, C. (1966). *J. Méd. Bordeaux*, **143,** 685.
MARGOLIES, M. P. (1951). *Medicine, Baltimore*, **30,** 357.
MUASSAM, M. G., KHALEQUE, K. A., and IBRAHIM M. (1960). *J. trop. Med. Hyg.*, **63,** 95.
NOLAN, C. M. and WHITE, P. C. (1978). *J. Am. med. Ass.*, **239,** 2352.
OWOR, R. (1964). *E. Afr. med. J.*, **41,** 251.
—— (1972). *E. Afr. med. J.*, **49,** 614.
PACHECO, G., WYKOFF, D. E., and JUNG, R. C. (1960). *Am. J. trop. Med. Hyg.*, **9,** 367.
PARNIS, R. O. (1964). *Trans. R. Soc. trop. Med. Hyg.*, **58,** 437.
PLOTNIKOV, N. N., KARNAUKHOV, V. K., ZALNOVA, N. S., ALEKSEEVA, M. I., BORISOV, I. A., and STROMSKAYA, T. F. (1965). *Medskaya Parazit.*, **34,** 725.
ROCHE, P. J. L. (1948). *Trans. R. Soc. trop. Med. Hyg.*, **41,** 819.
SADUN, E. H. (1975). *Am. J. Hyg.*, **62,** 81.
SEAH, S. K. K. (1973). *J. trop. Med. Hyg.*, **76,** 291.
SHAPER, A. G. (1974). In *Cardiovascular disease in the tropics* (ed. A. G. Shaper, M. S. R. Hutt and Z. Fejfar). p. 148. British Medical Association, London.
—— and PATEL, K. M. (1964). *E. Afr. med. J.*, **41,** 246.
SHERLOCK, S. (1975). *Diseases of the liver and biliary system.* 5th ed. p. 260, 727, and 771. Blackwell, Oxford.
STEMMERMANN, G. N. (1953). *Am. J. Path.*, **29,** 731.
STRAUSS, W. G. (1962). *Am. J. trop. Med. Hyg.*, **11,** 625.
TAILLEZ, R. and KORACH, S. (1970). *Annls Inst. Pasteur, Paris*, **118,** 330.
VAN DER SPUY, S. (1978). *S. Afr. med. J.*, **53,** 1030.
VIRANUVATTI, V. (1968). In *Proceedings of the third S.E. Asian Seminar on Parasitology and Tropical Medicine.* (ed. A. A. Sandosham and V. Zamon). p. 134. Singapore.
WAGNER, F. B. and SHEPHERD, A. (1976). *Papua New Guin. med. J.*, **19,** 156.
WANG, S-M, CHANG, K-N, SHEN, S-L, HUEI, P-L, CHOU, H-M, HSU, K-S, CHAO, C., WU, S-M, LAN, H-C, TS'AO, S-C, CHENG, S., LI, P-H, CHENG, C., and SUNG, H-Y. (1965). *China med. J.*, **84,** 748.
WEENS, H. S. (1945). *Ann. intern. Med.*, **22,** 182.
YAMAGATA, S., TAKANAKA, M., YAEGASHI, A., WARTANABE, S., ABE, T., and KANNO, T., (1964). *Jap. J. Parasit.*, **13,** 112.
YANG, S. C. H. and LOUBE, P. J. (1946). *Ann. Surg.*, **123,** 299.
YUE, P. C. K. (1974). *Aust. N.Z. J. Surg.*, **44,** 53.

Section 3 : The pancreas

15

The pancreas in the tropics

In temperate areas, both acute and chronic pancreatitis are frequently caused by alcohol (*Br. med. J.*, 1978); the former type is common in 'spree' drinkers. In 55 patients with chronic calcific pancreatitis mean daily alcohol intake was estimated at 175 g (Sarles, Sarles, Camatte, Muratore, Gaini, Guien, Pastor, and Le Roy, 1965), and in a further study at 150 g (Sarles, 1973).

Two main types of pancreatitis are seen in tropical countries. The acute form resembles that seen in temperate climates and is frequently associated with intermittent excessive alcohol consumption, which is a common problem in many parts of Africa. The chronic form, chronic calcific pancreatitis has certain features which differentiate it from chronic pancreatic disease seen in temperate zones (Avery Jones, Gummer, and Lennard-Jones, 1968) and which is usually a long-term result of alcohol (*Br. med. J.*, 1977). However many acute and chronic cases do not have an obvious aetiology and may result from virus infections. Acute haemorrhagic and suppurative pancreatitis are not often seen in tropical countries.

15.1. Acute pancreatitis (AP)

This is a severe acute abdominal condition often presenting as an acute emergency, in which there is intra-abdominal liberation of pancreatic enzymes. Pathology may be localized to one part of the organ, or may be generalized. Changes vary from acute oedema with cellular infiltration, to necrosis of the acinar cells, haemorrhage from necrotic blood vessels and intra- and extra-pancreatic fat necrosis.

Overall, acute pancreatic disease is uncommon in Africa. In Kampala, for example, it accounted for only four cases in 841 acute non-traumatic emergencies over a three-year period (McAdam, 1961). However in the Baragwanath Hospital, Johannesburg, the disease accounts for much acute abdominal pain and is the most common cause of non-traumatic abdominal emergencies (Lawson, 1962). In the Far east, liver flukes are responsible for many cases. Throughout the third world, ascariasis is an important cause.

15.1.1. Aetiology of AP

The majority of cases are currently labelled as idiopathic (The, 1977). However, many are undoubtedly alcoholically induced; that applies to tropical as well as temperate countries. Many are due to biliary tract disease, which although an uncommon problem in Africa, is a considerable problem in some

Far eastern countries. Less common causes in the western world—hyperparathyroidism, hyperlipidaemia, vasculitis, abdominal trauma, diabetes mellitus, and iatrogenic disease associated with corticosteroids and thiazide diuretics—seem to be unusual causes of the disease in Africa and Asia.

Pancreatic obstruction due to invasion of the duct by an adult *Ascaris lumbricoides* occasionally occurs. In children pancreatitis in association with ascariasis can be due to several factors: (i) blockage of the ampulla of Vater with bile regurgitation, (ii) introduction of enteric organisms into the pancreatic duct by the worm, and (iii) an acute necrotizing process surrounding the disintegrating worm (Edington and Gilles, 1976). Because the adult worm has entered the sphincter of Oddi, biliary obstruction is usually present concurrently with pancreatic obstruction. Inflammation producing both an acute pancreatitis, and pseudocyst formation has been reported (Evans, Lubben, and Whigham, 1953). Management of pancreatic obstruction is on similar lines to that for biliary obstruction (Chapter 14). Surgery is undertaken only when there is doubt about the diagnosis or where an expanding pseudocyst is present (Davey, 1968); that is treated by cyst-gastrostomy.

Infection with the oriental liver fluke (*Clonorchis sinensis*) (Chapter 14) may give rise to acute pancreatitis in the Far east, China, Japan, Korea, Taiwan, and Vietnam. The flukes enter the ampulla of Vater where they produce an obstruction (McFadzean and Yeung, 1966) and rarely an acute necrosis of the organ; adenomatous hyperplasia and periductal fibrosis occur. Squamous-cell metaplasia of the ductular epithelium may also occur.

Infection with *Opisthorchis felineus* and *O. viverrini* (Chapter 14) can similarly involve the pancreatic duct. Thailand, the Philippines, India, Japan, and Vietnam are affected.

Rarely tapeworms (Chapter 19) can enter the pancreatic duct producing obstruction and pancreatic necrosis.

It seems likely, although not proven, that viruses contribute to the pancreatitis seen in the third world; mumps. Coxsackie B, cytomegalovirus, and hepatitis B virus (Sherlock, 1975) have all been implicated in this disease. There is also evidence that *Mycoplasma pneumoniae* is associated with acute pancreatitis (Leinikki, Pantzar, and Tykka, 1973; Mårdh and Ursing, 1974; Freeman and McMahon, 1978). In the last of those studies, nine of 27 consecutive patients with acute pancreatitis had serological evidence of infection with *Mycoplasma pneumoniae*; however four of them also had gall-stones, which is of interest in view of a known affinity of myoplasma for cholesterol.

In young children the condition can occur in severe dehydration associated with acute gastroenteritis (Collins, 1958); inspissated secretions block the pancreatic duct.

15.1.2. Presentation of AP

Severe upper abdominal pain is the main symptom, and the condition is frequently mistaken for a surgical emergency. The pain is worsened by lying down, and improved by sitting up and leaning forward; radiation to the back is usual. Vomiting, sweating, and shock usually accompany the pain. There is a tachycardia, fever, hypotension, and clamminess of the skin. Abdominal tenderness and distension with ileus may be present. Mild jaundice is not uncommon. The main differential diagnosis is a posterior duodenal ulcer with penetration to the pancreas, or perforation. Most other acute abdominal and thoracic conditions may be mimicked. The mortality from acute pancreatitis is very high especially when hepatic, cardiovascular, or renal impairment are present.

15.1.3. Investigation of AP

A leucocytosis is usual. The serum amylase concentration is elevated in 90 per cent of cases within the first 24 hours; serum lipase rises more slowly. Urine amylase is elevated. Serum bilirubin and alkaline phosphatase concentrations may be elevated especially where there is an obstruction at the ampulla of Vater, as occurs in ascariasis. Hyperglycaemia and an abnormal glucose tolerance is common. Serum calcium is low especially after the fifth or sixth day; if tetany is present the prognosis is bad.

15.1.4. Treatment of AP

Continuous nasogastric suction and intravenous nutrition should be carried out. Atropine may be given as an antispasmodic. Aprotinin ('Trasylol'), 200 000 units six hourly, given intravenously for five days, should be started as soon as possible after diagnosis; that probably reduces mortality ($P < 0{\cdot}05$) (Trapnell, Rigby, Talbot, and Duncan, 1974) but there are many who doubt its efficacy. Plasma volume must be maintained with intravenous plasma, and hypocalcaemia with tetany should be treated with intravenous calcium gluconate. Broad-spectrum antibiotics are frequently administered but their value is unproved (Soergel, 1978). If *Mycoplasma pneumoniae* is in fact a significant factor in the aetiology of acute pancreatitis (see above) it is probably worthwhile to give antibiotics for that reason.

15.2. The pancreas in kwashiorkor

In severe kwashiorkor, pancreatic atrophy is one of the most impressive and constant findings at post-mortem (Trowell, Davies, and Dean, 1954); the entire gland is often in a state of autolysis, and is diminished in size due to shrinkage of the acinar cells.

15.3. Chronic calcific pancreatitis (CCP)

In the western world, alcoholism, hereditary pancreatitis, hypercalcaemia, and hyperlipoproteinaemia I, IV, and V are the usual causes of chronic pancreatitis. Alcohol is the only aetiological agent of these which assumes significance in third-world countries. Chronic relapsing pancreatitis seems to be unusual. Iron deposits occur in African siderosis (Chapter 8). A far more important entity, and one which can be counted a tropical disease, is *chronic calcific pancreatitis.* This constitutes the most common cause of overt malabsorption in many parts of the tropics, including tropical and South Africa. It is common in Indonesia (Zuidema, 1959), Uganda (Shaper, 1960; 1964; Banwell, Campbell, Blackman, Hutt, and Leonard, 1963; Banwell, Hutt, Marsden, and Blackman, 1964; Banwell, Hutt, Leonard, Blackman, Connor, Marsden, and

Campbell, 1967; Cook, 1967a; Cook and Kajubi, 1972), India (Mahadevan, 1961; Geevarghese and Pitchumoni, 1966), Zaire (Bourgoignie, Sonnet, and Dechef, 1962), Nigeria (Kinnear, 1963; Olurin and Olurin, 1969), and South Africa (Jackson, Marks, and Bank, 1966; Marks, Bank, and Louw, 1968). It has not been reported from south America. The disease as it occurs in east Africa has been reviewed by Kajubi, Shaper, and Owor (1972). Sixty-five per cent of patients with overt malabsorption had the disease. Eight per cent of patients attending the diabetic clinic at the Mulago Hospital, Kampala, had pancreatic calcification; below and above 45 years the percentages were 13 and 2·4 per cent respectively.

15.3.1. Aetiology of CCP

The largest clinical series to be reported from Uganda was by Banwell, *et al.* (1967); of 45 patients shown during a two-year period to be suffering from malabsorption, 30 had chronic exocrine pancreatic disease. Twenty-four were male and six female; 57 per cent were under 30 years of age. Seventeen of them had frank diabetes mellitus. Olurin and Olurin (1969) recorded 45 cases in Nigerians in Ibadan, Nigeria, during an 11-year period; sex incidence was equal, and young people were predominantly affected (69 per cent were 20 years or less, and four were 10 years old). Fifteen (33 per cent) had steatorrhoea. Diabetes, in 82 per cent, was the commonest reason for seeking medical attention. There was no history of alcohol excess; protein malnutrition was considered by the authors to be responsible for the pancreatic calcification in at least 90 per cent of the patients.

There are very marked local differences in incidence rates in Africa. During five years in Lusaka, Zambia, only two cases were seen despite a widespread search (Cook, 1974); the disease seems to be much more common however in northern Zambia (Lowenthal, Motola, Siddorn, and Parker, 1968). Although alcohol consumption is extremely common in the Zambian population, malnutrition is unusual in adults, and probably less usual in children than in many other parts of tropical Africa where the disease is common.

A significant impairment in intravenous glucose tolerance was demonstrated in a group of Ugandan children who had had kwashiorkor five to 12 years before, when compared with a control group taken from a similar environment (Cook, 1967b; 1968). In Jamaica, a similar result was obtained in 28 children who had had protein-calorie malnutrition six to 20 (mean 12) weeks before (James and Coore, 1970); in that study impaired oral glucose tolerance was also demonstrated, and furthermore, plasma insulin concentrations were significantly lower in the patients compared with controls. It was suggested by those investigators therefore that a permanent reduction in β-cell mass had resulted from severe malnutrition. Using oral glucose and intravenous glucagon and tolbutamide tests, Kajubi (1972a) has reported, however, that there was not a significant difference in the blood glucose concentration in 15 children who had had kwashiorkor nine to 16 years before, compared with a control group; in that study, although fasting plasma-insulin concentrations were significantly lower, growth hormone concentrations were significantly higher in the patients compared with the controls, and maximum insulin response was similar in both groups. It was concluded from that study that the functional β-cell mass in children who have recovered from kwashiorkor is identical with that of controls. There is thus some evidence to suggest that permanent pancreatic damage can persist after recovery from severe malnutrition, possibly of a chronic type, and that that might account for the high prevalence of chronic calcific pancreatic disease in many parts of the tropics. That would be consistent with the observations of Trowell, *et al.* (1954), that fibrosis follows atrophy of the pancreatic acinar cells in kwashiorkor. Malnutrition has also been suggested on clinical grounds to be the cause in Indonesia (Zuidema, 1959), Uganda (Shaper, 1960), and south India (Geevarghese and Pitchumoni, 1966). Malnutrition was also suggested to be aetiologically important by Ndugwa and Sebikari (1976) (see below). Barbezat (1967) has demonstrated that pancreatic exocrine function may become permanently impaired after chronic malnutrition.

In south India, where the disease is very common, alcohol does not seem to be important (Geevarghese and Pitchumoni, 1966). In South Africa however there seems no doubt that alcohol is an important aetiological factor (Jackson, *et al.*, 1966). Shaper (1964) considered that in 36 cases seen in Kampala during 1958–64, half had had bouts of heavy drinking on a background of malnutrition. In both Uganda and Nigeria alcohol seems a possible aetiological agent, but in the older and not the young age group.

A compromise hypothesis would be that malnutrition renders the pancreas more susceptible to the effect of alcohol. The possibility of virus diseases, e.g. cytomegalic disease, mumps (Chapter 1), viral hepatitis, or Coxsackie virus B (Chapter 7), being implicated has not been excluded. Viral hepatitis and mumps commonly produce acute pancreatitis and should be seriously considered as being important aetiological agents. In a limited study in Uganda, mucoviscidosis did not seem to be relevant to the problem (Bwibo, Rwabwogo-Atenyi, and Kagwa, 1972).

Toxic agents, especially hydrocyanic acid from cassava have also been suggested as possible causative agents (Pitchumoni and Thomas, 1973).

15.3.2. Presentation of CCP

The disease may occur as early as three years (Edington and Gilles, 1976); the youngest patient this author has seen was six years old. In a report of the condition from Uganda, seven children below the age of 10 years were described (Ndugwa and Sebikari, 1976); all had recurrent abdominal pain, five had pancreatic calcification, and one diabetes mellitus. All of them had evidence of malnutrition. There is a clear male preponderance; young men are the main group affected. The main clinical features of the disease are malabsorption, with steatorrhoea, and diabetes mellitus.

Abdominal pain is often extremely severe and may in fact drive sufferers to suicide; it is usually epigastric and radiates to the back but it is frequently atypical. Nausea, vomiting, and flatulence are common during severe attacks of pain. Loss of weight is often gross and evidence of severe malnutrition ('adult kwashiorkor') is often present. Some or all of the cutaneous and hair changes of kwashiorkor may be present. Parotid hypertrophy is common; this frequently increases as the diabetes is brought under control with insulin. Unexplained hypoglycaemic attacks are common, especially while on insulin treatment. Hypoalbuminaemic oedema is common. The incidence of obstructive jaundice, which is not usually associated with pancreatitis in temperate areas, is high (Davey, 1968; Owor, 1972). A family history is unusual.

The disease should be distinguished from other causes of overt malabsorption (Chapter 20), diabetes mellitus, pancreatic carcinoma, and cholestatic liver disease (Chapter 14), peptic ulcer and severe malnutrition.

Prognosis is bad and although the patient may survive for a number of years, the weight loss and severe abdominal pain can be extremely depressing.

15.3.3. Pathology of CCP

There is intralobular, perilobular, and perivascular fibrosis with disappearance of the islets of Langerhans. Calcification first appears in the ducts and ductules. It is still not clear whether the calcification begins as calculi. Eventually the organ becomes a fibrous cord, encrusted with calcium salts (Edington and Gilles, 1976). Siderosis can be demonstrated in liver-biopsy specimens but there is no evidence that cirrhosis is more common.

15.3.4. Investigation of CCP

Assessment of pancreatic function has been reviewed by Kajubi (1972b). Figure 15. 1. shows an abdominal radiograph of a Zambian woman with calcification of the entire pancreas. There may be fine dissemination of calcium in the body or tail of the pancreas, or large discrete calculi. All diabetic patients in the tropics should have a straight abdominal radiograph. Serum amylase, bilirubin, and alkaline phosphatase concentrations may be elevated during acute attacks. Glycosuria may be present; the glucose tolerance test may be abnormal. Evidence of malabsorption, which is often severe, can be demonstrated with appropriate tests (Chapter 20); steatorrhoea may be gross. Jejunal structure and function are maintained. Needle liver-biopsies show fat and an excess of iron in the hepatocytes; the cause of the increase in iron absorption in this condition and other forms of chronic pancreatitis is not clear. Cirrhosis is very unusual. Severe iron-deficiency anaemia is also very unusual in patients with this disease.

15.3.5. Treatment of CCP

This consists of (i) controlling the diabetes mellitus, for which insulin is usually required, and (ii) providing pancreatic extract (Pancreatin BPC, 6g orally with meals) to replace the exocrine function. It might be anticipated that management of the diabetes would be similar to that after total pancreatectomy and that 25 to 50 units of insulin daily would be required. In practice many require far more than that, but others have such a mild endocrine abnormality that oral hypoglycaemic agents are adequate for good control. Alcohol is best avoided.

Abdominal pain can be extremely severe and resistant to analgesics. The main object of surgery in chronic pancreatitis is to relieve pain. Mahadevan (1961) working in India, and Davey (1968) in Nigeria, have reported that following transduodenal division of the sphincter of Oddi (sphincterotomy),

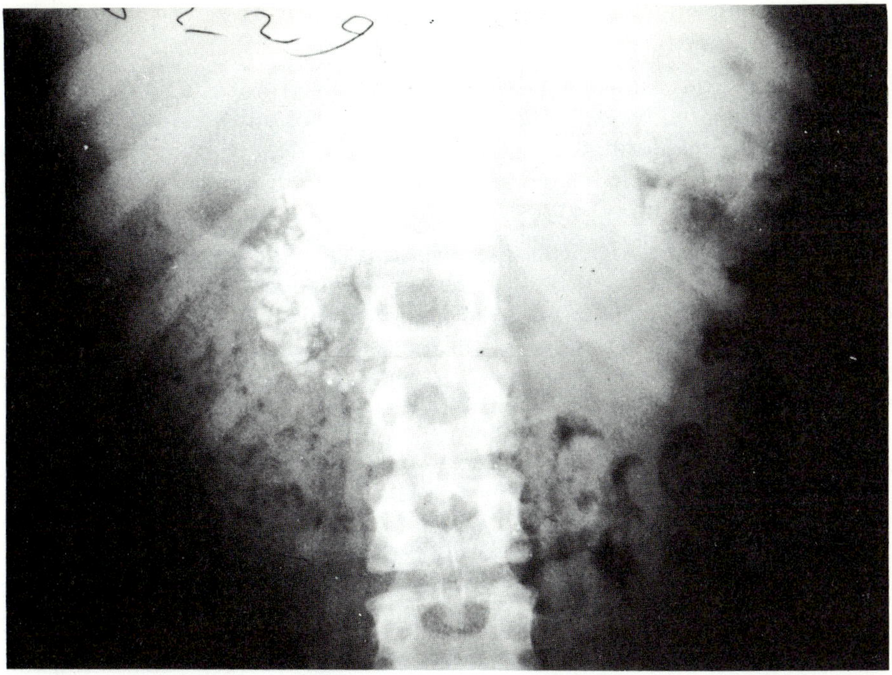

FIG. 15.1. Straight abdominal radiograph in a 22-year-old Zambian woman from the Nsenga tribe, who was admitted to hospital with upper abdominal pain. Gross pancreatic calcification is shown (chronic calcific pancreatitis). There was no history of alcohol excess. She had evidence of malabsorption and had an abnormal oral glucose-tolerance test.

and cholecystjejunostomy, together with drainage of the pancreatic duct, the pain disappears together with the pancreatic calcification. In east Africa, surgery is occasionally carried out to relieve increasing biliary tract obstruction; a cholecystjejunostomy may be necessary.

Although pancreatic resection is widely practised in Europe and the USA for chronic pancreatitis (*Br. med. J.*, 1977), it has not been carried out to any great extent in tropical countries. The operation carries a 20 per cent mortality within the following three to four years, despite a low immediate postoperative death rate. In a large series in Michigan, of 600 patients treated, three died postoperatively, and 30 later; however in that study, approximately 50 per cent of the operations produced a satisfactory result. Davey (1968) has reported successful results of caudal pancreatectomy with implantation of the body of the pancreas into the proximal jejunum, at Ibadan, Nigeria.

15.4. Other pancreatic infections in the tropics

Mumps and Coxsackie B. The pancreas is frequently involved in these two viral infections.

Viral hepatitis. Severe pancreatic involvement in viral hepatitis is probably much more common than is generally appreciated (Chapter 7).

Yellow fever. Haemorrhages into the pancreas occur as part of the bleeding diathesis in yellow fever (Chapter 7).

Schistosomiasis. Occasionally the pancreas is involved in *Schistosoma mansoni*, *S. japonicum*, and *S. haematobium* infections (Owor and Madda, 1977); ova with pseudotubercle formation and scarring can be demonstrated in histological sections. Pancreatic calcification has also been associated with *S. haematobium* infection (Olurin and Olurin, 1969).

Trichinellosis (Trichiniasis). This disease is caused by the nematode *Trichinella spiralis.* It is found in countries where raw or inadequately cooked pork is eaten. The pancreas may be involved along with many other organs, during larval invasion of human tissues; focal necroses and intense eosinophilic infiltrations occur. The infection is sometimes fatal, but involvement of organs other than the pancreas is usually responsible for that.

A marked eosinophilia, larval identification in a muscle biopsy, and intradermal and serological tests are of value in diagnosis.

Cysticercosis. Infection with cysticerci, a result of *Taenia solium* infection, occasionally involves the pancreas (Chapter 19). It is doubtful whether there are any clinical manifestations of that.

Hydatid disease. The pancreas, especially the head, is occasionally the site of an echinococcal infection (Chapter 12) (Carcassonne, Monfort, and Bensoussan, 1972; Galbiati, 1977).

15.5. Pancreatic carcinoma

This seems to be an unusual disease in most parts of the third world; it has a low incidence in cancer registries (Doll, Muir, and Waterhouse, 1970). I have seen occasional cases in east and central Africa, but the overall conclusion is that it is less common than in the western world. In a three-year period during which 1754 cases of gastrointestinal disease were admitted, there were six cases of pancreatic carcinoma at the Goroka Base Hospital, Papua New Guinea (Wagner and Shepherd, 1976).

Burkitt's lymphoma may produce single or multiple deposits in the pancreas.

15.6. The Zollinger–Ellison syndrome

The Zollinger-Ellison syndrome, in which there is a non-β-islet cell tumour, excessive gastrin secretion, and peptic ulceration has been reported in west Africans and in an African in South Africa (Bank, Marks, Sealy, Louw, and Silber, 1965).

References

AVERY JONES, F., GUMMER, J. W. P., and LENNARD-JONES, J. E. (1968). *Clinical gastroenterology.* 2nd ed. p. 742. Blackwell, Oxford, and Edinburgh.

BANK, S., MARKS, I. N., SEALY, R., LOUW, J. H., and SILBER, W. (1965). *Gut*, **6,** 279.

BANWELL, J. G., CAMPBELL, J., BLACKMAN, V., HUTT, M. V., and LEONARD, P. (1963). *E. Afr. med. J.*, **40,** 277.

——, Hutt, M. S. R., Marsden, P. D., and Blackman, V. (1964). *E. Afr. med. J.*, **41,** 188.
——, ——, Leonard, P. J., Blackman, V., Connor, D. W., Marsden, P. D., and Campbell, J. (1967). *Gut*, **8,** 388.
Barbezat, G. O. (1967). *S. Afr. med. J.*, **41,** 84.
Bourgoignie, J., Sonnet, J., and Dechef, F. (1962). *Annls Soc. belge. Méd. trop.*, **42,** 261.
Br. med. J. (1977). **1,** 255.
—— (1978). **2,** 381.
Bwibo, N. O., Rwabwogo-Atenyi, J., and Kagwa, A. (1972). *E. Afr. med. J.*, **49,** 128.
Carcassonne, M., Monfort, G., and Bensoussan, A. (1972). *Annls Chir. infant.*, **13,** 431.
Collins, J. (1958). *Archs Dis. Childh.*, **33,** 432.
Cook, G. C. (1967a). *Br. med. J.*, **1,** 613.
—— (1967b). *Nature, Lond.*, **215,** 1295.
—— (1968). *Metabolism*, **17,** 1073.
—— (1974). *Trans. R. Soc. trop. Med. Hyg.*, **68,** 419.
—— and Kajubi, S. K. (1972). In *Medicine in a tropical environment* (ed. A. G. Shaper, J. W. Kibukamusoke and M. S. R. Hutt). p. 364. British Medical Association, London.
Davey, W. W. (1968). *Companion to Surgery in Africa*. p. 196, 219. E. and S. Churchill, Edinburgh and London.
Doll, R., Muir, C., and Waterhouse, J. (1970). *Cancer in five continents*, 2. International Union against Cancer. Springer-Verlag, Berlin, Heidelberg and New York.
Edington, G. M. and Gilles, H. M. (1976). *Pathology in the tropics*. 2nd. ed. p. 101, 664. Edward Arnold, London.
Evans, S. S., Lubben, J. F., and Whigham, H. E. (1953). *Ann. Surg.*, **138,** 801.
Freeman, R. and McMahon, M. J. (1978). *Gut*, **19,** 367.
Galbaiti, E. (1977). *Minerva chir.*, **32,** 361.
Geevarghese, P. J. and Pitchumoni, C. S. (1966). In *Proceedings of the world congress on diabetes in the tropics* (ed. J. C. Patel and N. G. Talwalker). p. 223. Bombay, India.
Jackson, W. P. U., Marks, I. N., and Bank, S. (1966). In *Proceedings of the world congress on diabetes in the tropics* (ed. J. C. Patel and N. G. Talwalker). p. 230. Bombay, India.
James, W. P. T. and Coore, H. G. (1970). *Am. J. clin. Nutr.*, **23,** 386.
Kajubi, S. K. (1972a). *Am. J. clin Nutr.*, **25,** 1140.
—— (1972b). *E. Afr. med. J.*, **49,** 478.
——, Shaper, A. G. and Owor, R. (1972). In *Medicine in a tropical environment* (ed. A. G. Shaper, J. W. Kibukamusoke and M. S. R. Hutt). p. 380. British Medical Association, London.
Kinnear, T. W. G. (1963). *E. Afr. med. J.*, **40,** 288.
Lawson, H. H. (1962). *S. Afr. med. J.*, **36,** 542.
Leinikki, P., Pantzar, P., and Tykka, H. (1973). *Scand. J. Gastroent.*, **8,** 631.
Lowenthal, M. N., Motola, I., Siddorn, J., and Parker, P. (1968). *Med. Jl. Zambia*, **2,** 37.
McAdam, I. W. J. (1961). *E. Afr. med. J.*, **38,** 536.
McFadzean, A. J. S. and Yeung, R. T. T. (1966). *Trans. R. Soc. trop. Med. Hyg.*, **60,** 466.
Mahadevan, R. (1961). *Br. med. J.*, **1,** 626.
Mårdh, P-A, and Ursing, B. (1974). *Scand. J. Inf. Dis.*, **6,** 167.
Marks, I. N., Bank, S., and Louw, J. H. (1968). In *Progress in gastroenterology* (ed. G. B. J. Glass). **1,** 412. Grune and Stratten, New York.
Ndugwa, C. M. and Sebikari, S. R. K. (1976). *E. Afr. med. J.*, **53,** 475.
Olurin, E. O. and Olurin, O. (1969). *Br. med. J.*, **4,** 534.

Owor, R. (1972). *E. Afr. med. J.*, **49,** 614.
—— and Madda, J. P. (1977). *E. Afr. med. J.*, **54,** 137.
Pitchumoni, C. S. and Thomas, E. (1973). *Lancet*, **2,** 1397.
Sarles, H. (1973). *Digestion*, **9,** 389.
——, Sarles, J-C, Camatte, R., Muratore, R., Gaini, M., Guien, C., Pastor, J., and Le Roy, F. (1965). *Gut*, **6,** 545.
Shaper, A. G. (1960). *Lancet*, **1,** 1223.
—— (1964). *Br. med. J.*, **1,** 1607.
Sherlock, S. (1975). *Diseases of the liver and biliary system*. 5th ed. p. 117. Blackwell, Oxford.
Soergel, K. H. (1978). *Gastroenterology*, **74,** 620.
The, T. L. (1977). *W. Indian med. J.*, **26,** 175.
Trapnell, J. E., Rigby, C. C., Talbot, C. H., and Duncan, E. H. L. (1974). *Br. J. Surg.*, **61,** 177.
Trowell, H. C., Davies, J. N. P., and Dean, R. F. A. (1954). *Kwashiorkor*. p. 123, 125, 146 and 148. Edward Arnold, London.
Wagner, F. B. and Shepherd, A. (1976). *Papua New Guin. med. J.*, **19,** 156.
Zuidema, P. J. (1959). *Trop. geogr. Med.*, **11,** 70.

Section 4 : The spleen

16

The tropical splenomegaly syndrome (TSS) and other splenic diseases in the tropics

16.1. The spleen in the tropics

In western countries, the spleen weighs between 150 and 200g; the average weight in Africans in Africa is approximately twice that figure (Bruce-Chwatt, 1967). When dealing with splenomegaly in a tropical country, all aetiological factors acting in non-tropical areas must also be borne in mind; however in the great majority of cases, malaria is the responsible agent.

With greatly enlarged spleens a syndrome known as 'hypersplenism' is common; there is a reduction in circulating white and red blood cells and platelets. Hypersequestration of blood in the spleen is often very marked.

Splenectomy should never be undertaken lightly in tropical countries. Such populations are usually exposed to malaria, and the spleen is an extremely important line of defence in that disease. Following splenectomy it is often impossible to persuade patients that long-term prophylaxis is vital; also, short-term morbidity and mortality rates following splenectomy are often considerable, due largely to bacterial infection.

Table 16.1 summarizes the common causes of splenomegaly in tropical countries.

16.2. The tropical splenomegaly syndrome (TSS)

The most important feature of the tropical splenomegaly syndrome is marked, and often massive, splenomegaly which is usually associated with hepatomegaly, involving especially the left lobe; that occurs in people living in malarious areas (*Br. med. J.*, 1967; 1969). The spleen frequently weighs four kg or more. Children as well as adults are affected (Vanier, Hutt, and Cook, 1968). Anaemia, a grossly elevated serum IgM concentration, and an increased serum fluorescent malarial antibody titre are usually present.

Plasmodium malariae in peripheral blood is probably found more often than in a control population; although that is so in Uganda (Marsden, Hutt, Wilks, Voller, Blackman, Shah, Connor, Hamilton, Banwell, and Lunn, 1965), work in Papua New Guinea has not substantiated that observation (Crane and Pryor, 1971). Liver-biopsy histology shows hepatic sinusoidal-lymphocytosis. Much research into this disease has been carried out in Africa, particularly in Uganda, where it is known locally as 'big-spleen disease' (Leather, 1961; Hutt and Hamilton, 1972), and Papua New Guinea (Pryor, 1967a; Pitney, 1968; Crane, 1972).

Table 16.1. *Some causes of splenomegaly in the tropics*

Tropical splenomegaly syndrome (TSS)

Other infections
Viruses: infectious mononucleosis, viral hepatitis, and many other virus infections
Bacteria: typhoid fever, brucellosis, tuberculosis, bacterial endocarditis
Parasites: malaria, schistosomiasis, Kala azar, trypanosomiasis

Portal hypertension Chapter 11)

Diseases of the haemopoietic system
Haemolytic anaemias: sickle-cell disease, thalassaemia
Megaloblastic anaemia

Diseases of the reticuloendothelial system
Burkitt's lymphoma
Leukaemia
Reticuloses: reticulum-cell sarcoma, lymphosarcoma

Cysts and other neoplasia

Splenic abscess: unknown aetiology

Spontaneous haemorrhage and rupture

Miscellaneous: amyloidosis, lipid storage diseases

When spleen weights in tropical Africa are plotted there is a pronounced skewing towards the heavier spleens (Bruce-Chwatt, 1956; Shaper, 1969). In Kampala, there is a clear tribal difference in mean spleen weight; people from Rwanda and Burundi have significantly larger spleens than the Ganda (Shaper, 1969). TSS therefore comprises those people with spleens at the upper end of the distribution curve, most of whom are aware of the large dimension of the organ, and they often have evidence of hypersplenism. TSS seems to be distinct from the syndrome described by Banti (1883, 1894, 1937) and also the condition(s) described in India (Basu and Aikat, 1963; Boyer, Sen Gupta, Biswas, Pal, Basu Mallick, Iber, and Basu, 1967; Najak and Ramalingaswami, 1969) and China (McIntosh, 1932) as tropical splenomegaly; in both of those entities cirrhosis is usually present, albeit late in the disease, and the splenomegaly seems to be primarily a result of portal hypertension. It is nevertheless possible that all of those authors described a miscellaneous group of cases of marked splenomegaly some of which were, in fact, true TSS.

Edington and Gilles (1976) consider that the disease is not a homogeneous entity but probably constitutes a collection of syndromes; their evidence is that in some areas, portal hypertension and its complications, and in others 'hypersplenism' and haematological sequelae, predominate.

16.2.1. Distribution of TSS

The syndrome is only present in areas where malaria is endemic (Marsden and Crane, 1976). It is not seen in malaria-free areas, although Dacie, Brain, Harrison, Lewis, and Worlledge (1969) have reported splenomegaly with sinusoidal lymphocytosis in the United Kingdom; however other features of the syndrome were absent in those cases. Reports of the disease have been made from Ghana (Ratnesar, Hathorn, Lahiri, Younn, and Kovi, 1966), the Ivory Coast, Algeria (Charmot and Vargues, 1963), Uganda (Leather, 1961; Marsden, *et al.*, 1965), the Sudan (Mustafa, 1965), Nigeria (Edington, 1967), Zambia (Lowenthal and Hutt, 1968), Zaire, Madagascar, Papua New Guinea (Schofield, 1962; Pryor, 1967a; Crane, 1972), and Hong Kong (Cook, MacFadzean, and Todd, 1963).

The disease has very sharp geographical limitations; thus although common in northern Zambia (Lowenthal, Hamilton, Hutt, and Wilks, 1966) it is unusual in Lusaka, in the south of the country. The condition has been reported in a European woman in northern Zambia (Lowenthal and Hutt, 1970).

16.2.2. Aetiology of TSS

In the majority of people living in malarious areas, the reticuloendothelial system, and especially the spleen and liver, is repeatedly bombarded by malarial infections from early childhood (Chapter 5). Antibody concentrations increase, and malaria pigment is deposited throughout the reticuloendothelial system. After some years of such infections, active immunity is acquired and clinical attacks cease. The spleen becomes smaller and the pigment has dispersed by the early years of the second decade. High antibody titres are maintained by repeated subsequent parasitaemias. Patients with TSS have however deviated from the usual pattern, and development of splenomegaly is progressive.

Epidemiological data support a malarious origin for TSS (Marsden and Crane, 1976), and in areas where malaria has been eradicated the syndrome has disappeared (Hutt and Hamilton, 1972). There is some evidence that non-immunes arriving in a highly malarious area are particularly at risk; Rwandans are more often affected than the local Ganda, in Kampala (Hamilton, Hutt, Wilks, Olweny, Ndawula, and Mwanje, 1965). Elevated fluorescent-antibody titres are present. Antimalarial treatment results in a diminution of spleen size, a fall in serum IgM concentration, partial correction of the serological abnormalities and reduction in the sinusoidal lymphocytosis; the anaemia also improves. It is however unusual to find a parasitaemia.

There is some evidence that haemoglobin AS exerts some degree of protection from the syndrome. In Uganda, of 143 consecutive cases of TSS none had Hb AS (Hamilton, Morrow, Ziegler, Pike, Wood, Banyikidde, and Hutt, 1969).

The reason for a minority of individuals pursuing the course to TSS, rather than developing a straightforward immunity is not clear (Marsden and Crane, 1976); present evidence suggests an aberrant rather than a deficient immune response. The actual mechanism is however not understood, although numerous hypotheses have been advanced (Marsden and Crane, 1976). The tribal and familial distributions in Uganda (Hamilton *et al*., 1965; Shaper, 1969) and Papua New Guinea (Crane, 1972) suggest that genetic factors might be involved.

16.2.3. Presentation of TSS

The history is of a longstanding mass in the left hypochondrium dating from childhood or adolescence; that is in sharp contrast to recent splenic enlargement which follows clearly defined attacks of acute malaria. It is more common in women than men; the condition may be present at as early as four years of age (Cook and Hutt, 1967). It is most common in lower social groups. Discomfort in the left hypochondrium is the usual presenting symptom. Episodes of acute pain in the left hypochondrium, accompanied by transient guarding and rigidity are occasionally reported. A history of recurrent fevers over many years may be obtained. Symptoms referable to anaemia may also be present, especially after a recent acute haemolytic episode; adaptation to a chronic mild anaemia is usually complete.

Examination reveals a large, or very large, firm spleen usually with a prominent notch (Fig. 16.1); it is not infrequently enlarged to the right iliac fossa. The organ can often be detected visually before the abdomen is palpated; there are frequently scarification marks over the spleen—an indication of 'local' therapeutic activity. On auscultation, a murmur is often heard over the spleen, due to an augmented splenic circulation. Some degree of hepatomegaly, often involving the left lobe especially, is detected. Anaemia is always present. There is no lymphadenopathy. Mild jaundice due to haemolysis is a common feature, but is only deep during a haemolytic episode (often associated with pregnancy).

Peripheral vasodilatation and a low blood pressure are often detected. Mild cardiomegaly and dilated jugular veins are associated with a raised blood volume. Mild ankle oedema is occasionally present. Bacterial and viral infections are common.

Chronic leg ulcers, failure of development of secondary sexual characteristics, amenorrhoea, and dwarfism may complicate the clinical picture.

Diagnosis is usually reached by a process of exclusion. Haematology and results of liver-biopsy, together with the clinical findings are usually adequate. Many other studies, including a search for malarial parasites, barium meal, splenovenography, postsinusoidal wedge pressure, isotope studies, plasma volume estimation, immunological studies, and splenic smears have all at various times been carried out.

In a minority of people, the anaemia rapidly becomes more severe, the spleen size increases, and death follows within a few years. Overwhelming infection is the commonest cause of death. Haemorrhage and splenic rupture seem to be rare complications.

At Ibadan, Nigeria, the question of malignant transformation of TSS to leukaemia or lymphoma has been raised (Anand and Davey, 1965; Watson-Williams and Allan, 1968). There, high peripheral blood and bone marrow lymphocyte counts can create difficulty in the differentiation from chronic lymphocytic leukaemia. In Zambia (Lowenthal and Hutt, 1968) the possibility

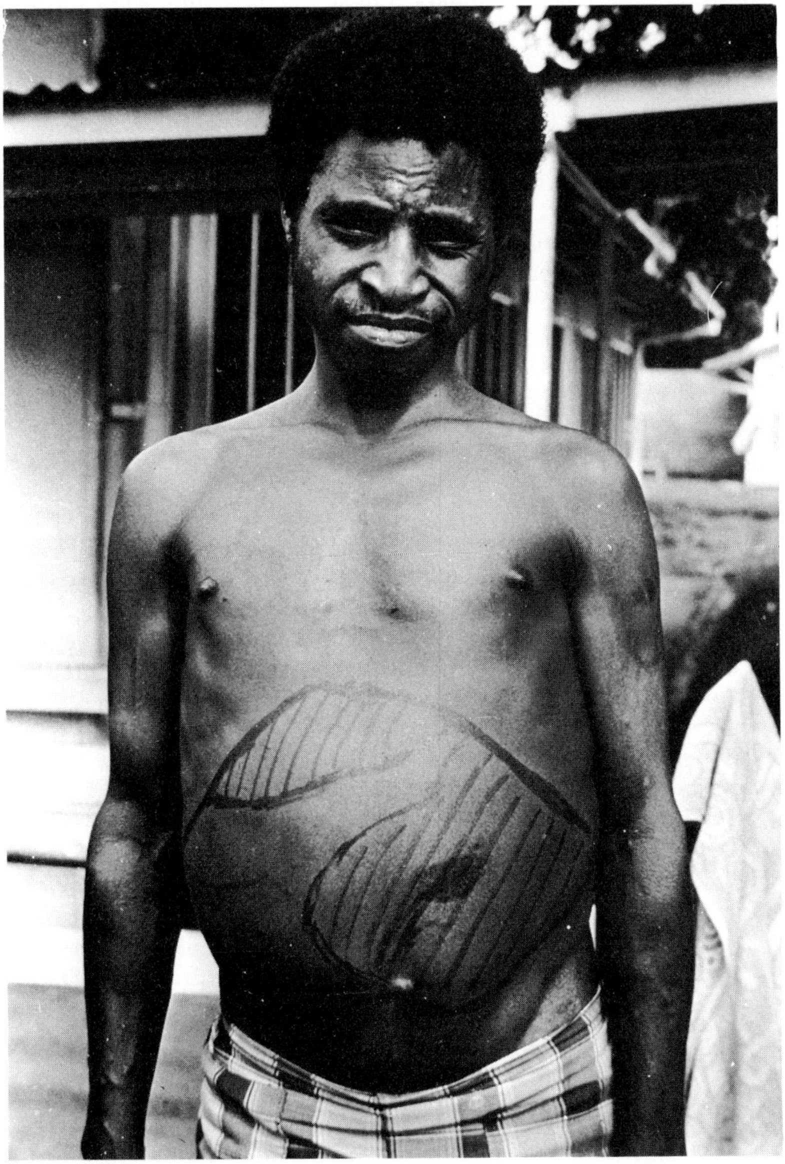

Fig. 16.1. A 20-year-old Papua New Guinean man with the tropical splenomegaly syndrome. The diagnosis was confirmed by liver-biopsy histology which showed marked sinusoidal lymphocytosis. Barium-swallow showed oesophageal varices.

of transformation to lymphoma (especially follicular lymphoma of the spleen) has also been suggested. Overall, however, there is no clear evidence for those events at present; in typical lymphatic leukaemia the lymphocytic infiltration is in the portal areas and not the sinusoids.

Other conditions in which gross splenomegaly is present should be excluded; they include kala-azar, sickle-cell anaemia, leukaemia, and portal hypertension due to other causes (Chapter 11). Appropriate diagnostic tests to exclude those entities are necessary. In kala-azar, Leishman-Donovan bodies are present in marrow or splenic smears. Sickle-cell disease is excluded by haemoglobin electrophoresis. Leukaemia and other malignancies of the lymphoreticular system produce characteristic changes in peripheral blood and bone-marrow. Cirrhosis can usually be diagnosed clinically, but can be confirmed by liver-biopsy; extrahepatic portal obstruction due to portal vein thrombosis is established by splenovenography; and an *S. mansoni* infection is diagnosed by examination of stools for ova, and from rectal and liver-biopsies. Other causes of splenomegaly, not necessarily diseases of the tropics, should also enter the differential diagnosis.

16.2.4. Haematology of TSS

Haematological abnormalities are in large part the result of hypersplenism; they are characterized by anaemia, leucopenia, and thrombocytopenia. Haemoglobin concentration is usually less than 10·0g per dl. The degree of anaemia is usually greater with the larger spleens. Peripheral blood shows a normochromic, normocytic anaemia with polychromasia and anisocytosis, and a high reticulocyte count. The reticulocyte count is usually between two and five per cent. Occasional nucleated red blood-cells are present in severe cases. There is usually a neutropenia with a lymphocytosis, which is often relative but may be absolute. The bone-marrow is hyperplastic and contains normal myeloid cells and megakaryocytes; it is never fibrotic.

There are three mechanisms in the pathogenesis of the anaemia (Pryor, 1967b): (i) a shortened red blood-cell survival, due to splenic destruction, (ii) pooling of red blood-cells in the spleen, and (iii) plasma volume expansion and production of a dilutional anaemia.

Occasional metamyelocytes and myelocytes are often present in the presence of severe neutropenia. There is a failure to produce a neutrophil leucocytosis in patients with infections such as pneumococcal pneumonia (Crane, Wells, and Hudson, 1972). Although thrombocytopenia is present in patients with very large spleens, it is rarely severe and serious bleeding is very unusual.

Plasma volume expansion is due largely to overproduction of the immunoglobulins IgG and IgM, with a secondary increase in albumin synthesis. A 'splenic shunt' is also a contributory factor (Crane, Wells, and Jones, 1975). There is indirect evidence that splenic 'constriction' occurs following exercise and stress; that would account for the surprisingly good exercise tolerance in very anaemic people with TSS. All of those changes are corrected by splenectomy (Hamilton, Richmond, Donaldson, Williams, Hutt, and Lugumba, 1967).

Acute haemolytic episodes which go on for some weeks untreated, are common in the course of the disease; they are often associated with pregnancy, and frequently begin with a febrile episode. Red-cell destruction is accompanied by a very high reticulocyte count, erythroid hyperplasia of the bone marrow, and an elevated serum bilirubin concentration. The Coombs' test is negative. Blood transfusion during an attack produces a mild transient rise in haemoglobin only, and occasionally precipitates intravascular haemolysis. Corticosteroids are of value in preventing haemolysis and sustaining the rise in haemoglobin concentration brought about by blood transfusion.

16.2.5. Biochemistry of TSS

Standard liver function tests are usually all normal. Serum bilirubin is raised if there is haemolysis. The prothrombin time may be prolonged, but that is usually readily corrected with vitamin K. Serum albumin is reduced, and globulin, especially the IgM component, is raised markedly; IgG is raised to a lesser extent (*Br. med. J.*, 1967; Sagoe, 1970; Ziegler and Stuiver, 1972). Serum uric acid is frequently raised in TSS in Uganda (Jagwe and Felitar, 1977); that is thought to be due to the proliferation of small lymphocytes.

16.2.6. Immunological investigations of TSS

High serum IgM concentrations have been demonstrated in TSS in Papua New Guinea, east and west Africa (Sagoe, 1970), Vietnam (Butler, Wilson, Sulzer, and Loan, 1973), and Ethiopia (Watkins and Butler, 1972). High serum IgM concentrations arise between six and 20 years of age, and that event takes place concurrently with the splenic enlargement (Crane, Pitney, Hobbs, and Gunn, 1971); that seems to depend on the intensity of malarial transmission, and in Papua New Guinea it is also dependent on altitude. The reason why high IgM concentrations are produced in only a small minority of subjects exposed to malaria is so far obscure. Antigenic variation within the parasite (Brown and Brown, 1965), failure or interference with T cell control of the switch from IgM to IgG production (Goidl and Marsden, 1974), or abnormal stimulation of B cells by a mitogen released from parasites (Greenwood, 1974), are suggested mechanisms.

High malaria antibody titres can be demonstrated by indirect fluorescence (Gebbie, Hamilton, Hutt, Marsden, Voller, and Wilks, 1964; Marsden, *et al.*, 1965; Butler, *et al.*, 1973). Using refinements of that technique, and homologous antigens to the three major human plasmodial species, in a study of 249 people with TSS, a correlation between IgM, but not IgG, and spleen size has been demonstrated in Papua New Guinea (Crane, Gardner, Hudson, Hudson, and Voller, 1977); no single species of malaria was predominantly involved. Serum IgG concentrations were also higher than in the 87 controls. That study indicates therefore that no single species of malarial parasite is involved in the production of TSS in Papua New Guinea.

Many other antibodies can be demonstrated in TSS (Marsden and Crane, 1976); they might arise as non-specific manifestations of massive IgM overproduction by different clones of immunocytes, or as crossreacting antibodies against plasmodial antigens. They include cold agglutinins, rheumatoid factor, and antibodies to thyroglobulin, antinuclear factor, and cryoproteins. Following treatment with long-term antimalarials, serum IgM concentration and antimalarial antibody titres show a significant reduction (Sagoe, 1970); occasional parasitaemia is presumably required for maintenance of high concentrations.

Circulating immune complexes might be involved in TSS (Ssebabi, Jagwe, Nzaro, and Amsel, 1975; Crane, 1977); in a study of the ultrastructure of the hepatic sinusoids in TSS, Fluck, Hutt, Fluck, and Stuiver (1973) considered that the appearances were consistent with such a reaction occurring there. However that probability remains hypothetical at present.

Systematic investigation of B and T cell function, and the consequences of reversing the disease by antimalarial therapy, have not yet been performed.

16.2.7. Histology of TSS

Hepatic sinusoidal lymphocytosis, which is often gross (Fig. 16.2), and round-cell infiltration of the portal tracts have been described (Leather, 1961; Hamilton, Hutt, Wilks, Olweny, Ndawula, and Mwanje, 1965; Marsden, Connor, Voller, Kelly, Schofield, and Hutt, 1967). The lymphocytosis, which superficially resembles extramedullary haemopoiesis, is the dominant feature. Many of the lymphocytes, which are small and mature, have the appearance of activated cells as judged from their ribosome content, expanded perinuclear space, and increase in mitochondria and endoplasmic reticulum. Although not absolute, spleen size shows a positive correlation with the degree of sinusoidal lymphocytosis (Hutt and Hamilton, 1972). The lymphocytes tend to disappear after antimalarial treatment; they are not related to extramedullary haemopoiesis, infectious mononucleosis, or lymphatic leukaemia (Marsden, *et al.*, 1967). Not all cases of TSS have a sinusoidal lymphocytosis; whether such cases form a basically different syndrome is not clear.

The hepatic sinusoids are lined with hyperplastic and hypertrophic Kupffer cells, and cells which although morphologically similar to Kupffer cells contain fewer mitochondria and less endoplasmic reticulum (Fluck, *et al.*, 1973). Those lining cells give fluorescent reactions indicating the presence of IgM, IgG, and complement. Those cells do not contain malarial pigment, although following marked haemolysis, haemosiderin may be present.

It seems unlikely that portal fibrosis occurs in TSS in either Uganda (Hamilton, *et al.*, 1965) or Papua New Guinea (Pitney, Pryor, and Tait Smith, 1968), despite an observed correlation between portal fibrosis and splenomegaly in a malarious Papua New Guinean village (Marsden and Connor, 1968); it seems much more likely that that fibrosis has other causes, for it is no more prominent than in livers of patients without TSS. Reticulin stains usually show normal architecture. There is no cholestasis or necrosis of hepatocytes. Portal tract fibrosis seems to be more common in India and Hong Kong; it is possible that the disease there is different.

Splenic pathology is non-specific; the histopathology has been described by Sagoe and Edington (1972). There is some degree of capsular thickening and there may be a perisplenitis; infarction is very unusual. The sinusoids containing grossly enlarged phagocytes, and evidence of reticuloendothelial hyper-

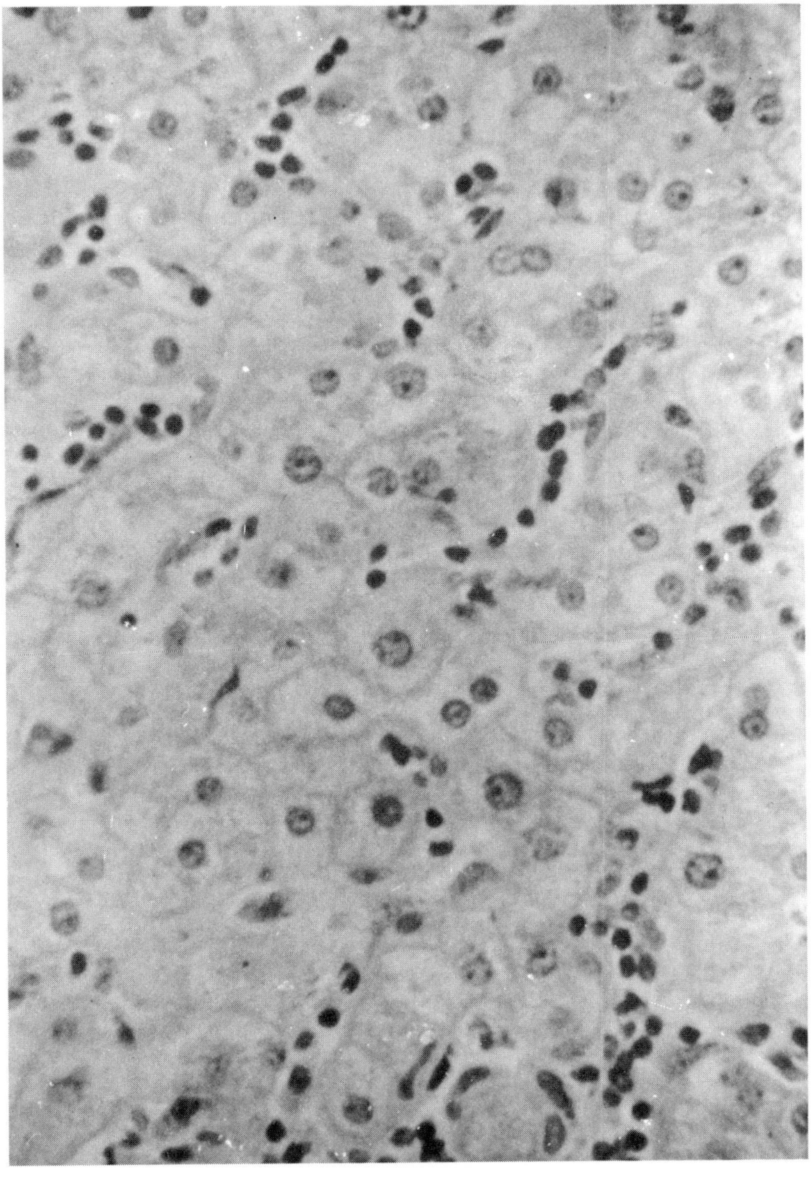

FIG. 16.2. Needle liver-biopsy section (haematoxylin and eosin) from a Papua New Guinean man with the tropical splenomegaly syndrome. The section shows moderately severe sinusoidal infiltration with small lymphocytes; there is no disturbance of architecture.

plasia, are widely dilated. Lymphocytes and plasma cells are present in large numbers. Because immunoglobulin production falls after splenectomy, it is probable that the round cells in the spleen are largely responsible for the overproduction of immunoglobulins (Crane, Pryor, and Wells, 1972).

16.2.8. Portal haemodynamics in TSS

Patients with TSS have a raised intrasplenic pressure (Leather, 1961), and frequently evidence of portal-systemic anastomoses (Marsden, *et al.*, 1965). Oesophageal varices are occasionally present and oesophageal bleeding is well documented. In both Uganda and Papua New Guinea, bleeding from oesophageal varices is an undoubted cause of death in TSS, although the actual incidence of that is impossible to ascertain at present. The mechanism of the portal hypertension is unclear (Chapter 11). Increased splenic flow has been suggested to be the main cause because up to 25 per cent of the total blood volume may be diverted though the spleen (Williams, Parsonson, Somers, and Hamilton, 1966). However, there is sometimes evidence of a pressure gradient across the liver consistent with some degree of obstruction of the portal blood flow (Harries, Forrester, Bhardwaj, and Bagshawe, 1965; Williams, *et al.*, 1966); portal fibrosis is not a feature of the disease and the explanation of that is not clear. It is possible however that the sinusoidal infiltrates are responsible; Williams, *et al.* (1966) were not able to demonstrate a correlation between the increase in presinusoidal resistance, which was present in six of 15 patients, and the presence and degree of hepatic sinusoidal or portal tract lymphocytic infiltration.

16.2.9. Treatment of TSS

The first report of the successful long-term use of an antimalarial agent (proguanil hydrochloride, 'Paludrine'), came from Nigeria (Watson-Williams and Allan, 1968). Further reports using both that compound and other antimalarials, have appeared from east and central Africa (Bagshawe, 1970; Lowenthal, O'Riordan and Hutt, 1971; Stuiver, Ziegler, Wood, Morrow, and Hutt, 1971), and Papua New Guinea (Crane, Hudson, and Hudson, 1973). Several antimalarials have been used over long periods. Proguanil, 100 mg daily, has been most widely used (Bagshawe, 1970; Sagoe, 1970; Crane, *et al.*, 1973), but chloroquine, 300 mg (base) weekly (Stuiver, Ziegler, Wood, Morrow, and Hutt, 1971; Crane, *et al.*, 1973), and cycloguanil, 350 mg at three to six monthly intervals, have also been tried (Crane, *et al.*, 1973; Lowenthal, *et al.*, 1971). However even with treatment lasting for several years, complete remission is not always achieved. After 12 months, 70 per cent of 266 Papua New Guinea patients showed a response (Crane, *et al.*, 1973); however only 25 per cent of the spleens became impalpable, and indeed after 2·5 years the larger spleens were still palpable. If treatment is discontinued while the patient is still exposed to mosquito bites a relapse occurs (Watson-Williams and Allan, 1968).

As the splenomegaly decreases, serum IgM declines and the haemoglobin concentration rises (Sagoe, 1970; Crane, *et al.*, 1973). Cold agglutinins (Crane, *et al.*, 1973), IgM malaria antibody titres, and hepatic sinusoidal lymphocytosis (Lowenthal and Hutt, 1968) all decrease. These facts strongly suggest that TSS is a result of repeated, usually mild, parasitaemias and that to bring about a cure it is necessary to eliminate such events.

Immunosuppressive therapy has been used in children with TSS in Uganda (Vanier, *et al.*, 1968), and also in adults in Vietnam (Buu-Hoi, Biu-Quoc-

Huong, Tran-Lu-Y, and Chau-Van-Tuong, 1962) and Zambia (Lowenthal and Jones, 1972). However, because it is difficult to follow-up and supervise patients with this disease in the third world, such treatment should be viewed with caution.

Stimulation of the immune response with repeated BCG injections seems to be beneficial to patients with active chronic hepatitis; such treatment might be of value in TSS and a controlled therapeutic trial seems to be indicated.

Splenectomy has been carried out (i) when the grossly enlarged spleen was giving rise to marked discomfort, and (ii) when there was no response to antimalarial therapy. The procedure was in fact carried out before recognition of the efficacy of antimalarial treatment, and initial results were encouraging (Hamilton, Richmond, Donaldson, Williams, Hutt, and Lugumba, 1967; Pryor, 1967c). Overall, however, splenectomy is associated with a high incidence of overwhelming infection, of both bacterial and malarial origin, and a high subsequent mortality rate. Three of six patients followed for five years in Uganda (Hamilton, Stuiver, and Zeigler, 1971), and seven of 18 Papua New Guineans followed for from 3·5 to 6 years (Crane, Pryor, and Wells, 1972), died. Splenectomy is not therefore recommended except possibly after failed antimalarial treatment.

Following splenectomy, serum immunoglobulin concentrations fall dramatically, the anaemia improves, and portal haemodynamics return towards normal (Williams, *et al.*, 1966; Hamilton, *et al.*, 1967).

In very acute haemolysis during pregnancy exchange blood transfusion may be required.

16.3. Other causes of splenomegaly in the tropics

Although the spleen is very commonly palpable in people who have been born and bred in tropical countries, the organ is rarely massively enlarged. Systemic leishmaniasis (kala-azar) (Chapter 8) is the only other condition which is likely to be confused clinically with TSS. However smaller degrees of splenomegaly have multiple causes. Most are a result of malarial infection. However, cirrhosis (Chapter 8) and *Schistosoma mansoni* and *S. japonicum* infection of the liver (Chapter 10) can produce moderate degrees of enlargement. Sickle-cell disease is another cause which is widespread in tropical Africa (Sprague and Paterson, 1958; Jenkins, 1963). Conditions which also occur in temperate areas must always be considered in the differential diagnosis, e.g. idiopathic thrombocytopenic purpura and congenital spherocytosis.

16.3.1. The spleen in portal hypertension

Portal hypertension in tropical countries is usually a result of either macronodular cirrhosis or hepatic schistosomiasis. Splenomegaly is frequently present in both of those conditions, especially when the disease is advanced. Other causes of portal hypertension are covered in Chapter 11.

Marked congestive change in the spleen may be seen in idiopathic cardiomegaly, right-sided endomyocardial fibrosis, and constrictive pericarditis which usually results from tuberculosis. In endomyocardial fibrosis splenic infarcts are fairly common.

16.3.2. Haematological causes

Anaemia. In anaemic states, splenomegaly may be present; that is often so in the anaemias of pregnancy.

Sickle-cell disease (SS). Splenomegaly is common in young children with this disease, but due to multiple infarctions, the spleen becomes small in later life due to fibrosis and scarring. However that is not always so in Africa. Splenic abscesses occasionally occur.

Sickle-cell trait (AS). Bearers of the sickle-cell trait suffer from splenic infarcts and may be unduly susceptible to splenic abscesses. Infarcts occur especially when the oxygen content of inspired air is lowered in, for example, unpressurized aircraft (Rotter, Luttgens, Peterson, Stock, and Motulsky, 1956). Splenic abscesses have been reported mainly from Nigeria and Zaire.

The spleen in this disease may vary in size from a few grams to 2000 g or more. In the child it is dark blue and rubbery, and the cut surface is dark red. The splenic pulp is packed with sickled erythrocytes and the sinusoids compressed; erythrophagocytosis and haemosiderin deposits may be present in the Kupffer cells and histiocytes. In older children, there may be fibrosis with iron and calcium salt deposition; areas of calcification may be visible on abdominal radiographs. As progressive fibrosis occurs the organ shrinks to small dimensions. Splenic infarction and abscesses may complicate the picture.

Thalassaemia major. There is usually moderate splenomegaly. A chronic haemolytic anaemia with generalized siderosis is present. Erythrophagocytosis by the reticuloendothelial system, and congestion of the splenic pulp with infarcts occur.

Haemoglobin-H disease. There may be splenomegaly in this disease which is caused by a 'fast-moving' haemoglobin.

16.3.3. Virus infections

The spleen is affected by most viral infections involving the reticuloendothelial system. Thus in yellow fever, dengue, and lassa fever (Chapter 7) for example, this organ is involved (Edington and Gilles, 1976).

16.3.4. Bacterial causes

Typhoid fever (salmonellosis). During the hyperaemic stage the spleen becomes involved; it is enlarged, hyperaemic and cherry-red. Typhoid nodules (Chapter 22), and marked proliferation of reticuloendothelial histiocytes in the sinusoids and germinal centres are present.

Brucellosis. Splenomegaly is a feature of this disease, which is caused by *Brucella abortus, Br. suis,* and *Br. melitensis*. The classical lesions are miliary granulomata resembling those due to tuberculosis and sarcoidosis (Chapter 5); there may be necrosis and suppuration, but never caseation. In extreme cases there may be 'hypersplenism'.

Pasteurella pseudotuberculosis. If death occurs in this disease (Chapter 23) numerous abscesses may be present in the liver and spleen; the causative organism can be cultured.

Clostridium welchii infection. Gas-filled cysts in the spleen and liver have been described in debilitated patients (Ashley, 1965).

Oroya fever (bartonellosis). Splenomegaly and hepatomegaly occur in this disease which is caused by *Bartonella bacilliformis* (Chapter 7). Areas of infarction and necrosis can be demonstrated; pulp cords are congested and erythrophagocytosis and hypertrophy of the sinusoidal lining cells, which contain the causative organisms, are apparent.

Relapsing fever. The spleen is enlarged in both tick-borne and louse-borne relapsing fever. It contains miliary lesions consisting of mononuclear cell infiltrates and congestion; numerous causative organisms, *Borrelia duttoni* or *B. recurrentis* are present. There are often infarcted areas also.

Tuberculoma. This is rarely found in the spleen.

16.4. Splenic abscess

In certain parts of Asia (Islam, 1967) and Africa, especially west Africa, splenic abscess is common. I have seen a number of cases in Lagos, Nigeria. Cockshott and Weaver (1962) have reported 6 cases from Ibadan, Nigeria. In Zimbabwe Rhodesia, also, the condition seems to be fairly common (Wallace, 1922; Gelfand, 1947a; b), although in Zambia I have not personally seen the condition at all in five years. It occurs rarely in Papua New Guinea.

The history is usually of two to three weeks duration. There is pain and swelling in the left hypochondrium, and pyrexia which may be severe. The 'tumour' is obviously in the spleen and is tender and fluctuant. Rarely, the condition becomes chronic and continues for years.

Chest and abdominal radiographs show gas in the abscess; early on, there may be a speckled appearance due to the trapping of gas in the walls of the abscess, and later a large bubble with a fluid level appears. Barium meal may also help to localize the lesion. Needling of the spleen is dangerous.

Owing to the fact that untreated splenic abscesses rupture into the peritoneal or pleural cavities, splenectomy should be undertaken without delay. If the patient is extremely ill, which is often the case, immediate drainage must be performed; that may result however in a sinus which takes a long time to heal. In the chronic condition, splenectomy is also the correct treatment.

The aetiology is unknown. Culture of the pus is always sterile; amoebiasis is not the cause. Owing to the epidemic nature of the cases described by Wallace (1922), a viral aetiology has been suggested but not proved. Cockshott and Weaver (1962) found that five of their six cases were carriers of the S (sickle-cell) gene; they postulated that the condition followed a splenic infarct, which was succeeded by necrosis and gas formation. However, in Zimbabwe Rhodesia, where the condition is also seen, the S gene is uncommon.

16.5. Splenic tumours

Tumours of the spleen are essentially tumours of the reticuloendothelial system. They are not uncommon throughout the tropics but the types of tumour differ from those in the western world. It is possible that multiple viral, bacterial, and parasitic infections influence the incidence and pattern of tumours. In one post-mortem study, tumours of the reticuloendothelial system were shown to be more common in patients with schistosomiasis compared with controls (Edington, von Lichtenberg, Nwabuebo, Taylor, and Smith, 1970).

Lymphosarcoma and reticulum-cell sarcoma are common in much of Africa (Edington and Gilles, 1976). Hodgkin's disease has a widespread distribution. Incidence rates of splenic tumours are available for Iran (Arnim, 1966) and Saudi Arabia (Taylor, 1963). The gross difference in type of tumour is the high prevalence of Burkitt's lymphoma.

Burkitt's lymphoma. Burkitt's lymphoma occurs most commonly in children, usually between two and 15 years of age; it is a malignant lymphoreticular disease which usually involves the facial bones and periorbital region (Chapter 1). However any part of the body may be affected, and the abdominal viscera may be principally infiltrated. The origin may be multicentric. The tumour was first described in 1904 by Cook (1945), and subsequently by Burkitt (1958) in Uganda; the pathology has been described by O'Conor and Davies (1960) and Wright (1963).

Distribution of the tumour is throughout tropical Africa, Papua New Guinea, and other tropical countries where temperature and humidity are high; it has also been described occasionally in temperate areas. The presence of stable *Plasmodium falciparium* malaria and the Epstein-Barr (EB) virus seems essential for its production; it is possible that altered immunological status brought about by malaria renders the EB virus oncogenic.

In the spleen, deposits of varying size and of soft consistency may be present. They are yellowish-white in colour. Histologically sheets of 'blast' cells are seen; they consist largely of a nucleus with a narrow rim of cytoplasm. Large histiocytes are scattered amongst the tumour cells. Phase contrast and tissue culture techniques may assist diagnosis.

Giant lymphangioma of the spleen. This condition may present with a huge splenic mass. A case in an Ethiopian woman has been described (Jain, 1975). Like most tumours of the spleen the condition is rare.

Primary sarcoma of the spleen. Three cases of this disease in Ugandan Africans have been described (Lee and Owor, 1972).

Leukaemia. Leukaemias occur in all tropical countries but probably less commonly than in most non-tropical ones.

Generally the presentation is the same, although in chronic lymphatic leukaemia, the spleen is often markedly enlarged with minimal or absent lymphadenopathy (Haddock, 1967).

16.6. Rupture of the spleen

When the frequency of very large spleens in the tropics is taken into account, a high incidence of traumatic rupture might be anticipated; however that is not the case (Davey, 1968). Most cases follow severe trauma (Patey, 1929; Manuwa, 1935; Fordyce, 1951; Iovetz-Tereshchenko, 1951; O'Connell, 1951): road accidents, stab and gunshot wounds, falls from palm trees, etc. However, there is a group in which rupture seems undoubtedly to be spontaneous (Leighton, 1921; Lubitz, 1949; Orloff and Peskin, 1958; Symes and Smyth, 1959; Bearn, 1961; Adesola and Elebute, 1964), but that is a rare event overall. Even then a previous injury, with delayed haemorrhage, undoubtedly explains some cases (Adesola and Elebute, 1964). Tortion of the spleen is a rare event, and few cases have been described in the tropics (Sheppard Wilson, 1958; Bowesman, 1960; Colin and Odhiambo, 1975).

After the foot of the bed has been raised for 10 to 15 min, it is usual for a patient with a ruptured spleen to experience referred pain in one or both shoulders, due to blood irritating the abdominal surface of the diaphragm.

Blood transfusion must be started and laparotomy performed as a matter of urgency. The commonest cause of death following splenectomy for ruptured spleen is haemorrhage from another abdominal organ, e.g. the liver, which the surgeon has overlooked (Davey, 1968).

References

Adesola, A. O. and Elebute, E. A. (1964). *W. Afr. med. J.*, **13,** 73.

Anand, S. V. and Davey, W. W. (1965). *Br. J. Surg.*, **52,** 335.

Arnim, K. (1966). *Proceedings of the International Academy of Pathology.* Kyoto, Japan. p. 176.

Ashley, D. J. B. (1965). *J. clin. Path.*, **18,** 170.

Bagshawe, A. F. (1970). *E. Afr. med. J.*, **47,** 622.

Banti, G. (1883). *Bull. N.Y. Acad. Med.*, **31,** 113.

—— (1894). *Med. Week, Paris.*, **2,** 364.

—— (1937). *Med. Class.*, **1,** 899.

Basu, A. K. and Aikat, B. K. (1963). *Tropical splenomegaly.* London, Butterworths.

Bearn, J. G. (1961). *Trans. R. Soc. trop. Med. Hyg.*, **55,** 242.

Bowesman, C. (1960). *Surgery and Clinical Pathology in the tropics.* p. 279. Livingstone, Edinburgh.

Boyer, J. L., Sen Gupta, K. P., Biswas, S. K., Pal, N. C., Basu Mallick, K. C., Iber, F. L., and Basu, A. K. (1967). *Ann. intern. Med.*, **66,** 41.

Br. med. J. (1967). **4,** 614.

—— (1969). **4,** 4.

Brown, K. N. and Brown, I. N. (1965). *Nature, Lond.*, **208,** 1286.

Bruce-Chwatt, L. J. (1956). *Bull. Wld Hlth Org.*, **15,** 513.

—— (1967). *Br. med. J.*, **2,** 311.

Burkitt, D. (1958). *Br. J. Surg.*, **46,** 218.

Butler, T., Wilson, M., Sulzer, A. J., and Loan, N. T. (1973). *Am. J. trop. Med. Hyg.*, **22,** 1.

Buu-Hoi, N. P., Bui-Quoc-Huong, Tran-Lu-Y. , and Chau-Van-Tuong. (1962). *Chemotherapia*, **4,** 31.

Charmot, G. and Vargues, R. (1963). *Sem. Hôp. Paris*, **39,** 1421.

Cockshott, W. P. and Weaver, E. J. M. (1962). *Br. J. Surg.*, **49,** 665.

Colin, J. F. and Odhiambo, P. B. (1975). *E. Afr. med. J.*, **52,** 596.

Cook, A. R. (1945). *Uganda memories*, Uganda Society, Kampala.

Cook, G. C. and Hutt, M. S. R. (1967). *Br. med. J.*, **3,** 454.

Cook, J., McFadzean, A. J. S., and Todd, D. (1963). *Br. med. J.*, **2,** 337.

Crane, G. G. (1972). *Papua New Guin. med. J.*, **15,** 3.

—— (1977). *Papua New Guin. med. J.*, **20,** 6.

——, Gardner, A., Hudson, P., Hudson, B. and Voller, A. (1977). *Trans. R. Soc. trop. Med. Hyg.*, **71,** 308.

——, Hudson, P. and Hudson, B. E. T. (1973). *Papua New Guin. med. J.*, **16,** 46.
——, Pitney, W. R., Hobbs, J. R. and Gunn, C. (1971). *Trans. R. Soc. trop. Med. Hyg.*, **65,** 795.
—— and Pryor, D. S. (1971). *Trans. R. Soc. trop. Med. Hyg.*, **65,** 315.
——, ——, and Wells, J. V. (1972). *Trans. R. Soc. trop. Med. Hyg.*, **66,** 733.
——, Wells, J. V. and Hudson, P. (1972). *Trans. R. Soc. trop. Med. Hyg.*, **66,** 724.
——, ——, and Jones, P. (1975). *Trans. R. Soc. trop. Med. Hyg.*, **69,** 212.
Dacie, J. V., Brain, M. C., Harrison, C. V., Lewis, S. M., and Worlledge, S. M. (1969). *Br. J. Haemat.*, **17,** 317.
Davey, W. W. (1968). *Companion to Surgery in Africa.* p. 205. E. and S. Livingstone, Edinburgh and London.
Edington, G. M. (1967). *Br. med. J.*, **1,** 715.
—— and Gilles, H. M. (1976). *Pathology in the tropics.* 2nd ed. pp. 216, 492 and 498. Edward Arnold, London.
——, Von Lichtenberg, F., Nwabuebo, I., Taylor, J. R. and Smith, J. H. (1970). *Am. J. trop. Med. Hyg.*, **19,** 982.
Fluck, D. J., Hutt, M. S. R., Fluck, D. M., and Stuiver, P. C. (1973). *Trans. R. Soc. trop. Med. Hyg.*, **67,** 638.
Fordyce, G. E. (1951). *Br. med. J.*, **2,** 852.
Gebbie, D. A. M., Hamilton, P. J. S., Hutt, M. S. R., Marsden, P. D., Voller, A., and Wilks, N. E. (1964). *Lancet*, **2,** 392.
Gelfand, M. (1947a). *Trans. R. Soc. trop. Med. Hyg.*, **40,** 789.
—— (1947b). *Lancet*, **2,** 904.
Goidl, E. A. and Marsden, P. D. (1974). *Lancet*, **1,** 690.
Greenwood, B. M. (1974). *Lancet*, **1,** 435.
Haddock, D. R. W. (1967). *J. trop. Med. Hyg.*, **70,** 60.
Hamilton, P. J. S., Hutt, M. S. R., Wilks, N. E., Olweny, C., Ndawula, R. L., and Mwanje, L. (1965). *E. Afr. med. J.*, **42,** 191.
——, ——, ——, ——, ——, and —— (1965). *E. Afr. med. J.*, **42,** 196.
——, Morrow, R. H., Zeigler, J. L., Pike, M. C., Wood, J. B., Banyikidde, S. K., and Hutt, M. S. R. (1969). *Lancet*, **2,** 109.
——, Richmond, J., Donaldson, G. W. K., Williams, R., Hutt, M. S. R., and Lugumba, V. (1967). *Br. med. J.*, **3,** 823.
——, Stuiver, P. C. and Ziegler, J. L. (1971). *J. trop. Med. Hyg.*, **74,** 230.
Harries, J. R., Forrester, A. T. T., Bhardwaj, V. B., and Bagshawe, A. F. (1965). *E. Afr. med. J.*, **42,** 575.
Hutt, M. S. R. and Hamilton, P. J. S. (1972). In *Medicine in a Tropical Environment* (ed. A. G. Shaper, J. W. Kibukamusoke, and M. S. R. Hutt). p. 306. British Medical Association, London.
Iovetz-Tereshchenko, N. N. (1951). *Br. med. J.*, **2,** 608.
Islam, N. (1967). *J. trop. Med. Hyg.*, **70,** 153.
Jagwe, J. G. M. and Felitar, V. A. (1977). *E. Afr. med. J.*, **54,** 74.
Jain, S. P. (1975). *E. Afr. med. J.*, **52,** 294.
Jenkins, T. (1963). *Med. Proc.*, **9,** 6.
Leather, H. M. (1961). *Br. med. J.*, **1,** 15.
Lee, J. O. and Owor, R. (1972). *E. Afr. med. J.*, **49,** 355.
Leighton, W. E. (1921). *Ann. Surg.*, **74,** 13.
Lowenthal, M. N. and Hutt, M. S. R. (1968). *E. Afr. med. J.*, **45,** 100.
—— and —— (1970). *Br. med. J.*, **3,** 262.
——, Hamilton, P. J. S., Hutt, M. S. R. and Wilks, N. E. (1966). *Cent. Afr. J. Med.*, **12,** 99.
—— and Jones, I. G. (1972). *Med. Jl. Zambia*, **6,** 155.
——, O'Riordan, E. C. and Hutt, M. S. R. (1971). *Br. med. J.*, **1,** 429.
Lubitz, J. M. (1949). *Blood*, **4,** 1168.

McIntosh, J. S. (1932). *China med. J.*, **46**, 992.
Manuwa, S. L. A. (1935). *W. Afr. med. J.*, **8**, 15.
Marsden, P. D. and Connor, D. H. (1968). *Trans. R. Soc. trop. Med. Hyg.*, **62**, 568.
——, ——, Voller, A., Kelly, A., Schofield, F. D., and Hutt, M. S. R. (1967). *Bull. Wld Hlth Org.*, **36**, 901.
——, and Crane, G. G. (1976). *Revta Inst. Med. trop. S. Paulo*, **18**, 54.
——, Hutt, M. S. R., Wilks, N. E., Voller, A., Blackman, V., Shah, K. K., Connor, D. H., Hamilton, P. J. S., Banwell, J. G. and Lunn, H. F. (1965). *Br. med. J.*, **1**, 89.
Mustafa, D. (1965). *J. trop. Med. Hyg.*, **68**, 183.
Najak, N. C. and Ramalingaswami, V. (1969). *Archs Path.*, **87**, 359.
O'Connell, T. C. J. (1951). *Br. med. J.*, **2**, 1404.
O'Conor, G. T. and Davies, J. N. P. (1960). *J. Pediat.*, **56**, 526.
Orloff, M. J. and Peskin, G. W. (1958). *Int. Abstr. Surg.*, **106**, 1.
Patey, D. H. (1929). *Br. med. J.*, **1**, 898.
Pitney, W. R. (1968). *Trans. R. Soc. trop. Med. Hyg.*, **62**, 717.
——, Pryor, D. S., and Tait Smith, A. (1968). *J. Path. Bact.*, **95**, 417.
Pryor, D. S. (1967 a). *Q. Jl. Med.*, **36**, 321.
—— (1967 b). *Q. Jl. Med.*, **36**, 337.
—— (1967 c). *Br. med. J.*, **3**, 825.
Ratnesar, V. C., Hathorn, M., Lahiri, H., Younn, S., and Kovi, J. (1966). *Ghana med. J.*, **5**, 109.
Rotter, R., Luttgens, W. F., Peterson, W. L., Stock, A. E., and Motulsky, A. G. (1956). *Ann. intern. Med.*, **44**, 257.
Sagoe, A. S. (1970). *Br. med. J.*, **3**, 378.
—— and Edington, G. M. (1972). *W. Afr. med. J.*, **21**, 168.
Schofield, F. D. (1962). *Trans. R. Soc. trop. med. Hyg.*, **56**, 60.
Shaper, A. G. (1969). *Trans. R. Soc. trop. Med. Hyg.*, **63**, 206.
Sheppard Wilson, W. (1958). *Cent. Afr. J. Med.*, **4**, 299.
Sprague, C. C. and Paterson, J. C. S. (1958). *Blood*, **13**, 569.
Ssebabi, E. C. T., Jagwe, J. G. M., Nzaro, E. and Amsel, S. (1975). *E. Afr. med. J.*, **52**, 680.
Stuiver, P. C., Ziegler, J. L., Wood, J. B., Morrow, R. H. and Hutt, M. S. R. (1971). *Br. med. J.*, **1**, 426.
Symes, W. D. and Smyth, F. G. (1959). *Papua New Guin. med. J.*, **3**, 103.
Taylor, J. W. (1963). *Cancer, N.Y.*, **16**, 1530.
Vanier, T. M., Hutt, M. S. R. and Cook, G. C. (1968). *Br. med. J.*, **2**, 649.
Wallace, A. F. (1922). *Med. Jl. S. Afr.*, **17**, 155.
Watkins, R. P., and Butler, W. T. (1972). *Proc. Soc. exp. Biol. Med.*, **141**, 708.
Watson-Williams, E. J. and Allan, N. C. (1968). *Br. med. J.*, **4**, 793.
Williams, R., Parsonson, A., Somers, K., and Hamilton, P. J. S. (1966). *Lancet*, **1**, 329.
Wright, D. H. (1963). *Br. J. Cancer*, **17**, 50.
Ziegler, J. L. and Stuiver, P. C. (1972). *Br. med. J.*, **3**, 79.

Section 5 : The small intestine

17

Acute bacterial and viral infections of the small intestine (excluding cholera and salmonellosis)

THIS group of diseases is extremely important in the third world (Hansen, Kaminsky, Bagg, Kapikian, Slack, and Sack, 1978). They are responsible for a great morbidity rate in adults, and an enormous mortality rate in children (Hocking, 1977; Cutting, 1979). A child at birth has a 50 per cent chance of dying before the age of seven years, primarily as a result of an acute diarrhoeal disease (Kretchmer, 1969). Climatic temperature has little to do with the problem; grossly neglected public health measures and poor sanitation are responsible. In fact the present position in the third world is probably comparable to that in the UK and USA a century ago.

Great advances have been made during the last decade in the identification of bacteria, and more importantly viruses, responsible for this group of diseases. However there are still many organisms which are of uncertain significance in acute diarrhoeal disease (Grady and Keusch, 1971). Undoubtedly many further advances will occur in the next decade.

The importance of malnutrition in these diseases is difficult to evaluate; there are many variables in a highly complex situation (*Lancet*, 1978a). The malnutrition-gastroenteritis cycle is undoubtedly of great importance, however, in developing countries, and especially in children. Malnutrition might render the small intestine more liable to invasion, and damage, by organisms which are not usually pathogenic (James, Drasar, and Miller, 1972; Heyworth and Brown, 1975; Rowland and McCollum, 1977). Epidemiological studies suggest that the magnitude of infection might be important; in many areas, diarrhoea and malnutrition become more common during the rainy season, when water supplies are more easily contaminated with faecal material. Some evidence suggests that the quantity of water ingested is more important than the quality (White, Bradley, and White, 1971), while other evidence indicates that the general level of hygiene in the home is more important than direct water-borne infection (Walker and Walker, 1978).

The gastrointestinal tract possesses several protective mechanisms (Williams and Drasar, 1972); gastric acid and gut motility are important in prevention of infection, and in the proliferation of anaerobes. It seems likely that gastric acid is important in protecting against acid-sensitive pathogens as with *V. cholerae* infections (Nalin, Levine, Levine, Hoover, Bergquist, McLaughlin, Libonati, Alam, and Hornick, 1978). Beer increases acid production (Nalin, Levine, Rhead, Bergquist, Rennels, Hughes, O'Donnell, and Hornick, 1978) and that probably explains many old clinical observations that alcohol consumption in tropical countries is associated with a lower incidence of acute gastrointestinal infection.

The role of iron in host-bacterial interrelations is becoming clearer (Payne and Finkelstein, 1978); the ability of potential pathogens to obtain iron may determine both the nature and also the virulence of the infection. Low serum iron in many third-world populations probably has a protective action against some bacterial infections.

17.1. Pathological basis for acute diarrhoea

It is now clear that there is a fairly sharp distinction between two groups of bacteria: those which act via a potent enterotoxin, and those which actively invade tissues. In the former group, which is exemplified by cholera (Chapter 18), are most of those which operate on the small intestine by way of cyclic AMP (cAMP) production; in them there is a fluid diarrhoea, and usually no blood or mucus in the stool. In the latter group tissue invasion occurs and the stool contains blood and mucus. That is especially severe in the large intestine; shigellosis (Chapter 24) is the best example. Table 17.1 summarizes some important clinical and pathological features of the common causes of diarrhoea and dysentery (Grady and Keusch, 1971; Rowland, 1978).

The area of the bowel which is principally involved by the enterotoxin or by tissue invasion influences the composition of the fluid required for replacement. Bicarbonate loss from the small intestine can, for example, be mitigated if the reabsorptive capacity of the colon is preserved.

Table 17.1. *Summary of some characteristics of common intestinal pathogens and their correlation with the main clinical features of the resulting disease*

Bacterium	Enterotoxin production	Mucosal invasion	Diarrhoea	Dysentery	Abdominal pain	Vomiting	Incubation period (hours)
*Vibrio cholerae**	+	0	+	0	0	±	24–72
Escherichia coli	+	0	+	0	±	0	24–72
	0	+	0	+	+	0	
Clostridium welchii	+	0	+	0	++	±	8–15
	0	±	+	+	++	+	18–48
Staphylococci	+	0	+	0	±	++	4–8
	+	±	+	+	+	±	intermediate
Salmonella spp.*	0	+	+	±	±	±	12–36
Shigella spp.*	+	+	+	+	+	±	24–72

* These infections are covered in Chapters 18, 22, and 24 respectively.

Handling of antigens by the enterocyte is now known to be a complex matter (Walker, 1978); previously held views that the small intestine was impenetrable have recently changed and dietary proteins, bacteria, and other antigens and toxins are known to pass into the portal system (Bjørneboe, Prytz, and Ørskov, 1972; Triger, Alp, and Wright, 1972) (Chapter 8).

17.1.1. Enterotoxin production

Table 17.2 summarizes some of the characteristics of bacterial enterotoxins (Grady and Keusch, 1971; Evans, 1979). A large number of bacteria as well as *V. cholerae* (Love, 1969; Field, Fromm, Al-Awqati, and Greenough, 1972; Banwell and Sherr, 1973; Sladen, 1973; DiBona, Chen, and Sharp, 1974) have now been shown to produce net water secretion to the jejunal lumen as a result of cAMP production (Turnberg, 1978). Among those are *Staphylococcus aureus* (Sullivan and Asano, 1971; Elias and Shields, 1976), *Escherichia coli* (Pierce and Wallace, 1972; Guerrant, Ganguly, Casper, Moore, Pierce, and Carpenter, 1973), *Clostridium welchii* (McDonel, 1974), *S. dysenteriae–1* (Rout, Formal, Giannella, and Dammin, 1975), and *Klebsiella pneumoniae* (Klipstein, Horowitz, Engert, and Schenk, 1975). In *S. dysenteriae–1* infections mucosal damage is also present (Binder and Whiting, 1977).

Table 17.2. *Characteristics of some bacterial enterotoxins*

Bacterium	Mean molecular weight	Optimum pH for toxicity	Inactivation at 60°C	Tropism*	Luminal fluid accumulation
V. cholerae	60 000	8	+	GI; ? C	++
E. coli	>10 000	7–8	+	GI	+
C. welchii	>10 000	6–9	+	GI; ? C	+
Staphylococci (enterotoxin B)	35 000	7–8	0	CNS; GI	+
S. dysenteriae–1	60 000	8	+	GI; ? CNS	+

* GI = gastrointestinal; CNS = central nervous system; C = capillaries

17.1.2. Mucosal invasion

The majority of pathogenic small-intestinal bacteria, although producing an enterotoxin, have some invasive properties also (Table 17.1); only *Vibrio cholerae* produces a severe illness without any mucosal invasion (Chapter 18). In the ileum, *Salmonella typhi* is invasive but only within the lymphoid (Peyer's) patches. At the large-intestinal level, the shigellae are primarily mucosal invaders, although at least one of the group, *S. dysenteriae–1*, also produces an enterotoxin.

17.1.3. Role of intestinal hormones

The importance of the intestine as an endocrine organ is only just beginning to be appreciated (Solcia, Polak, and Buffa, 1975; Grossman, 1977; Bloom, 1978). Vasoactive intestinal peptide (VIP) is elevated in the watery diarrhoea syndrome (Bloom, Polak, and Pearse, 1973).

17.2. Travellers' diarrhoea

The most common disorder by which travellers to tropical countries are afflicted is a transient diarrhoea, now usually known as 'Travellers' diarrhoea' (Turner, 1967). It is usually felt to be an unavoidable risk of travelling to the third world. Acute watery diarrhoea results from an infection with one of a variety of pathogens; no vaccine is available at present, but its subsequent introduction will revolutionize treatment of this disease. Many local variants have been described under many different names: 'Basrah belly', 'Casablanca crud', 'Delhi belly', 'Gyppi tummy', 'G.I. trots', 'Ho Chi Minhs', 'Hong Kong dog', 'Montezuma's revenge', 'Simla trots', 'Rangoon runs', 'Turista', etc.

17.2.1. Aetiology

The majority of cases are clearly infective in origin, and are caused by unusual serotypes of *E. coli* which are enterotoxigenic (Rowe, Taylor, and Bettelheim, 1970; Shore, Dean, Holik, and Davis, 1974; Gorbach, Kean, Evans, Evans, and Bessudo, 1975; Merson, 1975; Merson, Morris, Sack, Wells, Feeley, Bradley, Sack, Creech, Kapikian, and Gangarosa, 1976). The study by Rowe, *et al.* (1970) in British troops in Aden initiated much of the work on the role of *E. coli* in this disease. In a study of 39 American Peace Corps workers, 27 developed the disease soon after arrival in Kenya. Most were caused by enterotoxigenic *E. coli*, most of which were antibiotic sensitive, in contrast to nonenterotoxigenic *E. coli* (Sack, Kaminsky, and Sack, 1977). The enterotoxin is released by the organisms, which multiply in the small intestine, and attaches to ganglioside receptors on the intestinal villi. It stimulates adenylate cyclase production, which in turn increases the cyclic adenosine monophosphate (cAMP) concentration in the small-intestinal lumen (Evans, 1979). That results in hypersecretion, abdominal distension, and diarrhoea.

17.2.2. Presentation

The illness starts suddenly with up to 10 loose stools per day, and that is associated with nausea, vomiting, and abdominal colic. Fever is unusual. Untreated, the illness lasts for one to five days. There is no doubt that travellers' diarrhoea affects some individuals much more frequently than others; it can occur sporadically or in epidemics.

17.2.3. Treatment

Prophylaxis is based largely on using commonsense methods for avoiding infection; drinking water, together with water used for brushing teeth, and milk, should be boiled. All fruit and vegetables should be peeled and washed in chlorinated water; watercress should be avoided. Cooked food should have been prepared recently. Shellfish and ice-cream must always be viewed with suspicion.

Prophylactic antibiotics should be reserved for people who are especially susceptible to the disease, and should not be continued for long periods. Tablets containing streptomycin and sulphonamide, 'Streptotriad' (streptomycin 65 mg, sulphadimidine 100 mg, sulphadiazine 100 mg, and sulphathiazole 100 mg) may be taken in a dose of one or two daily, and will substantially reduce the incidence of travellers' diarrhoea (Turner, 1967). Neomycin and phthalylsulphathiazole have also been used. Because the pathophysiology of the disease is similar to that of cholera, and because the organism seems to be uniformly sensitive to tetracycline, a double-blind controlled trial of prophylactic doxycycline was carried out in Kenya (Sack, Kaminsky, Sack, Itotia, Arthur, Kapikian, Ørskov, and Ørskov, 1978); 9 of 21 individuals taking a placebo, and one of 18 taking doxycycline suffered from travellers' diarrhoea during the three-week period after arrival in Kenya ($P<0{\cdot}01$). Furthermore the protection seemed to persist for a week after withdrawal of treatment. It was concluded that doxycycline effectively prevents most episodes of travellers' diarrhoea. That agent should not be given in pregnancy or lactation, or in childhood, due to teeth-staining; it is also a photosensitizer (Newburger, 1978). Co-trimoxazole has not been adequately evaluated. Iodochlorahydroxyquin ('Vioform' or 'Enterovioform') is usually ineffective and is also toxic and should not be used (Kean, 1963; Oakley, 1973). A randomized double-blind trial of oral lactobacilli ('Lactinex') prophylaxis failed to reduce the incidence of travellers' diarrhoea (Pozo-Olano, Warram, Gómez, and Cavazos, 1978).

For the treatment of an attack, 'Streptotriad' can be given: two tablets twice daily for three days. A cautious approach should be taken however in the treatment of *E. coli* with antibiotics, for that not only encourages the development of resistant strains but also enterotoxic ones (see below).

Diphenoxylate hydrochloride ('Lomotil') (diphenoxylate 2·5 mg and atropine sulphate 0·025 mg) may be given in a dose of two tablets six hourly, to prevent severe abdominal colic; however that compound acts by impairing peristalsis, and it seems likely that that might favour continued small-intestinal bacterial colonization (Chapter 20). Probably the most effective agent in reducing the total weight of ileal content, and also water, sodium, and potassium is codeine phosphate (60 mg thrice daily) (Newton, 1978); in a study comparing ileostomy output after codeine phosphate and diphenoxylate hydrochloride (tab 2, t.d.s.), codeine phosphate was the more effective.

17.3. 'Pig bel' disease (enteritis necroticans)

Pig-bel disease (enteritis necroticans), which is common in the Papua New Guinea highlands, has been associated with infected pork eaten at large feasts (Murrell and Roth, 1963; Murrell, Egerton, Rampling, Samels, and Walker, 1966; Murrell, Roth, Egerton, Samels, and Walker, 1966). During a three-year period, 1973–6, a firm diagnosis of that disease was made in 52 adults at the Goroka Base Hospital in the Papua New Guinea highlands (Wagner and Shepherd, 1976); in the same period 74 children underwent operations for pig-bel disease. Those figures represented a significant decrease in incidence from a peak period, 1971–2. Pig feasts are held every three to 10 years; the animals are dissected under unhygienic conditions and are then partly cooked; the contaminated meat is subsequently distributed over several weeks (Murrell, 1966). However the disease occurs throughout the year, and in fact the highest incidence is during a period when pig-feasting is not at its height. It is associated with heat sensitive type-C strains, usually subtype 5, of *Cl. welchii.* Children are more often affected than adults, and mortality is highest between one and 10 years. The result varies from a mild gastroenteritis to severe dysentery, sometimes with intestinal obstruction (Murrell, *et al.*, 1966; Murrell, 1967; *Lancet*, 1977). There is necrosis in the jejunum, sometimes the ileum also, and occasionally sloughing and necrosis of the colon also takes place (Chapter 28). A fulminant form requires urgent removal of the devitalized necrotic intestine. There is a high overall mortality rate.

A severe haemorrhagic necrotizing jejunitis with bloody diarrhoea, shock, abdominal pain, and sometimes death ('Darmbrand') was recognized in Germany and other parts of Europe after World War II (Jeckeln, 1947; Zeissler and Rassfeld-Sternberg, 1949); that was almost certainly the same condition as 'pig-bel'.

A similar condition has been reported from Kampala, Uganda. Thirty patients, 23 of them children, and seven adults, were seen between 1961–8 (Wright and Stanfield, 1967; Musoke and Sekabunga, 1972); thirteen of them were diagnosed at laparotomy, four clinically, and three at post-mortem. The disease is not epidemic there as in the German and Papua New Guinean experience, although it seems very similar to the disease seen in all of those areas.

In Thailand, Headington, Sathornsumathi, Simark, and Sujatanond (1967) have described segmental small-intestinal infarcts associated with mesenteric adenitis in children; the cause is obscure, but it might be similar to that in pig-bel disease. The children present with watery diarrhoea, are febrile, and the faeces are strongly positive for occult blood. A necrotizing enteritis with a high mortality rate has also been reported in premature infants in Singapore (Tan, Tan and Wong, 1972). Surgery is usually indicated.

17.3.1. Aetiology

It has been suggested that the high incidence of the disease in the Papua New Guinea highlands is due to a low concentration of digestive proteases in the small-intestinal lumen, and that that allows the B toxin of *Cl. welchii* to cause the disease (Lawrence and Walker, 1976). However that does not seem to be the entire explanation, because there is often a lag of several days between meat ingestion and onset of the disease. Also, most samples of food examined do not contain clostridia. It seems likely that another factor within the gastrointestinal tract allows small-intestinal colonization with *Cl. welchii.* That might involve intestinal motility or alteration of colonic flora by another agent consumed at the same time as the suspect meat.

The condition seems in many respects similar to some cases of colitis in the newborn, necrotizing colitis, and antibiotic-induced colitis (Chapter 28).

17.3.2. Pathology

Loops of jejunum are distended, and the serosal surface is discoloured by inflammation, and sometimes haemorrhage (Wright, 1966) (Fig. 17.1). A

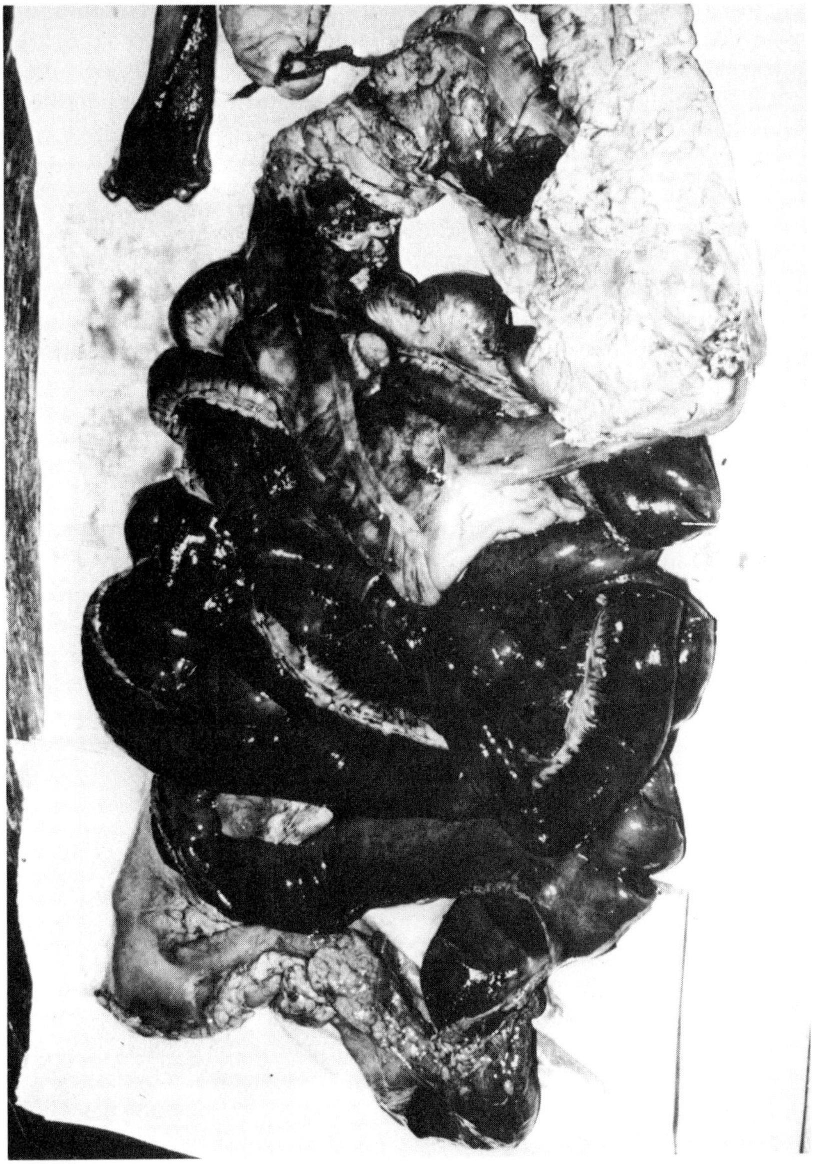

FIG. 17.1. The small intestine in pig-bel disease (enteritis necroticans). Post-mortem specimen from a child who died of that disease in Papua New Guinea. Extensive necrosis involving most of the small intestine is demonstrated.

fibrinopurulent exudate is present over the affected area, and sometimes there is peritonitis also. The duodenum may be involved, but usually the disease starts in the first few cm of the jejunum. The length affected varies from a few feet to the whole of the organ. The jejunal wall is thickened, and the affected area covered by bile-stained necrotic material. Necrotic areas in the ileum, and occasionally the colon also, may be present. The mesenteric lymph nodes are enlarged. Necrosis usually involves the full thickness of the mucosa; a slough, if present, contains large numbers of bacteria. Gas bubbles may be present in both the wall of the jejunum, and the mesenteric nodes. There may be histological evidence of healing, and later fibrosis.

17.3.3. Presentation

There is a male predominance. A sudden onset of severe colicky epigastric pain follows several days of fever. Anorexia, diarrhoea (often bloody), and vomiting occur. Abdominal distension, dehydration, toxaemia, and shock follow. The condition is diagnosed from those symptoms, together with the finding of an easily palpable, thickened segment of small bowel. The disease occurs, but is unusual, in pregnancy (Freedman and Gandionco, 1976). Amoebic colitis (Chapter 25) may be closely mimicked. Acute gastroenteritis, food-poisoning, peritonitis, acute intestinal obstruction, amoebic colitis, acute pancreatitis, mesenteric adenitis, hepatic abscess, and sickle-cell crisis should be included in the differential diagnosis.

In the Ugandan experience, 17 of 30 patients died; a further patient had subacute small-intestinal obstruction caused by jejunal stenosis after clinical recovery. Strictures (Fig. 17.2), fistulae, and malabsorption have been reported as long-term sequelae. Mortality rate may be as high as 85 per cent.

Cl. welchii is often isolated from the stool, intestinal content, or resected bowel segment (Foster, 1966). A neutrophil leucocytosis is usually present. Gaseous distension and fluid levels can often be seen on straight abdominal radiographs (Bassett, 1966).

17.3.4. Treatment

Fluid and electrolyte replacement are usually necessary; gastric suction and intravenous maintenance of fluid and electrolyte status are also often required. Chloramphenicol and ampicillin have been given with benefit. Penicillin and type C gas-gangrene antiserum are also of value in pig-bel disease. If there is no improvement in the patient's condition, laparotomy should be performed; the reasons for that are: (i) to confirm the diagnosis, and (ii) to resect the necrosed section of small intestine (Roth, 1966; Sekabunga, 1966). There is suggestive evidence from Papua New Guinea that with subacute cases a bypass procedure carries a lower mortality rate, at least in the short term, than resection and anastomosis. Surgical aspects of the disease in Papua New Guinea have been described by Smith (1969).

A controlled trial of specific immunization against *Cl. welchii*, type-C, has been carried out in the Chimbu province of Papua New Guinea. 5070 children from one to 15 years entered the trial. Over a 20-month period there were 16 cases of pig-bel disease, including one death, in the control group; there were two cases in the immunized group, and no fatalities. The disease which, untreated, has a very high mortality rate thus now seems to be largely preventable (Lawrence, Walker, and Shann, 1978; Lawrence, Shann, Freestone, and Walker, 1979).

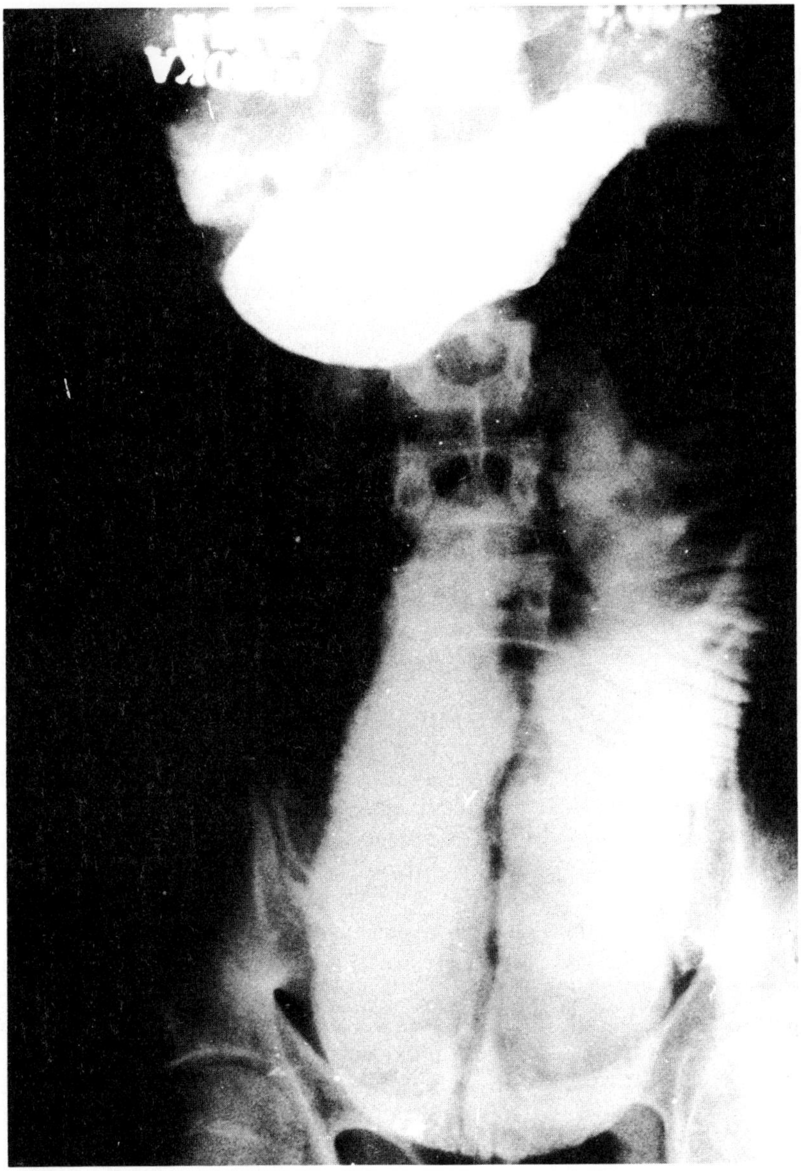

FIG. 17.2. Barium-meal in a patient who had recovered from pig-bel disease at Goroka in the Papua New Guinea highlands. The examination was made nine months after the acute jejunitis. Gross dilatation of a loop of jejunum is shown proximal to a stricture.

17.4. Other bacterial causes of 'food-poisoning'

Food poisoning is a rather vague term which is used in two different ways. First, it is used in a non-specific sense to describe a mild disturbance of gastrointestinal function which is not accompanied by pyrexia; that covers any acute attack of anorexia, nausea, vomiting, and diarrhoea attributed to an abnormality of ingested food, which may be of viral or bacterial origin, or associated with food intolerance, and poisoning by organic (e.g. mushrooms or shellfish) and inorganic (e.g. sodium nitrite) compounds. Alternatively, it can be used in a more specific sense, and covers diseases caused by various bacterial toxins of, for example, staphylococcal or clostridial origin, together with specific but mild acute gastro-intestinal infections with strains of cholera, *Escherichia coli*, salmonella, and shigella organisms.

The treatment is usually symptomatic and does not involve specific microbial agents; *mist. kaolin et morph.* is usually of value. Because it depresses peristalsis, it seems best to avoid diphenoxylate hydrochloride ('Lomotil') which is probably associated with an increase in small-intestinal bacterial colonization; fatal overdoses have also been reported with that agent (Penfold and Volans, 1977). Iodochlorahydroxyquin ('Vioform' or 'Enterovioform') should be avoided due to its neurological toxicity.

Fluid and electrolyte replacement may be necessary, and that can nearly always be achieved by the oral route. Hypovolaemic shock and respiratory embarrassment will have to be treated in a severe case. Bacteriological and toxicological examination of food and faeces should be carried out.

17.4.1. Escherichia coli gastroenteritis

Certain serotypes of *E. coli* are causative in epidemic infantile enteritis. Although they are now firmly accepted as causes of diarrhoea in children, their role in adult diarrhoea has only recently been accepted (*Lancet*, 1975a). Some pathogenic strains of *E. coli* elaborate an enterotoxin which is active only in the small intestine; however there are strains which do not produce an enterotoxin and are responsible for a dysenteric disease by way of mucosal invasion, which is similar to that caused by virulent shigellae (Sakazaki, Tamura, and Saito, 1967; Dupont, Formal, Hornick, Snyder, Libonati, Sheahan, LaBrec, and Kalas, 1971).

Various *in vitro* animal preparations have been used to study the two enterotoxins which are classified as 'heat-labile' (LT) and 'heat-stable' (ST). LT is more likely to produce diarrhoea in children, although that is not always the case (Ryder, Wachsmuth, Buxton, Evans, Dupont, Mason, and Barrett, 1976). Several reports from Bangladesh (Nalin, McLaughlin, Rahaman, Yunus, and Curlin, 1975) and Mexico (Gorbach, Kean, Evans, Evans, and Bessudo, 1975) indicate that both LT and ST play a part in travellers' diarrhoea in adults. LT acts by activating adenylcyclase in the same way as *Vibrio cholerae*. Adhesiveness to the enterocyte may be important with some strains (*Lancet*, 1975a).

Enterotoxin production by *E. coli* seems to have an association with antibiotic resistance. Echeverria, Verhaert, Ulyangco, Komalarini, Ho, Ørskov, and Ørskov (1978) have studied the antimicrobial sensitivities of 176 enterotoxigenic *E. coli* isolated from 57 children and adults in the Philippines, Korea, Taiwan, and Indonesia; 72 per cent of isolates were resistant to one or more, and 44 per cent to four or more, antibiotics. That, together with other observations, suggests that the widespread use of antibiotics will increase the distribution of enterotoxigenic *E. coli*, because genes coding for antibiotic resistance and enterotoxin production are frequently transferred together.

17.4.2. Staphylococcus

Cultures of *Staphylococcus aureus* were shown in 1930 to be capable of producing an enteritis (Dack, Carey, and Woolpert, 1930). The disease is usually caused by contaminated meat, and dairy and bakery products; potato salad containing mayonnaise is a good culture medium. It frequently occurs in groups of people who have eaten the same food. Edington and Gilles (1976) have recorded a choleraic-like epidemic of staphylococcal food-poisoning in Burma in which there was a considerable mortality rate. Fatal diarrhoea occasionally occurs, especially after abdominal surgery (Chapter 28); in most of those patients, broad-spectrum antibiotic therapy has been given. The organisms remain alive and multiply at between 4 and 36°C; a temperature of 60°C for one hour will sterilize food. Certain phage types, only, produce an enterotoxin which is heat-stable. The enterotoxin acts on gut receptors which transmit impulses to the medullary centres.

The incubation period is usually 1–8 hours. The onset is acute. Severe vomiting is often more prominent than the diarrhoea; there is no fever. Recovery usually takes place in 24–48 hours.

Fluid and electrolyte replacement is all that is required in the majority of cases.

17.4.3. Clostridium welchii

Rewarmed or cold cooked-meat dishes are usually responsible for this disease. *Cl. welchii* has been associated with food poisoning since the latter years of the nineteenth century. An enterotoxin is produced by the organism, and that causes hypersecretion into the small-intestinal lumen, by increasing the concentration of cyclic AMP. The enterotoxin is only produced by some strains of clostridium; therefore only some are enteropathogenic. In fulminant necrotizing enterocolitis, while *Cl. welchii* infections are frequently lethal (Egerton, 1966; Pedersen, Hansen, Halveg, and Christiansen, 1976; Kosloske, Ulrich, and Hoffman, 1978), *Cl. butyricum* are not (Howard, Flynn, Bradley, Noone, and Szawatkowski, 1977). Gas gangrene is also produced by this organism, and that is common in tropical countries.

The incubation period is usually 8–16 hours. Diarrhoea, of acute onset, is usually far more prominent than vomiting; there is no fever. Clostridium may be found in the food and faeces of the infected patient, in whom they may be present for a number of days after clinical recovery. Recovery without treatment is usual in one to four days.

17.4.4. Clostridium botulinum

Clostridium botulinum grows readily in tinned foods which have been badly packed, and also in vacuum-packed anaerobic foods; the tins are often swollen or have defective seals. A powerful exotoxin is produced (usually in types A, B, or E) which is absorbed from the upper small intestine, and blocks acetylcholine at neuromuscular junctions. Although not common it occurs in sporadic outbreaks (Merson, Hughes, Dowell, Taylor, Barker, and Gangarosa, 1974; Horwitz, Marr, Merson, Dowell, and Ellis, 1975). The incubation period is 24–96 hours, and the onset is usually with diplopia, dysphagia, dysphonia, and other neurological signs, especially in type E. Vomiting sometimes occurs, but diarrhoea is unusual; indeed there may even be constipation. Respiratory embarrassment and pharyngeal paralysis may be problems. There is no fever. The disease may be complicated by coma and delirium, and has a high mortality rate.

Toxin is present in food and serum, and is identified by mouse inoculation and specific antiserum. Cultures from the liver and spleen may be positive at post-mortem; toxin may also be recovered from the liver (Wilson and Miles, 1975).

A clear airway must be maintained; adequate ventilation is essential. Polyvalent botulinus antitoxin should be given intravenously immediately the diagnosis has been made; skin testing should be performed and, if negative, two vials of trivalent A, B, and E botulinus antitoxin given. Other persons who may have eaten the infected food should be contacted and investigated as soon as possible.

17.4.5. Vibrio parahaemolyticus, salmonella spp. and *shigella* spp.

Food-poisoning caused by these organisms is dealt with in the sections devoted to the more serious diseases: *Vibrio parahaemolyticus* (Chapter 18), *salmonella* spp. (Chapter 22) and *shigella* spp. (Chapter 24).

In addition to *V. parahaemolyticus*, other non-cholera vibrios (NCV) are important in man (Blake, Merson, Weaver, Hollis, and Heublein, 1979; Carpenter, 1979); Campylobacter (see below), *V. alginolyticus* and a lactose-fermenting (L+) vibrio are now known to be important in human disease, and they are also associated with ingestion of infected seafood.

During the incubation period, *S. typhi* bacilli multiply in the duodenum, where bile forms an excellent culture medium; they are present at high concentration in the jejunal lumen. There may be an inflammatory reaction which is either diffuse or granulomatous. An exudate consists of histiocytes, plasma cells, lymphocytes, and occasional polymorphonuclear cells; eosinophils and mast cells may also be increased (Sprinz, Gangarosa, and Williams, 1966). In the fully developed disease, although most lesions are in the distal ileum, the jejunum may also be affected.

In an examination of stools from 1187 food handlers in Nairobi, Kenya, 37 cases of shigellosis and 28 of salmonellosis were diagnosed (Itotia, Cruickshank, and Refai, 1978).

17.4.6. Campylobacter

Until recently campylobacter infections were considered to be rare causes of disease in man (*Lancet*, 1978b), although they were well known to be pathogenic in sheep and cattle. Campylobacter enteritis is a well known entity in domestic pets (Carpenter, 1979); that might form a reservoir for human infection.

The campylobacter constitute a large group of organisms resembling vibrios.

The group is heterogeneous and is made up of several serotypes. The organism does not produce an identifiable enterotoxin, nor does it destroy the intestinal mucosa. In fact, the mechanism by which it penetrates the mucosa is as yet unknown, but it may be similar to that of non-typhoid salmonellae, and yersiniae (Carpenter, 1979).

In Europe, most enteritic infections due to these organisms occur in children, although adults too can be affected. However, such infections seem to be very common in Africa (DeMol and Bosmans, 1978). In most cases the organisms are probably ingested in contaminated water. However, there is evidence that the disease is a zoonosis and that many species, including birds and dogs, can harbour the organisms.

Clinically, carriers seem to be relatively common. The incubation period is two to 10 days with a mean of about five days. The diarrhoea is usually of acute onset and lasts for several days; there may or may not be a fever. Vomiting, and fluid and electrolyte depletion may occur. Abdominal pain may be severe. The jejunum and ileum are maximally affected, and at laparotomy can be seen to be acutely inflamed. A septicaemia may occur, especially in immune-suppressed individuals.

Treatment of this form of enteritis consists of fluid replacement, and either furazolidone or erythromycin; a number of recent reports of erythromycin resistant campylobacters have however appeared (Brunton, Wilson, and MacRae, 1978). If there is a septicaemia, gentamycin should be given.

17.4.7. Anthrax of the small intestine

Ingestion of insufficiently cooked meat from infected animals—cattle, sheep, and goats—may produce this form of anthrax. In Kenya this is the most common form of the disease (Fendall and Grounds, 1965); it is also not uncommon in west Africa.

Clinically the disease may present in a way similar to that of enteritis necroticans (pig-bel disease) (see above).

The duodenum and jejunum are oedematous and there are haemorrhagic, necrotizing lesions in the mucosa; lesions may also be present in the associated lymph nodes.

17.5. Viral causes of acute enteritis

Until recently, pathogens could not be isolated from most cases of gastroenteritis (Cohen, Kalser, Arteaga, Yawn, Frazier, Leite, Ahearn, and Roth, 1967; Lawson and Curtis, 1967; Mata, Urrutia, and Gordon, 1967; *Lancet*, 1975b). Recently, however, many virus particles have been described in diarrhoeal faeces.

17.5.1. Rotavirus

Rotaviruses were first detected in 1973, in the duodenal epithelium of six infants with acute non-bacterial gastroenteritis (Bishop, Davidson, Holmes, and Ruck, 1973; *Br. med. J.*, 1977). Rotaviruses are RNA viruses, and are 65 nm in diameter; they are indistinguishable from reoviruses in size and appearance. Intestinal lactase may act as a receptor and uncoat the outer shell

(Chapter 21) (Schoub, Jenkins, and Robins-Browne, 1978). That these agents are responsible for disease is now widely accepted (Walker-Smith, 1978; Cutting, 1979); the evidence for that is at least comparable with that for toxigenic strains of *E. coli.*

In the third world these agents have been demonstrated in the stools of infants with diarrhoea in Bangladesh, India, Zimbabwe Rhodesia, Singapore, South Africa (Schoub, Koornhof, Lecatsas, Prozesky, Freiman, Hartman, and Kassel, 1975), Papua New Guinea (Wyatt, Hocking, Bishop, and Wyatt (1976), and in Australian aborigines (Davidson, Bishop, Townley, Holmes, and Ruck, 1975). In south India, rotaviruses were detected in the stools of 13 of 50 infants and young children with acute gastroenteritis, but all of 30 controls gave negative results (Maiya, Pereira, Mathan, Bhat, Albert, and Baker, 1977); 33 of them were found to have bacterial pathogens, of which enteropathogenic *E. coli*, salmonellae, and shigellae were the most common.

Children from six months to three years are especially susceptible, but the virus may be excreted by adults also. Clinically, the disease starts with diarrhoea which may occur in families or institutions. The incubation period is 48–72 hours. It seems to be more common in the colder, wet months of the year. Whereas in temperate areas there is a marked seasonal variation in rotavirus infections, in tropical countries they are important throughout the year. The diarrhoea may be prolonged with large stool volumes; oral fluid replacement is more likely to be required than with the diarrhoea due to *E. coli*. There may be respiratory signs also. Leucocytes are not present in the stool as they are in bacterial infections.

17.5.2. Other viral enteritides

The Norwalk virus is a 27 nm picorna virus which has caused epidemics and has also been shown to produce jejunal mucosal damage in volunteers (Schrieber, Blacklow, and Trier, 1973; *Lancet*, 1975b). Two antigenically separate viruses have been isolated.

A 22 nm DNA virus has also been demonstrated in human faeces (Paver, Caul, Ashley, and Clarke, 1973) but its actual significance is not yet clear.

In south India a large corona virus (100–400 nm) has been demonstrated in symptomatic and asymptomatic patients (Mathan, Mathan, Swaminathan, Yesudoss, and Baker, 1975).

17.5.3. Enteroviruses

This group includes the poliomyelitis, Coxsackie, Echo (enteric cytopathogenic human orphan), and Reo (respiratory and enteric orphan) viruses. They produce an acute enteritis, which is rarely severe, and are excreted in the faeces, occasionally in healthy carriers. They are most prevalent in tropical countries with substandard public health services (Assaad and Cockburn, 1971). Swimming pools in tropical countries constitute an important source of infection. Infection is usually acquired early in life in the third world.

The alimentary tract is the principal portal of entry of all members of this group of viruses. During the incubation period, the virus replicates in the lymphoid tissues of the intestine and mesenteric lymph glands; that is followed by a viraemia and involvement of other organs—in poliomyelitis, the central nervous system predominates.

Drinking-water is not always free of this group of viruses after routine processing (*Lancet*, 1978c); swimming baths and shellfish are other sources of infection.

17.5.4. Systemic virus infections

Not all gastrointestinal infections damage the gastrointestinal tract. In some that is merely the site of entry, and the major disease is caused in other organs. However, there are a number which are associated with small-intestinal mucosal damage (Sheehy, Artenstein, and Green, 1964).

In severe measles, extensive damage to the jejunal mucosa occurs; that may be associated with malabsorption (Chapter 20) and secondary disaccharidase deficiencies (Chapter 21).

Severe jejunal mucosal changes have been clearly demonstrated in viral hepatitis (Astaldi, Grandini, Poggi, and Strosselli, 1964; Conrad, Schwartz, and Young, 1964); malabsorption and secondary disaccharidase deficiencies may complicate the clinical picture.

Adenovirus infections may also give rise to diarrhoea (Gardner, McGregor, and Dick, 1960; Duncan and Hutchison, 1961).

17.6. Secondary hypolactasia

In many acute infections of the small intestine, there is damage to the brush-border of the enterocyte; depression of disaccharidases inevitably follows. Because lactase is present at a lower concentration than some of the other brush-border enzymes, including maltase and sucrase, it is often severely depressed (Chapter 21). During and after such infections, therefore, lactose intolerance can be an important clinical problem. Avoidance of milk and lactose containing foods is necessary.

Cow's milk-sensitive enteropathy (cow's milk protein intolerance) (Chapter 21) in infants can probably be precipitated by *E. coli* infections; presentation of the disease may be indistinguishable from *E. coli* enteritis (Harrison, Kilby, Walker-Smith, France, and Wood, 1976) and that organism can occasionally be isolated.

17.7. Oral fluid-replacement in non-cholera diarrhoea

Following the demonstration of glucose-mediated water and electrolyte transport in many forms of enteritis, the problem was how to apply that observation to the field situation (Cash, 1979). That applies to *E. coli* and other acute diarrhoeas as well as cholera (Hirshhorn, McCarthy, Ranney, Hirshhorn, Woodward, Lacapa, Cash, and Woodward, 1973).

Oral sugar-electrolyte solutions are now being used extensively in many types of severe diarrhoea in the same way as they are in cholera (Chapter 18) (Hirschhorn, *et al.*, 1973; Kielmann and McCord, 1977; Palmer, Koster, Islam, Rahman, and Sack, 1977; Field, 1977). The only contraindication for a glucose-containing fluid is when the degree of small-intestinal mucosal damage is so severe that monosaccharides cannot be absorbed. However, when sucrose is being used as the sugar the problem arises as to the adequacy of the sucrase concentration in the brush-border, which is already damaged by the bacterial or viral lesion. In practice, however, sucrose solutions seem satisfactory for oral rehydration (Chapter 18), not only in cholera but also in other small-intestinal infections. In mild diarrhoeal disease, much of which was a result of rotavirus infection in which some mucosal damage would be anticipated, an oral sucrose-electrolyte solution seemed just as effective as a glucose-electrolyte solution (Rahilly, Shepherd, Challis, Walker-Smith, and Manly, 1976; Chatterjee, Mahalanabis, Jalan, Maitra, Agarwal, Bagchi and Indra, 1977; Hutchins, Lawrie, Matthews, Manly, and Walker-Smith, 1978). In Bangladesh also, children with rotavirus diarrhoea do just as well on sucrose as glucose solutions (Sack, Chowdhury, Eusof, Ali, Merson, Islam, Black, and Brown, 1978). In Costa Rica, in children with various types of diarrhoea there was little to choose between sucrose and glucose (Nalin, Levine, Mata, de Cespedes, Vargas, Lizano, Loria, Simhon, and Mohs, 1978). Obviously therefore in most types of small-intestinal diarrhoea, sucrase concentrations must be adequate.

The possibility also exists that more complex compounds (disaccharides and polypeptides), which are hydrolysed within the enterocyte at either the brush-border or in the cytosol, will be associated with more rapid rehydration than monosaccharides and amino-acids (Nalin, Cash, Rahman, and Yunus, 1970) by producing an accelerated sodium and water absorption rate. Work on sucrose absorption is still progressing.

There is a risk of acidosis and hypokalaemia if potassium and bicarbonate are omitted from the fluid, i.e., if a simple glucose or sucrose, plus salt, solution is used (*Lancet*, 1978d; Mosley, 1978).

In some cases of diarrhoea mediated by the cyclic AMP system, prostaglandins have been implicated in the pathophysiology. Thus, aspirin may be of value in treatment (Mennie, Dalley, Dinneen, and Collier, 1975).

References

Assaad, F. and Cockburn, W. C. (1972). *Bull. Wld Hlth Org.*, **46**, 329.

Astaldi, G., Grandini, U., Poggi, C., and Strosselli, E. (1964). *Am. J. dig. Dis.*, **9**, 237.

Banwell, J. G. and Sherr, H. (1973). *Gastroenterology*, **65**, 467.

Bassett, D. (1966). *Papua New Guin. med. J.*, **9**, 60.

Binder, H. J. and Whiting, D. S. (1977). *Infect. Immunol.*, **16**, 510.

Bishop, R. F., Davidson. G. P., Holmes, I. H., and Ruck, B. J. (1973). *Lancet*, **2**, 1281.

Bjørneboe, M., Pyrtz, H., and Ørskov, F. (1972). *Lancet*, **1**, 58.

Blake, P. A., Merson, M. H., Weaver, R. E., Hollis, D. G., and Heublein, P. C. (1979). *New Engl. J. Med.*, **300**, 1.

Bloom, S. R. (1978). *Gut hormones.* Churchill Livingstone, Edinburgh and London.

——, Polak, J. M., and Pearse, A. G. E. (1973). *Lancet*, **2**, 14.

Br. med. J. (1977). **2**, 784.

Brunton, W. A. T., Wilson, A. M. M., and MacRae, R. M. (1978). *Lancet*, **2**, 1385.

Carpenter, C. C. J. (1979). *New Engl. J. Med.*, **300**, 39.

Cash, R. A. (1979). *Tropical Doctor*, **9**, 25.

Chatterjee, A., Mahalanabis, D., Jalan, K. N., Maitre, T. K., Agarwal, S. K., Bagchi, D. K., and Indra, S. (1977). *Lancet,* **1**, 1333.

Cohen, R., Kalser, M. H., Arteaga, I., Yawn, E., Frazier, D., Leite, C. A., Ahearn, D. G., and Roth, F. (1967). *J. Am. med. Ass.*, **201**, 835.

Conrad, M. E., Schwartz, F. D., and Young, A. A. (1964). *Am. J. Med.*, **37**, 789.

Cutting, W. A. M. (1979). *Tropical Doctor*, **9,** 16.
Dack, G. M., Carry, W. E., and Woolpert, O. (1930). *J. prev. Med.*, **4,** 167.
Davidson, G. P., Bishop, R. F., Townley, R. R. W., Holmes, I. H., and Ruck, B. J. (1975). *Lancet*, **1,** 242.
DeMol, P. and Bosmans, E. (1978). *Lancet*, **1,** 604.
Dibona, D. R., Chen, L. C., and Sharp, G. W. G. (1974). *J. clin. Invest.*, **53,** 1300.
Duncan, I. B. R. and Hutchison, J. G. P. (1961). *Lancet*, **1,** 530.
DuPont, H. L., Formal, S. B., Hornick, R. B., Snyder, M. J., Libonati, J. P., Sheahan, D. G., LaBrec, E. H., and Kalas, J. P. (1971). *New Engl. J. Med.*, **285,** 1.
Echeverria, P., Verhaert, L., Ulyango, C. V., Komalarini, S., Ho, M. T., Ørskov, F., and Ørskov, I. (1978). *Lancet*, **2,** 589.
Edington, G. M. and Gilles, H. M. (1976). *Pathology in the tropics.* 2nd ed. p. 520. Edward Arnold, London.
Egerton, J. R. (1966). *Papua New Guin. med. J.*, **9,** 55.
Elias, J. and Shields, R. (1976). *Gut*, **17,** 527.
Evans, N. (1979). *Tropical Doctor*, **9,** 10.
Fendall, N. R. E., and Grounds, J. G. (1965). *J. trop. Med. Hyg.*, **68,** 77.
Field, M. (1977). *New Engl. J. Med.*, **297,** 1121.
——, Fromm, D., Al-Awqati, Q., and Greenough, W. B. (1972). *J. clin. Invest.*, **51,** 796.
Foster, W. D. (1966). *E. Afr. med. J.*, **43,** 559.
Freedman, D. and Gandionco, R. (1976). *Papua New Guin. med. J.*, **19,** 173.
Gardner, P. S., McGregor, C. B., and Dick, K. (1960). *Br. med. J.*, **1,** 91.
Gorbach, S. L., Kean, B. H., Evans, D. G., Evans, D. J., and Bessudo, D. (1975). *New Engl. J. Med.*, **292,** 933.
Grady, G. F. and Keusch, G. T. (1971). *New Engl. J. Med.*, **285,** 831 and 891.
Grossman, M. I. (1977). *Fedn Proc. Fedn Am. Socs exp. Biol.*, **36,** 1930.
Guerrant, R. L., Ganguly, U., Casper, A. G. T., Moore, E. J., Pierce, N. F., and Carpenter, C. C. J. (1973). *J. clin. Invest.*, **52,** 1707.
Hansen, D. P., Kaminsky, R. G., Bagg, L. R., Kapikian, A. Z., Slack, R. C. B., and Sack, D. A. (1978). *Am. J. trop. Med. Hyg.*, **27,** 609.
Harrison, M., Kilby A., Walker-Smith, J. A., France, N. E., and Wood, C. B. S. (1976). *Br. med. J.*, **1,** 1501.
Headington, J. T., Sathornsumathi, S., Simark, S., and Sujatanond, W. (1967). *Lancet*, **1,** 802.
Heyworth, B. and Brown, J. (1975). *Archs Dis. Childh.*, **50,** 27.
Hirschhorn, N., McCarthy, B. J., Ranney, B., Hirschhorn, M. A., Woodward, S. T., Lacapa, A., Cash, R. A., and Woodward, W. E. (1973). *J. Pediat.*, **83,** 562.
Hocking, B. (1977). *Papua New Guin. med. J.*, **20,** 71.
Horwitz, M. A., Marr, J. S., Merson, M. H., Dowell, V. R., and Ellis, J. M. (1975). *Lancet*, **2,** 861.
Howard, F. M., Flynn, D. M., Bradley, J. M., Noone, P., and Szawatkowski, M. (1977). *Lancet*, **2,** 1099.
Hutchins, P., Lawrie, B., Matthews, T. H. J., Manly, J., and Walker-Smith, J. A. (1978). *Lancet*, **1,** 1211.
Itotia, J. N., Cruickshank, B., and Refai, M. (1978). *E. Afr. med. J.*, **55,** 366.
James, W. P. T., Drasar, B. S., and Miller, C. (1972). *Am. J. clin. Nutr.*, **25,** 564.
Jeckeln, E. (1947). *Dt. Med. Wschr.*, **72,** 105.
Kean, B. H. (1963). *Ann. intern. Med.*, **59,** 605.
Kielmann, A. A. and McCord, C. (1977). *J. trop. Pediat.*, **23,** 197.
Klipstein, F. A., Horowitz, I. R., Engert, R. F., and Schenk, E. A. (1975). *J. clin. Invest.*, **56,** 799.
Kosloske, A. M., Ulrich, J. A., and Hoffman, H. (1978). *Lancet*, **2,** 1014.
Kretchmer, N. (1969). *Pediatrics*, **43,** 4.

Lancet (1975a). **2,** 1131.
—— (1975b). **1,** 257.
—— (1977). **2,** 1113.
—— (1978a). **2,** 616.
—— (1978b). **2,** 135.
—— (1978c). **2,** 1352.
—— (1978d). **2,** 300.
LAWRENCE, G. (1978). *Papua New Guin. med. J.*, **21,** 113.
——, SHANN, F., FREESTONE, D. S., and WALKER, P. D. (1979). *Lancet*, **1,** 227.
—— and WALKER, P. D. (1976). *Lancet*, **1,** 125.
LAWSON, J. S. and CURTIS, P. G. (1967). *Med. J. Aust.*, **1,** 101.
LOVE, A. H. G. (1969). *Gut*, **10,** 63.
MCDONEL, J. L. (1974). *Infect. Immunol.*, **10,** 1156.
MAIYA, P. P., PEREIRA, S. M., MATHAN, M., BHAT, P., ALBERT, M. J., and BAKER, S. J. (1977). *Archs Dis. Childh.*, **52,** 482.
MATA, L. J., URRUTIA, J. J., and GORDON, J. E. (1967). *Trop. geogr. Med.*, **19,** 247.
MATHAN, M., MATHAN, V. I., SWAMINATHAN, S. P., YESUDOSS, S., and BAKER, S. J. (1975). *Lancet*, **1,** 1068.
MENNIE, A. T., DALLEY, V. M., DINNEEN, L. C., and COLLIER, H. O. J. (1975). *Lancet*, **2,** 942.
MERSON, M. H. (1975). *New Engl. J. Med.*, **292,** 969.
——, HUGHES, J. M., DOWELL, V. R., TAYLOR, A., BARKER, W. H., and GANGAROSA, E. J. (1974). *J. Am. med. Ass.*, **229,** 1305.
——, MORRIS, G. K., SACK, D. A., WELLS, J. G., FEELEY, J. C., BRADLEY SACK, R., CREECH, W. B., KAPIKIAN, A. Z., and GANGAROSA, E. J. (1976). *New Engl. J. Med.*, **294,** 1299.
MOSLEY, W. H. (1978). *Lancet*, **1,** 991.
MURRELL, T. G. C. (1966). *Papua New Guin. med. J.*, **9,** 39.
—— (1967). *Australas. Ann. Med.*, **16,** 4.
——, EGERTON, J. R., RAMPLING, J. R., SAMELS, J., and WALKER, P. D. (1966). *J. Hyg., Camb.*, **64,** 375.
—— and ROTH, L. (1963). *Med. J. Aust.*, **1,** 61.
——, ——, EGERTON, J. R., SAMELS, J., and WALKER, P. D. (1966). *Lancet*, **1,** 217.
MUSOKE, L. K. and SEKABUNGA, J. G. (1972). In *Medicine in a tropical environment* (ed. A G. SHAPER, J. W. KIBUKAMUSOKE, and M. S. R. HUTT). p. 395. British Medical Association, London.
NALIN, D. R., CASH, R. A., RAHMAN, M., and YUNUS, M. (1970). *Gut*, **11,** 768.
——, LEVINE, M. M., MATA, L., DE CESPEDES, C., VARGAS, W., LIZANO, C., LORIA, A. R., SIMHON, A., and MOHS, E., (1978). *Lancet,* **2,** 277.
——, LEVINE, R. J., LEVINE, M. M., HOOVER, D., BERGQUIST, E., MCLAUGHLIN, J., LIBONATI, J., ALAM, J., and HORNICK, R. B. (1978). *Lancet*, **2,** 856.
——, ——, RHEAD, J., BERGQUIST, E., RENNELS, M., HUGHES, T., O'DONNELL, S., and HORNICK, R. B. (1978). *Lancet*, **2,** 859.
——, MCLAUGHLIN, J. C., RAHAMAN, M., YUNUS, M., and CURLIN, G. (1975). *Lancet*, **2,** 1116.
NEWBURGER, P. E. (1978). *New Engl. J. Med.*, **299,** 261.
NEWTON, C. R. (1978). *Gut*, **19,** 377.
OAKLEY, G. P. (1973). *J. Am. med. Ass.*, **225,** 395.
PALMER, D. L., KOSTER, F. T., ISLAM, A. F. M. R., RAHMAN, A. S. M. M., and SACK, R. B. (1977). *New Engl. J. Med.*, **297,** 1107.
PAVER, W. K., CAUL, E. O., ASHLEY, C. R., and CLARKE, S. K. R. (1973). *Lancet*, **1,** 237.
PAYNE, S. M. and FINKELSTEIN, R. A. (1978). *J. clin. Invest.*, **61,** 1428.
PEDERSEN, P. V., HANSEN, F. H., HALVEG, A. B., and CHRISTIANSEN, E. D. (1976). *Lancet*, **2,** 715.

PENFOLD, D. and VOLANS, G. N. (1977). *Br. med. J.*, **2,** 1401.
PIERCE, N. F. and WALLACE, C. K. (1972). *Gastroenterology*, **63,** 439.
POZO-OLANO, J. DE D., WARRAM, J. H., GÓMEZ, R. G., and CAVAZOS, M. G. (1978). *Gastroenterology*, **74,** 829.
RAHILLY, P. M., SHEPHERD, R., CHALLIS, D., WALKER-SMITH, J. A., and MANLY, J. (1976). *Archs Dis. Childh.*, **51,** 152.
ROTH, L. (1966). *Papua New Guin. med. J.*, **9,** 51.
ROUT, W. R., FORMAL, S. B., GIANNELLA, R. A., and DAMMIN, G. J. (1975). *Gastroenterology*, **68,** 270.
ROWE, B., TAYLOR, J., and BETTELHEIM, K. A. (1970). *Lancet*, **1,** 1.
ROWLAND, H. A. K. (1978). *Trans. R. Soc. trop. Med. Hyg.*, **72,** 289.
ROWLAND, M. G. M. and MCCOLLUM, J. P. K. (1977). *Trans. R. Soc. trop. Med. Hyg.*, **71,** 199.
RYDER, R. W., WACHSMUTH, I. K., BUXTON, A. E., EVANS, D. G., DUPONT, H. L., MASON, E., and BARRETT, F. F. (1976). *New Engl. J. Med.*, **295,** 849.
SACK, D. A., CHOWDHURY, A. M. A. K., EUSOF, A., ALI, M. A., MERSON, M. H., ISLAM, S., BLACK, R. E., and BROWN, K. H. (1978). *Lancet*, **2,** 280.
——, KAMINSKY, D. C., and SACK, R. B. (1977). *Johns Hopkins med. J.*, **141,** 63.
——, ——, ——, ITOTIA, J. N., ARTHUR, R. R., KAPIKIAN, A. Z., ØRSKOV, F., and ØRSKOV, I. (1978). *New Engl. J. Med.*, **298,** 758.
SAKASAKI, R., TAMURA, K., and SAITO, M. (1967). *Jap. J. med. Sci. Biol.*, **20,** 387.
SCHOUB, B. D., KOORNHOF, H. J., LECATSAS, G., PROZESKY, O. W., FREIMAN, I., HARTMAN, E., and KASSEL, H. (1975). *Lancet*, **1,** 1093.
——, JENKINS, T., and ROBINS-BROWNE, R. M. (1978). *Lancet*, **1,** 328.
SCHRIEBER, D. S., BLACKLOW, N. R., and TRIER, J. S. (1973). *New Engl. J. Med.*, **288,** 1318.
SEKABUNGA, J. G. (1966). *E. Afr. med. J.*, **43,** 541.
SHEEHY, T. W., ARTENSTEIN, M. S., and GREEN, R. W. (1964). *J. Am. med. Ass.*, **190,** 1023.
SHORE, E. G., DEAN, A. G., HOLIK, K. J., and DAVIS, B. R. (1974). *J. infect. Dis.*, **129,** 577.
SLADEN, G. E. (1973). *Gut*, **14,** 671.
SMITH, F. (1969). *Aust. N.Z. J. Surg.*, **38,** 199.
SOLCIA, E., POLAK, J. M., and BUFFA, R. (1975). In *Gastrointestinal hormones* (ed. J. C. Thompson). p. 155. University of Texas Press, Austin.
SPRINZ, H., GANGAROSA, E. J., and WILLIAMS, M. (1966). *Am. J. dig. Dis.*, **2,** 615.
SULLIVAN, R. and ASANO, T. (1971). *Am. J. Physiol.*, **220,** 1793.
TAN, K. L., TAN, A. Y. O., and WONG, T. T. T. (1972). *Clin. Pediat.*, **11,** 44.
TRIGER, D. R., ALP, M. H., and WRIGHT, R. (1972). *Lancet*, **1,** 60.
TURNBERG, L. A. (1978). *Clin. Sci. molec. Med.*, **54,** 337.
TURNER, A. C. (1967). *Br. med. J.*, **4,** 653.
WAGNER, F. B. and SHEPHERD, A. (1976). *Papua New Guin. med. J.*, **19,** 156.
WALKER, A. R. P. and WALKER, B. F. (1978). *Lancet*, **2,** 639.
WALKER, W. A. (1978). *Archs Dis. Childh*, **53,** 527.
WALKER-SMITH, J. (1978). *Archs Dis. Childh.*, **53,** 355.
WHITE, G. F., BRADLEY, D. J., and WHITE, A. U. (1971). *Drawers of water.* p. 151. Univ. of Chicago Press, Chicago and London.
WILLIAMS, R. and DRASAR, B. (1972). In *recent advances in gastro-enterology* (ed. J. Badenoch and B. Brooke) p. 31. Churchill Livingstone, London.
WILSON, G. S. and MILES, A. A. (1975). In *Principles of bacteriology, virology and immunity.* 6th ed. Edward Arnold, London.
WRIGHT, D. H. (1966). *E. Afr. med. J.*, **43,** 544.
—— and STANFIELD, J. P. (1967). *J. Pediat.*, **71,** 264
WYATT, G. B., HOCKING, B., BISHOP, R., and WYATT, J. L. (1976). *Papua New Guin. med. J.*, **19,** 134.
ZEISSLER, J. and RASSFELD-STERNBERG, L. (1949). *Br. med. J.*, **1,** 267.

18

Cholera

CHOLERA is the best example of a disease which causes classical small-intestinal diarrhoea. The causative organism is non-invasive and produces its effect solely by enterotoxin production.

The disease is associated with poverty, overcrowding, and low socio-economic status. It is characterized by severe watery diarrhoea, dehydration, and vascular collapse; renal failure may supervene. There has been a significant spread of the disease over the last two decades (*Lancet*, 1976). The causative organism is classically *Vibrio cholerae*, although in recent outbreaks the *El Tor* biotype of that organism has usually been responsible. The bioecology of *V. cholerae* is largely obscure (*Lancet*, 1976); it is not clear where the organism retreats to during interepidemic and interseasonal periods. Infection is confined to the small intestine, where functional changes in electrolyte and fluid transfer lead to a net movement of fluid towards the lumen; the organism is not found in blood or urine.

Untreated, the clinical disease has a mortality rate ranging from 20 to 80 per cent; with prompt and competent treatment, that figure should be under one per cent.

The disease has a long history (Pollitzer, 1959). The epidemiological study by Doctor John Snow in London is well known (Snow, 1855); an epidemic in 1854 was localized to contaminated water drawn from the Broad Street pump in Soho and, after removing the handle of the pump, he was able to show a rapid decline in new cases of the disease. That *V. cholerae* was the responsible pathogen did not rapidly become clear; Koch had suspected in 1883 that it was (Koch, 1884), but the German bacteriologists Pettenkofer and Emmerich were doubtful to the extent that they drank a culture of the bacillus which almost killed one of them, and caused marked discomfort in the other (Grady and Keusch, 1971).

18.1. Distribution of cholera

Cholera occurs endemically in India, Pakistan, Bangladesh, Afghanistan and many parts of the Far east (Barua, 1972); although epidemics periodically occur in the Middle east and tropical Africa (Cox, 1972; Mngola, 1972; Roberts, 1972; Radojcic, 1973; Mhalu, Mmari, and Ijumba, 1979) they have in general been seasonal and self-limiting. Classical cholera due to *V. cholerae* is now virtually limited to the India-Pakistan subcontinent—especially in the deltas of the Ganges and Brahmaputra. Elsewhere the *El Tor* biotype is responsible for the disease; that originated in Indonesia (Barua, 1972; *Lancet*, 1973a), and since 1961 has spread in pandemic form from that focus. The disease has a seasonal pattern. In Calcutta, it has a peak incidence during the hot dry season and ends with the onset of the rains; in Dacca it follows the monsoon and slowly disappears during the hot dry season. The disease can today be transferred by air-travel; in the past it followed population movements, and was associated with caravan routes and pilgrimages such as the great annual Islamic Hadj to Mecca, Saudi Arabia. An outbreak of cholera affected 43 air travellers from Britain to Australia and New Zealand in 1972 (*Lancet*, 1973a); the origin of infection was contaminated seafood prepared in a Middle-eastern country and served on board the aeroplane. An outbreak in Israel in 1970 was caused by vegetables manured with human faeces (Swartz, 1972; Gerichter, Sechter, and Cahan, 1972).

A carrier state lasting a few weeks can occur and gall-bladder foci have been identified (Wallace, Pierce, and Anderson, 1967), as in typhoid fever. Symptomless carriers are therefore important.

18.2. Bacteriology and pathophysiology

Cholera vibrios are curved, Gram-negative, flagellated rods, 1·5–2 μm in length and 0·5–0·6 μm in breadth, which are so motile that they appear to vibrate. Infection is by the oral-faecal route; although rapidly killed at 55°C the organism can survive for several days on moist clothing, and several weeks in contaminated water.

The two biotypes are *V. cholerae* and *El Tor*; each type contains three serotypes: Inaba, Ogawa, and Hikojima. The *El Tor* biotype was named after a quarantine station of that name in Egypt, where it was first isolated in 1921; that type can be distinguished by its ability to haemolyse goat and sheep red-cells.

Following ingestion, vibrios rapidly multiply within the intestinal lumen. The vibrios do not invade the mucosa or enter the portal circulation; neither do they alter the morphology or ability of the mucosa to absorb nutrients. A close contact between *V. cholerae* and the small-intestinal mucosa is important (*Lancet*, 1977). The organisms secrete a toxin which attaches tightly to the enterocyte and increases the activity of adenylate cyclase (Sharp and Hynie, 1971) and consequently the 3′,5′- cyclic monophosphate (cyclic AMP) (cAMP) concentration (Shafer, Lust, and Sircar, 1970; Field, 1971); adenyl cyclase converts adenosine triphosphate (ATP) into cAMP (Evans, 1979). The clinical manifestations of the disease are a result of this increase in cAMP synthesis (Carpenter, 1971; *Lancet*, 1972). That intermediaries rather than the enterotoxin of *V. cholerae* are responsible for the diarrhoea was suggested by experiments which showed that when *V. cholerae* was placed in a small, surgically separated intestinal loop, diarrhoea resulted from the remaining bowel (Vaughan Williams, Dohadwalla, and Dutta, 1969).

Cholera enterotoxin has a molecular weight of approximately 60 000, an optimum pH of 8, and is inactivated at 60°C. At pH 6 it is far less active in evoking fluid transfer (Finkelstein, Atthasampunna, and Chulasamaya, 1966; Grady, Madoff, and Duhamel, 1968; Duhamel, Talbot, and Grady, 1970). As cAMP accumulates in the enterocytes, sodium chloride absorption is inhibited in the villus cells, and secretion of chloride and bicarbonate is stimulated, especially in the secretory cells of the crypts of Lieberkühn. The overall equilibrium between absorption and secretion of electrolytes and fluid is therefore grossly deranged, leading to a massive net secretion towards the lumen; the relative roles played by derangements in absorption and secretion are difficult to evaluate, and the precise dynamics are not yet clear (Phillips, 1964; Sladen and Dawson, 1969; Love, Phillips, Rohde and Veall, 1972).

The protein concentration of intestinal fluid in cholera is less than two per cent of the serum value. Gordon (1962), using intravenous ^{131}I-labelled polyvinylpyrrolidone, showed that in patients with cholera there is no more loss into the lumen than in normal subjects. Except for being excessive in volume, the fluid pouring into the lumen remains iso-osmotic and reflects the chloride-bicarbonate ratio characteristic of that area of bowel; thus the bicarbonate concentration increases as the ileum is reached. When the reabsorptive capacity of the colon is overwhelmed, diarrhoea becomes torrential. Excessive potassium loss exacerbates the metabolic acidosis. The subsequent effect is the production of severe dehydration with haemoconcentration and circulatory collapse. Renal changes, of tubular necrosis, are sometimes associated with anuria and uraemia.

Glucose does not interfere with the specific effects of cAMP on active ion transport, but independently stimulates salt and water absorption.

Histologically the mucosa is morphologically intact (Gangarosa, Beisel, Benyajati, Sprinz, and Piyaratn, 1960; Fresh, Versage, and Reyes, 1964) and able to absorb electrolytes and water normally from solutions containing glucose and glycine, and that is consistent with the view that the diarrhoea is dominated by abnormal secretion towards the lumen. Following animal work *in vitro*, human ileal preparations were shown to be able to maintain sodium transport in the presence of cholera toxin, provided the mucosal surface was exposed to actively transported sugars and amino-acids (Grady, Madoff, Duhamel, Moore, and Chalmers, 1967). Following that, *in vivo* studies showed that the stool volume of patients with cholera decreased significantly when intragastric glucose was given (Hirschhorn, Kinzie, Sachar, Northrup, Taylor, Ahmad, and Phillips, 1968).

Despite its non-invasiveness, *V. cholerae* does induce serum bactericidal and agglutinating antibodies, albeit not as well as shigellae which penetrate the mucosa.

Gastric juice has for long been known to destroy *V. cholerae* (Crendiropoulo, 1921). A high proportion of patients with cholera has hypochlorhydria (Gitelson, 1971; Sack, Hennessey, and Mitra, 1970; Sack, Pierce, Hennessey, Mitra, Sack, and Muzumder, 1972). Hypochlorhydria has been clearly shown to predispose to severe cholera (Nalin, Levine, Levine, Hoover, Bergquist, McLaughlin, Libonati, Alam, and Hornick, 1978); in that study, normal gastric acid was shown to be vibriocidal, whereas that in hypochlorhydric subjects had no effect on *V. cholerae*. Smoking of *Cannabis indica*, widely practised on the Indian subcontinent, has been shown to be associated with a low acid output, and that may predispose to severe cholera (Nalin,

Levine, Rhead, Bergquist, Rennels, Hughes, O'Donnell, and Hornick, 1978).

A claim has been made in the Philippines that blood group O is associated with a higher infection rate than group A (Barua and Paguio, 1977).

18.3. Presentation of cholera

The incubation period is from a few hours to five days and there are no prodromal symptoms. The disease takes a similar course whichever biotype is responsible (Wallace, Carpenter, Mitra, Sack, Khanra, Werner, Duffy, Oleinick, and Lewis, 1966) and it is similar in adults and children. When clinical cholera due to the *El Tor* biotype develops it is indistinguishable from that caused by *V. cholerae* (Bart, Huq, and Khan, 1970); however a higher proportion of patients is asymptomatic. A broad spectrum of clinical severity exists (*Lancet*, 1973a), from a subclinical illness (which in most epidemics accounts for most cases) to rapid death in untreated cases.

The highest rates of infection occur in family contacts of clinical cases (McCormack, Mosley, and Fahimuddin, 1969); however nosocomial transmission in Dacca, where patients with cholera were lying side-by-side with visiting relations, was unusual (Benenson, Ahmed, and Oseasohn, 1965). It is possible that food is an important intermediary, because the secondary attack rate is higher when the woman of the house, and not the man, is the index case (Oseasohn, Ahmad, and Islam, 1966). Seafood is an important source of infection.

Onset is sudden. Diarrhoea is at first mild, but soon increases with the painless passage of large volumes of opalescent liquid, the classical 'rice-water' stools (Cash, Music, Libonati, Snyder, Wenzel, and Hornick, 1974); the volume may be up to 24 litres per 24 hours. The stools contain very high concentrations of vibrios. Blood may be present in the stool later in the disease. Vomiting usually starts after the diarrhoea and consists of material similar to the stool; it is also teeming with vibrios. Thirst, muscle cramps, hoarseness, and anuria follow. This continues for three to four days, during which dehydration may become extremely severe, with dry mouth and tongue, loss of skin turgor, sunken eyes, and hollow cheeks. With progressive dehydration, the blood pressure falls and circulatory failure ensues. Body temperature is often mildly elevated, but to a greater extent later in the disease. Muscle cramps and tetanic spasms may become very severe. Confusion and disorientation may be troublesome. Hypoglycaemic convulsions are common in children. Oliguria gives rise to anuria and acute renal failure; the kidneys may show ischaemic tubular necrosis and hypokalaemic nephropathy (Benyajati, Keoplug, Beisel, Gangarosa, Sprinz, and Sitprija, 1960; Hinman, Saha, Walker, and Carpenter, 1963). Rapid development of cataracts has been reported in the presence of severe dehydration (Wilcocks and Manson-Bahr, 1972). The rapidity of death depends on the severity of dehydration. Mortality rate in a cholera epidemic is often 50 per cent or more, and even higher in children and old patients. If effective treatment is instituted early, recovery is dramatic, and mortality should be very low. Protection occurs after the disease, but is short-lived.

An hypothesis has been presented which suggests that repeated cholera exposures predispose to development of the Mediterranean lymphoma (ML)

(Al-Saleem, 1978) (Chapter 23); that is based on the recent extension of endemic cholera territory, and that seems to correlate with an increase in ML.

18.4. Investigation of cholera

Diagnosis is usually straightforward, especially in epidemics; other causes of severe acute diarrhoea with vomiting (Chapters 17 and 24), and algid malaria (*Plasmodium falciparum*) should be excluded by appropriate investigations.

The stool volume is up to 24 litres per day. Stools are isotonic with a low protein concentration of approximately 10 g per litre; pH is approximately 7·5 and electrolyte concentrations are approximately: sodium 139, potassium 24, chloride 106, and bicarbonate 48 mmol per litre (Pollitzer, 1959; Greenough, 1965). Cholera stool contains a high concentration of immunoglobulin IgA (Grady and Keusch, 1971). Vibrios are easily identified in specimens of stool or vomit; specimens should be transported to the laboratory as rapidly as possible in alkaline peptone water at pH 9·0. Serological identification is important.

In classical cholera the vibrios can be found in the faeces during the incubation period and for up to five days after onset of the attack, but they may disappear within the first 12 hours; with the *El tor* variety however, the organism can occasionally persist for several weeks or months. A simple method for the rapid diagnosis of cholera using immersion dark-ground illumination and a miniature microscope should prove of value in remote areas (McArthur, 1977).

Serum immunoglobulins IgA and IgM are elevated, the former being notably higher in the *El Tor* biotype (Goldstein, 1966; Felsenfeld, Felsenfeld, and Greer, 1966).

18.5. Treatment

18.5.1. General measures

The disease can easily be prevented by applying basic sanitation and public health procedures which require a modicum of organization, goodwill, and money (*Lancet*, 1972); however that seems to be more difficult to achieve than an understanding of the pathophysiology of the disease at a cellular level.

Prophylactically, vaccination with dead vibrios renders some protection; two injections of 0·5 and 1·0 ml separated by one week should be given, with a 0·5 ml booster dose every six months. Cholera vaccination was introduced in 1884 by Ferran, and used with success in India in 1892 by Haffkine (*Lancet*, 1973b). In the Philippines, Inaba and Ogawa parenteral vaccines gave 60 and 70 per cent protection rates against those two serotypes, for four months (Azurin, Cruz, Pesigan, Alvero, Camena, Suplido, Ledesma, and Gomez, 1967); incidence of cholera in villages with simple sanitary facilities was reduced by 70 per cent in three years. Two investigations at Dacca, Bangladesh (Sommer, Khan, and Mosley, 1973; Sommer and Mosley, 1973) showed no appreciable difference in incidence of infection in two groups of contacts of cholera patients; one group was given monovalant Inaba vaccine, and the other a placebo. Mass vaccination campaigns seem therefore to be of little value. The 26th assembly of the WHO (1973) recommended that cholera vaccination should not be compulsory in any country, due to its limited public-health value. However, many countries, including those of the Middle east, still make it compulsory for all travellers, and some have recently tightened their regulations. Overall, vaccines are disappointing and do not offer a sufficient degree or duration of protection (Mosley, McCormack, Fahimuddin, Aziz, Rahman, Chowdhury, Martin, Feeley, and Phillips, 1969; Mosley, Aziz, Rahman, Chowdhury, and Ahmed, 1973), but they do offer a degree of protection to individual travellers and should be made available to those particularly exposed to infection.

Administration of one gram of tetracycline daily for five days has been advocated for the treatment of infected people, and prevention of secondary cases (*Lancet*, 1973a, b; Sommer, Khan, and Mosley, 1973). It is of proved efficacy in shortening the duration of the diarrhoea, and clearing the stool of vibrios in the *El tor* variety; it is usual to start treatment three hours after replacement therapy has commenced, i.e. when the vomiting has stopped. However there are doubts as to the justification for mass chemotherapy with tetracycline in infected areas (Benčić, Witjaksono, Hondro, and de Witt, 1976). Rapidly developing resistance to tetracycline, and a slow onset of resistance to chloramphenicol, nitrofurantoin, neomycin, ampicillin, and sulphadimidine has been observed in an *El tor* epidemic in Tanzania (Mhalu, *et al*., 1979).

An increase in cAMP, which results from the effect of cholera toxin on the enterocyte, can also be produced by prostaglandins. It is well known that aspirin prevents the synthesis of prostaglandins and their effect on cAMP; the suggestion has been made therefore that aspirin should be tried in cholera (Bennett, 1971).

Analgesics may be necessary for severe muscle cramps, and intravenous calcium gluconate for tetany.

Treatment of the disease is aimed at repleting the water and electrolyte balance and correcting the acidosis, if present. Other measures should be directed to the accompanying shock and anuria.

The diarrhoea is usually controlled within 48 hours. Careful nursing is necessary; contacts should be vaccinated and great care taken over disposal of faeces and bed linen, and the sterility of water supplies.

18.5.2. Fluid replacement

Fluid replacement has been revolutionized by the awareness over the last decade that water and electrolytes, when given orally, can be absorbed very well from the small intestine in cholera, if given in the form of a glucose solution of the correct molar concentration (glucose stimulated membrane-transport) (Phillips, 1964; Hirschhorn, *et al.*, 1968; Nalin, Cash, Islam, Molla, and Phillips, 1968; Nalin and Cash, 1974; Cash, 1979). The sodium-glucose carrier system is not affected by cAMP. If one litre of isotonic saline is given orally to a patient with cholera, his stool output will increase by approximately one litre; if however, an iso-osmotic solution containing sodium and glucose is given, the glucose, and also much of the salt and water, will be absorbed. If enough of this solution is given faecal loss can be fully replaced, although that does not necessarily decrease the stool volume. It has been suggested that the discovery of enhanced water and electrolyte absorption from an oral solution containing the correct concentration of glucose is potentially the most important medical advance during the twentieth century (*Lancet*, 1978).

An oral solution containing:

Sodium chloride	3·5 g
Sodium bicarbonate	2·5 g
Potassium chloride	1·5 g
Glucose	20·0 g

and made up to one litre, will in all but the most severe case produce rapid rehydration. The volume of fluid given is based on stool fluid loss, which should be measured every two hours; 20 litres or more of fluid may be lost in 24 hours. Cachets of preweighed glucose-electrolyte components, for rapid dilution in drinking water, are now available commercially; they can be mixed with water in field conditions with the saving of numerous lives. Examples are: (i) a UNICEF preparation (15–611–00), and (ii) 'Dioralyte' (Armour, England).

The presence of an underlying systemic infection, which is very common in the third world, does not influence water absorption rate from a glucose solution (Cook, 1979).

A controversy has arisen concerning the value of sucrose, instead of glucose, solutions for oral rehydration. Obviously sucrose is more readily available, but it seems possible that some patients in tropical countries have a depressed sucrase concentration due to mucosal damage (Nalin, 1975), although that should not present a particular problem in cholera. In practice sucrose seems to be satisfactory (Palmer, Koster, Rafiqul Islam, Mizanur Rahman, and Bradley Sack, 1977); in that double-blind study, sucrose was shown to be an effective replacement for glucose in patients over five years old with cholera. Two other trials indicate that sucrose solutions give results comparable with glucose solutions in acute diarrhoeal disease (Chapter 17). An Indonesian group has achieved good results by substituting sucrose for a similar concentration of glucose in the above formula (Moenginah, Suprapto, Soenarto, Bachtin, Sutrisno, Sutaryo, and Rohde, 1975).

For initial rehydration, intravenous fluids are necessary in a severe case. The correct composition of such fluids has for long been recognized (O'Shaughnessy, 1831; Latta, 1831; MacKintosh, 1836) but they have not been introduced on a large scale until recently. Solutions currently vary in their composition; one example, which has been used in Dacca, Bangladesh (Greenough, Gordon, Rosenberg, Davies, and Benenson, 1964; Mackay, 1979), contains:

Sodium chloride	5·0 g
Sodium bicarbonate	4·0 g
Potassium chloride	1·0 g

made up to one litre. Such fluids reach a very small fraction of people afflicted with the disease only (*Lancet*, 1976). The state of hydration must be assessed clinically, on the basis of general appearance, skin turgor, and intraocular tension. As a rough guide, in an average case, one-tenth of the bodyweight (in kilograms) of fluid (in litres) should be given initially, i.e. for a 50 kg patient, five litres are necessary; the first litre should be given in 10 minutes.

18.6. Vibrio cholerae food-poisoning

Vibrio parahaemolyticus (Sakazaki, Iwanami, and Fukumi, 1963) is another member of the cholera group, which can produce an acute gastroenteritis; infection is common wherever raw seafood is commonly consumed (Barker, 1974; Ellner and Johnson, 1978). It is largely a marine organism and is able therefore to live in a high salt concentration. This organism makes a seasonal appearance, which has been associated with the cyclic appearance of zooplankton in the water column (Kaneko and Colwell, 1975); that observation might provide a clue to the missing link in the bioecology of *V. cholerae* (*Lancet*, 1976).

It is particularly important in Japan, where it is a common cause of food-poisoning, due presumably to the custom of eating raw fish (sushi); it was responsible for 45 per cent of the cases of food-poisoning there in 1965–6 (Grady and Keusch, 1971). Infection has also been recorded in many other Asian countries, including Bangladesh (Hughes, Boyce, Aleem, Wells, Rahman, and Curlin, 1978). It has been reported in the UK (*Br. med. J.*, 1973); frozen shrimps and prawns imported from Malaysia, Indonesia, Taiwan, and Bangladesh are usually the source of infection.

That this organism is a gastrointestinal pathogen has been appreciated since 1956 (Takikawa and Fujisawa, 1956; Sakazaki, Iwanami, and Fukumi, 1963).

Other marine vibrios also, have been implicated in outbreaks of diarrhoea associated with shellfish (Grady and Keusch, 1971). In addition, *V. alginolyticus* and a recently discovered lactose-fermenting (L+) vibrio are important in acute intestinal disease in man (Carpenter, 1979).

Hypersecretion is due to increased cAMP in the small intestine; there may also be some mucosal invasion.

The incubation period is 24 to 72 hours. There is an abrupt onset of diarrhoea (occasionally bloody), usually in an area which is endemic for cholera; vomiting may be present but there is no fever. A history of having eaten crabs or other seafoods is usual; groups are usually affected. The severity of the illness is variable. Stool and food cultures are positive.

Untreated, recovery is usual in one to three days. As for cholera, prompt replacement of fluids and electrolytes is necessary. Tetracycline shortens the length of time over which vibrios are excreted.

References

AL-SALEEM, T. I. (1978). *Lancet*, **2,** 709.

AZURIN, J. C., CRUZ, A., PESIGAN, T. P., ALVERO, M., CAMENA, T., SUPLIDO, R., LEDESMA, L., and GOMEZ, C. Z. (1967). *Bull. Wld Hlth Org.*, **37,** 703.

BARKER, W. H. (1974). *Lancet*, **1,** 551.

BART, K. J., HUQ, Z., and KHAN, M. (1970). *J. infect. Dis.*, **121,** Suppl. 17.

BARUA, D. (1972). *Proc. R. Soc. Med.*, **65,** 423.

—— and PAGUIO, A. S. (1977). *Ann. Hum. Biol.*, **4,** 489.

BENČIĆ, Z., WITJAKSONO, H., HONDRO, S., and DE WITT, W. E. (1976). *Tropical Doctor*, **6,** 2.

BENENSON, A. S., AHMED, S. Z., and OSEASOHN, R. O. (1965). *Proceedings of the Cholera Research Symposium, Honolulu, Hawaii, 1965.* p. 332. Government Printing Office, Washington, D.C.

BENNETT, A. (1971). *Nature, Lond.*, **231,** 536.

BENYAJATI, C., KEOPLUG, M., BEISEL, W. R., GANGAROSA, E. J., SPRINZ, H., and SITPRIJA, V. (1960). *Ann. intern. Med.*, **52,** 960.

Br. med. J. (1973). **2,** 562.

CARPENTER, C. C. J. (1971). *Am. J. Med.*, **50,** 1.

—— (1979). *New Engl. J. Med.*, **300,** 39.

CASH, R. A. (1979). *Tropical Doctor*, **9,** 25.

——, MUSIC, S. I., LIBONATI, J. P., SNYDER, M. J., WENZEL, R. P., and HORNICK, R. B. (1974). *J. infect. Dis.*, **129,** 45.

COOK, G. C. (1979). *Acta trop.*, in press.

COX, P. S. V. (1972). *E. Afr. med. J.*, **49,** 440.

CRENDIROPOULO, M. (1921). *Bull. Off. int. Hyg. publ.*, **13,** 247.

DUHAMEL, R. C., TALBOT, P., and GRADY, G. F. (1970). *J. infect. Dis.*, **121,** suppl., 85.

ELLNER, P. D. and JOHNSON, E. (1978). *New Engl. J. Med.*, **299,** 261.

EVANS, N. (1979). *Tropical Doctor*, **9,**10.

FELSENFELD, O., FELSENFELD, A. D., and GREER, W. E. (1966). *J. infect. Dis.*, **116,** 329.

FIELD, M. (1971). *New Engl. J. Med.*, **284,** 1137.

FINKELSTEIN, R. A., ATTHASAMPUNNA, P., and CHULASAMAYA, M. (1966). *J. Immun.*, **96,** 440.

FRESH, J.W., VERSAGE, P. M., and REYES, V. (1964). *Archs Path.*, **77,** 529.

GANGAROSA, E. J., BEISEL, W. R., BENYAJATI, C., SPRINZ, H., and PIYARATN, P. (1960). *Am. J. trop. Med. Hyg.*, **9,** 125.

GERICHTER, C. B., SECHTER, I., and CAHAN, D. (1972). *Israel J. med. Sci.*, **8,** 531.

GITELSON, S. (1971). *Israel J. med. Sci.*, **7,** 663.

GOLDSTEIN, H. B. (1966). *Proc. Soc. exp. Biol. Med.*, **121,** 425.

GORDON, R. S. (1962). *SEATO conference on cholera.* p. 54. Bankok, Thailand, SEATO.

GRADY, G. F. and KEUSCH, G. T.(1971). *New Engl. J. Med.*, **285,** 831 and 891.

——, MADOFF, M. A., and DUHAMEL, R. C. (1968). *J. infect. Dis.*, **118,** 263.

——, MADOFF, M. A., DUHAMEL, R. C., MOORE, E. W., and CHALMERS, T. C. (1967). *Gastroenterology*, **53,** 737.

GREENOUGH, W. B. (1965). *Lancet*, **2,** 991.

——, GORDON, R. S., ROSENBERG, I. S., DAVIES, B. I., and BENENSON, A. S. (1964). *Lancet*, **1,** 355.

HINMAN, E. J., SAHA, T. K., WALKER, W. G., and CARPENTER, C. C. J. (1963). *Bull. Calcutta Sch. trop. Med. Hyg.*, **11,** 154.

HIRSCHHORN, N., KINZIE, J. L., SACHAR, D. B., NORTHRUP, R. S., TAYLOR, J. O., AHMAD, S. Z., and PHILLIPS, R. A. (1968). *New Engl. J. Med.*, **279,** 176.

HUGHES, J. M., BOYCE, J. M., ALEEM, A. R. M. A., WELLS, J. G., RAHMAN, A. S. M. M., and CURLIN, G. T. (1978). *Am. J. trop. Med. Hyg.*, **27,** 106.

KANEKO, T. and COLWELL, R. (1975). *Appl. Microbiol.*, **29,** 269.

KOCH, R. (1884). *Br. med. J.*, **2,** 403, 453.

Lancet (1972). **2,** 167.

—— (1973a). **2,** 601.

—— (1973b). **1,** 1369.

—— (1976). **2,** 1283.

—— (1977). **1,** 1293.

—— (1978). **2,** 300.

LATTA, T. A. (1831). *Lancet*, **1,** 173.

LOVE, A. H. G., PHILLIPS, R. A., ROHDE, J. E. and VEALL, N. (1972). *Lancet*, **2,** 151.

MCARTHUR, J. (1977). *J. trop. Med. Hyg.*, **80,** 99.

MCCORMACK, W. M., MOSLEY, W. H., and FAHIMUDDIN, M. (1969). *Am. J. Epidemiol.*, **89,** 393.

MacKay, D. M. (1979). *Tropical Doctor*, **9**, 31.
Mackintosh, J. (1836). *Principles of Pathology and Practice of Physic.*
Mhalu, F. S., Mmari, P. W., and Ijumba, J. (1979). *Lancet*, **1**, 345.
Mngola, E. N. (1972). *E. Afr. med. J.*, **49**, 151.
Moenginah, P. A., Suprapto, Soenarto, J., Bachtin, M., Sutrisno, D., Sutaryo, and Rohde, J. E. (1975). *Lancet*, **2**, 323.
Mosley, W. H., Aziz, K. M. A., Rahman, A. S. M. M., Chowdhury, A. K. M. A., and Ahmed, A. (1973). *Bull. Wld Hlth Org.*, **49**, 381.
——, McCormack, W. M., Fahimuddin, M., Aziz, K. M. A., Rahman, A. S. M. M., Chowdhury, A. K. M. A., Martin, A. R., Feeley, J. C., and Phillips, R. A. (1969). *Bull. Wld Hlth Org.*, **40**, 177.
Nalin, D. R. (1975). *Lancet*, **1**, 1400.
—— and Cash, R. A. (1974). In *Cholera* (ed. D. Barua and W. Burrows). p. 253. W. B. Saunders Co., Philadelphia, London and Toronto.
——, ——, Islam, R., Molla, M., and Phillips, R. A. (1968). *Lancet*, **2**, 370.
——, Levine, R. J., Levine, M. M., Hoover, D., Bergquist, E., McLaughlin, J., Libonati, J., Alam, J., and Hornick, R. B. (1978). *Lancet*, **2**, 856.
——, Levine, M. M., Rhead, J., Bergquist, E., Rennels, M., Hughes, T., O'Donnell, S., and Hornick, R. B. (1978). *Lancet*, **2**, 859.
Oseasohn, R., Ahmad, S., and Islam, M. A. (1966). *Lancet*, **1**, 340.
O'Shaughnessy, W. B. (1831). *Lancet*, **1**, 227.
Palmer, D. L., Koster, F. T., Rafiqul Islam, A. F. M., Mizanur Rahman, A. S. M., and Bradley Sack, R. (1977). *New Engl. J. Med.*, **297**, 1107.
Phillips, R. A. (1964). *Fedn Proc. Fedn Am. Socs exp. Biol.*, **23**, 705.
Pollitzer, R. (1959). *Monograph Ser. W.H.O.*, No. 43.
Radojcic, V. (1973). *E. Afr. med. J.*, **50**, 696.
Roberts, J. M. D. (1972). *E. Afr. med. J.*, **49**, 159.
Sack, G. H., Hennessey, K. N., and Mitra, R. C. (1970). *Clin. Res.*, **18**, 682.
——, Pierce, N. F., Hennessey, K. N., Mitra, R. C., Sack, R. B., and Muzumder, D. N. G. (1972). *Bull. Wld Hlth Org.*, **47**, 31.
Sakazaki, R., Iwanami, S., and Fukumi, H. (1963). *Jap. J. med. Sci. Biol.* **16**, 161.
Shafer, D. E., Lust, W. D., and Sircar, B. (1970). *Proc. Natl Acad. Sci.*, **67**, 851.
Sharp, G. W. G. and Hynie, S. (1971). *Nature, Lond.*, **229**, 266.
Sladen, G. E. and Dawson, A. M. (1969). *Gut*, **10**, 82.
Snow, J. (1855). *On the mode of communication of Cholera*. 2nd ed. Churchill, London.
Sommer, A., Khan, M., and Mosley, W. H. (1973). *Lancet*, **1**, 1230.
—— and Mosley, W. H. (1973). *Lancet*, **1**, 1232.
Swartz, T. A. (1972). *Proc. R. Soc. Med.*, **65**, 428.
Takikawa, J. and Fujisawa, T. (1956). *Shokuhin Eisei Kenkyn*, **6**, 15.
Vaughan Williams, E. M., Dohadwalla, A. N., and Dutta, N. K. (1969). *J. infect. Dis.*, **120**, 645.
Wallace, C. K., Pierce, N. F., and Anderson, P. N. (1967). *Lancet*, **1**, 865.
——, Carpenter, C. C. J., Mitra, P. P., Sack, R. B., Khanra, S. R., Werner, A. S., Duffy, T. P., Oleinick, A., and Lewis, G. W. (1966). *Br. med. J.*, **2**, 447.
WHO (1973). *Press release WHA/18*. May 23.
Wilcocks, C. and Manson-Bahr, P. E. C. (1972). *Manson's tropical diseases*. 17th ed. p. 867. Baillière Tindall, London.

19

Small-intestinal parasites, excluding those which are associated with malabsorption

THIS chapter is dominated by two nematode infections: those caused by the hookworm and the roundworm. Everyone who has any knowledge of medicine in a tropical country will appreciate the very great importance of these two parasitic infections; in most areas, the vast majority of people are infected, and although mortality is not usually a direct result of infection, there is an enormous morbidity rate. Even though nutritional status might appear reasonably good, working efficiency, exercise tolerance, powers of concentration, and intellectual ability are all impaired. Hookworms undergo a cycle of development in the soil; the resulting larvae are infective and penetrate the intact skin; the distribution of this group of diseases is therefore limited by requirements of the developing larvae for warmth and humidity. Roundworms, however, merely survive in the soil in the form of ova which must be *ingested* for their life-cycle to continue; they are not therefore so susceptible to temperature changes and are common in temperate regions, also.

Both infections depend for survival on the state of hygiene and sanitation within a community: defaecation on to the ground, and the use of untreated night-soil as an agricultural fertilizer are both important factors in their transmission.

The treatment of these diseases has been reviewed by Davis (1973) and Gilles (1978).

19.1. Ancylostomiasis (hookworm disease) (HW)

Most people living in tropical countries of the third world are infected with either *Ancylostoma duodenale* or *Necator americanus*. In a study in western Nigeria (Gilles, Watson-Williams, and Ball, 1964), for example, 90 per cent of the men and 82 per cent of the women were found to be infected with *N. americanus*. One estimate is that 1000 million people (approximately one quarter of the world's population) have hookworm infections (Peters and Gilles, 1977). The areas dominated by *A. duodenale* were originally the Mediterranean littoral and parts of the Far east. *N. americanus* (literally, the American aggressor) used to be the more common parasite in America and tropical Africa; however both parasites are now widely distributed in both the tropics and subtropics. In Tanzania, for example, one recent study has shown that 70 per cent of hookworm infections are due to *N. americanus*, and 30 per cent to *A. duodenale* (Rep and Shaba, 1976). *Necator* is in fact less pathogenic than *Ancylostoma*.

The disease can occur in small outbreaks. During a game of 'Kabaddi' during which there is extensive skin contact with the ground, 27 young men in one village in India developed a severe dermatitis and pulmonary symptoms, which were followed by abdominal discomfort and anaemia after several months (Koshy, Raina, Sharma, Mithal, and Tandon, 1978). *A. duodenale* was responsible and all made a complete recovery after treatment of that disease.

19.1.1. Parasitology and pathology of HW

The adult worms live in, and attach themselves to, the duodenal and jejunal villi by suction with their buccal cavities; they are 8–10 mm in length. Symptoms and signs depend on the worm load (Douglas and Tamanika, 1973; Zigas, 1973); with a heavy infection, anaemia and hypoproteinaemia occur, because blood oozes from the anchor sites. Intensity of infection depends very largely on the defaecation behaviour of the local population; that has been clearly shown in rural Bengal, India (Kochar, Schad, Chowdhury, Dean, and Nawalinski, 1976). It has been estimated that a single *A. duodenale* can withdraw approximately 0·2 ml blood daily; *N. americanus* on the other hand withdraws only some 0·05 ml. Assuming that each worm removes 0·15 ml of blood daily, iron loss from one, or even 10 worms, is negligible; however the loss from 1000 worms is an entirely different matter (150 ml per day); iron deficiency anaemia ensues (Lozoff, Warren, and Mahmoud, 1975). It has been suggested, but not proved, that bearers of the sickle-cell trait have a decreased susceptibility to hookworm disease.

After fertilization, ova which are approximately 60 μm in length, are produced by the female worms, and are passed in the faeces; one female ancylostoma can produce approximately 30,000 ova, and one necator 9000 ova, daily. If they fall on most soil, larvae are produced and they remain in the soil until human skin is contacted; in suitable conditions they can survive for several months. Thus, anyone not wearing shoes, and that applies to most people, and especially children in third-world countries, is prone to infection. After skin penetration the larvae migrate to the right side of the heart, through the lungs, and up the major bronchi and trachea, to be swallowed. They end up, some three to five days after skin penetration, in the duodenum and jejunum where development to adult worms occurs. Ancylostoma infection can also take place by the oral route; vegetables contaminated by larvae are thus a further source of infection. As far as is known, necator can only infect by the cutaneous route.

19.1.2. Presentation of HW

The first manifestation of infection is a local erythematous dermatitis ('ground itch'), at the site of the initial infection; that may be macropapular or vesicular, and usually passes unnoticed. As the larvae pass from the small pulmonary vessels to the alveoli and small bronchioles, there may be a transient illness (as in ascariasis) which consists of a cough with bloody sputum; that however is also not usually noticed. If the infection is sizeable, some two to four weeks later abdominal symptoms begin. They consist usually of mild abdominal discomfort, flatulence, and occasional diarrhoea; at that stage the worms are attaching themselves to the small-intestinal mucosa.

The most common sequel is anaemia (Fig. 19.1) and that may be followed by hypoproteinaemia; those symptoms occur after some three to six months, and also depend on the size of the hookworm load. The anaemia is usually hypochromic, and microcytic, and is often superimposed upon a nutritional anaemia; a combined iron and folate deficiency picture may thus be seen. The severity of the anaemia is dependent on three indices (Edington and Gilles, 1976): (i) the iron content of the human diet, (ii) the state of the iron reserves, and (iii) the intensity and duration of infection. A super-added folate-deficient megaloblastic anaemia is sometimes masked by the severity of the iron-deficiency, and that only becomes overt after a partial haematological response to oral iron (Daftary and Bhende, 1956; Borrero, Restrepo, Botero, and Latorre, 1961). Folate deficiency may be due to dietary deficiency, defective absorption, or increased demand, in for example infancy and pregnancy. Hypoproteinaemia is due mainly to loss of blood and lymph into the intestinal lumen, but also to depressed albumin synthesis, caused usually by chronic infections.

The reason why only a proportion of an infected population develops severe symptoms is complex; individual immunity is probably at least as important as the intensity of the worm load. Serum IgE concentrations are raised (Kojima, Yokogawa, and Tada, 1972); there is evidence that adults have a higher antibody level than children to hookworm antigens in endemic areas (Soulsby and Gilles, 1974).

19.1.3. Complications of HW

If the anaemia is severe, and that is likely if 500 or more worms are present, there may be cardiac failure. However, oedema is more often due to hypoproteinaemia alone. Rarely, massive intestinal haemorrhage can occur (Naik, Mitra, and Mehta, 1976); although that is usually in children, cases in adults have been reported. Stunting of growth occurs in children. Although frequently suggested, there is no good evidence that malabsorption results from hookworm infections (Gilles, *et al*., 1964; Aziz and Siddiqui, 1968; Tandon, Kholi, Saraya, Ramachandran, and Prakash, 1969; Cook, Kajubi, and Lee, 1969; Cook, 1974; Koshy *et al*., 1978); suggestions that that can occasionally occur have been made more often for ancylostoma than necator infections.

19.1.4. Investigation of HW

Characteristic ova can be identified in faeces; there are a number of different techniques for quantitation of ova. A hypochromic, microcytic anaemia is usually present; the severity of that depends on the size of the worm load (see above). An eosinophilia is usually present in the early months of infection, i.e. during the invasive stage. The stool gives a positive result when tested for occult blood.

19.1.5. Treatment of HW

A good diet and iron supplements are necessary. In very severe cases, intravenous iron or blood transfusion may be required, but in this author's experience that is very rarely indicated. The anaemia is longstanding and complete cardiac adaptation has occurred. There is a great tendency for newly

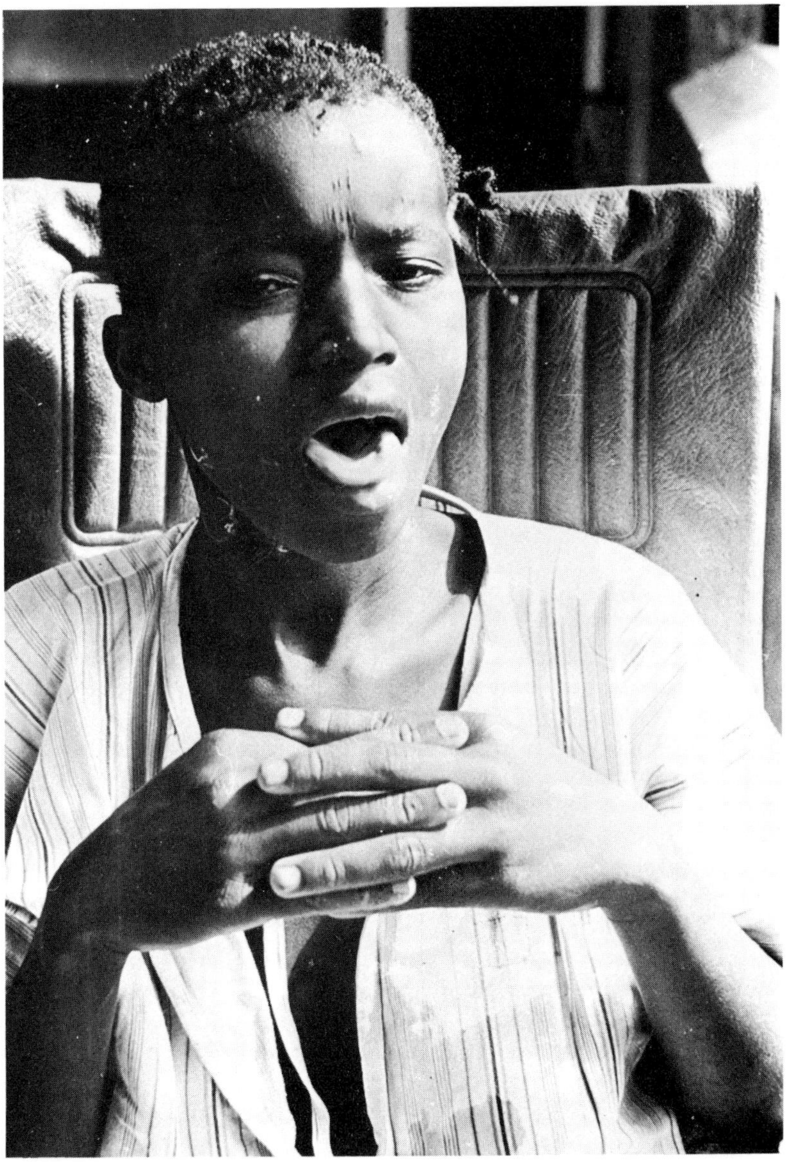

FIG. 19.1. A 22-year-old Zambian woman at the University Teaching Hospital, Lusaka with a severe hypochromic anaemia caused by a heavy hookworm infection. The tongue and nail beds were very pale. Haemoglobin was 3·0 g per dl. Response to oral iron was rapid after eradication of the infection.

arrived and inexperienced doctors in tropical countries to give blood transfusions unnecessarily, with the not infrequent precipitation of cardiac failure. With haemoglobin concentrations as low as 2·0 g per dl, the response to oral iron is perfectly satisfactory and after an initial reticulocyte response has been observed, treatment can be continued at home. The hazards of transfusion cannot be overemphasized. Apart from overloading the circulation (Ofori Atta, 1958), transfusion reactions are common; in Ghana the incidence has been given as six per cent (Edington, 1956). Furthermore, there is the problem of producing a local thrombophlebitis or cellulitis due to lack of sterile precautions, and also the danger of introducing diseases from the donor blood, of which viral hepatitis is the most important. If transfusions must be given, packed red blood-cells should be given together with a potent diuretic such as intravenous frusemide ('Lasix') or ethacrynic acid (Harrison and Lawson, 1966). In Uganda, 29 patients with hookworm disease were treated with intraperitoneal blood transfusions (Fowler, Knight, and Patel, 1968). Using a ^{51}Cr-labelled red-cell technique, it was shown that from 35–100 per cent of the blood was absorbed in 6–10 days. If it is essential to raise the haemoglobin level rapidly, which is very rarely the case, intraperitoneal transfusion is probably safer therefore than intravenous infusion. It is important to appreciate, however, that repletion of iron in iron-deficient people predisposes them to certain infections including malaria, tuberculosis, and brucellosis (Murray, Murray, Murray, and Murray, 1978a); those authors suggested that iron-deficiency in some groups, such as the Somali nomads whom they studied, may be part of an ecological compromise permitting optimum co-survival of host and infecting agent.

Bephenium hydroxynaphthoate ('Alcopar') is the therapeutic agent of choice; it is more effective against *A. duodenale* than *N. americanus.* Five grammes are given orally on three consecutive days following overnight fasts; in children a proportionately lower dose, in the form of a syrup, may be given. It is bitter and occasionally produces nausea and vomiting. An alternative agent, and one which is of value if there is a coincidental *Ascaris lumbricoides* infection, is mebendazole (methyl-5-benzoylbenzimidazole-2-carbamate) ('Vermox'); 100 mg should be given twice daily for three days. There are no side-effects. Mebendazole affects glucose uptake and increases the utilization of endogenous glycogen in nematodes (hookworm, ascaris, *Enterobius,* and *Trichuris*) and cestodes (Van den Bosshe, 1978). It also affects mitochondrial malate-induced phosphorylation in those parasites. There are other effects also, and it seems probable that it is a combination of them which accounts for the antihelminthic activity. In a report from Bangkok, Thailand, mebendazole (100 mg thrice daily for three days) has been shown to be effective in *N. americanus* infections (Migasena, Suntharasamai, and Harinasuta, 1978); a reduction in egg count of 97 per cent was recorded at three weeks, and 70 per cent were completely cured. Corresponding percentages with tetrachlorethylene (0·1 ml per kg) were 99 and 77 respectively. Pyrantel embonate given as a single dose of 1·1 g has been shown to be more effective than bephenium in *N. americanus* infections in Mauritius (Mawdsley and Barr, 1975). In a study in Cairo, Egypt, using single dose therapy, levamisole ('Ketrax') (150 mg) produced a 93 per cent, pyrantel embonate ('Combantrin') (750 mg) a 78 per cent, and bephenium hydroxynaphthoate (5 g) an 81 per cent cure rate in hookworm infections (Farid, Bassily, Miner, Hassan, and Laughlin, 1977). The cost of therapeutic agents is often a limiting factor in the third world in the treatment of large sections of the population. Tetrachlorethylene (TCE) is a much cheaper agent; 0·12 ml per kg bodyweight (to a maximum dose of five ml) should be given after an overnight fast. Two or more doses at four-day intervals may be necessary. The recommendation is usually made that the ascaris infection is treated before TCE is given. The side-effects are nausea, vomiting, epigastric discomfort, and rarely drowsiness, vertigo, and hypotension. TCE should not be given if there is evidence of liver disease.

19.2. Ascariasis (roundworm infection) (RW)

With the exception of hookworm disease, infection with *Ascaris lumbricoides* is probably the most common intestinal helminthic disease in man. It is common throughout the world, and involves hundreds of millions of people, especially in warm climates and countries where the standards of public health and personal hygiene are low. The ova can survive in cold climates. In many tropical countries, infection-rates of 70–80 per cent in the indigenous populations have been reported (Stoll, 1947; Goodwin and Standon, 1958; Gilles, 1964). Susceptibility to infection seems to be greatest in children, and declines as adult life is reached. Serum antibodies to ascaris have been demonstrated early in the infection (Lejkina, 1965). An inverse association between ascariasis and malaria has been demonstrated (Murray, Murray, Murray, and Murray, 1978b); following treatment of their ascaris infections a group of children were shown to be unusually susceptible to malaria. Those authors suggested that severe ascariasis, by lowering the nutritional status, protects against malaria; furthermore that may represent an ecological balance for optimum co-survival of the host and his two parasites.

19.2.1. Parasitology and pathology of RW

The adult worms, which are brownish-yellow, may reach 30 to 40 cm in length; males are slightly smaller than females. They live in the small-intestine of man, from duodenum to the ileocaecal valve; the vast majority however live in the mid-jejunum. They can live for a year or more, lying free in the lumen. As many as 1000 worms, weighing up to four kg have been extracted from a single patient (Gilles, 1978). After fertilization, the females produce up to 200 000 ova daily; they are passed in the faeces and will remain viable in moist soil. The ova, which may remain viable for one year are resistant to cold and most disinfectants; they are killed by direct sunlight, and temperatures above 45°C. When conditions are suitable, the ova become infective, and contain an active larva in 10 to 14 days.

Man is infected by food and drink contaminated with faeces and not via the skin, as in hookworm disease; in children dirty fingers are very important. Pigs may be a serious source of infection with *A. lumbricoides* in rural Papua New Guinea (Jones, 1976). When they reach the small-intestine the ova come under the influence of digestive enzymes, and motile rhabditiform larvae are released. They pass through the intestinal mucosa and into the mesenteric lymphatics and portal system, from whence they reach the right atrium; from there they pass to the lungs, and after burrowing through the alveolar walls migrate up the bronchial tree to the pharynx. They are then swallowed and pass back to the small-intestine; some 60 to 75 days after ingestion the larvae have matured, and ova production begins. That is the usual cycle, but occasionally they pass to the left side of the heart from the pulmonary capillaries; they may enter the systemic circulation and can reach any part of the body. Many complications have been recorded. In the respiratory system, lung abscess, empyema, and tracheal obstruction may occur. Mesenteric vein obstruction with strangulation, is a rare event. Granulomatous nodule formation in the peritoneum is unusual (Cooray and Panabokke, 1960). In the genitourinary system, urethral involvement and urinary retention have been recorded.

19.1.2. Presentation of RW

During their passage through the lungs, some four to 16 days after infection, the larvae damage the capillary and alveolar walls as they force their way through. That may give rise to a fever, and pneumonitis or pneumonia. A febrile illness, cough, haemoptyses, and crepitations may result. Larvae may be found in the sputum. It is at this invasive stage that a peripheral eosinophilia occurs; the term Loeffler's syndrome may be applied. The bronchioles may contain polymorphonuclear leucocytes most of which are eosinophils, and Charcot-Leyden crystals (El Hashmi, 1971). Hepatomegaly may also occur during the migratory stage (Chapter 5). After passage through the lungs some larvae go astray and end up in the skin, kidney, brain, eye, meninges, spinal cord, myocardium, etc.

It is impossible to assess the frequency and importance in terms of morbidity of the migratory stage, because most people in tropical countries do not present with trivial symptoms. It is possible that death occasionally follows the pulmonary complications; that is apparently a problem in Saudi Arabia (Gelpi and Mustafa, 1968).

The vast majority of patients with a few adult ascaris in their small-intestine are completely asymptomatic.

The pneumonitis is similar to that caused by hookworm and strongyloides infections; tropical eosinophilia and bronchial asthma are differential diagnoses. Urticaria may occur in the invasive stage.

19.2.3. Complications of RW

With heavy infections, abdominal discomfort and colic may occur. They may be partly the result of a mesenteric lymphadenopathy (Tukomo, 1956). The incidence rate of serious complications (Ajao and Ajao, 1979) is however surprisingly low. Worms may be coughed up, vomited, or passed through the nose; rarely they may cause asphyxia in children. With a high parasite load and a low protein intake, malnutrition may be a complication (Tripathy, González, Lotero, and Bolaños, 1971; Tripathy, Duque, Bolaños, Lotero, and Mayoral, 1972). However, if overall nutritional status is adequate, that is a most unusual event (Blumenthal and Schultz, 1976); in that study, although serum albumin and ascorbic acid concentrations were lower in infected individuals, they were not present at inadequate levels. A claim that protein absorption is impaired in children has been made (Venkatachalam and Patwardhan, 1953). There is no clear evidence however that ascariasis is associated with malabsorption; its effect on small-intestinal bacterial flora has not been assessed. Occasionally, worms become hooked to a jejunal biopsy-capsule and a long wriggling ascaris emerges from the patient's mouth in spectacular fashion; I have on two occasions experienced that, only to be thanked most profusely by a grateful patient. Alternatively, they may force themselves into the common bile-duct (Chapter 14), pancreatic duct (Chapter 15), appendix (Chapter 27) (Milwidsky, 1945), and other diverticula. Adult ascaris may appear at any ectopic site (Bustamante-Sarabia, Martuscelli-Q, and Tay, 1977). Intestinal obstruction (Crane, Pak, and Lee, 1965) and intussusception may occur, especially in children (Ajao and Ajao, 1979). Obstruction is most common in the ileum, which is the narrowest part of the small-intestine, but can occur anywhere. Purgation occasionally seems to precipitate obstruction. Pain and vomiting are often accompanied by a mild fever (Davey, 1968); a mass of worms is palpable per abdomen in over 50 per cent of patients and that is usually in the umbilical region, but occasionally in the iliac fossae. Because a patient has ascariasis, intestinal obstruction must not be assumed to be the result of that infection; other causes, e.g. volvulus and intussusception are also common in tropical countries. With complete obstruction, surgery is indicated; resection of a segment of small intestine is occasionally necessary. Obstruction of a Meckel's diverticulum with resulting perforation has been reported. Ascaris have caused perforation of Peyer's patches in typhoid fever; they may be found lying free in the abdominal cavity at operation (Qassab and Al-Khateeb, 1966). Whether ascaris can perforate the normal small-intestine is not clear; according to Davey (1968), most experienced surgeons in Africa have found at least one worm free in the peritoneal cavity, without finding an explanation for its presence. The disease can certainly cause fatalities (Piggott, Hansbarger, and Neafie, 1970); in that study, 38 of 437 patients with ascariasis had either serious or fatal illnesses.

19.2.4. Investigation of RW

During the invasive stage an eosinophilia is often present, and a chest radiograph may show pulmonary infiltration. While migrating through the lungs, larvae, eosinophils, and Charcot-Leyden crystals are occasionally found in the sputum.

Ascariasis is usually diagnosed by demonstrating ova in the stool; they are usually found easily in direct smears, but concentration techniques are available. Adult worms are occasionally passed spontaneously in the stool. They are sometimes outlined by barium during radiological examinations (Middlemiss, 1961); barium coats the exterior of the worm, and also outlines its gut (Fig. 19.2). A straight radiograph of the abdomen may reveal a single worm, or a conglomerated mass of worms, in outline; in the presence of obstruction, fluid levels and dilated loops of small-intestine can be visualized.

Serological tests are available, but at present none is adequate for diagnostic purposes.

19.2.5. Treatment of RW

Piperazine (given in the form of citrate, phosphate, or adipate) ('Antepar' or 'Entacyl') is the drug of choice (Bell and Nassif, 1971); the dose is 75 mg per kg bodyweight. An adult with a heavy infection should receive a single dose of 4·0 g, and children correspondingly smaller doses, on a weight basis. The treatment may have to be repeated after one week. Headaches, dizziness, and visual disturbances occasionally occur. Convulsions have rarely been reported in children. Piperazine should not be given if there is a history of epileptic fits or of hepatic or renal impairment. The broad spectrum antihelminthic agent, mebendazole ('Vermox'), 100 mg twice daily for three days, is usually effective (Wolfe and Wershing, 1974). Mebendazole is free of toxic effects. That compound also eliminates hookworms which are frequently present coincidentally.

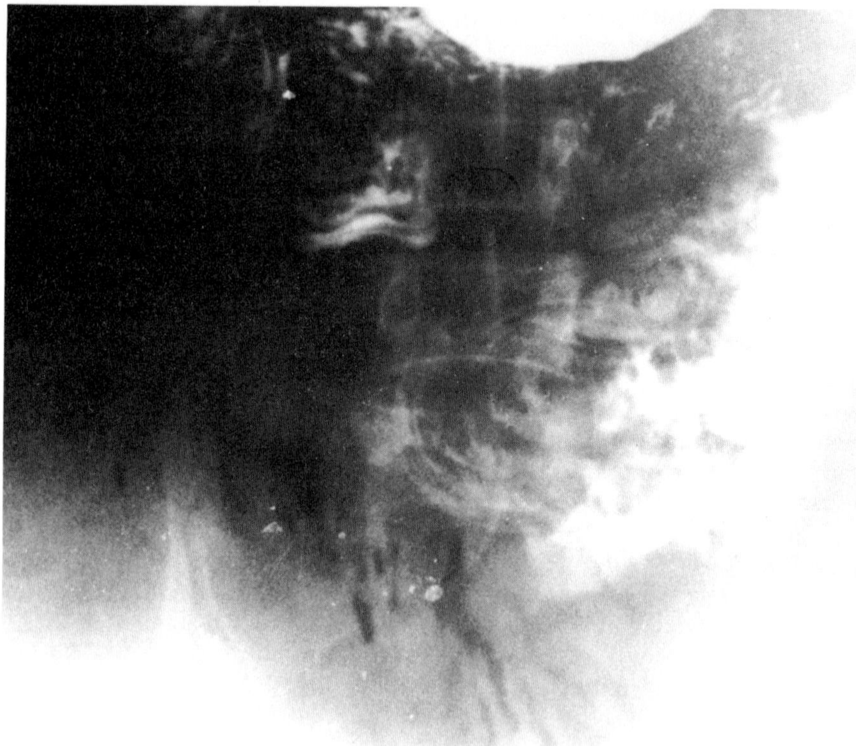

FIG. 19.2. Barium-meal in a Papua New Guinean woman with a heavy roundworm (*Ascaris lumbricoides*) infection. Several adult worms have been outlined by the barium.

In terms of rapid action, tolerance and low dosage, levamisole ('Ketrax') is also a satisfactory agent for treatment of ascariasis (Van den Bosshe, 1978); that is given in a single oral dose of 2·5 mg per kg bodyweight. Nausea, vomiting, abdominal discomfort, headache, and dizziness occur in approximately one per cent of patients. Levamisole and tetramisole act on the neuromuscular system of immature and adult nematodes; an initial stimulation of ganglionic structures is followed by a depolarizing type of neuromuscular inhibition. Administration to heavily infected African schoolchildren led to almost complete elimination of ascaris, and also the excretion of hookworm ova; *Strongyloides stercoralis* larvae were also reduced by 77 and 78 per cent one year later (Gatti, Krubwa, Vandepitte, and Thienpont, 1972). In Egypt, using single dose therapy, levamisole (150 mg) produced a 100 per cent, pyrantel embonate ('Combantrin') (750 mg) a 90 per cent, and bephenium hydroxynaphthoate (5 g) a 73 per cent cure rate in ascaris infections (Farid, Bassily, Miner, Hassan, and Laughlin, 1977). In central Iran, a single oral dose of 10 mg of pyrantel embonate per kg bodyweight was given in a mass eradication campaign. Ascaris infection rates were reduced from 87 to 95 per cent, to one to eight per cent in six villages using that regime (Arfaa and Ghadirian, 1977); all age groups and both sexes responded similarly. Serial faecal examinations after treatment indicated that by one year the prevalence of infection had returned to the pretreatment level, although the average stool ova-counts were lower.

19.3. Other nematode infections

19.3.1. Ternidens diminutus

In parts of east and central Africa, infection with the monkey hookworm is relatively common (Peters and Gilles, 1977); the parasite can be found at all levels of the small and large intestine. In most cases the infection is asymptomatic and the ova, which can be demonstrated in faeces, are usually mistaken for those of hookworms; however the adult worms, which are passed after the usual course of treatment for hookworm disease, are characteristic.

19.3.2. Gnathostomiasis

Infection is caused by the nematode *Gnathostoma spinigerum*. A wide range of animals form a reservoir. It is common in Israel, the Sudan, India, and the Far east; most cases have been reported from Thailand.

Gastrointestinal symptoms may be prominent at presentation, but usually in association with haemoptyses, haematuria, and angioneurotic oedema. The brain is principally involved, however, and that accounts for a high mortality rate.

Diagnosis is by finding an eosinophilia and identifying the immature worms. Cutaneous and precipitin tests are available for diagnosis.

19.3.3. Trichinellosis (Trichiniasis)

This disease, caused by the nematode *Trichinella spiralis* is found in those tropical countries where pork is eaten; it is a parasite of the bush pig. Gastrointestinal disturbances occur in the early, migratory, phase of the illness. There may be an enteritis with petechial haemorrhages, oedema, and mild ulceration. Fever may have the characteristics of that associated with typhoid fever. Manifestations in other systems, including the cardiac, respiratory, muscular, ocular, and central nervous systems, usually dominate the clinical picture (Edington and Gilles, 1976).

An eosinophilia is usually present. Encysted larvae are found most easily in muscle biopsies. Intradermal and serological tests are of value in diagnosis.

19.3.4. Trichostrongyliasis

These parasites are occasionally present in the digestive tract of man; they are in fact parasitic in the digestive tract of herbivorous animals. Maturing and adult worms attach to the small-intestinal mucosa, and mild anaemia may ensue in heavy infections. Treatment is the same as that for hookworm infections.

19.4. Trematode infections

19.4.1. Fasciolopsiasis (intestinal-fluke infections)

The large, fleshy, small-intestinal fluke *Fasciolopsis buski*, occurs commonly as a parasite of man and pigs in the Far east, China, Taiwan, south-east Asia and India (Plaut, Kampanart-Sanyakorn, and Manning, 1969). In some parts of north-east Thailand, almost the entire population of some villages is affected. One estimate is that 10 million people are infected in the Far east (Cross, 1969). The adult *F. buski* is the largest parasitic trematode of man, and may reach a length of 7·5 cm. Other species, *Heterophyes heterophyes* and *Metagonimus yokagawai*, occur in the Far east, Indonesia, the Philippines, south China, India, Egypt and Tunisia; they are less common and rarely produce symptoms, however, and will not be considered further.

Ova, which are passed in the stool of man and the pig, hatch on reaching water to produce free-living miracidia. They penetrate, and develop in snails, from which cercariae escape and encyst on various species of water plant; raw water chestnut plants which are peeled by children with their teeth, and caltrops, which are harvested and eaten raw, are often fertilized with human faeces. If these are ingested by man, he becomes infected. Larvae are liberated from encysted cercariae, and the adult flukes live in the small-intestine either attached to the mucosa, causing foci of inflammation, or enmeshed in mucous secretions; they live on duodenal secretions and mature in about three months. Egg output per worm averages 25 000 per day.

Many infections are initially symptomless. A few months later, epigastric and hypogastric pain, diarrhoea which is sometimes intermittent with constipation, anorexia, and nausea occur. Intestinal stasis, ulceration, and obstruction have been reported. Anaemia, oedema and ascites occur later. Death occasionally occurs from cachexia or intercurrent infection. Prognosis after treatment is usually good.

A diagnosis is made by finding ova, and occasionally flukes, in the stool. An eosinophilia, usually accompanied by a leucocytosis, is common.

The drug of choice is crystalline hexyl-resorcinol in a dose of one gramme orally, after an overnight fast; purgation should be given two hours later. A proportionately lower dose should be given to children. As with taeniasis (see below) results of treatment seem to be better if the compound is given through a duodenal tube. The treatment should be repeated after 3 or 4 days. An alternative agent is tetrachlorethylene, which should be given in the same dosage as for hookworm disease (Suntharasamai, Bunnag, and Tejavanij, 1974).

19.4.2. Schistosomiasis

In *Schistosoma mansoni* and *S. japonicum* infections the small-intestine is in rare cases affected to a greater extent than the large-intestine (Edington and Gilles, 1976). With progressive fibrosis, stenosis may occur. If the muscular layer and serosa are involved, pseudotubercles may produce a focal exudative peritonitis and intestinal adhesions. In *S. haematobium* infections, ova with pseudotubercle formation, and scarring, can occur in the small-intestine; they are asymptomatic.

19.4.3. Paragonimiasis

The lung fluke, *Paragonimus westermani*, penetrates the jejunal wall during its life cycle, and passes through the peritoneal cavity *en route* for the diaphragm and lungs; the adult fluke usually lives in the lungs. Ulceration of the intestine with presence of ova in the stool sometimes occurs; a fibrous exudate containing ova and eosinophils may be present. Adhesions, with symptoms of intestinal obstruction, and appendicitis, occasionally result.

This infection occurs focally throughout the Far east, south-east Asia, the Pacific islands, west Africa, and parts of south America.

Ova may be found in the sputum or stool. There is usually an eosinophilia. Serological tests are of some value in diagnosis.

19.5. Cestode (tapeworm) infections (TW)

19.5.1. Parasitology and pathology of TW

Adult tapeworms consist of a scolex (head), neck, and a chain of proglottids (segments); each proglottid contains both male and female reproductive organs. Six species, four of which are widely distributed throughout the world, frequently infect man.

The two most common, which are also two of the largest, are the beef (*Taenia saginata*) and pork (*T. solium*) tapeworms; they can reach lengths of 10 and seven metres in length, respectively. *T. saginata* is found especially commonly in the Middle east, Kenya (Nelson, Pester, and Rickman, 1965), and Ethiopia. Two dwarf worms, which are also common, are *Hymenolepis nana* (the dwarf tapeworm) and *H. diminuta* (the rat tapeworm); they reach lengths of 2·5 to 4, and 20 to 30 cm respectively. A third, *Drepanidotaenia lanceolata* rarely infects man. *H. nana* is common in south America, India, and the USA; it is usually a disease of children. *H. diminuta* is primarily a disease of rats and mice; human infection usually involves children, and is acquired accidentally (see below). The fish tapeworm (*Diphyllobothrium latum*), which is found not only in cold and temperate lake-regions throughout the world, but also in the Middle east, east and southern Africa, Japan, the Philippines, Chile, and both the USA and Europe, can also reach a length of 10 metres. The dog tapeworm (*Dipylidium caninum*) is occasionally found in children, sometimes in Europe and America.

Segments of adult *T. saginata, T. solium,* and *D. latum* which live in the small intestine of man are passed in the faeces either before or after ova have been released. The intermediate hosts for the former two parasites are usually infected while grazing in pastures which have either been fertilized with human faeces, or flooded with sewage-laden water. *T. saginata* and *T. solium* ova, when ingested by cattle and pigs, respectively, release embryos which penetrate the small-intestinal wall and are transported to various organs, including the skeletal muscles, where they encyst as cysticerci. If raw or undercooked beef which contains viable cysticerci of *T. saginata* is eaten by man, he becomes infected and an adult worm matures in his intestine. However, if he eats raw or undercooked pork, the larvae of *T. solium* may find their way to various parts of his body, chiefly the muscles, brain and subcutaneous tissues, where they encyst as cysticerci. Infection with *T. solium* can take place by autoinfection, i.e. faecal to mouth infection, regurgitation of ova from the small-intestine to the stomach, or by person-to-person transmission, i.e. in water and food contaminated with infected faeces. Cysticerci are small white bodies; their size varies and can be up to 20 mm. They may be oval or spherical. The life-span is from a few months to 35 years (Dixon and Lipscomb, 1961). The intermediate host of *D. latum* is various species of fish, e.g. salmon and pike, and freshwater crustaceans (*Cyclops* or *Diaptomus*); infection occurs from faecal contamination of fresh water. Human infection follows eating raw or under-cooked fish. The adult *D. latum* usually lives in the lower ileum and thus differs from the others in its localization; most reside in the jejunum. Man usually harbours one or two of the adults of the larger worms, only.

The life cycles of *H. nana* and *H. diminuta* are different. In the case of *H. nana*, both larval and adult stages are found in the human intestine; transmission is usually from man to man directly, but rats and mice can also be infected, and food contaminated with their faeces can be a source of infection. *H. diminuta* has an intermediate host in various arthropods—rat fleas, beetles, cockroaches, and other insects; human infection occurs when food contaminated by them is eaten accidentally. When infected, it is usual for many of these smaller worms to be present in the human intestine, commonly the upper ileum. *D. lanceolata* infects birds and man, and is found on rare occasions as an accidental infection.

D. caninum infections occur usually in young children living closely with infected dogs and cats; transmission is by swallowing infected intermediate hosts—various fleas and lice.

19.5.2 Presentation of TW

Organic symptoms are unusual and consist of mild abdominal discomfort; worm phobia is however common. The patient either notices segments of the adult worm in the stool, or occasionally on clothing or bedding. The worms are dependent nutritionally on their host's diet, and carbohydrate, protein, and vitamins of the B complex are avidly ingested (Chandler, 1943); in experimental undernutrition, worm load and ova production are reduced (Burlingame and Chandler, 1941). A small proportion, probably about one per cent, of people infected with *D. latum* in Scandinavia suffer from a B_{12} deficient megaloblastic anaemia; the adult worm ingests dietary vitamin B_{12}. Heavy infections with *H. nana* may cause diarrhoea, abdominal pain, anorexia, weight loss, and nervous manifestations in children.

19.5.3. Complications of TW

The most serious complication is cysticercosis, which occurs with *T. solium* infections.* Whereas the larvae usually migrate to muscles or connective tissues, where they slowly die and calcify, occasionally they enter the brain (where they calcify very slowly) and produce a variety of neurological sequelae, including fits, raised intracranial pressure, nerve palsies, etc. The subcutaneous tissues, heart, eye, liver, lung, pancreas, parotid gland, and peritoneum may also be involved (Dixon and Lipscomb, 1961).

A mass of worms can occasionally produce intestinal obstruction; perforation and a secondary peritonitis have been reported. Prolonged watery diarrhoea has also been described. Appendicitis is a rare complication.

19.5.4. Investigation of TW

Segments of the adult worms, which are passed in the stool, can be identified microscopically; species differentiation is facilitated by compressing the segments between two glass slides and observing the uterus. Ova may also be detected by stool microscopy. There may be a mild eosinophilia or lymphocytosis. A haemagglutination test is positive in about 50 per cent of patients with cysticercosis. In cysticercosis, calcified cysticerci can be demonstrated by radiological examination of muscles; calcification of cysticerci in the brain takes place much more slowly. Skin and complement fixation tests are available in diagnosing cysticercosis (Biagi and Tay, 1958; Rydzewski, Chisholm, and Kagan, 1975); the haemagglutination test gives an 85 per cent positivity rate in that condition. A vitamin B_{12} deficient megaloblastic anaemia is occasionally found with *D. latum* infections.

19.5.5. Treatment of TW

Treatment has been reviewed by Davis (1973). Eradication of *T. solium* is important because of the possibility of cysticercosis of the brain; the other species are harmless, except in rare instances.

Mepacrine hydrochloride ('Quinacrine') is the therapeutic agent of choice; it is given after an overnight fast, preferably down an intraduodenal tube, at a dose of 900 mg for an adult. Due to the possibility of vomiting and regurgitation of ova in the case of *T. solium* infections, chlorpromazine or phenobarbitone should be given simultaneously. Two hours later a saline purge is given, and the scolex of the worm searched for in the strained stool; proof of a cure depends on identifying the scolex. Mepacrine may produce acute haemolysis in the presence of glucose-6-phosphate dehydrogenase deficiency. Niclosamide ('Yomesan') and bunamidine are also of value. The antischistosomal drug, praziquantel, is effective in a single dose against mature cestodes (Van den Bosshe, 1978). In a study in Costa Rica, 37 patients with *T. solium*, and 4 with *T. saginata* were treated with mebendazole for three to six days (Chavarria, Villarejos, and Zeledon, 1977); the optimum effective dose was 300 mg twice daily for three days. Within 48 hours, most patients had eliminated long

* That disease has recently become a major problem in Irian Jaya (Subianto, 1978; Tjahjadi, 1978).

chains of lifeless proglottids. Monthly follow-up for four or five months showed that with the optimum dose there was a 100 per cent cure rate; with lower dose regimes cure rate was only approximately 70 per cent. However, Vakil, Dalal, and Enjetti (1975) found that proglottids of *T. saginata* invariably appeared two to three months after that treatment. Mebendazole and other benzimidazoles are also effective, and active, against the larval stage of *E. granulosus.* Paromomycin, one gramme given in four doses over one day, is effective in *T. solium* and *T. saginata* infections (Botero, 1970); in *H. nana* infections, 45 mg per kg, for five to seven days should be given. Although gastrointestinal side-effects are common, they are not severe.

Heavy *H. nana* infections may require treatment. In an investigation in Egypt, three groups of 20 patients with *H. nana* infections were given either: niclosamide ('Yomesan') (60 mg per kg bodyweight, followed by 15 mg per kg body weight for six days), mepacrine (15 mg per kg bodyweight for one day) or thiabendazole (25 mg per kg bodyweight twice daily for two days) (El-Masry, Farid, and Bassily, 1974); after two weeks, 85, 60, and 20 per cent of patients in those three groups were free of ova, and after five weeks the percentages were 70, 15, and five respectively.

There is no specific treatment for cysticercosis; benzimidazole compounds are being tested in experimental animals. Anticonvulsive agents may be required for epilepsy.

19.6. Protozoal infections

These very rarely produce small-intestinal disease. Coccidiosis, which may be associated with malabsorption, is dealt with in Chapter 20.

19.6.1. Eosinophilic granuloma of the small intestine

This disease is thought to be a result of granulomatous formation in response to a parasitic infection, probably the nematode *Eustoma rotundatum* (Chapters 4 and 27). There is a diffuse or focal eosinophilic infiltration; polypoid lesions may be present. Although the commonest site is in the pyloric antrum, the small-intestine may also be affected.

19.6.2. Malaria

Gastrointestinal symptoms are very common in acute malaria, especially in children; they clear rapidly after treatment has been started. It has been suggested that capillary stasis, with necrosis and haemorrhage are responsible; epithelial desquamation has been reported in the algid type of malaria. Although some evidence for malabsorption in the presence of malaria parasitaemia has been presented, that has not been substantiated (Chapter 20).

19.6.3. Leishmaniasis (Kala azar)

Involvement of the gastrointestinal tract seems to be a relatively minor feature of this disease; the reticuloendothelial system, including the liver (Chapter 5) and spleen (Chapter 16), are heavily involved.

The lamina propria, of the duodenum and jejunum, may contain histiocytes in which Leishman-Donovan bodies can be demonstrated. Villi are enlarged and swollen and there may be ulceration. In the presence of small-intestinal involvement, parasites have been detected in the stool. Severe involvement has been described as a terminal event when large numbers of parasites can be demonstrated in smears from the jejunum (Sati, 1962); in that report, an intractable diarrhoea due to small-intestinal involvement was felt to be a significant factor leading to death. I am not aware of any study in which malabsorption has been adequately demonstrated in this infection.

References

AJAO, O. G. and AJAO, A. O. (1979). *Tropical Doctor*, **9,** 33.

ARFAA, F. and GHADIRIAN, E. (1977). *Am. J. trop. Med. Hyg.*, **26,** 866.

AZIZ, M. A. and SIDDIQUI, A. R. (1968). *Gastroenterology*, **55,** 242.

BELL, W. J. and NASSIF, S. (1971). *Am. J. trop. Med. Hyg.*, **20,** 584.

BIAGI, F. F., and TAY, J. (1958). *Am. J. trop. Med. Hyg.*, **7,** 63.

BLUMENTHAL, D. S. and SCHULTZ, M. G. (1976). *Am. J. trop. Med. Hyg.*, **25,** 682.

BORRERO, J., RESTREPO, A., BOTERO, D., and LATORRE, G. (1961). *Am. J. trop. Med. Hyg.*, **10,** 735.

BOTERO, D. R. (1970). *Am. J. trop. Med. Hyg.*, **19,** 234.

BURLINGAME, P. L. and CHANDLER, A. C. (1941). *Am. J. Hyg.*, **33,** 1.

BUSTAMANTE-SARABIA, J., MARTUSCELLI-Q, A., and TAY, J. (1977). *Am. J. trop. Med. Hyg.*, **26,** 568.

CHANDLER, A. C. (1943). *Am. J. Hyg.*, **37,** 121.

CHAVARRIA, A. P., VILLAREJOS, V. M., and ZELEDON, R. (1977). *Am. J. trop. Med. Hyg.*, **26,** 118.

COOK, G. C. (1974). *Trans. R. Soc. trop. Med. Hyg.*, **68,** 419.

——, KAJUBI, S. K. and LEE, F. D. (1969). *J. Path.*, **98,** 157.

COORAY, G. H. and PANABOKKE, R. G. (1960). *Trans. R. Soc. trop. Med. Hyg.*, **54,** 358.

CRANE, P. S., PAK, Y. H., and LEE, H. K. (1965). *Ann. Surg.*, **162,** 34.

CROSS, J. H. (1969). *Proceedings of the fourth South east Asian Seminar on Parasitology and Tropical medicine, schistosomiasis and other snail-transmitted helminthiases (ed.* C. Harinasuta), p. 177. Bangkok, Thailand.

DAFTARY, V. G. and BHENDE, Y. M. (1956). *J. postgrad. Med.*, **2,** 44.

DAVEY, W. W. (1968). *Companion to Surgery in Africa.* p. 219. E. and S. Livingstone. Edinburgh and London.

DAVIS, A. (1973). *Drug treatment in intestinal helminthiases.* p. 15, 52 and 95. World Health Organization, Geneva.

DIXON, H. B. F. and Lipscomb, F. M. (1961). *Spec. Rep. Ser. med. Res. Coun.*, **299,** 58.

DOUGLAS, J. and TAMANIKA, M. (1973). *Papua New Guin. med. J.*, **16,** 54.

EDINGTON, G. M. (1956). *W. Afr. med. J.*, **5,** 71.

—— and GILLES, H. M. (1976). *Pathology in the tropics.* 2nd ed. pp. 91, 114 and 162. Edward Arnold, London.

EL-HASHMI, W. (1971). *Am. J. Path.*, **65,** 311.

EL-MASRY, N. A., FARID, Z., and BASSILY, S. (1974). *E. Afr. med. J.*, **51,** 532.

FARID, Z., BASSILY, S., MINER, W. F., HASSAN, A., and LAUGHLIN, L. W. (1977). *J. trop. Med. Hyg.*, **80,** 107.

FOWLER, J. M., KNIGHT, R., and PATEL, K. M. (1968). *Br. med. J.*, **3,** 220.

GATTI, F., KRUBWA, F., VANDEPITTE, J., and THIENPONT, D. (1972). *Annls Soc. belge Méd. trop.*, **52,** 19.

GELPI, A. P. and MUSTAFA, A. (1968). *Am. J. Med.*, **44,** 377.

GILLES, H. M. (1964). *Akufo: an environmental study of a Nigerian village community.* University Press, Ibadan.

—— (1978). *Tropical Doctor*, **8,** 62.

——, Watson-Williams, E. J. and Ball, P. A. J. (1964). *Q. Jl. Med.*, **33,** 1.
Goodwin, L. G. and Standon, O. D. (1958). *Br. med. J.*, **1,** 131.
Harrison, K. A. and Lawson, J. B. (1966). *Lancet*, **2,** 905.
Jones, H. I. (1976). *Papua New Guin. med. J.*, **19,** 153.
Kochar, V. K., Schad, G. A., Chowdhury, A. B., Dean, C. G., and Nawalinski, T. (1976). *Medical anthropology* (ed. F. X. Grollig and H. B. Haley). p. 287. Mouton, The Hague and Paris.
Kojima, S., Yokogawa, M., and Tada, T. (1972). *Am. J. trop. Med. Hyg.*, **21,** 913.
Koshy, A., Raina, V., Sharma, M. P., Mithal, S., and Tandon, B. N. (1978). *Am. J. trop. Med. Hyg.*, **27,** 42.
Lejkina, E. S. (1965). *Bull. Wld Hlth Org.*, **32,** 699.
Lozoff, B., Warren, K. S., and Mahmoud, A. A. F. (1975). *J. infect. Dis.*, **132,** 606.
Mawdsley, J. H. and Barr, R. D. (1975). *E. Afr. med. J.*, **52,** 1.
Middlemiss, H. (1961). *Tropical Radiology.* Heinemann, London.
Migasena, S., Suntharasamai, P., and Harinasuta, T. (1978). *Ann. trop. Med. Parasit.*, **72,** 199.
Milwidsky, H. (1945). *Acta med. orient.*, **4,** 370.
Murray, M. J., Murray, A. B., Murray, M. B., and Murray, C. J. (1978a). *Br. med. J.*, **2,** 1113.
Murray, J., Murray, A., Murray, M., and Murray, C. (1978b). *Am. J. clin. Nutr.*, **31,** 1363.
Naik, S. R., Mitra, S. K., and Mehta, S. (1976). *J. trop. Med. Hyg.*, **79,** 2.
Nelson, G. S., Pester, F. R. N., and Rickman, R. (1965). *Trans. R. Soc. trop. Med. Hyg.*, **59,** 507.
Ofori Atta, S. B. G. (1958). *Archs Dis. Childh.*, **33,** 202.
Peters, W. and Gilles, H. M. (1977). *A colour atlas of Tropical Medicine and Parasitology.* p. 161 and 170. Wolfe Medical Publications Ltd, London.
Piggott, J., Hansbarger, E. A., and Neafie, R. C. (1970). *Am. J. clin. Path.*, **53,** 223.
Plaut, A. G., Kampanart-Sanyakorn, C., and Manning, G. S. (1969). *Trans. R. Soc. trop. Med. Hyg.*, **63,** 470.
Qassab, K. and Al-Khateeb, A. K. (1966). *J. Fac. Med. Baghdad.*, **8,** 62.
Rep, B. H. and Shaba, J. K. (1976). *E. Afr. med. J.*, **53,** 160.
Rydzewski, A. K., Chisholm, E. S., and Kagan, I. G. (1975). *J. Parasit.*, **61,** 154.
Sati, M. H. (1962). *Sudan med. J.*, **1,** 216.
Soulsby, E. J. L. and Gilles, H. M. (1974). *J. Parasit.*, **51,** 2.
Stoll, N. R. (1947). *J. Parasit.*, **33,** 1.
Subianto, D. B. (1978). *Trop. geogr. Med.*, **30,** 275.
Suntharasamai, P., Bunnag, D., and Tejavanij, S. (1974). *S. E. Asian J. trop. Med. Publ. Hlth*, **5,** 556.
Tandon, B. N., Kohli, R. K., Saraya, A. K., Ramachandran, K., and Prakash, O. (1969). *Gut*, **10,** 293.
Tjahjadi, G. (1978). *Trop. geogr. Med.*, **30,** 279.
Tripathy, K., Duque, E., Bolaños, O., Lotero, H., and Mayoral, L. G. (1972). *Am. J. clin. Nutr.*, **25,** 1276.
——, González, F., Lotero, H., and Bolaños, O. (1971). *Am. J. trop. Med. Hyg.*, **20,** 212.
Tukumo, A. (1956). *Hiroshima J. med. Sci.*, **5,** 21.
Vakil, B. J., Dalal, N. J., and Enjetti, E. (1975). *J. trop. Med. Hyg.*, **78,** 154.
Van den Bosshe, H. (1978). *Nature, Lond.*, **273,** 626.
Venkatachalam, P. S. and Patwardhan, V. N. (1953). *Trans. R. Soc. trop. Med. Hyg.*, **47,** 169.
Wolfe, M. S. and Wershing, J. M. (1974). *J. Am. med. Ass.*, **230,** 1408.
Zigas, V. (1973). *Papua New Guin. med. J.*, **16,** 51.

20

Malabsorption in the tropics

MALABSORPTION exists, when, due to either a functional defect in the small intestine or a major digestive gland, one or more substances (either nutrients or test compounds) are inadequately transferred from the lumen of the bowel to the portal venous system. Reviews of malabsorption in temperate (Dawson, 1965; Dyer and Dawson, 1968; Frazer, 1968; Shingleton and Dobbins, 1968; Floch, 1969; Jeffries, Weser, and Sleisenger, 1969; Losowsky, Walker, and Kelleher, 1974) and tropical (Cook, 1967; 1974a; Cook and Kajubi, 1972) countries are available.

20.1. Small-intestinal structure and function in the tropics

20.1.1. Tropical enteropathy

The jejunal mucosa of people living under tropical conditions (tropical enteropathy) differs slightly from that of those in temperate areas. Finger-shaped villi (Warwick and Williams, 1973) are rare and leaf-shaped villi are usual (Cook, Kajubi, and Lee, 1969); ridges are common, but convolutions are unusual.

Tropical enteropathy is the usual state for most Africans in Uganda (Banwell, Hutt, and Tunnicliffe, 1964; Cook and Kajubi, 1966; Cook, Kajubi, and Lee, 1969), Zambia (Cook, Asp, and Dahlqvist, 1973), Nigeria (Falaiye, 1971), and Zimbabwe Rhodesia (Thomas, Clain, and Wicks, 1976). It is also usual in Thailand (Sprinz, Sribhibhadh, Gangarosa, Benyajati, Kundel, and Halstead, 1962), south India (Baker, Ignatius, Mathan, Vaish, and Chacko, 1962), Bangladesh (Lindenbaum, Alam, and Kent, 1966), Pakistan (Russell, Aziz, Ahmad, Kent, and Gangarosa, 1966), Puerto Rico (Angel, Guerra, Martinez, and Plough, 1963), and Haiti (Klipstein, Samloff, and Schenk, 1966). A recent report from Peru (Perea, Fernan-Zegarra, Cruz, Ballon, and Picoaga, 1978) documents similar changes in Peruvian Indians; postinfective tropical malabsorption (TM) (see below) is apparently not seen in Peru.

20.1.2. Aetiology of tropical enteropathy

Many suggestions have been put forward to explain the mild small-intestinal changes; genetic factors, nutritional status, luminal parasites, ambient temperature, thyroid status, and various bacterial and viral infections have all been suggested (Cook and Kajubi, 1972). The most likely explanation seems to be that tropical enteropathy results from repeated bacterial and viral infections involving the small-intestine (Cook, Kajubi, and Lee, 1969); that suggestion is supported by the observation that the severity of the abnormalities is greater in Africans from low, compared with high, socioeconomic strata (Thomas, Clain, and Wicks, 1976). Tropical enteropathy is thus related to living conditions in which most of the indigenous populations of tropical countries exist. That has been confirmed by studies in Peace Corps workers in Pakistan, who lived under those conditions (Lindenbaum, Kent, and Sprinz, 1966). The vast majority of them had mild gastrointestinal complaints; severe symptoms, together with steatorrhoea and megaloblastic anaemia are uncommon in tropical enteropathy, but are very common in TM (see below). Although malabsorption of xylose and B_{12} were common (39 and 52 per cent respectively), steatorrhoea was unusual. Two of 114 individuals in that study developed clinical evidence of tropical malabsorption (TM).

It has been suggested (Cook, 1967; Klipstein, 1968; Klipstein, Samloff, Smarth, and Schenk, 1968) that TM represents the severe end of the spectrum of tropical enteropathy. Some of the cases described by Falaiye (1970), Moshal, Hift, Kallichurum, and Pillay (1973) and Thomas and Clain (1976) as '*tropical sprue*' in Africa, were probably examples of tropical enteropathy. Baker (1972a) and Baker and Mathan (1972) have however challenged the view that those are closely related entities, and have assembled epidemiological data showing that they are entirely separate. Whether or not tropical enteropathy predisposes in some subtle way to TM must at present remain *sub judice*; the low incidence of that disease in Africa suggests that it does not.

The jejunal mucosa has limited ways in which it can respond to injury; jejunal mucosal appearances in some cases of TM, three to four months after the onset of the disease (England and O'Brien, 1966), are similar to those in tropical enteropathy. The effect of treatment on tropical enteropathy has not been adequately studied (Lindenbaum, 1973).

20.1.3. Subclinical malabsorption

A number of studies in tropical countries have indicated that abnormal D-xylose tests, and flat blood-glucose curves after oral glucose, are very common in indigenous people (Lindenbaum, Alam, and Kent, 1966; Cook, Kajubi, and Lee, 1969; Falaiye, 1971; Lindenbaum, 1973).

Malabsorption of D-xylose and B_{12} are common in both Africa (Banwell, Campbell, Blackman, Hutt, and Leonard, 1963; Cook, Kajubi, and Lee, 1969; Falaiye, 1969; 1971; Cook, 1972; 1974a; Thomas, Clain, and Wicks, 1976) and Asia (Baker, *et al.*, 1962; Sprinz, *et al.*, 1962; Angel, *et al.*, 1963; Lindenbaum, 1965; Klipstein, *et al.*, 1966; Lindenbaum, *et al.*, 1966; Russell, *et al.*, 1966; Baker and Mathan, 1972; Baker, 1976). The D-xylose test has been shown to give a high proportion of abnormal results in normal members of those populations. Kajubi and Okel (1973) have shown that vitamin B_{12} absorption takes place slowly in healthy Ugandans, despite the fact that serum concentrations are normal; that might be associated with the mild mucosal changes, and explains a high frequency of abnormal Schilling tests in that population. Fleming (1968) has shown that Nigerian serum has a greater B_{12} binding capacity than that of Europeans, and that might be associated with the high serum globulin concentrations. Fat absorption may also be impaired, but in the absence of symptoms.

Jejunal glucose absorption rate from a 200 mM solution has been compared in well-nourished rural Africans in Zambia, in urban Arabs in Saudi Arabia, and in a group of patients of northern European origin (G. C. Cook, *unpublished*); mean rate was significantly lower in the Africans than either the Saudi Arabians or the Europeans. That indicates that most rural Africans in Africa have a significant reduction in their jejunal absorptive capacity for glucose. Those functional abnormalities are widespread, and might have a practical value in nutrition in the third world. They do not seem to correlate simply with jejunal-mucosal morphology (*tropical enteropathy*) but have a more complex basis. Various factors have been suggested to explain them (see below).

20.1.4. Aetiology of subclinical malabsorption

Mucosal changes (tropical enteropathy). As already indicated, the surface area of the jejunal mucosa is diminished in tropical populations compared with Europeans in Europe (Banwell, Hutt, and Tunnicliffe, 1964; Klipstein, 1968; Cook, Kajubi, and Lee, 1969; Falaiye, 1969; 1971; Lindenbaum, 1973). However, normal D-xylose absorption after an oral load, and glucose absorption-rate from the jejunum using a double-lumen tube perfusion system, are possible in people with the histological and dissecting-microscopic appearances of *tropical enteropathy* (Cook, 1971a; 1971b; 1972). A comparison has been made, using the D-xylose absorption test, between groups of urban Zambians, English, and Saudi Arabians who, although all hospital in-patients, had no evidence of an organic disease, malnutrition, a systemic disease, diabetes mellitus, or severe anaemia (Cook, 1979a); the Zambians had the typical jejunal mucosal appearances of Africans living in Africa. Mean xylose excretion was very similar in the three groups. Undue emphasis has undoubtedly been placed on those minor morphological changes, which *per se* do not account for significant subclinical malabsorption. The morphological changes of tropical enteropathy are compatible with normal xylose absorption; the high incidence of abnormal xylose absorption tests in indigenous people in tropical countries must be due to other, perhaps environmental, factors.

Systemic bacterial infections. Gastrointestinal infections influence small-intestinal absorption; they do so by damaging the enterocyte (Chapter 17), and by producing enzyme deficiencies. The effect, however, of systemic infections such as lobar pneumonia or pulmonary tuberculosis on intestinal absorption has only recently been studied.

The association between infection and nutritional status is complex. Poskitt (1972) has demonstrated, in Uganda, that there is a correlation between the time of onset of kwashiorkor and the incidence of both systemic (bronchopneumonia, malaria, and measles) and gastrointestinal infections; the association was much more clearcut than that between kwashiorkor and the seasonal availability of food. That is partly explained by increased energy demands, and hypercatabolism associated with infections, but impaired absorption is also important.

In Zambia, xylose and glucose absorption have been measured in groups of patients, some of whom had acute bacterial pneumonia or pulmonary tuberculosis, and others who had no evidence of an infection; all were clinically well-nourished and they did not have evidence of gastrointestinal disease. Mean xylose excretion after a 25g oral load was significantly lower in those with acute and chronic infections, compared with those without infections (Cook, 1972). Using a jejunal perfusion system, absorption rates were measured from solutions of glucose (56, 139, and 278 mM) in three similar groups; at concentrations of 139 and 278 mM, those with infections had a significant impairment of glucose absorption, compared with those without infections (Cook, 1971a). Furthermore, a significant correlation between glucose absorption rate and xylose excretion was demonstrated, indicating that glucose absorption rate from a jejunal segment, bears a significant relationship to overall monosaccharide absorption from the small-intestine (Cook and Carruthers, 1974). In 18 Zambian Africans without evidence of an infection, a significant *inverse* correlation between glucose absorption rate (from a 200 mM solution), and serum gamma-globulin (Cook, 1973a) and immunoglobulin IgG (Cook, 1974b) concentrations was demonstrated. D-xylose excretion after a 25 g oral load has also been shown to correlate *inversely* with serum gamma-globulin and IgG in Zambian patients (Cook, 1974b; 1977a). There were no significant correlations, however, between glucose absorption rate and xylose excretion, and other serum globulin fractions, immunoglobulins IgA, IgM, or IgD, or albumin. Absorption, and nutritional status (assessed by serum albumin concentration) were not significantly related. Those findings suggest that carbohydrate, upon which most people in the third world subsist, is poorly absorbed in the presence of systemic infections.

Using the same technique, an impairment of crystalline folic acid absorption has been demonstrated in the presence of similar systemic infections (Cook, Morgan, and Hoffbrand, 1974).

Further studies have been carried out using the amino-acid, glycine (Cook, 1973b); the perfusion solutions contained 50, 100, 150, and 250 mM glycine. In patients with acute infections, a significant *increase* in the absorption rate was demonstrated; absorption was not affected by chronic infections. Studies with L-histidine (100 mM) also showed a significantly higher absorption rate in the presence of acute infections (Cook, 1977b). A significant positive correlation between glycine absorption rate (from a 100 mM solution) and serum gamma-globulin concentration, was demonstrated in patients who did not have systemic infections (Cook, 1973b). Using the dipeptide glycylglycine, systemic infections have been shown to have no significant effect on absorption rate from a 50 mM solution (Cook, 1974c); furthermore, there was not a significant correlation between absorption rate, and gamma-globulin concentration. Amino-acids and dipeptides use separate jejunal transfer mechanisms (Matthews, 1971; Cook, 1973c, 1974d, 1976a); these observations are consistent with the now accepted views that external factors influence the absorption rates of amino-acids but not dipeptides.

Folate depletion and anaemia. Hypochromic anaemia, usually caused by hookworm disease (Chapter 19), and megaloblastic anaemia, resulting from dietary folate-deficiency, are common throughout the tropics. Iron is poorly absorbed in some tropical countries; diets contain high phytate and phosphate concentrations, which form insoluble complexes with iron salts, with the impairment of absorption (Foy and Kondi, 1956).

Jejunal absorption is normal in hypochromic anaemia (Butterworth, Perez-Santiago, Martinez de Jesus, and Santini, 1959; Cook, 1976b). Investigations of absorption in the presence of nutritional megaloblastic anaemia have however given conflicting, and sometimes contradictory, results (Butterworth *et al.*, 1959; Lindenbaum, 1973; Halsted, 1975). In patients with folate deficiency associated with alcoholism, absorption defects are associated with mucosal changes (Hermos, Adams, Liu, Sullivan, and Trier, 1971), and they are probably a direct effect of alcohol. In untreated Addisonian pernicious anaemia, there seems to be a definite absorption defect also (Lindenbaum, Pezzimenti, and Shea, 1974); xylose absorption returns to normal, however, after treatment (Bezman, Kinnear, and Zamcheck, 1959).

In nutritional folate deficiency, Foy and Kondi (1971) showed a decreased xylose excretion after a 5g load, but suggested that that might be a manifestation of defective metabolism or excretion. Forshaw (1969) and Dawson (1971) demonstrated xylose malabsorption in nutritional folate deficiency; that returned to normal after treatment with folic acid. Winawer, Sullivan, Herbert, and Zamcheck (1965) were unable to detect an abnormality. In Kuala Lumpur, Tasker (1961) found that the mean xylose excretion after a 5g oral load was 0·71 g per five hours in 36 patients with nutritional megaloblastic anaemia, compared with 1·43g in 21 controls. In Singapore, Siang, England, and O'Brien (1966) found xylose malabsorption in only two of eight patients with nutritional megaloblastic anaemia. Reynolds, Hallpike, Phillips, and Matthews (1965) demonstrated reduced xylose excretion in two patients with megaloblastic anaemia, in both of whom serum folate concentration was low, and in one of whom serum B_{12} concentration was also reduced; xylose absorption improved after treatment. Winawer, *et al.* (1965) studied six patients with dietary folate deficiency and megaloblastic anaemia. Although changes in jejunal morphology were minimal, xylose excretion tended to be low (5·1g per five hours or less, in four of six patients); fat absorption was normal. An investigation in Zambia showed that Africans with untreated megaloblastic anaemia, caused by dietary folate depletion, had a significant impairment of D-xylose excretion (mean 3·6 g per five hours) compared with those with other types of anaemia (Cook, 1976b); furthermore, D-xylose absorption in some of them correlated significantly with the jejunal glucose absorption rate ($P < 0{\cdot}02$). Those with severe hypochromic anaemia had mean values for D-xylose absorption from a 25g load, and jejunal absorption rates of glucose and glycine, which were normal for that population. Folic acid absorption rates, in the presence of both megaloblastic and hypochromic anaemia, were not significantly different from those in controls who were neither anaemic nor had systemic infections.

There is therefore a clear indication that although anaemia *per se* does not affect absorption, folate depletion (which may be accompanied by a megaloblastic anaemia) is associated with monosaccharide malabsorption; the possibility that that is related to subcellular changes in the enterocyte has not been excluded.

Marginal malnutrition. Marginal malnutrition has been considered a probable cause of subclinical malabsorption (Mayoral, Tripathy, Garcia, and Ghitis, 1966; 1967; Mayoral, Tripathy, Garcia, Bolaños, and Ghitis, 1968; Tandon, Magotra, Saraya, and Ramalingaswami, 1968; Halsted, Sheir, Sourial, and Patwardhan, 1969; Falaiye, 1971; Mahalanabis, Jacobs, Banwell, Mukherji, and Bose, 1972).

Falaiye (1971) studied eight patients, most of whom had low serum albumin and folate concentrations, in Nigeria; xylose absorption improved in four after the intravenous administration of amino-acids, which raised serum albumin concentrations to normal. However, a marked fall in serum total globulin concentrations also occurred. In four, who were treated with tetracycline, there was not a significant change in either the serum albumin concentration (which was normal in two) or xylose absorption. Tandon, *et al.* (1968) demonstrated an improvement in jejunal morphology and absorptive capacity in 14 adults with protein malnutrition and anaemia, after three months on a high protein diet. Cook (1974e) has shown that in six malnourished Zambian adults, whose disease was due to a variety of causes (four had serum albumin concentrations of 20g per 1 or less), not only was dissecting microscopic and histological examination of the jejunal mucosa normal, but there was also normal absorption of xylose, and jejunal absorption rates of glucose, glycine and glycylglycine, when compared with controls from the same population. Furthermore, no significant correlations have been found between jejunal absorption rates for glucose, glycine and glycylglycine, and serum albumin concentration in adult Zambians (Cook, 1973a; b; 1974f). Neither has it been possible to find a significant relationship between D-xylose absorption and serum albumin concentration (G. C. Cook, *unpublished*).

Apart from some severe cases of kwashiorkor in children, therefore, it seems unlikely that malnutrition *per se* predisposes to subclinical malabsorption.

Pellagra. In India, Mehta, Kaur, Avasthi, Wig, and Chhuttani (1972) reported that 22 of 24 patients with pellagra had evidence of malabsorption. Impairment of xylose, fat, and B_{12} absorption was demonstrated in some of them; improvement was noted after treatment. It seems likely, however, that insufficient attention was given in that study to controls from the same population, many of whom also had evidence of malabsorption. A high incidence of mucosal abnormalities and xylose malabsorption in pellagra has also been documented in Egypt; however those changes did not seem to be worse than in controls or patients with hookworm disease (Halsted, *et al.*, 1969). In Johannesburg, Van Heerden, Grieve, and Metz (1966) showed that fat absorption was normal in patients with pellagra. In 12 Zambian patients with classical pellagra, D-xylose absorption was normal in 11, and jejunal morphology was normal in the nine who were studied (Cook, 1976c). However, in that investigation there was a significant *inverse* correlation between D-xylose excretion after a 25g load and serum immunoglobulin IgG concentration (see above).

Malaria. In simian malaria models, decreased splanchnic flow has been observed (Edington and Gilles, 1976). Impaired xylose absorption has been reported in acute *P. falciparum* malaria (Olsson and Johnston, 1969); eight of 10 soldiers with acute malaria had impaired D-xylose excretion after an oral load, but lactose-tolerance tests were normal in 11 of 12 tested. Jejunal biopsies showed minimal vascular congestion and oedema of the lamina propria. Those findings were interpreted as being consistent with decreased splanchnic flow. In Taiwan, Karney and Tong (1972) have demonstrated impaired absorptive function in 11 patients with acute *P. falciparum* infections; nine had impaired D-xylose absorption, six decreased B_{12} absorption, and five a low serum carotene concentration. Some of those results improved after recovery; mean D-xylose excretion increased from 3·5 to 4·9g per 5 hours. Mild jejunal mucosal changes, which also reverted to normal after treatment, were also reported. In Zambia, only two of 15 patients with a malaria parasitaemia had a D-xylose excretion of less than 5·0g per five hours after a 25g oral load, and there was not a significant change after treatment (Cook, 1975); mean values were 6·2 and 6·6g per five hours, respectively. However, significant inverse correlations between D-xylose excretion, and serum gamma-globulin and IgG concentrations were demonstrated (see above). That study suggests that impaired absorption does not result from malarial parasitaemia, but that it bears a relationship to chronic infection, and correlates with elevated serum gamma-globulin and IgG concentrations.

20.1.5. Practical importance of subclinical malabsorption

In populations with a high incidence of systemic infections, a substantial proportion of ingested carbohydrate is presumably absorbed slowly from the small-intestine. That obviously has a potential importance in the presence of marginal malnutrition (Cook, 1967; 1974a; 1974f). Glucose absorption rates from the jejunum in healthy rural Africans in Zambia are often comparable to those in European patients with TM (G. C. Cook, *unpublished*); that observation lends support to a nutritional importance of subclinical malabsorption in the third world.

Subclinical folate deficiency is extremely common in many parts of the tropics; that is largely of dietary origin, and is exacerbated by pregnancy and the puerperium. Folic acid absorption is impaired in the presence of systemic infections (Cook, Morgan, and Hoffbrand, 1974); that might be important in setting up a vicious circle leading to a severe deficiency.

Although further work is required, the evidence at present available suggests that systemic infections are probably more important than subclinical malnutrition in the pathogenesis of carbohydrate and folic acid malabsorption (Cook, 1974a; 1974f); protein absorption is differently affected. Those findings re-emphasize the importance of eliminating systemic infections from developing countries if improved nutritional status is to be achieved.

Before too many practical conclusions are drawn from those observations, however, it should be appreciated that the small-intestine has a substantial functional reserve; even if 'concertina-ing' of the small-intestine, which takes place in the perfusion studies cited above, is taken into account (Cook and Carruthers, 1974), it is still difficult to assess the overall absorptive deficit. Also, the importance of the colon in absorption is far from clear (Chapter 29). It is thus difficult to assess accurately the overall nutritional importance of these observations at present.

The importance of absorption *rates* in nutrition has received very little attention; it seems likely that abnormal xylose absorption parallels the absorption rate of dietary carbohydrate (Cook, 1976d; 1977c). Coronary atheroma is very uncommon in most people in the third world; they also have a relatively slow carbohydrate absorption rate. High serum insulin concentrations are probably atherogenic (*Lancet*, 1977a); they occur far less commonly in people living in developing countries than in the western world.

20.2. Causes of severe malabsorption in the tropics

Some causes of malabsorption are far more common in tropical that temperate areas of the world (Table 20.1). A disease, or more accurately a group of diseases, known since 1880 as *tropical sprue*, has not only dominated malabsorption, but also gastroenterology, in the tropics over many years. There are numerous other causes of malabsorption in tropical countries however, and it must never be forgotten that most of the aetiological factors responsible in temperate areas can also operate in the tropics. Therefore, a differential diagnosis must always include those diseases. Failing absorptive function associated with ageing (Montgomery, Haeney, Ross, Sammons, Barford, Balakrishnan, Mayer, Culank, Field, and Gosling, 1978; Warren, Pepperman, and Montgomery, 1978) is unlikely to create problems in the third world for some time, because life-expectancy is still greatly impaired.

Considerable confusion has surrounded the nosology of tropical malabsorption, much of which stems from the fact that since the term was first adopted in 1880 by Sir Patrick Manson, *tropical sprue* has been used to cover virtually all of the causes of malabsorption which start in tropical countries. It is now clear that most cases of malabsorption originating in those areas result from an acute intestinal infection, which for some yet unknown reason continues at a subacute level; chronic malabsorption results from persisting small-intestinal bacterial colonization. For that reason that disease will be referred to as post-infective tropical malabsorption (TM) (see below) and not as *tropical sprue* which is considered to have little to commend it.

TM is a disease with an acute or subacute onset, and is characterized by diarrhoea and clinical and laboratory evidence of malabsorption (Tomkins, James, Walters, and Cole, 1974). It is sometimes a sequel to 'travellers' diarrhoea' (Rowe, Taylor, and Bettelheim, 1970; Merson, Morris, Sack, Wells, Feeley, Bradley Sack, Creech, Kapikian, and Gangarosa, 1976) which is followed by persisting bacterial colonization of the small-intestine (Banwell and Gorbach, 1969; Klipstein, Holdeman, Corcino, and Moore, 1973; Tomkins, Drasar, and James, 1975; *Lancet*, 1977b) probably due to stasis (Cook, 1978a). There is sometimes an associated *Giardia lamblia* (Schultz, 1975;

Eastham, Douglas, and Watson, 1976; Tandon, Tandon, Satpathy, and Shriniwas, 1977; Wright, Tomkins, and Ridley, 1977) or *Strongyloides stercoralis* infection, but the role of those parasites in the pathogenesis of the malabsorption is not yet clear (see below).

Table 20.1. *Some causes of malabsorption*

Digestive disorders	
Gastric	gastrectomy, gastrojejunostomy, Zollinger–Ellison syndrome
* Pancreatic	Chronic calcific pancreatitis, mucoviscidosis
* Bile-salt deficiency	cirrhosis, ileal disease, and trauma
Absorptive disorders	
* Short bowel syndrome	trauma or surgery
Mucosal damage	gluten-induced enteropathy
*Bacterial colonization of small intestine	postinfective tropical malabsorption (TM), 'blind-loop' syndrome', enteritis necroticans ('pig-bel' disease), *Pneumatosis (Cystoides) intestinalis.*
* Viral and bacterial infections	viral hepatitis, measles, Norwalk agent, tuberculosis
* Parasitic infections	*Giardia lamblia, Strongyloides stercoralis, Coccidia, Capillaria philippinensis.*
Inflammation and infiltration	Crohn's disease, systemic sclerosis, amyloidosis
* Malignant conditions	Burkitt's and other lymphomas (including the Mediterranean lymphoma)
* Venous and lymphatic obstruction	Right-sided endomyocardial fibrosis, constrictive pericarditis, idiopathic tropical cardiomegaly (Chapter 8).
Miscellaneous causes	
Drugs	neomycin, para-amino salicylic acid, phenindione, phenolphthalein.
Isolated malabsorption	
* Enzyme deficiency	hypolactasia (primary and secondary) (Chapter 21)
Monosaccharide malabsorption	
Addisonian pernicious anaemia	

* indicates causes which are more common in tropical than temperate zones.

Detailed investigations of small-intestinal flora have occasionally been carried out in tropical countries, and there are also reports of stool concentrations (Hill, Crowther, Drasar, Hawksworth, Aries, and Williams, 1971); in that study lower counts of bacteroides, and higher counts of enterococci were found in Ugandan Africans, compared with residents of the UK and the USA.

20.2.1. Pancreatic and hepatic causes

Pancreatic causes, which are dominated by *chronic calcific pancreatitis* are dealt with in Chapter 15. Hepatic causes of malabsorption are covered in Chapters 7, 8, and 13.

20.2.2. Bile-salt deficiency

In the upper small intestine bile-salt deficiency is associated with inadequate micelle formation, which produces mildly abnormal triglyceride absorption; absorption of fat-soluble vitamins may, however, be seriously affected. Two common situations in tropical countries in which there is a bile-salt deficiency are cirrhosis, usually of macronodular type (Badley, Murphy, and Bouchier, 1969) (Chapter 8), and disease or resection of the ileum (Chapter 23). The high incidence rates for HB_sAg suggest that viral hepatitis is an important aetiological factor in cirrhosis in Kenya (Bagshawe, Parker, and Jindani, 1971), Uganda (Anthony, Vogel, Sadikali, Barker, and Peterson, 1972), and Zambia (Lowenthal, Banatvala, Chrystie, Jones, Nag, Mohelsky, and Hutt, 1973), for example. In those studies, 20, 33, and 50 per cent positive HB_sAg incidence rates, respectively, were found in patients with cirrhosis; corresponding rates in controls, who did not have cirrhosis, for the same populations were 6, 3, and 13 per cent. Alcohol is relevant in some cases; however malnutrition is of no importance (Chapter 13) (Cook and Hutt, 1967). Severe disease of the ileum is usually due to tuberculosis; trauma or resection of lengths of small intestine may follow hernia, volvulus, or intussusception (Chapter 23). Anaerobic bacteria, by deconjugating bile-salts, constitute a further and possibly the most important cause of diarrhoea and malabsorption (see below).

20.2.3. Loss of small-intestinal absorptive area

Ileocaecal tuberculosis is not only an important cause of malabsorption in tropical countries, but is also not infrequently seen in immigrants in the UK and USA, and other parts of the western world. As well as being associated with severe pathological strictures, ileal-resection is often necessary in that disease, and for that reason also, the absorptive area may be reduced, with consequent malabsorption. Trauma, caused by road traffic accidents, and knife and gunshot wounds, also leads to resection of lengths of small-intestine in the third world (Chapter 23). Volvulus of the small- and large-intestine similarly is sometimes followed by resection; that is especially common in some African tribes. Intussusception, usually thought of as a disease of childhood, occurs commonly in some adult Africans.

In Papua New Guinea, Uganda, and probably many other parts of the tropics also, *Clostridium welchii* infections give rise to a necrotizing enteritis (pig-bel disease) (Chapter 17); by causing severe pathological changes, and also because considerable lengths of small-intestine sometimes have to be resected, that disease is a further cause of decreased surface area and malabsorption.

20.2.4. Undernutrition

The role of undernutrition in malabsorption is not easy to delineate (see above); however it seems likely that *severe* malnutrition, especially kwashiorkor in infancy and childhood, is occasionally responsible.

Steatorrhoea has been reported in five children with kwashiorkor, and that was probably due to subnormal concentrations of conjugated bile-salts (Mahalanabis, Jacobs, Banwell, Mukherji, and Bose, 1972). In *severe* kwashiorkor, marked jejunal mucosal morphological changes have been demonstrated (Burman, 1965; Stanfield, Hutt, and Tunnicliffe, 1965); they are often accompanied by defects in the absorption of mono- and di-saccharides (James, 1968; Wharton, Howells, and Phillips, 1968). Similarly, in Iranian children dying of marasmus, severe mucosal changes have been observed (Creamer, Dutz, and Post, 1970). Those changes are probably a result of bacterial contamination of the upper small-intestine (Gracey, Suharjono, Sunoto, and Stone, 1973). After recovery from kwashiorkor, the changes resolve, and several years later the jejunum is morphologically normal for the population studied (Cook and Lee, 1966); twenty children who had had kwashiorkor four to 10 (mean 5·7) years previously had a jejunal mucosa which was similar to that of the vast majority of adult Ugandan Africans (Cook, Kajubi, and Lee, 1969).

20.2.5. Gluten-induced enteropathy

Coeliac disease seems to be rare in tropical countries. There are important differences between this disease, which is related to gluten ingestion, and TM. Diarrhoea is far more common in TM than in coeliac disease. Jejunal biopsy-specimens show gross changes in coeliac disease, but only mild ones in TM. In coeliac disease the proximal small-intestine is mainly involved, whereas in TM the whole small intestine is abnormal. Osteomalacia is common in coeliac disease and rare in TM. Vitamin B_{12} deficiency is rare in coeliac disease and common in TM. Whereas broad-spectrum antibiotics are ineffective in coeliac disease, they are of great value in TM; similarly, folic acid is ineffective in coeliac disease but of great value in the treatment of TM.

Coeliac disease has been reported in India; two reports from New Delhi (Misra, Kasthuri, and Chuttani, 1966; Walia, Sidhu, Tandon, Ghai, and Bhargava, 1966) have documented gluten-induced enteropathy in local children. Until recently, however, there was no reliable report of coeliac disease from Africa. Seven children with the disease, two of whom were siblings, have now been recorded in northern Sudan (Suliman, 1978). All were of high socioeconomic status. They all had severe mucosal abnormalities with abnormal absorption tests. There was marked improvement on a gluten free diet; one patient had a relapse when gluten was reintroduced.

20.2.6. Other causes of severe malabsorption

Severe jejunal changes associated with malabsorption have been demonstrated in various viral infections, including viral hepatitis (Conrad, Schwartz, and Young, 1964).

Diarrhoea and abdominal pain are very common in measles, especially in children. Severe jejunal mucosal changes have been described (Dossetor and Whittle, 1975), leading to secondary hypolactasia (Chapter 21). Kwashiorkor may be precipitated. In addition, a severe necrotizing gastroenteritis has been demonstrated at post-mortem in that disease (Williams and Osotimehin, 1970).

The Norwalk agent, a 27 nm picorna virus, has been shown to produce mucosal damage and malabsorption (Schreiber, Blacklow and Trier, 1973).

Malabsorption has also been associated with other systemic infections and malignancies (Hindle and Creamer, 1965; Deller, Murrell, and Blowes, 1967; Dymock, MacKay, Miller, Thomson, Gray, Kennedy, and Adams, 1967; Klipstein and Smarth, 1969); in most studies that has been related to severe intestinal morphological abnormalities. Hindle and Creamer (1965) reported malabsorption in a patient with generalized glandular tuberculosis. Although they found abnormal B_{12} and D-xylose absorption in the presence of malignant disease, Klipstein and Smarth (1969) reported normal jejunal morphology. In none of those studies were serum protein or immunoglobulin concentrations measured (see above).

Falaiye and Oladapo (1971) have stressed the importance of excluding diabetic enteropathy as a cause of malabsorption in Nigeria.

20.3. Postinfective tropical malabsorption (TM)

The term *postinfective tropical malabsorption* (TM) is considered preferable to *tropical sprue* to describe a clinical syndrome of malabsorption, which usually follows an acute intestinal infection (sometimes with bloody stools). Severe malabsorption, with steatorrhoea, has for long been known to occur commonly in some parts of the tropics (see below). Although many people develop the disease after many years in the tropics, it may occur very soon after the first tropical exposure, or may even start in a temperate country.

The world distribution has also been recognized to be of great interest for many years; it is common in India and the Far east, and very often starts in Nepal and Afghanistan. The West Indies are also the site of origin of some cases. However, it is uncommon in Africa. The incidence seems to depend on the underlying prevalence of acute intestinal disease. The reason why some people develop TM after an acute intestinal infection, which in some is undoubtedly travellers' diarrhoea (Chapter 17) is unknown, but that seems to be related to a reduction in small-intestinal motility, and that leads to a persisting bacterial overgrowth (Cook, 1978a). At the cellular level, absorption is probably impaired by bacterial toxins.

The role of parasites in TM is still not clear. Although *Giardia lamblia* and *Strongyloides stercoralis* may be present in the small-intestine, there seem to be no differences in the clinical picture, investigations, or luminal flora compared with TM in the absence of those parasites; all degrees of severity may occur in both circumstances.

The disease at present does not have a precise clinical or pathological definition. If that proposed by Baker (1974) is accepted, i.e. 'malabsorption of two or more substances in people in the tropics when other known causes have been excluded', the disease is exceedingly common throughout the third world. In *subclinical tropical malabsorption* (see above), xylose and B_{12} are often abnormally absorbed; flat glucose tolerance curves and low serum folate concentrations are also common in indigenous people in the tropics, but symptoms, steatorrhoea, and megaloblastic anaemia are uncommon. A definition should now include reference to small-intestinal bacterial colonization, although obviously it is not practicable to obtain small-intestinal fluid before starting treatment in every case. Degrees of severity have been defined on the basis of the number of abnormal investigations, i.e. grade I if one substance, usually xylose, is malabsorbed: two substances, usually xylose and fat (grade II); and three substances, xylose, fat, and B_{12} (grade III) (Tomkins, James, Walters, and Cole, 1974; Cook, 1978a).

20.3.1. History of TM

Investigation of disease in tropical countries was until recently difficult; therefore many early descriptions of TM were made in England on people who had returned from India and the Far east (Martin, 1856; Fayrer, 1881).

Hillary (1766) gave what is considered to be the first accurate account of the disease (Booth, 1964). Between 1747 and 1751, in Barbados, he saw one case of the disease, then three more in the next three years, and some scores in the following four years. Most early writers stressed the insidious*, or slow, onset of the disease. Pringle (1764) appreciated that dysentery could proceed to chronic diarrhoea and the '*white flux*', in which 'the aliment will pass through the intestines with little alteration'; he also recognized that oral aphthae could be associated features. Twining (1835) was aware that the onset could be acute, with dysentery and bloody stools. Grant (1854) gave a clear description of a disease with an acute onset, which was called *hill diarrhoea*. Goodeve (1866) drew a sharp distinction between the white flux of the plains of India, and hill-diarrhoea, which could also progress to a fatal *diarrhoea alba*; he was aware of an associated arthropathy, scorbutic patches, corneal ulcerations, and terminal fluid retention; he stressed the risk of relapse. Unlike most of his contemporaries, he did not consider that liver involvement was important in the pathogenesis of the disease.

The term *sprue* was first used in the English language by Manson in 1880 whilst working in Amoy, China; he adopted it from the Dutch word *spruw*, which had for long been applied to oral aphthous ulceration in children, and was then in use in Java. He described a chronic diarrhoeal syndrome, associated with aphthous ulcers, which he regarded as a specific entity. Oral changes and diarrhoea were periodic, and the 'great wasting was altogether out of proportion to the amount of diarrhoea'. He considered that patients with the disease could seldom say when it began, and that it was 'exceedingly insidious in onset, and very slow in its progress'; however, he cited a case (Manson, 1880) which began after acute dysentery. He was also aware that in Manila and the Straits the course of the disease was more rapid than in Amoy. Manson's description served to emphasize the potential gravity of the disease, which had a substantial mortality when untreated, but whether he was justified in considering it to be a single entity must be seriously questioned (Cook, 1977d; 1978b). By 1898, Manson's experience of the disease had increased and he was of the opinion that it had been 'more or less recognised for many years'. Although *Strongyloides stercoralis* and *Entamoeba histolytica* were sometimes

* The use of the term *insidious* to describe the onset of the disease is probably a source of confusion in interpretation of the early literature. Insidious is defined (*Concise Oxford Dictionary*) as: treacherous, crafty; proceeding secretly or subtly.' That does not necessarily imply the opposite of acute in describing the onset of a disease, as it often does today. During the nineteenth century the notion of treachery or low cunning was probably dominant; since then the word has increasingly conveyed the idea of slow concealed working or gradual operation (P. Considine, *personal communication*).

present in the stool, he did not regard them as aetiologically important. The disease usually started slowly, but on a basis of months or years of bowel irregularity which began soon after arrival in the tropics; he was by then quite clear however that it could start with an attack of dysentery (with bloody stools) or acute enterocolitis. He recognized a great variability in the rate of progression of the disease; the course varied between a year or two, and ten or fifteen years.

Most nineteenth and early twentieth century reports stressed the oral changes (Chapter 1). The clinical picture of TM was usually dominated by diarrhoea, with grey-white stools at some stage or other, but that was not always severe. A feature of most reports was of diarrhoea in the early hours of the morning, which subsided by about midday (Chevers, 1886; Thin, 1897; Brown, 1908; Rogers, 1913; Low, 1928). Brown (1908) differentiated the severe initial diarrhoea from the chronic diarrhoea of advanced disease. Bahr (1915) gave examples of 24-hour stool weights in 'chronic sprue'; they were 259, 303, and 605 g, respectively, in contrast to 174 and 135 g in two healthy subjects. Anaemia was emphasized by most workers; latterly it became clear that it was macrocytic (Thin, 1897; Bahr, 1915; Low, 1928; Brown, 1908). Rogers (1913), like later workers, considered that the severity of anaemia was dependent on the length of history, and was always marked in fatal cases; 15 of 28 cases had anaemia, which was severe in two, in under one year. Dyspepsia was common (Brown, 1908). Oesophageal pain was emphasized by many writers (Manson-Bahr and Willoughby, 1930) and morphological changes similar to those involving the tongue and mouth were described by Thin (1890), Brown (1908), Begg (1912), and Rogers (1913). Hillary (1766) stressed the 'burning heat about the cardia, or upper mouth of the stomach'. Rogers (1913) and Brown (1908) mentioned shallow ulcers and congestive patches in the stomach.

Most observers were aware of changes in the small-intestine, although most expressed caution in that they might be due to post-mortem change (Brown, 1908). Cantlie (1905), Brown (1908), Rogers (1913), and others described thinning of the mucous membrane with extensive atrophy of the villi and the 'tube glands', together with small-cell inflammatory infiltration; in chronic cases, there were fibrotic changes in the mucous coat, and sometimes superficial ulcers also. Changes in the ileum were stressed by Thin (1890; 1897), Manson (1898) and Begg (1912). Begg (1912) demonstrated numerous bacteria in the ileal region, and was convinced that that was the basis of the disease; Thin (1897) considered that high faecal bacterial counts were of aetiological importance. Rogers (1913) felt that the disease had a bacterial or protozoal basis. Enlarged and hardened mesenteric glands were recorded by Fayrer (1881), Goodeve (1866), and Manson (1898).

Colonic pathology, including ulceration, was described by several writers. Brown (1908) and Rogers (1913) considered that the large-intestine exhibited changes similar to, but less severe than, those in the small-intestine. Ulceration and sloughing at a late stage of the disease were recorded, but the appearances were considered to be unlike those of dysentery (Brown, 1908). An atrophic colonic mucous membrane was recorded in the chronic cases studied by Manson-Bahr and Willoughby (1930).

Most early reports stressed hepatic changes; atrophy was associated with a small pale, constricted capsule. Rogers (1913) considered that the liver was often mildly enlarged during the early stages of the disease, but atrophied later; post-mortem evidence was felt to confirm the clinical impression of hepatic atrophy (MacLean, 1886; Fayrer, 1881). Liver weight was reduced; figures of 1·0, 0·8 and 0·7 kg, compared with a mean normal weight of 1·4 kg were given by Brown (1908). Jaundice did not occur (Begg, 1912), and histology (Brown, 1908) and liver-function tests were normal (Low, 1928). Most writers (Brown, 1908) considered the hepatic changes, probably correctly, to be of nutritional origin.

Most of the cases reported by Rogers (1913) were admitted between six and twelve months after onset; in a quarter, the disease had lasted for up to eight years. Most cases seen by Low (1928) had had symptoms for four to eight months. Rogers (1913) was of the opinion that prognosis regarding complete recovery was very unfavourable; of 45 cases, only two, one of whom was in hospital for 383 days, were discharged cured, and another returned with 'sprue' several months later. Twenty-six of the 45 showed no improvement after hospital treatment, and six died while under observation. Most deaths, usually caused by intercurrent infection, occurred during the first six to twelve months; early cases did no better than late ones. Of 150 cases described by Low (1928), in London, ten ultimately died; most of them were more than fifty years old. Seven of 200 cases seen by Manson-Bahr and Willoughby (1930), also in London, died.

The early phase of clinical investigation of TM was dominated by the work of Fairley and his colleagues, who published numerous papers in the 1920s and 1930s. The disease was thought to be infective although the causative organism was unknown. In Bombay, India, TM was common, but often in a minor form (Fairley and Mackie, 1926), and was rare in Indians (Megaw and Gupta, 1927). Long residence in Bombay, and preceding malaria and dysentery were thought to be outstanding predisposing factors. An adverse climate and malaria were considered to undermine the constitution, and the prevalent diseases to damage the alimentary tract. Several hospital admissions with debility and enteritis often preceded the classical picture of TM with sore tongue and white, gaseous, bulky stools; anaemia dominated the clinical picture in other cases. However, some had a clearly defined acute onset with fever for two to three days (Fairley, 1936). Gross intestinal ulceration and involvement of the terminal ileum were described. In a more detailed account of anatomical changes, Mackie and Fairley (1929) concluded that 'the changes in the intestine are most marked in the ileum, but are present to some degree throughout the whole tract'. Later, however, Fairley (1936) considered, on very limited evidence, that those appearances were largely a result of post-mortem change. The changes described were degeneration and aplasia of the small-intestinal mucosa, and there was ultimately 'almost complete disappearance of the absorptive and secretory epithelium'. They also felt that there was ante-mortem invasion of the intestinal wall by bacteria as 'in conditions of malnutrition due to vitamin deficiency'. Duodenal contents were found to be rich in bacteria. Searches for specific bacteria continued to be unrewarding (Mackie,

Goré, and Wadia, 1928), and protozoa, including amoebae and flagellates, were excessively rare, possibly, they considered, due to the high faecal acidity. By 1930, Manson-Bahr and Willoughby concluded that despite the large amount of work which had been expended upon the aetiology of the disease from a bacteriological standpoint, the bulk of the evidence was negative.

With the advantage of hindsight it seems likely that that disease often started as travellers' diarrhoea or hill-diarrhoea (Green, 1854) and that differed therefore from Manson's concept of sprue.

Several detailed reports on large numbers of cases of TM were published during World War II (1939–45). The disease usually started with acute diarrhoea, but there were inconsistencies regarding its being a sequel to dysentery. Leishman (1945) described his experience of TM in many hundreds of soldiers. It occurred in the fly-season, when dysentery was common; three-quarters were during the first two years of service, and in some very soon after arrival in the tropics. It was uncommon in west Africans. The onset was usually acute; nine per cent gave a history of frank dysentery (4 per cent amoebic, and 3·5 per cent bacillary). In more than 50 per cent, disease was fully developed two months after the onset of diarrhoea. Leishman referred also to a 'marasmic syndrome' in Indians; that seems more like Manson's chronic sprue. He attributed TM to a disturbance of bacteriological equilibrium in the small-intestine, possibly due to stagnation. Keele and Bound (1946) reported their experience of TM in India between 1942 and 1944. Forty-five per cent of cases occurred after one to two years in India, after which the incidence declined. Peak incidence in both plains and hills was highest in May and June, when the hills are cool and the plains hot. Although epidemiological evidence suggested that the peak occurred earlier in the year than that for dysentery and diarrhoea, in some individuals amoebic and bacillary dysentery undoubtedly preceded the onset of steatorrhoea. Many had an *acute* onset which was related to dysentery, usually amoebic; there was some evidence of colonic involvement. Malaria was thought to be a further aetiological agent, and recovery occurred after treatment; giardiasis and *tabes mesenterica* were excluded. Diarrhoea preceded a sore tongue by about six weeks in 80 per cent of cases; the reverse association was rare. Stefanini (1948) reported 1069 cases of TM in 12 500 Italian prisoners of war in the Himalayan foothills. The disease followed the rainy season, and in 73 per cent began with a sudden onset of explosive diarrhoea (five to 15 stools daily); bacillary dysentery was rife, and there was also much amoebic dysentery and malaria. Previous illnesses seemed to favour onset of the disease. A mild continuous fever was noted in 12 per cent of cases; associated symptoms, including deficiency signs and macrocytic anaemia, followed between two and four weeks after onset of the diarrhoea. Ninety per cent developed glossitis; the edges and tip of the tongue were first reddened, to be followed after a few days by small aphthae. Gastric mucosa showed patches of atrophy, purpuric spots, and signs of inflammation and oedema; most had hypochlorhydria. Sigmoidoscopy showed a reddened and congested mucosa which progressed to a greyish, atrophic mucosa in the chronic case. In five who died, the intestinal mucosa was pallid and atrophic. Elder (1947) described 400 cases of TM in British soldiers in Bengal, Assam, and Burma; the disease also occurred in Indians. In many, the illness began after a short stay in the tropics, and was sometimes of sudden onset, although in most it was insidious; fifteen per cent started with an attack of dysentery. Up to 20 or 30 stools were passed daily. Three hundred and ninety-three had glossitis, and many also had angular stomatitis and cheilosis. Twenty-two per cent had a macrocytic anaemia. Walters (1947) reported 42 cases of malabsorption in Indian soldiers; three-quarters of a battalion under investigation were Jats, who were vegetarians, and one-quarter were Rajputana Mussulmans, who were meat-eaters. Thirty-nine Jats and three Mussulmans developed severe TM. They had had diarrhoea (in six), frank dysentery (bacillary in 16 and amoebic in five) or malaria (in 10) in the preceding two to three months, and had an acute onset of disease. Skin changes were common. Twenty-eight had demonstrable steatorrhoea, 37 macrocytic anaemia, and 64 per cent had a peripheral neuropathy. In six of 14, sigmoidoscopy showed a thin mucosa with a granular surface. There were two deaths. TM developed, therefore, in vegetarians after an acute infection which was usually bacillary dysentery. Ayrey (1948) also considered from his experience in Burma, that the disease was basically a disease of malnutrition, although diarrhoea could precipitate its occurrence. In a retrospective study comparing the histories of 47 patients with 'sprue' with 100 suffering from non-diarrhoeal diseases, Woodruff (1949) concluded that organisms which produce frank dysentery and enteritis 'apparently do not predispose to sprue', however, most cases occurred when amoebic dysentery and other intestinal infections were prevalent.

Both Stannus (1942) and Leishman (1945) suggested that the condition was caused by an infection which upset the intestinal bacterial flora, and that that led to the impaired biosynthesis of B vitamins; that theme was the subject of an hypothesis by Manson-Bahr (1953).

Was hill-diarrhoea the same as Manson's sprue? Most workers after Grant (1854) considered 'sprue' and hill-diarrhoea to be separate entities (Chevers, 1886; Bahr, 1915). However, some (Crombie, 1880; Fayrer, 1881; Begg, 1912) felt that they were modifications of a single disease. Rogers (1913) considered that only neglected cases of hill-diarrhoea developed into 'sprue', and Manson-Bahr and Willoughby (1930) supported that association.

Can dysentery proceed to TM? Progression of acute dysentery, with bloody stools, to the '*white flux*' was recognized long before Manson; Pringle (1764) was well aware of that complication of dysentery. Twining (1835) considered that dysentery could proceed to a condition in which the 'stools are sometimes a copious, paste-like, brown mass, in a state of fermentation; occasionally they are frothy, with a subalbid, or pale-grey sediment, like a mixture of chalk and beer'.

Fayrer (1881), Thin (1897), and Rogers (1913) were amongst others to recognize the progression of dysentery to TM. Fever and repeated dysentery were striking features in several case histories of TM reported by Fayrer (1881). Thin (1897) recognized that patients who had suffered from severe attacks of dysentery were liable, even after return to temperate climates, to a form of diarrhoea and dyspepsia, but they did not get 'the very specific eruption (in the mouth) which characterized psilosis'. He also recognized cases of 'psilosis' in which the disease set in 'by severe diarrhoea from the first'. Brown (1908) had often seen dysentery give way to TM, but was not convinced that there was a causal relationship. Rogers (1913) concluded that five of his 50 cases of 'sprue' followed dysentery. In view of the fact that 91 of 150 cases had a history of debilitating disease (dysentery, diarrhoea, or malaria in most), Low (1928) arrived at the conclusion that 'prolonged residence in the endemic area, diseases of the alimentary canal such as hill-diarrhoea and dysentery, in short any debilitating disease may bring it out'. MacLean (1866) considered that progression was dependent upon whether the lesions were bounded by the ileocaecal valve or passed into the small-intestine.

There is no doubt, therefore, that fatty stools can follow dysentery (*Lancet*, 1944). In 1944, Howat reported steatorrhoea in a corporal in the British Army, following Sonne dysentery; that patient developed his diarrhoea in east Africa, where TM is uncommon, but there are no details as to whether he had served also in Asia. King and Joske (1960) described two patients with a 'sprue-like illness' following severe intestinal infections; both were in good health before the infection. In Bangladesh, Lindenbaum (1965) demonstrated, in previously healthy subjects with shigellosis, cholera, and staphylococcal food-poisoning, that malabsorption of D-xylose, folic acid, and B_{12} was usual during the diarrhœic period; during the week after the diarrhoea had finished, malabsorption of D-xylose and B_{12} was present in approximately 70 per cent of them, and the prevalence of that was higher in those who presented with severe symptoms and dehydration. There was no relation to the causative organism; the cholera cases seemed however to be less severely affected. Some still had evidence of malabsorption 378 days, for D-xylose, and 196 days, for B_{12}, after the diarrhoea had stopped; one had lost weight.

Can travellers' diarrhoea and hill-diarrhoea proceed to TM? Grant (1854) was responsible for the first detailed report of hill-diarrhoea, although it had apparently been well recognized long before that. The disease started with fluid stools (from 4 to 12 daily), which were not usually bloody but which contained air bubbles. That condition frequently started soon after reaching a hill-station, was often epidemic, and sometimes proceeded to chronic *diarrhoea alba*. Hill-diarrhoea often started with headache, and nausea and vomiting, as well as severe diarrhoea; in addition, a fever up to 39°C, and rigors were frequent accompaniments (Brown, 1908). There was much speculation on the cause of hill-diarrhoea. A water-borne infection was favoured by some (Grant, 1854; Dickson, 1871; Fayrer, 1881; MacLean, 1886), but not all (Morehead, 1860; Crombie, 1880; Moore, 1886; Rogers, 1913). The possible role of mica in the water supply was raised (Moore, 1886; Duncan, 1905) but never proved. Galloway (1905a; b) concluded that both hill-diarrhoea and 'sprue' were caused by a specific micro-organism. Begg (1912) was convinced that TM was caused by a micro-organism which was probably water-borne; his use of santonin in its treatment was given in support of that view. Yeasts were also suggested (Nicholls, 1919). Most of the cases of TM reported from London by

Low (1928) seemed to be post infective, and he felt that a gastrointestinal toxin would 'best explain the real cause of the disease'.

Further examples of acute diarrhoea proceeding to TM have been given by Montgomery, Beale, Sammons, and Schneider (1973) and Haeney, Montgomery, and Schneider (1974). Young adults who have made overland journeys across central Asia, and have had acute diarrhoea in Afghanistan or Nepal, frequently develop TM (Tomkins, James, Walters, and Cole, 1974). Some, at least, start as travellers' diarrhoea (Rowe, Taylor, and Bettelheim, 1970).

Differences between the 'entity' described by Manson and TM. Today, most cases of TM have an acute onset; although the start of the disease is not always clearly demarcated, most patients can trace the disease to a bout of severe diarrhoea. Buccal changes, which often used to precede intestinal changes (Hillary, 1766; Rogers, 1913) are today very unusual, except in severe and very chronic cases; aphthous ulceration is not seen. Severe anaemia is also unusual, although in chronic cases of long duration, a folate deficient megaloblastic anaemia is sometimes present.

20.3.2. Geographical distribution of TM

For a very long time, one of the most fascinating aspects of TM has been its geographical distribution (Cook, 1974a). Although common in most of Asia and the Caribbean, it is very unusual in Africa. Although Manson (1898) included tropical Africa in the areas where sprue (psilosis) was especially common, subsequent experience has very largely disproved that; a mere handful of cases has been recorded from the continent, whereas there have been numerous reports from Asia. Trowell (1960) concluded that 'tropical sprue is almost absent among Europeans in Africa', and he also considered that reports of sprue in southern Africa were unacceptable; the only case he had seen was in a European who had, for long, lived in Asia. Gardner (1958) remarked on the rarity of sprue in Africa, despite increases in air travel. Recently, a few reports of TM in indigenous Africans have appeared; however, the majority are unlike the classical cases described in Asia, and few have had symptoms.

It would be most remarkable if the disease did not exist in Africa; it has even been reported in a 34-year-old woman in Birmingham who had never left England; she came from a poor background, had a classical clinical presentation, and biochemical findings which apart from a normal serum B_{12} concentration, were consistent (Drummond and Montgomery, 1970). TM usually resolves in a temperate climate.

Early reports were based on clinical observations without many investigations; the competence of the clinician was thus of paramount importance. In many reports, other causes of malabsorption were not positively ruled out. The most convincing of early cases was that described by Manson-Bahr (1928). He described a 28-year-old civil servant, whom he saw in London, who had been resident in Blantyre, Nyasaland (now Malawi), for nearly 10 years; it is not clear whether he had travelled further afield. The history and response to treatment are consistent with the diagnosis, although he did not have oral changes. Begg (1912) reported two cases of steatorrhoea from the upper Congo (Zaire), but did not give a clear indication of the cause; they were both women, who had been included in a consecutive series of 100 cases. They had 14-month and three-year histories, respectively; both were presumably expatriates. They were subsequently cured. Taute (1919) described three cases of 'sprue' in German East Africa (Tanzania). Gelfand (1947) described three cases of steatorrhoea in Europeans in Salisbury, Rhodesia (now Zimbabwe Rhodesia), over a six-year period; they had all been resident in the colony for many years. Two were women, and one a man, of 61, 72, and 57 years, respectively. Although other causes of malabsorption were not excluded, the histories are suggestive. There were no oral changes, but all were anaemic. They all recovered on bed rest and a 'sprue diet'. Limbos (1956) described a 41-year-old woman in Matadi, Belgian Congo (Zaire), who may have had TM.

With newer diagnostic methods the search for TM in Africa was intensified. In 1964, Harries reported two cases of malabsorption in Nairobi, Kenya. The first, a 34-year-old Mkamba man, had a two-month history of abdominal pain and diarrhoea, had lost weight, and had a smooth tongue. He had a megaloblastic anaemia and steatorrhoea; serum folate and D-xylose absorption were not measured. He responded to a high-protein diet and folic acid. The second was a 39-year-old Kikuyu man, who had a five-month history of abdominal pain, diarrhoea, weight-loss, and steatorrhoea. He had a low serum folate concentration. He responded well to a high-protein diet and vitamin B complex. The first patient died subsequently of tuberculosis, and the latter was not followed up. A brief report of two prisoners, on an abnormal diet, with steatorrhoea, was made by Banwell, Hutt, Leonard, Blackman, Connor, Marsden, and Campbell (1967) from Kampala, Uganda; they had glossitis and a severe megaloblastic anaemia. Folic acid produced an improvement.

The first detailed report of possible TM in an African, in Africa, was made by Falaiye (1970); he described nine Nigerians who had had recurrent diarrhoea, consisting of four to six stools per day for a mean of 21 (6–60) months, together with cramps, borborygmi, and weight-loss, which had not responded to antidiarrhœic or antiamoebic agents. All were anaemic, and three of four bone-marrows were megaloblastic; there were no buccal changes. Six of eight had a raised faecal fat; D-xylose excretion after a 25 g load was low in seven of them. Five had a low serum folate concentration; crystalline folic acid absorption was impaired in five in whom it was measured. Serum B_{12} concentration was normal in all of them. Jejunal biopsies showed more severe changes than in Nigerian controls; in one there was a convoluted pattern. The five who were treated responded clinically to tetracycline; xylose and fat absorption also showed an improvement in most re-tested. Many of those abnormal investigations are compatible with tropical enteropathy, but the clinical picture and high incidence of megaloblastic anaemia suggests TM. That disease is different from TM in Asia where, after the first few months, low serum B_{12} concentrations and very abnormal biopsies would be expected (England and O'Brien, 1966); it is possible that the local diet contained adequate vitamin B_{12}. Moshal (1970), and Moshal, Hift, Kallichurum, and Pillay (1973) described 24 cases in Durban, South Africa, selected from 71 patients with malabsorption. They all had partial villous atrophy. Nine were post-partum women with megaloblastic anaemia; all except one had a low serum folate concentration, and one had a low serum B_{12} concentration. One had a high faecal fat excretion, and seven a low D-xylose excretion; four had an abnormal Schilling test, using intrinsic factor. There was evidence of improvement in two after folic acid, and two after an antibiotic. Only four presented with diarrhoea. Those cases are probably similar to those with folate-deficient megaloblastic anaemia and malabsorption described by Foy and Kondi (1971). A further eight were not post-partum, and had no gastrointestinal symptoms, weight loss, or buccal changes; they all had megaloblastic anaemia. Three had a high faecal fat excretion; all had an abnormal D-xylose test. Serum folate and serum B_{12} concentrations were low in four of them; seven of eight Schilling tests were abnormal. Those patients had asymptomatic, subclinical malabsorption, together with a megaloblastic anaemia, which was due presumably to a combination of folate and B_{12} deficiencies. Four were treated with antibiotics, and they showed clear evidence of improvement; four did not respond to folate. Some cases of megaloblastic anaemia with low serum B_{12} concentrations, reported by Foy and Kondi (1971), responded to antibiotics; response of tropical enteropathy to antibiotic therapy has not been adequately investigated. The remaining seven presented with gastrointestinal symptoms, although only four had diarrhoea. Six had a megaloblastic bone-marrow; two of those had oral changes, and four complained of weight loss. Only three of them, all of whom presented with diarrhoea, had a raised faecal fat excretion; the dietary fat content was not stated. Six had a low serum folate concentration, and all had an abnormal D-xylose test. Serum B_{12} concentration was low in one, and two of six had an abnormal Schilling test. Two of the three with steatorrhoea had a normal blood glucose rise after oral glucose. Three showed evidence of recovery with either tetracycline, or folic acid and tetracycline. A minority of patients in that study may have had TM; the majority were probably also cases of megaloblastic anaemia associated with low dietary folate, or subclinical tropical malabsorption, or both; the incidence of symptoms was low. Keeton (1972) reported two cases of steatorrhoea in African men of 18 and 21 years respectively, in Durban; one had a *Giardia lamblia* infection, and was not anaemic; there was no report of D-xylose absorption, or of serum folate or B_{12} concentration or bone-marrow examination. The second case may have had TM, but other causes of malabsorption were not excluded. A report by Weir, Bank, Novis, and Marks (1972), also from South Africa, of a 22-year-old African woman who presented three weeks after delivery with anaemia and puerperal sepsis, may have had TM; she had a megaloblastic anaemia and malabsorption, but at laparotomy, she had large mesenteric lymph glands which contained chronic inflammatory cells and eosinophils. Tomkins, *et al.* (1974), recorded TM in three patients, who had travelled overland in Africa, seen in London during a five-year period; whether they had also travelled in Asia or the Middle east is not stated.

Thomas and Clain (1976), described 31 African patients who were seen at Salisbury, Zimbabwe Rhodesia, during a 15-month period. They were drawn from 48 patients who presented with megaloblastic anaemia, and three with diarrhoea and weight-loss. Details of diet are given, and that did not differ significantly from a control group. Only 48 per cent had diarrhoea, and three per cent a sore tongue. Twenty-six of them had an abnormal jejunal-biopsy; in most, convolutions were present. Twelve had steatorrhoea, all had B_{12} malabsorption, and 28 had impaired xylose absorption. Three had a *G. lamblia* infection. Most responded to conventional therapy. That group is similar to Asian cases of chronic sprue, in that jejunal mucosal changes are severe, but nutritional megaloblastic anaemia and tropical enteropathy presumably account for some of them. I have not personally seen a florid case of TM, with a classical clinical presentation, during 10 years in Africa.

TM exists in Africa, therefore, but a florid presentation, which is usual in Asia in both indigenous and expatriate populations (Baker, 1972; 1974; Baker and Mathan, 1972), is unusual. There are very few reports of cases of TM in Africa associated with severe symptoms, and even fewer with mortality.

The European population of Africa has always been less dense than in Asia; that could be an important factor in the scarcity of reports in expatriates in Africa. The most important predisposing factor to TM is probably a high incidence of acute diarrhœal disease in the local environment; that is much less common in many parts of Africa than in those parts of Asia where TM is a major problem. A notable exception is Lagos, where an illness resembling TM has been recorded (Falaiye, 1970); the studies of Falaiye (1970), and Moshal, *et al.* (1973), were carried out in Lagos and Durban, both of which are at sea level and have a hot humid climate, which is similar to that in other areas where TM has been reported. Ethnic factors can be ruled out, because large numbers of Europeans, and Asians from all parts of Asia, have now lived in tropical Africa for long periods. The very high incidence of tropical enteropathy in Africa suggests that it does not predispose to TM. The nutritional status of most adult Africans is relatively good; the staple diet often contains large amounts of folate. Klipstein (1969) has shown that TM is more often associated with megaloblastic anaemia in areas with a high incidence of malnutrition. However, there are areas where dietary folate depletion occurs, and that has a seasonal incidence. In Zambia, alcohol consumption is high, and folate depletion and megaloblastic anaemia are common. In India, reheating of food is commonly carried out, and the incidence of malabsorption is higher in vegetarians than in those who eat meat (Walters, 1947).

Two questions regarding the low incidence of TM in Africa are: (i) why is there a lower incidence of acute diarrhœal disease compared with Asia, and furthermore, why does cholera not become established in Africa; does that merely reflect the population density, public health facilities, and quality of the water supplies? (ii) Why do only a small minority of cases of acute gastrointestinal disease progress to TM; is that dependent solely on transit rate, and is folate status important? Experience with severe folate depletion and megaloblastic anaemia in Africa suggests that folate is not the answer; serum folate concentration tends to be low in healthy Nigerians (Falaiye, 1969) and Zambians (G. C. Cook and A. V. Hoffbrand, *unpublished*).

20.3.3. Pathology and bacteriology of TM

In the early stages, malabsorption of xylose, glucose, fat, B_{12}, and folate occurs; both the jejunum and ileum are thus presumably affected. After four months or thereabouts, the intestinal mucosa (both jejunal and ileal) shows 'partial villous atrophy'; a fall in serum B_{12} and folate has by then usually occurred (O'Brien and England, 1966). Severe morphological changes, as seen in adult coeliac disease, are extremely unusual; the changes are non-specific, do not correlate well with the severity of malabsorption, and can be observed in other conditions also (Collins, 1965). Folate deficiency and megaloblastic anaemia do not always occur (Sheehy, Cohen, and Brodsky, 1963; Sheehy, Cohen, Wallace, and Legters, 1965). Booth and Mollin (1964), have recorded subacute combined degeneration of the spinal cord in very chronic cases. In severe cases also, serum calcium and magnesium, and serum fat soluble vitamin concentrations are reduced; the prothrombin index is prolonged.

Hypoproteinaemia is due to: diminished protein intake, defective protein absorption, diminished albumin synthesis in the liver, and a protein-losing enteropathy (Garcia Lopez, Milanes, Spies, Lopez Toca, Aramburu, and Lopez, 1949; Baker, 1957).

There is often a depression of gastric acid secretion (Chapter 4). If mucosal damage is severe, secondary hypolactasia is present (Chapter 21).

Deaths from the disease should now be rare, but when they occur they are most common at the extremes of life (Edington and Gilles, 1976). At post-mortem, the body is grossly emaciated with an absence of subcutaneous fat. The skin is dry, with irregularly scattered areas of pigmentation; sometimes petechial haemorrhages are present. The heart shows brown pigmentation. There is often a diffuse increase in the bone-marrow due to megaloblastic hyperplasia, or it may be replaced by pale, fat-free gelatinous tissue; osteoporosis and osteomalacia may be present. Intestinal villi are shortened and thickened (O'Brien and England, 1966), but the changes are non-specific; the mucosa is thin with a predominance of plasma-cells, histiocytes, lymphocytes, and eosinophils in the lamina propria. Histiocytes containing PAS-positive granules can be demonstrated at the tips of the villi. The mitotic index is increased in the crypt epithelial cells; the goblet cells are increased. Adenosine triphosphatase can be demonstrated in the surface-epithelium; lipoid vacuoles are present in the thickened basement membrane, which separates the surface epithelium from the lamina propria. Ceroid (a lipofuscin pigment) may be present in the smooth muscle of the gastrointestinal tract, blood-vessels, prostate, uterus, urinary bladder, and lymph-nodes (lipofuscinosis or the brown-bowel syndrome) in the presence of significant malabsorption; that is also present in many people in northern Thailand in the absence of significant malabsorption (Troncale, Miller, Keusch, Comer, Chittayasothorn, Petchkit, and Nye, 1968). The significance of ceroid deposition is thus not clear; it has been suggested that it is caused by vitamin E deficiency, and a high intake of unsaturated fat.

Much recent work on TM has been dominated by morphological studies; that approach has doubtless retarded research in this area, because jejunal mucosal changes are non specific, usually not very severe, and never diagnostic.

High counts of enterotoxin producing coliform organisms have repeatedly been demonstrated in mid-jejunal aspirates (Banwell and Gorbach, 1969; Klipstein, Holdeman, Corcino, and Moore, 1973; Tomkins, Drasar, and James, 1975). They are undoubtedly responsible for the functional disturbances of TM. The possibility that a specific viral agent is implicated in the aetiology of tropical sprue has not yet been entirely eliminated. The demonstration of viral particles in the faeces in northern India, led Mathan, Mathan, Swaminathan, Yesudoss, and Baker (1975), to suggest that such agents might be relevant to the production of mild intestinal abnormalities and malabsorption seen there; those agents bore a resemblance to orthomyxo- and coronaviruses. In view of the high incidence of TM in 'hippies' travelling overland in Asia (Tomkins, *et al.*, 1974), in whom there is a high incidence of viral hepatitis, a virus spread by contaminated syringes could be important; severe jejunal mucosal changes are associated with viral hepatitis, and a survey of serum HB_sAg in this disease would be of interest.

20.3.4. Aetiology of TM

There can now be no reasonable doubt that the major precipitating factor in tropical sprue is a severe, usually acute, gastrointestinal infection; the epidemic nature of the disease, and its occurrence in 'sprue houses' makes that certain. Whether a vector is ever involved is unknown.

The small-intestine in TM is colonized by coliform bacilli (see above); obligate anaerobes are not found. High concentrations of *enterobacteria* are present in the small-intestinal lumen (Gorbach and Banwell, 1969; Gorbach, Banwell, Mitra, Chatterjee, Jacobs, and Guha Mazumder, 1969; Klipstein, *et at.*, 1973; Tomkins, *et al.*, 1975). It seems clear that that event often follows an acute attack of diarrhoea, which is probably often travellers' diarrhoea (O'Brien and England, 1971; Jones, Dean, and Parker, 1972). The main questions to be asked in the aetiology of TM therefore are: (i) why does small-intestinal colonization continue after the acute diarrhoeal attack in a minority of people, and (ii) how do those bacteria produce malabsorption? The answer to the first seems to be that there is a relative stasis in the small-intestine in patients with TM (Cook, 1978a); in that study, a breath-hydrogen technique was used to measure the mouth-caecum transit rate in patients with TM, and controls. Those with TM had a significant prolongation ($P < 0{\cdot}001$) in transit rate, and that was not dependent on gastric emptying. That observation confirmed the clinical impressions of Drew, Dixon, and Samuel (1947), O'Brien (1967) and Baker and Mathan (1971), and is of particular interest in view of the fact that small-intestinal motility is usually increased by the presence of bacteria (Abrams and Bishop, 1966; 1967; Gorbach, Plaut, Nahas, Weinstein, Spanknebel, and Levitan, 1967). A limited number of patients in that study had colonic disease, without significant malabsorption, and they also had prolonged transit compared with the controls; it seems possible therefore, that in some patients with an acute intestinal infection, which may be primarily colonic, peristaltic activity is depressed, and that predisposes to bacterial overgrowth in the small-intestine. The importance of decreased motility of the small intestine in bacterial colonization has repeatedly been demonstrated in animal experiments; thus opiates (Kent, Formal, and LaBrec, 1966), ganglion blocking agents (Dixon and Pauley, 1963), antiperistaltic pouches (Bishop, 1963), and ligation (Abrams and Bishop, 1966) have all been shown to predispose to massive bacterial overgrowth, with excessive deconjugation of bile-salts (Rosenberg, 1969). Regarding the second question, one possibility is that the bacteria adhere to the enterocyte, where they secrete an enterotoxin, which at high concentration damages the functional integrity of those cells. Many bacteria, including *E. coli, Salmonella typhimurium*, and *Vibrio cholerae* have been shown to possess adhesive properties (*Lancet*, 1977b) which are mediated by a transmissible plasmid. That possibility has received support from Tomkins, *et al.* (1975) who demonstrated a higher concentration of *Enterobacteria* in relation to the enterocyte, than in the luminal fluid in TM. The strains of coliforms which colonize the small-intestine might be particularly virulent, in that their enterotoxins induce a very marked secretion (Klipstein, Engert, and Short, 1978; Klipstein and Engert, 1978); in those studies enterotoxigenicity of *Klebsiella pneumoniae, Enterobacter cloacae*, and *E. coli* was tested by in-vitro perfusion of the rat jejunum; both heat-labile and heat-stable enterotoxins were involved.

It seems likely that hypochlorhydria predisposes sufferers to invasion of the small-intestine with acid-sensitive organisms; cholera is more severe in hypochlorhydric subjects (Nalin, Levine, Levine, Hoover, Bergquist, McLaughlin, Libonati, Alam, and Hornick, 1978) (Chapter 18). TM is very common in overlanders to Nepal, Afghanistan, and other Asian countries; many of them smoke *Cannabis indica* which has been shown to decrease gastric acidity (Nalin, Levine, Rhead, Bergquist, Rennels, Hughes, O'Donnell, and Hornick, 1978). Many of the trans-Asian travellers who are currently seen in the UK at present, actually undertake their journey to obtain hard drugs.

The role of the colon in TM is by no means clear. Many of the nineteenth and early twentieth century reports were of diseases which started with obvious colonic pathology; that organ was frequently severely diseased at post-mortem. The possibility of small-intestinal bacterial colonization from a diseased colon should be considered more seriously than hitherto.

Recent investigations have shown an impairment of glucose (Cook, 1971a; 1973a) and folic acid (Cook, Morgan, and Hoffbrand, 1974) absorption in patients with systemic infections (see above); those observations might be important in the pathogenesis of TM.

Relation to megaloblastic anaemia. Working in Puerto Rico, Castle, Rhoads, Lawson, and Payne (1935) and Suarez (1938) concluded that the primary defect in 'sprue' was haematological rather than small-intestinal, and that that was due primarily to a nutritional factor. Megaloblastic anaemia in east Africa (Foy, Kondi, and Hargreaves, 1952; Foy and Kondi, 1958), and in other tropical areas has been well documented. It occurs commonly in both sexes, although the majority of cases are associated with pregnancy and the puerperium. It has a seasonal incidence, and is undoubtedly related to a low folate intake; in Mombasa, Kenya, there is an increased incidence during the hot season when vegetables are scarce; most cases occur in association with pregnancy, and all respond to folic acid (Foster, 1968). A similar situation exists in Zambia (L. J. Cardozo and G. C. Cook, *unpublished*) where the seasonal incidence, and association with pregnancy and the puerperium, are also striking. During a 72-month period, 85 cases of megaloblastic anaemia were seen in Lusaka; 68 were in women, most of whom were pregnant. None had symptoms suggestive of TM, and only one man had significant evidence of malabsorption. Low serum folate concentrations are also common in the Sepik, Watut, and Markham Valley regions of Papua New Guinea (Pitney and Jones, 1966; Powell, Soatt, and Booth, 1970); TM is very rarely, if ever, seen there.

The anaemia is often severe, is accompanied by a low serum folate concentration, and D-xylose excretion correlates with the severity of the anaemia; folic acid absorption is normal (Foy and Kondi, 1971; H. Foy, *Personal communication*; Cook, 1976b). Most patients appear well nourished, and steatorrhoea is not a feature (Foy and Kondi, 1971).

Presentation is with symptoms referable to the anaemia; intestinal symptoms and signs, oral changes, and weight loss are absent. Response to folic acid is rapid. Improvement occurs with oral antibiotics; the mechanism is unknown (Foy and Kondi, 1971). Chronic infection, especially tuberculosis, can also induce a megaloblastic anaemia.

Despite associated malabsorption, there is no evidence that the condition is related to TM. However, some of the reports of 'sprue' in Africa by Moshal, Hift, Kallichurum, and Pillay (1973) and by Thomas and Clain (1976) probably fall into that category. In about half, Baker (1967) reported spontaneous improvement in B_{12} absorption, without treatment. O'Brien (1967) considered that B_{12} malabsorption was similar to that in the blind-loop syndrome; eight of ten cases had a raised urinary indican, probably due to abnormal ileal flora. In some, bacterial colonization of the ileum was probably related to B_{12} malabsorption and steatorrhoea, and was followed by improvement after antibiotics; in those who did not respond, invasion of the ileum was thought to be by tetracycline insensitive bacteria.

Vitamin B_{12} deficiency, in the absence of TM, is unusual in tropical countries despite the fact that dietary intake is often low. In both Singapore (Wells, 1958) and India (Wokes, Badenoch, and Sinclair, 1955) the disease does however exist, but usually in vegans. A rare type of megaloblastic anaemia in tropical countries responds to pyridoxine, but not to folic acid or vitamin B_{12}. Addisonian pernicious anaemia is rare in most indigenous people in tropical countries (Chuke, Traub, and Patel, 1972; Carmel and Johnson, 1978).

20.3.5. Presentation of TM

The dominant clinical feature of TM is usually continuing diarrhoea, with large, pale, fatty stools and excessive flatulence, after an acute intestinal infection; the associated weight-loss may be gross (Fig. 20.2).

The disease is usually endemic, but epidemics occasionally occur; Mathan, Ignatius, and Baker (1966) have reported such an event from south India.

Baker (1967) and O'Brien (1967) and their respective colleagues have described cases of TM with an acute onset. Most cases described by Klipstein

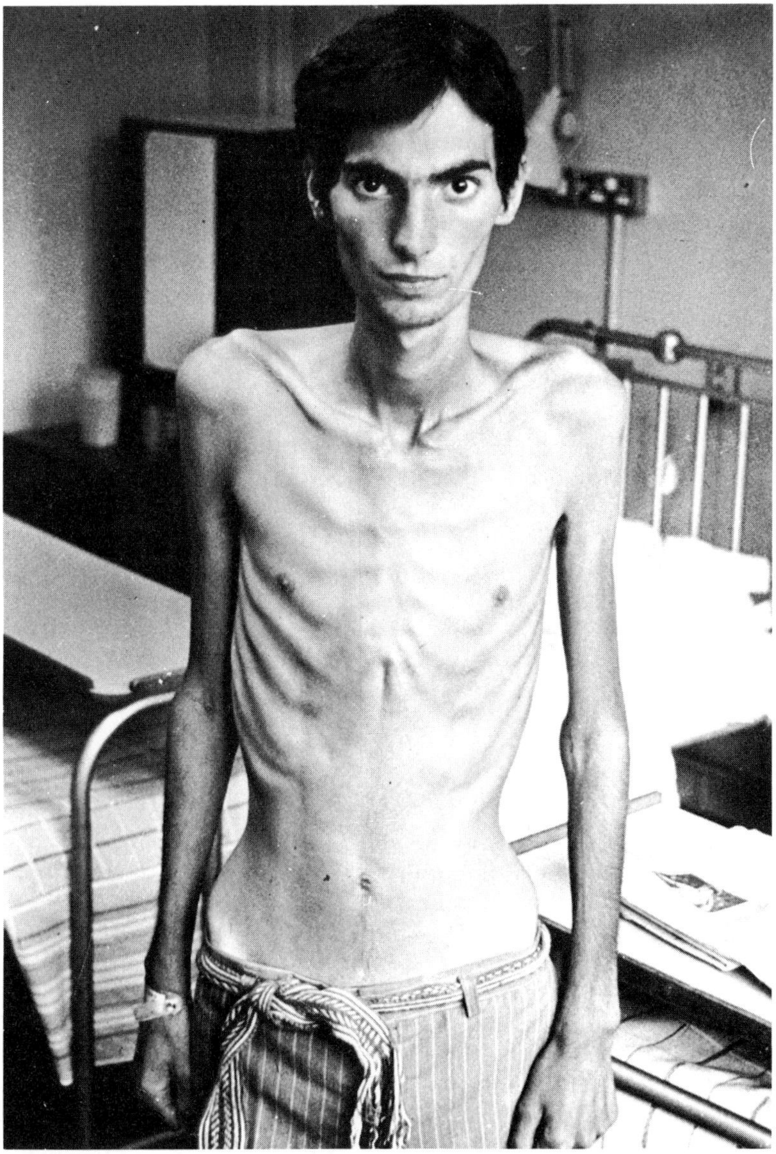

FIG. 20.1. A 19-year-old Englishman who had just returned to London after an overland journey to Afghanistan and Nepal. During his travels he had developed severe diarrhoea, which had become chronic, with large, pale, bulky stools, accompanied by weight-loss of approximately 20 kg. He was investigated at the Hospital for Tropical Diseases, London. Investigation revealed gross malabsorption (TM); D-xylose, fat, and B_{12} were all poorly absorbed. After treatment with tetracycline and folic acid, recovery was rapid.

(1971) also seem to have suffered from a disease of acute onset. Those reported in Indians by Baker from Madras, had a very acute onset (Baker and Mathan, 1968); the incubation period was usually five to six days. Diarrhoea (96 per cent), vomiting (50 per cent), and fever (at least 30 per cent) were common; adults were affected more often than children. O'Brien (1967) described 64 English servicemen with TM during a five-year period; in most, the disease had started in Borneo. Watery diarrhoea and colic started suddenly; it was worst at night in 11 of them. Six presented with glossitis and megaloblastic anaemia; they did not have diarrhoea. The Indians (Baker, 1967) had been poorly nourished. Most of the Englishmen (O'Brien, 1967) had lived on tinned food, and they usually developed symptoms as soon as they returned to fresh rations; the explanation for that is not clear. Fifty per cent of the cases described by Baker (1967) had glossitis, which was associated with folate deficiency. Anaemia, hypoproteinaemia, and vitamin A deficiency were common; the severely anaemic patients had splenomegaly.

A disease with a slow, or *insidious*, onset now seems much less common than was envisaged by Manson (1880). Of recent reports, those from London by Mollin (1967) and Mollin and Booth (1971) seem to be most closely related, on clinical grounds, to Manson's sprue. Mollin (1967) described 13 Europeans and Anglo-Indians with TM, which started in India or south-east Asia, some of whom had a very chronic condition, which had lasted up to 22 years. They had gastrointestinal symptoms and a folate-deficiency anaemia, which sometimes started after they had left the tropics. Folic acid, as well as fat, xylose, and B_{12} was malabsorbed. Jejunal morphological changes were usually mild and ileal changes were often more severe, especially in those who did not respond to folic acid. Therapeutic response was obtained after folic acid, B_{12}, or broad-spectrum antibiotics. Recovery after antibiotics suggested that the condition was related to intestinal bacterial colonization, but the slow response suggested that it was not a direct simple relationship. *S. stercoralis* has been clearly implicated in TM (see below), and it seems likely that much disease described by Manson and others, in China and the Far east, was associated with that parasite, which although common at that time was not regarded as a pathogen. General factors, such as chronic infections (including malaria) and vitamin deficiencies, were thought to be important in the *diarrhoea alba* of the plains of India; the role of chronic malnutrition is still difficult to evaluate. People who have repeated infections, both intestinal and systemic, frequently find it difficult to associate a specific attack with the onset of an illness. Some patients with an insidious onset of diarrhoea might fall into this group.

In the individual patient a careful dietary history is necessary, because the end-result of TM is clinically similar to severe malnutrition. If an adult presents with severe malnutrition (adult kwashiorkor), without other evidence of a cause, TM, ileocaecal tuberculosis and chronic calcific pancreatitis are often responsible. Sometimes, TM seems to start after the patient has left the tropics; that is not surprising because cases have been reported in people who have never left temperate climes. Diarrhoea is usually present in TM (see above), but may not be gross; blood in the stool is unusual. Diarrhoea is sometimes watery. Abdominal distension, excessive flatulence, abdominal colic, and excessive borborygmi and bowel movements are common in a severe case; those symptoms are often worsened by milk ingestion, due to a secondary hypolactasia (Chapter 21). If there is severe pain, chronic calcific pancreatitis should be suspected. Vomiting is unusual.

Apathy, depression, weight-loss, anaemia, glossitis with aphthous ulceration (Chapter 1), bone disease (usually osteomalacia), and fluid retention may be present in a severe case. Excessive tiredness and restlessness often result from a magnesium deficiency. Severe weight loss is often a result of anorexia rather than gross steatorrhoea. Nocturnal diuresis and hypothermia are common in a severe case. Amenorrhoea and infertility are also encountered. There is a loss of subcutaneous tissue and muscle mass. Anaemia is common. The hair is soft and lacks elasticity. Cheilosis, angular stomatitis, and glossitis may be present. Hypotonia is common. There may be tetany in a severe case. Oedema, hypotension, and pigmentation are present in an advanced case. The stools are classically bulky, offensive and pale; they float due to the presence of air-bubbles. If there is blood, pus, or mucus in the stool it is likely that dysentery has given rise to TM, although investigation for other large-intestinal pathology should be undertaken.

In children, in whom TM is less common than in adults (Grant, 1854; Crombie, 1880; Rogers, 1913), failure to grow, affecting weight more than height—is common. Kwashiorkor may be mimicked.

20.3.6. Investigation of TM

Investigation of malabsorption is often extremely difficult in tropical countries; few laboratories in the third world have the necessary facilities and techniques (Cook, 1967). Most diets in tropical countries contain a low fat content; that should always be taken into account in faecal fat estimations.

Investigations do not differ from those in other malabsorption states in temperate areas of the world (Losowsky, Walker, and Kelleher, 1974).

Investigations should, if possible, include the following: a xylose absorption test (after either 5 or 25 g xylose, given orally), 72-hour faecal fat estimation, a Schilling test, a jejunal-biopsy, and a search for stool parasites. Both 5 and 25 g xylose loads give reliable results; the latter dose is obviously more expensive and occasionally gives rise to nausea and vomiting, although I have found that to be an extremely unusual event. A one-hour blood xylose concentration seemed to give reliable information on absorptive status (Haeney, Culank, Montgomery, and Sammons, 1978). D-xylose is partly metabolized by bacterial action in the small-intestine of patients with TM; that has been clearly shown using a breath-hydrogen technique after oral xylose ingestion in that disease (Cook, 1979b). In tropical countries, a microscopic method for the determination of faecal fat gives valuable qualitative information (Cook, 1967). In addition, serum B_{12} and red blood-cell folate concentrations should be estimated if possible. Results of absorption tests depend on the severity of the disease; that applies to xylose, faecal fat, and Schilling tests, and also to serum vitamin B_{12}, red blood-cell folate, and serum albumin and globulin concentrations. Hypoalbuminaemia is usual in a severe case. Hypogammaglobulinaemia has occasionally been demonstrated (Jarnum,

Jeejeebhoy, and Singh, 1968; Mehta, Naik, Krishnan, Nain, and Sehgal, 1978).

Using a jejunal perfusion technique, a significant reduction in glucose absorption rate from the jejunum, from a 200 mM solution, has been demonstrated in TM (G. C. Cook, *unpublished*); some of those subjects also had a *G. lamblia* infection. However, glycine absorption rate from a 100 mM solution was not depressed in patients with TM; that result differs from those in two other investigations, which have demonstrated a reduction in the absorption rates of glycine and other amino acids, when given at a concentration of 20 mM (Klipstein and Corcino, 1975; Hellier, Radhakrishnan, Ganapathy, Mathan, and Baker, 1976). The explanation for that difference is not clear; it is not, however, dependent on the fact that glycine is near V_{max} when perfused at that rate and concentration (Cook, 1973b). It seems probable that bacterial enterotoxins are responsible for those abnormalities (Sack, 1976).

Blood glucose estimations after oral lactose (50 g), followed the next day by glucose (25 g) + galactose (25 g) have also been performed (Cook and Kajubi, 1972; Cook, 1978c). The value of assessing the jejunal lactase concentration in TM has, however, recently been assessed (Cook, 1978c). Lactase is not depressed in TM unless the disease is severe; mucosal damage is frequently mild in that disease, in contrast to gluten-induced enteropathy, and secondary lactase deficiency (Chapter 21) is present in only a proportion of cases. Also, many people exposed to TM suffer from genetically-determined adult hypolactasia. Using the hydrogen breath-test, it was concluded that assessments of lactase concentration are of no value, either in detecting the condition or in assessing its severity (Cook, 1978c). Serial lactase determinations (either direct or indirect) are thus of very limited value in TM.

Barium meal examination shows dilated loops of small-intestine, often with a clumping of barium which indicates malabsorption. The small-intestinal transit rate is decreased. Figures 20.2 and 20.3 show barium-meal radiographs in a patient with TM, and after treatment.

The anaemia of TM is usually caused by folate deficiency, and responds to folic acid (O'Brien, 1967); after two months the bone-marrow shows megaloblastic change. In a series described by Baker (1967), 50 per cent also had a low serum B_{12} concentration which was not associated with intrinsic factor deficiency; although most also had a low serum folate concentration, and 68 per cent had megaloblastic anaemia, folate malabsorption was uncommon. O'Brien (1967) considered that folate deficiency was progressive and was associated with folate malabsorption; after one month serum folate was usually less than 3 μg per l, and at four months most had megaloblastic anaemia. Vitamin B_{12} malabsorption was not dependent on an ileal lesion, and was rapidly corrected by oral broad-spectrum antibiotics.

Pathology and enzyme estimations of jejunal-biopsy specimens may be undertaken, and bacteriological studies of those specimens and jejunal fluid (see above) may give added information. Jejunal-biopsies show various grades of abnormality, the severest change being convolutions, which O'Brien (1967) considered occurred after about three months of the disease; a submucosal infiltration with lymphocytes and plasma cells is usually present. In O'Brien's

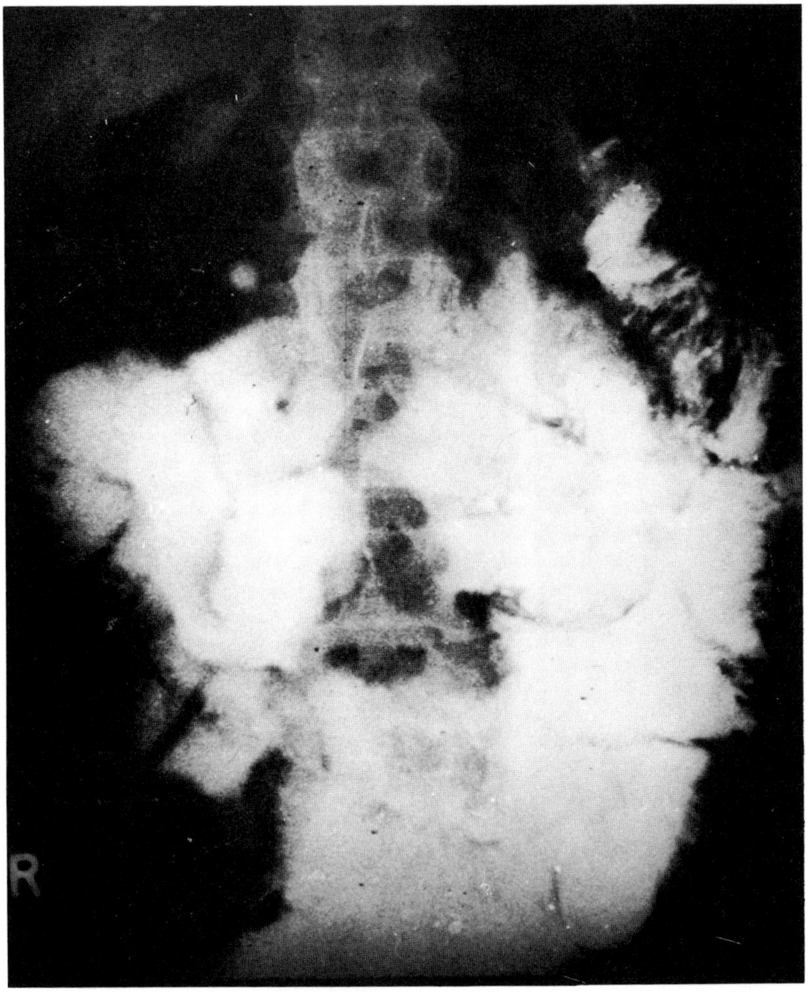

FIG. 20.2. Barium meal in a 24-year-old Englishman with tropical malabsorption (TM); all absorption tests were abnormal. Marked dilatation of the small-intestine, and loss of the mucosal pattern are shown; in addition, the small-intestinal transit rate for barium was impaired.

investigation the ileum was also examined; changes were less severe than those in the jejunum. Changes in the stomach, consisting of gastritis and gastric atrophy, and in the colon, an increased cellularity in the *lamina propria*, were reported by Baker (1967). Sigmoidoscopy shows a hyperaemic mucosa in some cases.

Having found evidence of significant malabsorption, it is important to ascertain that it is of small-intestinal origin, and furthermore to be sure that the condition is TM. Ileocaecal tuberculosis can be difficult to differentiate (Cook, 1974a) (Chapter 23); barium meal or enema, and sometimes laparotomy are often necessary for a firm diagnosis. Chronic calcific pancreatitis (Chapter 15) should be easily recognized; calcification is obvious on a plain abdominal radiograph. Chronic liver disease can be diagnosed from the clinical picture, tests of liver function, and if necessary a needle-biopsy of the liver (Chapter 8). Serum transaminase concentrations are often mildly elevated in severe cases of TM. Not infrequently viral hepatitis is also present in patients with TM contracted in Asia, who are seen later in the UK.

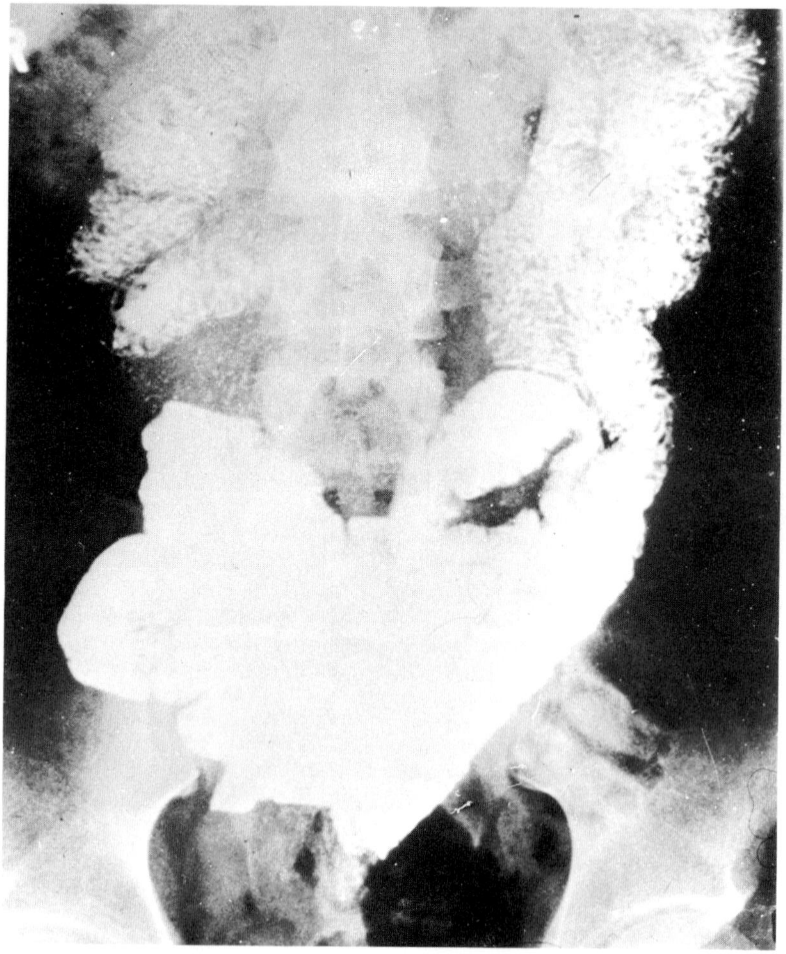

FIG. 20.3. Barium meal from the same patient as that in FIG. 20.2, six weeks later. He was symptomatically much improved and had gained weight; tests of absorption had almost returned to normal. There is less dilatation of the small-intestinal lumen, the mucosal pattern has returned, and the transit rate was then normal.

Ultrastructural changes in the jejunum in TM. There are few studies of ultrastructure of the jejunum in TM. Peters, Jones, Wells, and Cook (1978) have applied a subcellular fractionation technique, in conjunction with enzyme microanalysis, in a study of organelle pathology. There was no detectable difference between patients with TM who did, and did not also have, giardiasis; in one patient brush-border enzymes returned to normal after treatment, despite the fact that *G. lamblia* was still present in the jejunal-biopsy specimen. A significant reduction in brush-border enzymes, which return to normal after treatment, has been established; quantitative rather than qualitative alterations in the brush-border membrane are present, and that is unlike the situation in coeliac disease. There was no reduction in lysosomes, peroxisomes, and mitochondrial enzymes, in the patients with TM; however, the organelles were significantly more fragile. Endoplasmic reticulum was unchanged in TM. The enzyme 5-nucleotidase was assayed in the basal-lateral (plasma) membrane; a significant reduction was noted in TM, and that persisted after recovery; that might reflect an underlying abnormality in the enterocytes of individuals susceptible to TM.

Intestinal permeability. This has not been investigated in tropical malabsorption; in coeliac disease the small-intestinal mucosa has been shown to be abnormally permeable to protein macromolecules (Kivel, Kearns, and Liebowitz, 1964; Diamond, 1978; Hemmings and Williams, 1978) and disaccharides (Menzies, 1972). A test which takes those observations into account may be of value in diagnosis (Cobden, Dickinson, Rothwell, and Axon, 1978).

Gut hormones in TM. Gut hormones were studied in a group of patients with TM, before and after a standard breakfast, and compared with those in a control group (Besterman, Cook, Sarson, Christofides, and Bloom, 1978); in patients with TM, fasting concentrations of motilin and enteroglucagon were significantly elevated, and after the meal motilin increased slightly but enteroglucagon remained at the fasting concentration. The high enteroglucagon concentrations were related, possibly causally, to small-intestinal stasis (Besterman, Cook, Sarson, Christofides, Bryant, Gregor, and Bloom, 1979). Those with TM had a markedly reduced postprandial rise in gastric inhibitory polypeptide. Release of gastrin and pancreatic polypeptide were similar to that in the controls.

20.3.7. Treatment of TM

Treatment consists of an adequate diet, which is high in protein and contains added vitamins, together with antibiotics and/or folic acid supplements. Initially, symptomatic treatment may be required for the diarrhoea. Tetracycline should be given at a dose of 250 mg thrice daily for two weeks, and folic acid, five mg thrice daily, for four weeks. Recovery virtually always occurs, unless treatment is delayed until very late in the course of the disease. Of the cases described by Baker (1967) one-third, however, died, and most of the survivors recovered spontaneously; untreated, some 15 per cent went on for a year or more. Recovery takes place rapidly after treatment with oral tetracycline, but much more slowly after oral folic acid has been started. Diarrhoea and stool weight decrease and bodyweight increases. Biochemical tests of malabsorption improve: the xylose test, faecal fat excretion, and the Schilling test return to normal.

Symptomatic treatment is often required in the acute stage of the disease. Kaolin and morphine mixture, BPC, 15 ml may be given thrice daily. Alternatively, codeine phosphate, 30 mg thrice daily, or propantheline bromide, 15–30 mg four times daily, may be given.

If parasites which have been implicated in tropical malabsorption have been demonstrated in the stool or jejunal fluid (see below), the appropriate therapeutic agent should be given.

Symptomatically also, lactose intolerance may be important during both the acute illness and the convalescent period; that is due to secondary hypolactasia (Chapter 21). Viral hepatitis, which is sometimes present in patients with TM, may also produce mucosal damage and secondary hypolactasia. Avoidance of milk and lactose-containing foods is necessary.

20.4. Giardiasis and tropical malabsorption

Throughout the tropics, intestinal parasites are very common and it is difficult to assess their true role in malabsorption. Most evidence for an association has been produced for *Giardia lamblia* and *Strongyloides stercoralis*. *Capillaria philippinensis* and coccidia have also been clearly incriminated (Lindenbaum, 1973) (see below). The problem of the cause-effect relationship is exemplified by the possible role of hookworm infection in malabsorption (Chapter 19), which has repeatedly been raised (Sheehy, Meroney, Cox, and Soler, 1962); due to the frequency of mild absorption abnormalities in most people in the tropics, it is difficult to give a dogmatic answer to that problem. However, if it is ever associated with malabsorption that is unusual; Layrisse, Blumenfeld, Carbonell, Desenne, and Roche (1964) studied 22 patients with heavy infections and found that three had steatorrhoea, one of 18 had abnormal xylose absorption, and serum B_{12} was abnormal in one of them. Gilles, Williams, and Ball (1964) were not able to demonstrate malabsorption in hookworm disease in Ibadan, Nigeria; only one of 11 patients studied had steatorrhoea. In India, Tandon, Das, Saraya, and Deo (1966) found abnormal fat absorption in nine, and abnormal xylose absorption in three of 22 patients with hookworm infections. Tandon, Saraya, Ramachandran, and Sama (1969) showed that abnormal fat and xylose absorption occurred in 32 and 29 per cent, respectively, of 104 patients studied; they concluded that malabsorption was related to the severity of the accompanying hypoalbuminaemia. Although *Ascaris lumbricoides* (Chapter 19) is not considered by most investigators to play a role in malabsorption, abnormal fat and xylose absorption in four and three, respectively, of seven children studied, has been reported in one investigation (Tripathy, Duque, Bolaños, Lotero, and Mayoral, 1972). In Costa Rica, Kotcher, Mario Miranda, Esquivel, Peña-Chavarría, Donohugh, Baldizón, Acosta, and Apuy (1966) found no evidence of malabsorption in patients with either hookworm disease, giardiasis, or strongyloidiasis.

G. lamblia is frequently identified in the stool, duodenal aspirate, or jejunal biopsy of patients with TM (Wright, Tomkins, and Ridley, 1977). It seems possible that the outbreak of TM described by Hillary (1766), in Barbados, in the eighteenth century was associated with that parasite. It is also possible that some epidemics of hill-diarrhoea in the nineteenth century were associated with *G. lamblia*; the descriptions of diarrhoea of acute onset with excessive flatulence which started in the early hours of the morning, are consistent with giardiasis. An acute onset of diarrhoea with excessive flatulence and abdominal distension, reported in outbreaks of giardiasis in Colorado (Moore, Cross,

McGuire, Mollohan, Gleason, Healy, and Newton, 1969) and Leningrad (Brodsky, Spencer, and Schultz, 1974; Jokipii and Jokipii, 1977) is very similar to those nineteenth century descriptions; significant malabsorption occurred in many. Stool microscopy was widely used in the latter nineteenth century, however, and it seems unlikely that that parasite would have been missed; however, awareness of its probable pathogenicity was not apparent until the early twentieth century, and it might have been dismissed as being unimportant. Castellani (1905), in Ceylon, was of the opinion that flagellates were important in producing diarrhoea, if present in large numbers; he added, however, that they also occurred in normal people, especially natives. *G. lamblia* was associated with severe diarrhoea in soldiers during World War I (1914–18), in both the Middle east and Indo-China (Porter, 1916; Fantham, 1916).

Apart from its widespread distribution in tropical countries, giardiasis is now probably the most common human parasitic infection in the United Kingdom (*Lancet*, 1974). Recently, large outbreaks have also occurred in the USA (Wolfe, 1975; Schultz, 1975; Hartong and Arvanitakis, 1977), Australia (Simpson, 1975), and other European countries (Willcox, 1975; Eastham, Douglas, and Watson, 1976; Jokipii and Jokipii, 1977). Seven per cent of the inhabitants of Holland who have not travelled abroad have *G. lamblia* ova in the stool; 21 per cent of stool specimens from children between 5 and 9 years are positive (Meuwissen, Tongeren, and Werkman, 1977). In Glasgow, 13·3 per cent of Scottish, 10·2 per cent of Asian, and 1·1 per cent of Chinese and African children are infected with *G. lamblia* (Goel, Shanks, McAllister, and Follett, 1977).

Giardiasis is largely a disease of travellers, however (*Br. med. J.*, 1977), and is being increasingly reported in them (Babb, Peck, and Vescia, 1971; Sterner, Lantorp, and Lidman, 1971; Walzer, Wolfe, and Schultz, 1971). In one study in India, 23 per cent of 300 patients with non-dysenteric diarrhoea were found to be infected (Antia, Desai, and Jeejeebhoy, 1966).

In most outbreaks the organism has been isolated from water supplies (*Lancet*, 1974), including mountain-stream water (Barbour, Nichols, and Fukushima, 1976); that is of interest in the context of hill-diarrhoea.

20.4.1. Parasitology and pathology

G. lamblia was first detected in a stool-specimen by Van Leeuwenhoek, in Delft, in 1681; he detected the trophozoite, microscopically, in his own stool (Dobell, 1920). *G. lamblia* is a flagellated protozoan which lives in close proximity to, and might actually invade, the jejunal mucosal cells (Brandborg, Tankersley, Gottlieb, Barancik, and Sartor, 1967; Morecki and Parker, 1967; Saha and Ghosh, 1977). The trophozoites, which measure 12–18 μm in length, live in the duodenum and jejunum; they are found in the mucus adherent to the mucous membrane of the small-intestine. *G. lamblia* reproduces by binary fission. The cysts are oval and contain two nuclei initially, and four after division in the mature cyst. As it descends the gastrointestinal tract it encysts, and it is in that form that it is most likely to be detected in the stool. It is possible to confuse degenerated cysts of *G. lamblia* in the stool with isospora (Collins,

Keller, and Brown, 1978). The organism can be cultivated in artificial media. The cyst form is resistant to the usual chlorine concentrations in tapwater.

Although jejunal morphological changes have been associated with the organism, they are inconstant; villi may be shortened and stunted, and there may be an increase of mitoses in the enterocytes (Alp and Hislop, 1969). Acute inflammatory lesions are often superimposed upon a non-specific chronic inflammatory exudate in the mucosa (Yardley, Takano, and Hendrix, 1964). Partial villous atrophy and an increase in the size and number of goblet cells in the villi have been recorded.

The bile-ducts and gall-bladder are occasionally invaded. The degree of mucosal damage seems to bear very little correlation with symptoms; mild degrees of damage can often be associated with severe malabsorption. A patient in whom coeliac disease was excluded had total villous atrophy (Levinson and Nastro, 1978); after a single course of metronidazole, the biopsy became, and remained, normal.

It has for long been known that *G. lamblia* infection of the small-intestine can be associated with diarrhoea and malabsorption (Cortner, 1959) in children. Similarly in hypogammaglobulinaemia where there is impaired immunity, this organism has been associated with abnormal small-intestinal structure and function (Ament and Rubin, 1972; Brown, Butterfield, Savage, and Tada, 1972). The possible ways in which *G. lamblia* might produce malabsorption have been summarized (Tandon, Tandon, Satpathy, and Shriniwas, 1977): (i) a mechanical barrier to absorption, (ii) mucosal injury without invasion, (iii) mucosal invasion, and (iv) bacterial overgrowth with subsequent bile-salt deconjugation.

Amini (1963) demonstrated steatorrhoea in three of eight adults with giardia infestations, and that recovered after treatment. Ament and Rubin (1972) demonstrated both steatorrhoea and mucosal lesions in four of seven patients; they also tended to recover after treatment. Petersen (1972), in a review of giardiasis, concluded that malabsorption occasionally, but by no means always, occurs in infected adults. However, although the association is common, the causal role of *G. lamblia* in the pathogenesis of malabsorption is still unclear (Yardley, *et al.*, 1964) and many patients with giardiasis are completely asymptomatic. Although there is now evidence that the organism invades the duodenal and jejunal mucosa (see above), it is difficult to understand how a flagellated protozoan can penetrate tissues. The concentration of giardia trophozoites in the ileal region is difficult to assess; in practice, attempts to isolate the organism are usually directed at finding trophozoites in the upper jejunum, and the cysts in the stool. Some patients with giardiasis have a significant overgrowth of enterobacteria in the small-intestinal lumen (Tomkins, Wright, Drasar, and James, 1976) and free bile-acids in the duodenal aspirate (Tandon, Tandon, Satpathy, and Shriniwas, 1977). Giardia, and/or enterobacteria living in association with it, might cause bile-sale deconjugation, and subsequent malabsorption (Cook, 1977d). *G. lamblia* infections are common in Africa; however TM is very unusual on that continent. Those observations are consistent with the probability that the parasite merely alters the internal milieu of the lumen, which is subsequently colonized by bacterial over growth. Malabsorption is cured with metronidazole in most cases (see below); however, that compound also eradicates anaerobic bacteria, which can themselves deconjugate bile-salts and cause diarrhoea. The role of *G. lamblia per se* in the production of malabsorption is therefore not yet clear. The mechanism of the malabsorption might very well be similar to that in TM (see above).

20.4.2. Presentation

The incubation period is usually about two weeks, but may be as long as several months. Diarrhoea, which is usually worst in the mornings, and is watery, explosive, and sometimes bulky and offensive, but without blood or pus, is characteristic. Weakness, abdominal distension and discomfort, anorexia, nausea, weight-loss, flatulence, vomiting, belching, depression, and failure to thrive in children, are important symptoms. The acute stage may last from a few days to several months. Wright, *et al.* (1977) have reported 40 patients with clinical giardiasis; symptoms had been present for up to five years, and 23 had evidence of malabsorption. The reason why some people do not develop symptoms is unknown; that seems to have no relationship to the parasite load. Differences in host susceptibility may be important. Diagnosis of giardiasis is made from a history of diarrhoea, often alternating with constipation, colic, and typical malabsorption stools with excessive flatus; it often starts with an acute onset, and is frequently epidemic. The overall clinical presentation is usually identical to that of TM, and any grade of severity may be encountered; the presence and severity of malabsorption can be demonstrated with appropriate biochemical investigations as in TM. However, many people harbour this parasite for many years without experiencing any symptoms, or get at most mild abdominal discomfort and occasional morning diarrhoea. Death has however been attributed to giardiasis, as a result of acute ulceration of the jejunum (McGrath, O'Farrell, and Boland, 1940). Although *G. lamblia* is a parasite of a number of animals, those reservoirs seem to play little part in human infections.

20.4.3. Investigation

The trophozoites can frequently be demonstrated in jejunal fluid; plugs or threads of mucus should be stained on a glass microscope-slide with Giemsa, without centrifugation. Alternatively, they can be demonstrated in jejunal biopsy samples (Fig. 20.4). The 'string test', in which a string containing a weight at the distal end is swallowed and positioned in the jejunum, and to which trophozoites of *G. lamblia* sometimes adhere, and are identified microscopically, is occasionally of value (Beal, Viens, Grant, and Hughes, 1970). Cysts can be identified in stool specimens by microscopy.

Presence of *G. lamblia* cysts or trophozoites in the stool is erratic, and the patient may be symptomatic for several weeks before parasites are detectable (Jokipii and Jokipii, 1977); the finding of parasites in duodenal or jejunal fluid is a more satisfactory, but time-consuming, method of diagnosis.

Circulating antibody to *G. lamblia* (Ridley and Ridley, 1976) can be detected, and probably indicates increased jejunal mucosal permeability with the absorption of parasite antigen.

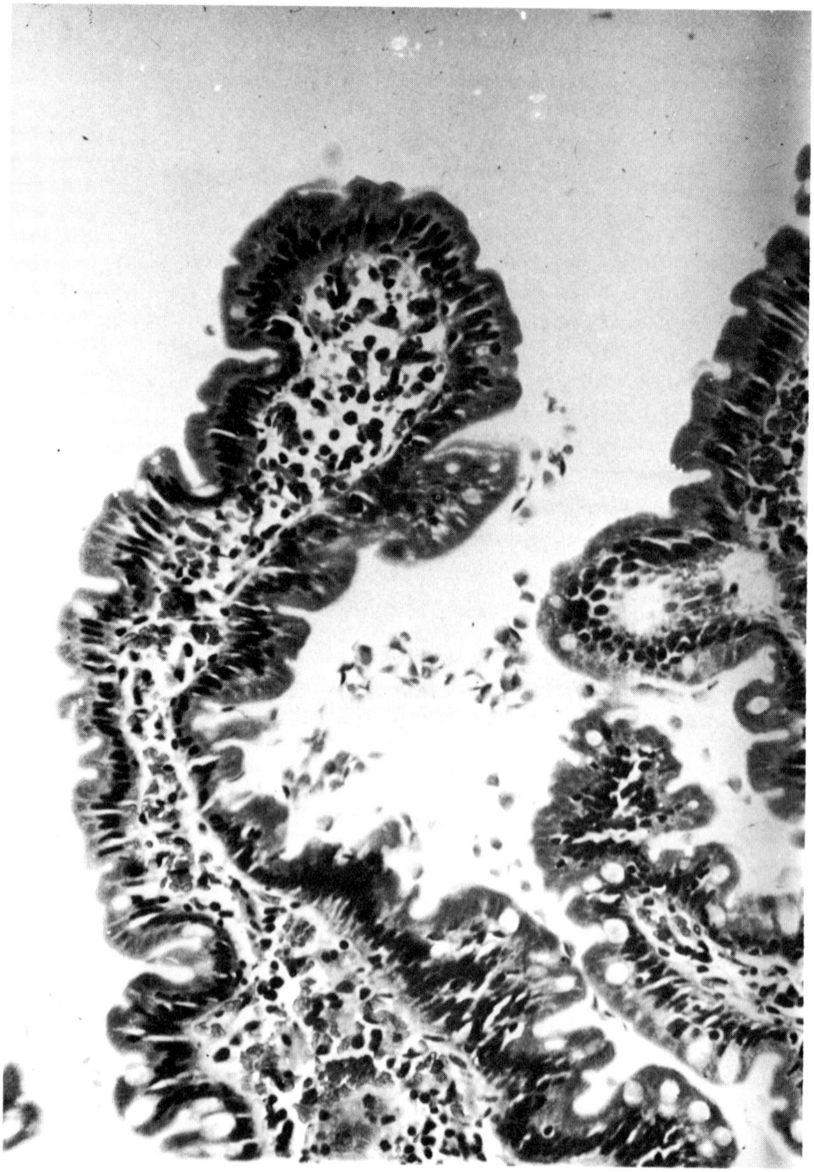

FIG. 20.4. Jejunal-biopsy specimen from a patient with TM associated with a *Giardia lamblia* infection. Absorption tests were severely abnormal. The villous architecture is relatively normal, but there is a cellular infiltrate in the lamina propria. Trophozoites of *G. lamblia* can be seen in the mucus in proximity to the enterocytes.

Malabsorption of varying degrees can be detected with the appropriate investigations (see above).

Other members of the household should be tested for infection.

20.4.4. Treatment

Treatment of giardiasis is either with metronidazole ('Flagyl'), or mepacrine (Bassily, Farid, Mikhail, Kent, and Lehman, 1970). Metronidazole should be given either as a 10-day course at a dose of 200 mg twice daily, or a three-day course of 2 g daily; the latter regime probably gives a slightly higher cure rate. Alcohol should be strictly avoided during treatment with metronidazole due to the possibility of a confusional state. The dose of mepacrine is 100 mg thrice daily for 10 days. Acute haemolysis may be produced by that agent in the presence of glucose-6-phosphate dehydrogenase deficiency. In one study, mepacrine 300 mg daily for 10 days cured 63 per cent, and metronidazole, 2 g daily for three days, 91 per cent of infections (Wright, *et al.*, 1977).

An alternative agent is tinidazole, in a dose of 150 mg twice daily for seven days, or as a single 2·0 g dose, orally (Pettersson, 1975); in a report from the Sudan (Salih and Abdalla, 1977) that agent eradicated the parasite in 32 of 33 symptomatic patients; the only failure was in a patient given the single dose regime. Nausea, skin-rash, and worsening of abdominal pain and diarrhoea were reported in some patients on the seven-day course. In a report from Egypt (El Masry, Farid, and Miner, 1978), a single 2·0 g dose cured 53 of 55 patients with heavy *G. lamblia* infections. A single 2·0 g dose was also used in a study in Iran (Farahmandian, Sheiban, and Sanati, 1978); a reduction of 94·5 per cent in positive stool tests was claimed. Forty-five patients with symptomatic giardiasis were treated with tinidazole by Jokipii and Jokipii (1978); 150 mg twice daily for 7 days, cured 14 of 19 (74 per cent), and a single dose of 2·0 g, 24 of 26 (92 per cent). Mild side-effects were noted after the higher dose. Most treatment failures were detected a few weeks after therapy, and that stresses the importance of long follow-up periods.

One hundred and seventy-two patients in Brazil were treated with either furazolidone, nimorazole, metronidazole, or tinidazole (Levi. de Ávila, and Neto, 1977); cure rates were 72, 94, 87, and 97 per cent, respectively, while in an untreated group the rate was 35 per cent. The only significant side-effects were with furazolidone.

An adequate diet with added protein and vitamins, is important in improving the nutritional status.

20.5. Strongyloidiasis and tropical malabsorption

Malabsorption in the tropics is often associated with the nematode worm *Strongyloides stercoralis* (O'Brien, 1975). Such infections are common in many tropical and subtropical areas throughout the world, including the south-eastern states of the USA.

S. stercoralis was frequently found during the nineteenth century in patients with TM, and was at one time thought to be the cause of 'sprue' (Manson, 1898). Brown (1908) claimed that 'about 30 per cent of cases of "sprue" in Cochin China, Siam and Malaya had intestinal parasites in the stool, one of the commonest being *S. stercoralis*'; that agent was 'considered by Normand in 1876 to be the aetiological agent in the epidemic diarrhoea of Cochin China, but its presence is now known to be merely adventitious, and to have no essential significance in the causation of the disease'. It now seems probable that that agent was in fact responsible for a significant number of cases of TM in Cochin China (Cook, 1978b). Manson (1898) was of the opinion that sprue there was more chronic than in India, and that observation is consistent with *S. stercoralis* infections, which due to autoinfection, are known to be associated with a very chronic clinical course.

Evidence for a role for this parasite in tropical malabsorption is overall somewhat contradictory. Milner, Irvine, Barton, Bras, and Richards (1965) recorded four infected patients, ranging from 13 to 28 years, with malabsorption, and Mayoral, Tripathy, Garcia, Bolaños, and Ghitis (1968) also stressed the importance of strongyloidiasis in that condition. A number of reports (Stemmermann and Nakasone, 1960; Alcorn and Kotcher, 1961; Paola, de Dias, and da Silva, 1962; Milner, *et al*., 1965), but not all (Cook, Kajubi, and Lee, 1969) indicate that it is associated with changes in jejunal morphology. Kotcher, Miranda, Esquivel, Peña-Chavarría, Donohugh, Baldizón, Acosta, and Apuy (1966) found normal fat and carbohydrate absorption, however, in patients harbouring that parasite. Garcia, Sessions, Strum, Schweistris, Tripathy, Bolaños, Lotero, Duque, Ramelli, and Mayoral (1977) are of the opinion that severe malnutrition causes mild enteropathy and malabsorption (Mayoral, Bolaños, Lotero, and Duque, 1975; Duque, Bolaños, Lotero, and Mayoral, 1975; Duque, Lotero, Bolaños, and Mayoral, 1975), and furthermore that in spite of moderate to severe symptoms, well-nourished patients with *S. stercoralis* infections do not suffer from malabsorption. They consider, therefore, that the malabsorption which occurs in a proportion of cases of *S. strongyloides* infection is related not to the parasite, but to the accompanying malnutrition. Despite that conclusion, the bulk of work incriminates the parasite in some cases of malabsorption, but like *G. lamblia* that is inconstant and its effect may depend on a change in the luminal milieu, and colonization with enteropathogenic bacteria.

20.5.1. Parasitology and pathology

This nematode, the adult of which can survive for five years, attaches itself to, and invades, the duodenal and jejunal mucosa where the female worm lays her eggs *within* the tissues. Adult worms may be up to 2·2 mm (female) and 0·7 mm (male) in length. The mechanism of the absorption defect which sometimes accompanies their presence, is not clear (see below). Rhabditiform larvae develop and are passed in human faeces. These free-living larvae develop after three months into infective filariform larvae, which can survive in warm moist soil; however their resistance is low, and they require optimal conditions of moisture and temperature for survival. Under certain circumstances they penetrate intact human skin, traverse the right heart, and escape into the alveoli via the pulmonary vessels. Some pass over the trachea to enter the small-intestine where they invade the mucosa. Filariform larvae travel to the lungs where they produce ova and rhabditiform larvae. The time between skin penetration and egg-laying is approximately four weeks. Filariform larvae sometimes develop during their passage down the lower intestine; they then invade the anal mucosa or skin, and cause an autoinfection (Hartz, 1946; Grove and Elsdon-Dew, 1958). The infection may thus persist in people who have left an endemic area for many years; in a recent study, Gill, Bell, and Reid (1977) have demonstrated a high incidence of strongyloides infection in men who were imprisoned by the Japanese in the Far east during World War II (1939–45).

There may be mild inflammatory changes in the lamina propria of the jejunum; the larvae and adult worms are often difficult to find, but are usually present within the mucosa or crypts. Ova may also be found in the mucosa of the duodenum and jejunum. There may be a mild eosinophilia, and lymphocytic infiltration. There is often stunting of the villi which return to normal after treatment (De Paola, 1961; Beker, Rivas Gómez, Valencia-Parparcén, and Moncada, 1963); Da Costa (1971) has suggested that the high epithelial-cell turnover might result in excessive loss of endogenous protein, and that that leads to malnutrition and hypoproteinaemia, especially in patients with hyper-infection.

Larvae may be found in any part of the bowel, and also the pyloric and abdominal lymph glands, which may be enlarged and hyperaemic; they have been described in the lymphatics and portal venous channels. Granulomatous lesions with giant cells and necrosis may be present; there may be ulceration. The ileum may be a site of larval reinvasion; tuberculoid foci may be seen, with necrosis and occasionally a degenerating ovum at the centre. Scattered larvae may be found in almost any organ in the body in the hyperinfection syndrome. The liver (Chapter 5) and large intestine (Chapter 27) may be involved.

20.5.2. Presentation

Little is known about primary immunity to *S. stercoralis*; there is some resistance to reinfection. A skin eruption ('creeping eruption') usually on the back, which is characterized by blotchy, erythematous and urticarial features, may occur during the migratory stage. Malaise, fever, anorexia, and cough may also be present during that stage. During pulmonary migration, respiratory symptoms of varying severity may occur. After a few weeks, abdominal pain, often diffuse and colicky, and alternating diarrhoea and constipation may occur. If infection is heavy, diarrhoea may be persistent, with malabsorption, lassitude, nausea, vomiting, and weight loss. Cholecystitis and asthma have been recorded. Presentation with necrotizing jejunitis has been reported (Craven, Cantrell, and Lewis, 1971).

The clinical picture of the established infection is related to the degree of malabsorption, which is sometimes gross (Napier, 1949). A period of 36 years between infection and diagnosis has been claimed in one case (Brown and Perna, 1958).

Fatal and overwhelming infections can occur (Ophüls, 1929; Willis and Nwokolo, 1966; Rivera, Maldonado, Vélez-García, Grillo, and Malaret, 1970; Adam, Morgan, Persaud, and Gibbs, 1973; Dwork, Jaffe, and Leiberman, 1975), especially in immunosuppressed and debilitated individuals, and particularly children. It is often associated with high dose corticosteroid treatment

(Purtilo, Meyers, and Connor, 1974). Hyper-infection has also been recorded in patients with leprosy and malignant lymphomas. In most cases that seems to be associated with autoinfection (Hartz, 1946; Bras, Richards, Irvine, Milner, and Ragbeer, 1964; Poltera, 1974; Wilson and Thompson, 1964).

Filariform larvae, which have already developed in the intestine, invade the perianal region with creeping eruption and wheal formation. A recurrent Loeffler's syndrome, with pulmonary symptoms and eosinophilia, may follow (Poltera, 1972; Nwokolo and Imohiosen, 1973).

During the invasive stage, hookworm 'ground-itch' and 'creeping-eruption' due to *Ancylostoma braziliense* give similar dermatological manifestations. Later, other causes of transient pneumonitis, urticaria and gastrointestinal symptoms should be considered.

20.5.3. Investigation

Motile larvae can sometimes be found in a 'direct smear' of fresh stool (Fig. 20.5); however, repeated stool samples are usually negative. Jejunal fluid is sometimes of value, and the 'string test' occasionally gives diagnostic results. It is unusual to find ova in the stool, even with severe diarrhoea.

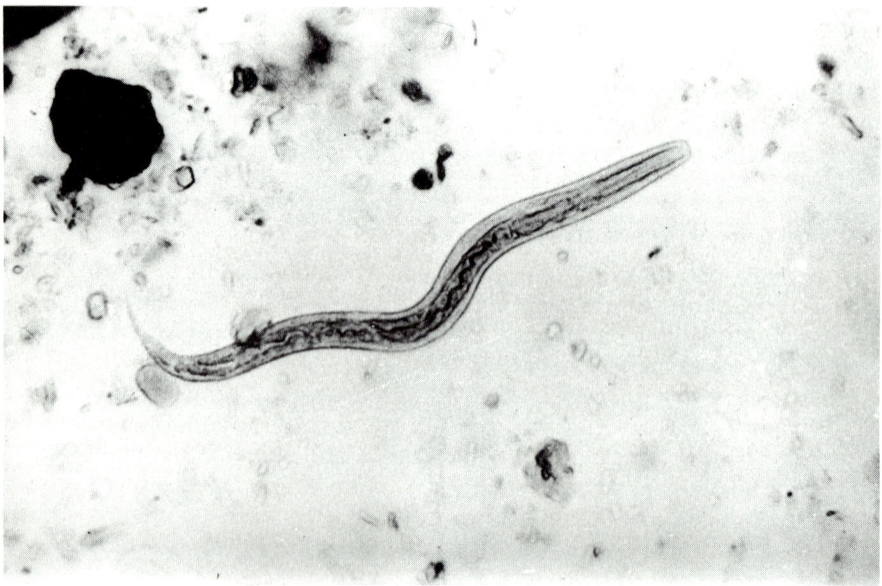

FIG. 20.5. Larva of *Strongyloides stercoralis* in a stool of a patient with mild malabsorption after a journey across Asia. Absorption tests were mildly abnormal.

Jejunal-biopsy specimens may show ova and larvae embedded in the mucosa and crypts. Malabsorption is often present (Toh and Chow, 1969); there may be atrophy of villi. Tests of absorption may be grossly abnormal; however, in some patients no abnormalities can be detected.

An eosinophilia, sometimes of massive proportions, is often found in the peripheral blood. There may be evidence of blood loss in heavy infections.

Radiological examination may reveal an 'irritability' or deformity of the duodenum (Beker, *et al.*, 1963).

Serological tests are of limited value.

The complement-fixation test for filariasis often gives a cross-reaction with strongyloides.

S. stercoralis can occasionally be found in sputum during pulmonary migration.

20.5.4. Treatment

Treatment is with thiabendazole ('Mintezol') at a dose of 25 mg per kg bodyweight twice daily for three days (maximum dose, 3 g daily). Side-effects are nausea, vomiting, diarrhoea, and giddiness; they are severe in about 30 per cent of patients, but are said to be lessened by taking the compound after meals. Drowsiness, pruritis, xanthopsia, bradycardia, and hypotension are rare side-effects. Crystalluria, leucopenia, and erythema multiforme have been reported rarely. Mebendazole (100 mg twice daily, for four days) is an alternative therapeutic agent. The hyperinfection syndrome also seems to respond to mebendazole (Boyd, Campbell, and Trudeau, 1978); in that report, thiabendazole was not used, due to severe renal failure, but a successful result was achieved with mebendazole. Dithiazanine iodide is effective but is potentially toxic (Stemmermann and Nakasone, 1960); manufacture has ceased.

20.5.5. Species other than S. stercoralis

Infection with *S. fülleborni* has been reported from Zambia (Hira and Patel, 1977), where it accounts for 10 per cent of strongyloides infections. In the Western Province of Papua New Guinea, a syndrome occurs in children consisting of pot-belly, diarrhoea, steatorrhoea, and wasting, with occasional deaths. It has also been attributed to *S. fülleborni* (Kelly and Voge, 1973; Kelly, Little, and Voge, 1976; Ashford, Vince, Gratten, and Miles, 1978). In Zaire, it seems likely that infection with *S. fülleborni* can take place via human breast milk (Brown and Girardeau, 1977); that would account for the peak incidence of the disease in infancy and childhood in both Zaire and Papua New Guinea. *S fülleborni* is common in monkeys, apes, and baboons in Africa and Asia. It is known to infect man in Zambia (Buckley, 1946), and Zimbabwe Rhodesia (Blackie, 1932), and is also common in east Africa. Although *S. fülleborni* infections are common in Papua New Guinea (Kelly, *et al.*, 1976), non-human primates have never inhabited that country and the origin of the parasite there is thus obscure.

Nippostrongylus brasiliensis is an intestinal nematode which infects mice and rats. Its behaviour is very similar to that of *S. strongyloides* in man, and it has therefore been used in experiments designed to throw light on human strongyloidiasis. Impairment of rejection of *N. brasiliensis* has been demonstrated in iron and protein deficient rats (Cummins, Duncombe, Bolin, Davis, and Kelly, 1978); that probably results from a suppressed immune response. Using the mouse as an experimental model, evidence has been produced which suggests that marginal protein-energy malnutrition causes a decrease in the intensity of immunological rejection mechanisms, impairing the clearance of *N. brasiliensis*

(Tomkins, Madi, and Ogilvie, 1978). Those observations might partly explain why only some individuals with *S. strongyloides* infections have mucosal damage and malabsorption. They are also consistent with the parasite being an opportunist organism.

20.6. Other small-intestinal parasites associated with malabsorption

Other parasites also, have been implicated in tropical malabsorption, but less commonly than the two already mentioned. The two well-established organisms to be associated with malabsorption are: *Capillaria philippinensis* which is confined to the north Philippines and Thailand, and coccidia (*Isospora belli* and *I. hominis*) which occurs sporadically, in patchy distribution, throughout the tropics.

20.6.1. Capillaria philippinensis

This nematode occurs in a limited area of Central Luzon, which includes the north Philippines, near the South China sea. Although there are over 200 nematodes of the species, only *C. philippinensis* (Chitwood, Valesquez and Salazar, 1968) has been incriminated in human disease; the organism is related to *Trichuris trichiura*.

The life cycle is unknown, but infection is probably obtained by ingesting one of three species of marine fish. Infection can occur in epidemics. The adult worms live in the upper small-intestine where they invade the mucosa. An autoinfection cycle, similar to that in strongyloidiasis, can occur in man (Cross, Banzon, Clarke, Basaca-Servilla, Watten, and Dizon, 1972). A resulting malabsorption state develops in a heavy infection and is occasionally fatal; diarrhoea (Dizon and Watten, 1969), followed by muscle wasting and oedema, 1969).

Adult nematodes and ova can be found in the stool. Abdominal pain and diarrhoea (Dizon and Watten, 1969) followed by muscle wasting and oedema can lead to death within two to four months. There may be severe malabsorption and a protein-losing enteropathy (Watten, Beckner, Cross, Gunning, and Jarimillo, 1972). More than 1000 cases and over 100 deaths have been reported (Watten, *et al.*, 1972).

Fluid and electrolyte replacement are vital, and prolonged treatment with thiabendazole should be undertaken (Whalen, Rosenberg, Strickland, Gutman, Cross, Watten, Uylangco, and Dizon, 1969); the dose is thiabendazole, 12·5 mg per kg orally twice daily for 30 days. It seems probable that that agent should be continued for one to two months (Whalen, Rosenberg, Gutman, Cross, Fresh, Strickland, and Uylangco, 1971). There is a high incidence of side-effects, most of a gastrointestinal nature, and a high relapse-rate, especially after short courses of treatment. Recently, mebendazole has been shown to be effective in a dose of 100 mg four times daily for 20 days (Singson, Banzon, and Cross, 1975); there are no side-effects, and it seems at present to be the drug of choice.

20.6.2. Coccidiosis (Isosporosis)

Infection results from the ingestion of viable cysts of *Isospora belli* and *I.*

hominis. They are common in many parts of the tropics, including the Middle and Far east (Smitskamp and Oey-Muller, 1966); high incidence rates have also been reported from Rumania, Holland, and Chile. The protozoa multiply in human small-intestinal mucosa.

Most cases are asymptomatic, but in some, mild fever, lassitude, malaise, abdominal discomfort, and diarrhoea develop after approximately one week (Limbos, Fain, and de Mulder, 1965; Jarpa Gana, 1966). The disease is usually self-limiting after one or two weeks, but persistent diarrhoea, malabsorption (French, Whitby and Whitfield, 1964; Brandborg, Goldberg, and Breidenbach, 1970), and occasional deaths have been reported.

Stool concentration techniques are necessary to demonstrate the immature cysts of *I. belli* and the mature sporocysts of *I. hominis*; they may not be detected by routine laboratory stool examination (Henderson, Gillepsie, Kaplan, and Steber, 1963; Smitskamp and Oey-Muller, 1966). Serial sectioning of jejunal-biopsies is of value in identifying the various stages of the life cycle in the enterocyte (Brandborg, *et al.*, 1970). There may be morphological damage (Pout, 1967). A peripheral eosinophilia is present in up to 50 per cent of cases (Jarpa Gana, 1966).

There is no specific treatment at present.

20.6.3. Cryptosporidium

Cryptosporidia are protozoan parasites which inhabit the brush-border of the enterocyte in a variety of animals. To date this seems to be a rare infection of man. The possibility exists that *Cryptosporidium* can produce malabsorption (Meisel, Perera, Meligro, and Rubin, 1976) although clear evidence of that is lacking at present; in that study, an opportunistic infection with that organism occurred in an immunosuppressed patient. Diarrhoea occurred which was associated with small-intestinal abnormalities.

20.7. Pneumatosis (cystoides) intestinalis and malabsorption

This rare cause of malabsorption, in which unexplained cysts are present in the small intestine and ascending colon, has been reported in a 45-year-old Kikuyu man in Kenya (Miller, 1964). A similar disease can be produced in germ-free rats if *Cl. welchii* are injected into the peritoneal cavity, distal small-intestine or caecum (Yale, Baligh, and Wu, 1974). It seems possible therefore, that the condition results from clostridial toxins, and is thus comparable to enteritis necroticans (pig-bel disease) (Chapter 17).

References

Abrams, G. D. and Bishop, J. E. (1966). *J. Bact.*, **92,** 1604.

—— and —— (1967). *Proc. Soc. exp. Biol. Med.*, **126,** 301.

Adam, M., Morgan, O., Persaud, C., and Gibbs, W. N. (1973). *Br. med. J.*, **1,** 264.

Alcorn, M. O. and Kotcher, E. (1961). *Sth. med. J., Nashville*, **54,** 193.

Alp, M. H. and Hislop, I. G. (1969). *Australas. Ann. Med.*, **18,** 232.

Ament, M. E. and Rubin, C. E. (1972). *Gastroenterology*, **62,** 216.

Amini, F. (1963). *J. trop. Med. Hyg.*, **66,** 190.

Angel, C. R., Guerra, R., Martinez, J., and Plough, I. C. (1963). *Fedn Proc. Fedn Am. Socs exp. Biol.*, **22,** 550.

ANITA, F. P., DESAI, H. G., and JEEJEEBHOY, K. N. (1966). *Indian J. med. Sci.*, **20,** 471.
ANTHONY, P. P., VOGEL, C. L., SADIKALI, F., BARKER, L. F., and PETERSON, M. R. (1972). *Br. med. J.*, **1,** 403.
ASHFORD, R. W., VINCE, J. D., GRATTAN, M. J., and MILES, W. E. (1978). *Trans. R. Soc. trop. Med. Hyg.*, **72,** 554.
AYREY, F. (1948). *Trans. R. Soc. trop. Med. Hyg.*, **41,** 377.
BABB, R. R., PECK, O. C., and VESCIA, F. G. (1971). *J. Am. med. Ass.*, **217,** 1359.
BABOUR, A. G., NICHOLS, G. R. and FUKUSHIMA, T. (1976). *Am. J. trop. Med. Hyg.*, **25,** 384.
BADLEY, B. W. D., MURPHY, G. M. and BOUCHIER, I. A. D. (1969). *Lancet*, **2,** 400.
BAGSHAWE, A. F., PARKER, A. M., and JINDANI, A. (1971). *Br. med. J.*, **1,** 88.
BAHR, P. H. (1915). *A report on researches on sprue in Ceylon 1912—1914*. University Press, Cambridge.
BAKER, S. J. (1957). *Indian J. med. Sci.*, **11,** 687.
—— (1967). In *Tropical Medicine Conference, 1967* (ed. J. H. Walters). p. 65. Pitman Medical Publishing Co. Ltd., London.
—— (1972). *Br. med. Bull.*, **28,** 87.
—— (1974). In *The small intestine* (ed. B. Creamer). p. 115. Heinemann, London.
—— (1976). *Bull. Wld Hlth Org.*, **54,** 485.
——, IGNATIUS, M., MATHAN, V. I. VAISH, S. K. and CHACKO, C. C. (1962). In *Intestinal biopsy*. Ciba Foundation Study Group, no. 14 (ed. G. E. W. Wolstenholme and M. P. Cameron). p. 84. Churchill, London.
—— and MATHAN, V. I. (1968). *Am. J. clin. Nutr.*, **21,** 984.
—— and —— (1971). In *Tropical sprue and megaloblastic anaemia*, p. 189. Churchill Livingstone, Edinburgh and London.
—— and —— (1972). *Am. J. clin. Nutr.*, **25,** 1047.
BANWELL, J. G., CAMPBELL, J., BLACKMAN, V., HUTT, M. V., and LEONARD, P. (1963). *E. Afr. med. J.*, **40,** 277.
—— and GORBACH, S. L. (1969). *Gut*, **10,** 328.
——, HUTT, M. S. R., LEONARD, P. J., BLACKMAN, V., CONNOR, D. W., MARSDEN, P. D. and CAMPBELL, J. (1967). *Gut*, **8,** 388.
——, ——, and TUNNICLIFFE, R. (1964). *E. Afr. med. J.*, **41,** 46.
BARBOUR, A. G., NICHOLS, G. R., and FUKUSHIMA, T. (1976). *Am. J. trop. Med. Hyg.*, **25,** 384.
BASSILY, S., FARID, Z., MIKHAIL, J. W., KENT, D. C., and LEHMAN, J. S. (1970). *J. trop. Med. Hyg.*, **73,** 15.
BEAL, C. B., VIENS, P., GRANT, R. G. L., and HUGHES, J. M. (1970). *Am. J. trop. Med. Hyg.*, **19,** 349.
BEGG, C. (1912). *Sprue: its diagnosis and treatment*. p. 112. Wright and Sons, Bristol.
BEKER, S., RIVAS GÓMEZ, A., VALENCIA-PARPARCÉN, J., and MONCADA, P. R. (1963). *G.E.N., Caracas*, **17,** 285.
BESTERMAN, H. S., COOK, G. C., SARSON, D. L., CHRISTOFIDES, N. D., and BLOOM, S. R. (1978). *Gut*, **19,** A438.
——, ——, ——, ——, BRYANT, M. G., GREGOR, M. and BLOOM, S. R. (1979). *Br. med. J.*, **2,** 1252.
BEZMAN, A., KINNEAR, D. G., and ZAMCHECK, N. (1959). *J. Lab. clin. Med.*, **53,** 226.
BISHOP, R. F. (1963). *Br. J. exp. Path.*, **44,** 189.
BLACKIE, W. K. (1932). *Med. Mem. Ser., London School of Hygiene and Tropical Medicine*, **5,** 91.
BOOTH, C. C. (1964). *Gut*, **5,** 45.
—— and MOLLIN, D. L. (1964). *Am. J. dig. Dis.*, **9,** 770.
BOYD, W. P., CAMPELL, F. W., and TRUDEAU, W. L. (1978). *Am. J. trop. Med. Hyg.*, **27,** 39.
BRANDBORG, L. L., GOLDBERG, S. B., and BREIDENBACH, W. C. (1970). *New Engl. J. Med.*, **283,** 1306.

——, Tankersley, C. B., Gottlieb, S., Barancik, M., and Sartor, V. E. (1967). *Gastroenterology*, **52,** 143.
Bras, G., Richards, R. C., Irvine, R. A., Milner, P. F. A., and Ragbeer, M. M. S. (1964). *Lancet*, **2,** 1257.
Br. med. J., (1977). **2,** 538.
Brodsky, R. E., Spencer, H. C., and Schultz, M. G. (1974). *J. infect. Dis.*, **30,** 319.
Brown, H. W. and Perna, V. P. (1958). *J. Am. med. Ass.*, **168,** 1648.
Brown, R. C. and Girardeau, M. H. F. (1977). *Am. J. trop. Med. Hyg.*, **26,** 215.
Brown, W. C. (1908). *Sprue and its treatment*. John Bale, Sons and Danielsson, London.
Brown, W. R., Butterfield, D., Savage, D., and Tada, T. (1972). *Gut*, **13,** 441.
Buckley, J. J. C. (1946). *J. Helminth.*, **21,** 111.
Burman, D. (1965). *Archs Dis. Childh.*, **40,** 526.
Butterworth, C. E., Perez-Santiago, E., Martinez de Jesus, J., and Santini, R. (1959). *New Engl. J. Med.*, **261,** 157.
Cantlie, J. (1905). *Br. med. J.*, **2,** 1281.
Carmel, R. and Johnson, C. S. (1978). *New Engl. J. Med.*, **298,** 647.
Castellani, A. (1905). *Br. med. J.*, **2,** 1285.
Castle, W. B., Rhoads, C. P., Lawson, H. A., and Payne, G. C. (1935). *Archs intern. Med.*, **56,** 627.
Chevers, N. (1886). *A commentary on the diseases of India*. p. 561. Churchill, London.
Chitwood, M. P., Valesquez, C., and Salazar, N. G. (1968). *J. Parasit.*, **54,** 368.
Chuke, P. O., Traub, N. E., and Patel, I. C. (1972). *E. Afr. med. J.*, **49,** 681.
Cobden, I., Dickinson, R. J., Rothwell, J., and Axon, A. T. R. (1978). *Br. med. J.*, **2,** 1060.
Collins, J. R. (1965). *Am. J. clin. Path.*, **44,** 36.
Collins, J. P., Keller, K. F., and Brown, L. (1978). *Am. J. trop. Med. Hyg.*, **27,** 835.
Conrad, M. E., Schwartz, F. D., and Young, A. A. (1964). *Am. J. Med.*, **37,** 789.
Cook, G. C. (1967). *Br. med. J.*, **1,** 613.
—— (1971a). *Gut*, **12,** 1001.
—— (1971b). *J. Physiol., Lond.*, **217,** 61.
—— (1972). *Am. J. clin. Nutr.*, **25,** 490.
—— (1973a). *Nature, Lond.*, **241,** 284.
—— (1973b). *Br. J. Nutr.*, **29,** 377.
—— (1973c). *Br. J. Nutr.*, **30,** 13.
—— (1974a). *Trans. R. Soc. trop. Med. Hyg.*, **68,** 419.
—— (1974b). *Br. med. J.*, **4,** 200.
—— (1974c). *Br. J. Nutr.*, **32,** 163.
—— (1974d). *J. Physiol., Lond.*, **237,** 187.
—— (1974e). *Br. J. Nutr.*, **32,** 503.
—— (1974f). *Gut*, **15,** 239.
—— (1975). *Trans. R. Soc. trop. Med. Hyg.*, **69,** 143.
—— (1976a). *Gut*, **17,** 252.
—— (1976b). *Gut*, **17,** 604.
—— (1976c). *Trans. R. Soc. trop. Med. Hyg.*, **70,** 349.
—— (1976d). *Br. med. J.*, **1,** 688.
—— (1977a). *Am. J. Gastroent., N.Y.*, **67,** 570.
—— (1977b). *Am. J. clin. Nutr.*, **30,** 1994.
—— (1977c). *Scand. J. Gastroent.*, **12,** 733.
—— (1977d). In *1976—7 Annual Report. London School of Hygiene and Tropical Medicine*, London. p. 65.
—— (1978a). *Br. med. J.*, **2,** 238.
—— (1978b). *Jl. R. Coll. Phycns.*, **12,** 329.
—— (1978c). *Trans. R. Soc. trop. Med. Hyg.*, **72,** 277.

—— (1979a). *Trop. geogr. Med.*, **31,** 93.
—— (1979b). *Am. J. clin. Nutr.*, in press.
——, Asp, N-G and Dahlqvist, A. (1973). *Gastroenterology*, **64,** 405.
—— and Carruthers, R. H. (1974). *Gut*, **15,** 545.
—— and Hutt, M. S. R. (1967). *Br. med. J.*, **3,** 454.
—— and Kajubi, S. K. (1966). *Lancet*, **1,** 725.
—— (1972). In *Medicine in a tropical environment* (ed. A. G. Shaper, J. W. Kibukamusoke, and M. S. R. Hutt). p. 364. British Medical Association, London.
——, ——, and Lee, F. D. (1969). *J. Path.*, **98,** 157.
—— and Lee, F. D. (1966). *Lancet*, **2,** 1263.
——, Morgan, J. O. and Hoffbrand, A. V. (1974). *Lancet*, **2,** 1416.
Cortner, J. A. (1959). *Am. J. Dis. Child.*, **98,** 311.
Craven, J. L., Cantrell, E. G., and Lewis, M. G. (1971). *Trans. R. Soc. trop. Med. Hyg.*, **65,** 532.
Creamer, B., Dutz, W., and Post, C. (1970). *Lancet*, **1,** 18.
Crombie, A. (1880). *Indian med. Gaz.*, **15,** 313.
Cross, J. H., Banzon, T., Clarke, M. D., Basaca-Servilla, V., Watten, R. H., and Dizon, J-J (1972). *Trans. R. Soc. trop. Med. Hyg.*, **66,** 819.
Cummins, A. G., Duncombe, V. M., Bolin, T. D., Davis, A. E., and Kelly, J. D. (1978). *Gut*, **19,** 823.
Da Costa, L. R. (1971). *Br. med. J.*, **3,** 281.
Dawson, A. M. (1965). *Abstr. Wld Med.*, **38,** 361.
Dawson, D. W. (1971). *J. clin. Path.*, **24,** 131.
Deller, D. J., Murrell, T. G. C., and Blowes, R. (1967). *Australas. Ann. Med.*, **16,** 236.
De Paola, D. (1961). *Patologia da Estrongiloidiase.* Clinica da Faculdade de Medicina, Rio de Janeiro.
Diamond, J. M. (1978). *Nature, Lond.*, **271,** 111.
Dickson, W. P. (1871). *Indian med.Gaz.*, **6,** 47.
Dixon, J. M. S. and Paulley, J. W. (1963). *Gut*, **4,** 169.
Dizon, J. J. and Watten, R. H. (1968). *J. Philipp. med. Ass.*, **45,** 5.
Dobell, C. (1920). *Proc. R. Soc. Med.*, **13,** 1.
Dossetor, J. F. B. and Whittle, H. C. (1975). *Br. med. J.*, **2,** 592.
Drew, R., Dixon, K., and Samuel, E. (1947). *Lancet*, **1,** 129.
Drummond, M. B. and Montgomery, R. D. (1970). *Br. med. J.*, **2,** 340.
Duncan, A. (1905). *Br. med. J.*, **2,** 1283.
Duque, E., Bolaños, O., Lotero, H., and Mayoral, L. G. (1975). *Am. J. clin. Nutr.*, **28,** 901.
——, Lotero, H., Bolaños, O. and Mayoral, L. G. (1975). *Am. J. clin. Nutr.*, **28,** 914.
Dwork, K. G., Jaffe, J. R., and Leiberman, H. (1975). *N.Y. St. J. Med.*, **75,** 1230.
Dyer, N. H. and Dawson, A. M. (1968). *Br. med. J.*, **2,** 161 and 225.
Dymock, I. W., Mackay, N., Miller, V., Thomson, T. J., Gray, B., Kennedy, E. H., and Adams, J. F. (1967). *Br. J. Cancer*, **21,** 505.
Eastham, E. J. Douglas, A. P., and Watson, A. J. (1976). *Lancet*, **2,** 950.
Edington, G. M. and Gilles, H. M. (1976). *Pathology in the tropics.* 2nd ed. p. 31 and 528. Edward Arnold, London.
Elder, H. H. A. (1947). *J. trop. Med. Hyg.*, **50,** 212.
El Masry, N. A., Farid, Z., and Miner, W. F. (1978). *Am. J. trop. Med. Hyg.*, **27,** 201.
England, N. W. J. and O'Brien, W. (1966). *Gut*, **7,** 128.
Fairley, N. H. (1936). *Trans. R. Soc. trop. Med. Hyg.*, **30,** 9.
—— and Mackie, F. P. (1926). *Indian J. med. Res.*, **14,** 105.
Falaiye, J. M. (1969). *W. Afr. med. J.*, **18,** 71.
—— (1970). *J. trop. Med. Hyg.*, **73,** 119.
—— (1971). *Br. med. J.*, **4,** 454.

—— and Oladapo, J. M. (1971). *W. Afr. med. J.*, **20,** 265.
Fantham, H. B. (1916). *Lancet*, **1,** 1165.
Farahmandian, I., Sheiban, F., and Sanati, A. (1978). *J. trop. Med. Hyg.*, **81,** 139.
Fayrer, J. (1881). *Tropical dysentery and chronic diarrhoea.* p. 127. Churchill, London.
Fleming, A. F. (1968). *W. Afr. med. J.*, **17,** 25.
Floch, M. H. (1969). *Am. J. clin. Nutr.*, **22,** 327.
Forshaw, J. (1969). *J. clin. Path.*, **22,** 551.
Foster, R. M. (1968). *E. Afr. med. J.*, **45,** 673.
Foy, H. and Kondi, A. (1956). *Lancet*, **1,** 423.
—— and —— (1958). *Trans. R. Soc. trop. Med. Hyg.*, **52,** 46.
—— and —— (1971). In *Tropical sprue and megaloblastic anaemia.* p. 261. Churchill Livingstone, Edinburgh and London.
——, ——, and Hargreaves, A. (1952). *Trans. R. Soc. trop. Med. Hyg.*, **46,** 327.
Frazer, A. C. (1968). *Malabsorption syndromes.* Heinemann, London.
French, J. M., Whitby, J. L., and Whitfield, A. G. W. (1964). *Gastroenterology*, **47,** 642.
Galloway, D. J. (1905a). *Br. med. J.*, **2,** 1284.
—— (1905b). *J. trop. Med. Hyg.*, **8,** 289.
Garcia, F. T., Sessions, J. T., Strum, W. B., Schweistris, E., Tripathy, K., Bolaños, O., Lotero, H., Duque, E., Ramelli, D., and Mayoral, L. G. (1977). *Am. J. trop. Med. Hyg.*, **26,** 859.
Garcia Lopez, G., Milanes, F., Spies, T. D., Lopez Toca, R., Aramburu, T., and Lopez, H. (1949). *Am. J. med. Sci.*, **218,** 660.
Gardner, F. H. (1958). *New Engl. J. Med.*, **258,** 791.
Gelfand, M. (1947). *Trans. R. Soc. trop. Med. Hyg.*, **41,** 109.
Gill, G. V., Bell, D. R., and Reid, H. A. (1977). *Br. med. J.*, **1,** 1007.
Gilles, H. M., Williams, E. J. W., and Ball, P. A. J. (1964). *Q. Jl. Med.*, **33,** 1.
Goel, K. M., Shanks, R. A., McAllister, T. A., and Follett, E. A. C., (1977). *Br. med. J.*, **1,** 676.
Goodeve, E. (1866). In *A system of medicine* (ed. J. R. Reynolds). **1,** p. 82. Macmillan, London.
Gorbach, S. L., Banwell, J. G., Mitra, R., Chatterjee, B. D., Jacobs, B., and Guha Mazumder, D. N. (1969). *Lancet*, **1,** 74.
——, Plaut, A. G., Nahas, L., Weinstein, L., Spanknebel, G., and Levitan, R. (1967). *Gastroenterology*, **53,** 856.
Gracey, M., Suharjono, Sunoto, and Stone, D. E. (1973). *Am. J. clin. Nutr.*, **26,** 1170.
Grant, A. (1854). *Indian Annls med. Sci.*, **1.** 2nd ed. p. 311. Calcutta and London.
Green, W. A. (1854). *Indian Annls med. Sci.*, **1,** 516.
Grove, S. S. and Elsdon-Dew, R. (1958). *Sth. Afr. J. Lab. clin. Med.*, **4,** 55.
Haeney, M. R., Culank, L. S., Montgomery, R. D., and Sammons, H. G. (1978). *Gastroenterology*, **75,** 393.
——, Montgomery, R. D., and Schneider, R. (1974). *Gut*, **15,** 377.
Halsted, C. H. (1975). *Nutr. Rev.*, **33,** 33.
——, Sheir, S., Sourial, N., and Patwardhan, V. N. (1969). *Am. J. clin. Nutr.*, **22,** 744.
Harries, J. R. (1964). *E. Afr. med. J.*, **41,** 180.
Hartong, W. A. and Arvanitakis, C. (1977). *J. Am. med. Ass.*, **237,** 1078.
Hartz, P. H. (1946). *Archs Path.*, **41,** 601.
Hellier, M. D., Radhakrishnan, A. N., Ganapathy, V., Mathan, V. I., and Baker, S. J. (1976). *Gut*, **17,** 511.
Hemmings, W. A. and Williams, E. W. (1978). *Gut*, **19,** 715.
Henderson, H. E., Gillepsie, G. W., Kaplan, P., and Steber, M. (1963). *Am. J. Hyg.*, **78,** 302.
Hermos, J., Adams, W., Liu, Y., Sullivan, L., and Trier, J. (1971). *Clin. Res.*, **19,** 394.

HILL, M. J., CROWTHER, J. S., DRASAR, B. S., HAWKSWORTH, G., ARIES, V., and WILLIAMS, R. E. O. (1971). *Lancet*, **1,** 95.
HILLARY, W. (1766). *Observations on the changes of the air and the concomitant epidemical diseases, in the island of Barbadoes.* 2nd. ed. p. 276. Hawes, Clarke and Collins, London.
HINDLE, W. and CREAMER, B. (1965). *Br. med. J.*, **2,** 455.
HIRA, P. R. and PATEL, B. G. (1977). *Am. J. trop. Med. Hyg.*, **26,** 640.
HOWAT, H. T. (1944). *Lancet*, **2,** 560.
JAMES. W. P. T. (1968). *Lancet*, **1,** 333.
JARNUM, S., JEEJEEBHOY, K. N., and SINGH, B. (1968). *Br. med. J.*, **4,** 416.
JARPA GANA, A. (1966). *Biológica, Santiago*, **39,** 3.
JEFFRIES, G. H., WESER, E., and SLEISENGER, M. H. (1969). *Gastroenterology*, **56,** 777.
JOKIPII, A. M. M. and JOKIPII, L. (1977). *Lancet*, **1,** 1095.
—— and —— (1978). *Am. J. trop. Med. Hyg.*, **27,** 758.
JONES, T. C., DEAN, A. C., and PARKER, G. W. (1972). *Am. J. Epidemiol.*, **95,** 111.
KAJUBI, S. K. and OKEL, R. M. (1973). *Afr. J. med. Sci.*, **4,** 403.
KARNEY, W. W. and TONG, M. J. (1972). *Am. J. trop. Med. Hyg.*, **21,** 1.
KEELE, K. D. and BOUND, J. P. (1946). *Br. med. J.*, **1,** 77.
KEETON, G. R. (1972). *S. Afr. med. J.*, **46,** 1170.
KELLY, A., LITTLE, M. D., and VOGE, M. (1976). *Am. J. trop. Med. Hyg.*, **25,** 694.
—— and VOGE, M. (1973). *Papua New Guin. med. J.*, **16,** 59.
KENT, T. H., FORMAL, S. B., and LA BREC, E. H. (1966). *Archs Path.*, **81,** 501.
KING, M. J. and JOSKE, R. A. (1960). *Br. med. J.*, **1,** 1324.
KIVEL, R. M., KEARNS, D. H., and LIEBOWITZ, D. (1964). *New Engl. J. Med.*, **271,** 769.
KLIPSTEIN, F. A. (1968). *Gastroenterology*, **54,** 275.
—— (1969). *Blood*, **34,** 191.
—— (1971). In *Tropical sprue and megaloblastic anaemia.* p. 129. Churchill Livingstone, Edinburgh and London.
—— and CORCINO, J. J. (1975). *Gastroenterology*, **68,** 239.
—— and ENGERT, R. F. (1978). *Gastroenterology*, **75,** 255.
——, ——, and SHORT, H. B. (1978). *Lancet*, **2,** 342.
——, HOLDEMAN, L. V., CORCINO, J. J., and MOORE, W. E. C. (1973). *Ann. intern. Med.*, **79,** 632.
——, SAMLOFF, I. M., and SCHENK, E. A. (1966). *Ann. intern. med.*, **64,** 575.
——, ——, SMARTH, G., and SCHENK, E. (1968). *Am. J. clin. Nutr.*, **21,** 1042.
—— and SMARTH, G. (1969). *Am. J. dig. Dis.*, **14,** 887.
KOTCHER, E., MIRANDA, M., ESQUIVEL, R. R., PEÑA-CHAVARRÍA, A., DONOHUGH, D. L., BALDIZÓN, C., ACOSTA, G. A., and APUY, J. L. (1966). *Gastroenterology*, **50,** 366
Lancet (1944). **2,** 630.
—— (1974). **2,** 1493.
—— (1977a). **1,** 1347.
—— (1977b). **1,** 1293.
LAYRISSE, M., BLUMENFELD, N., CARBONELL, L., DESENNE, J., and ROCHE, M. (1964). *Am. J. trop. Med. Hyg.*, **13,** 297.
LEISHMAN, A. W. D. (1945). *Lancet*, **2,** 813.
LEVI, G. C., DE ÁVILA, C. A., and NETO, V. A. (1977). *Am. J. trop. Med. Hyg.*, **26,** 564.
LEVINSON, J. D. and NASTRO, L. J. (1978). *Gastroenterology*, **74,** 271.
LIMBOS, P. (1956). *Annls Soc. belge Méd. trop.*, **36,** 151.
——, FAIN, A., and DE MULDER, P. (1965). *Trop. geogr. Med.*, **17,** 169.
LINDENBAUM, J. (1965). *Br. med. J.*, **2,** 326.
—— (1969). *Ann. intern. Med.*, **70,** 1277.
—— (1973). *Gastroenterology*, **64,** 637.
——, ALAM, A. K. M. J., and KENT, T. H. (1966). *Br. med. J.*, **2,** 1616.
——, KENT, T. H., and SPRINZ, H. (1966). *Ann. intern. Med.*, **65,** 1201.

——, PEZZIMENTI, J. F., and SHEA, N. (1974). *Ann. intern. Med.*, **80,** 326.
LOSOWSKY, M. S., WALKER, B. E., and KELLEHER, J. (1974). *Malabsorption in clinical practice.* Churchill Livingstone, Edinburgh and London.
LOW, G. C. (1928). *Q. Jl. Med.*, **21,** 523.
LOWENTHAL, M., BANATVALA, J. E., CHRYSTIE, I. L., JONES, I. G., NAG, J., MOHELSKY, V., and HUTT, M. S. R. (1973). *Trop. geogr. Med.*, **25,** 39.
McGRATH, J., O'FARRELL, P. T., and BOLAND, S. J. (1940). *Irish J. med. Sci.*, **6,** 802.
MACKIE, F. P. and FAIRLEY, N. H. (1929). *Indian J. med. Res.*, **16,** 799.
——, GORÉ, S. N., and WADIA, J. H. (1928). *Indian J. med. Res.*, **16,** 95.
MACLEAN, W. C. (1886). *Diseases of tropical climates.* p. 157. MacMillan, London.
MACLEAN, W. E. (1866). In *A system of medicine* (ed. J. R. Reynolds). **1,** p. 106. Macmillan, London.
MAHALANABIS, D., JACOBS, B., BANWELL, J. G., MUKHERJI, K. L., and BOSE, S. K. (1972). *Annls Inst. Chld Hlth Calcutta*, **1,** 15.
MANSON, P. (1880). *China. Imperial Maritime Customs II—Special series* No. 2. Medical Reports for the half year ended 31st March, 1880. p. 33. 19th issue. Statistical department of the Inspectorate General, Shanghai.
—— (1898). *Tropical Diseases. A manual of the diseases of warm climates.* p. 322. Cassell and Co. Ltd., London.
MANSON-BAHR, P. H. (1928). *Trans. R. Soc. trop. Med. Hyg.*, **22,** 81.
—— (1953). *Lancet*, **2,** 389.
—— and WILLOUGHBY, H. (1930). *Q. Jl. Med.*, **23,** 411.
MARTIN, J. R. (1856). *The influence of tropical climates on European constitutions.* p. 496. Churchill, London.
MATHAN, M., MATHAN, V. I., SWAMINATHAN, S. P., YESUDOSS, S., and BAKER, S. J. (1975). *Lancet*, **1,** 1068.
MATHAN, V. I. and BAKER, S. J. (1968). *Am. J. clin. Nutr.*, **21,** 1077.
——, IGNATIUS, M., and BAKER, S. J. (1966). *Gut*, **7,** 490.
MATTHEWS, D. M. (1971). *J. clin. Path.*, **24,** Suppl. **5,** 29.
MAYORAL, L. G., BOLAÑOS, O., LOTERO, H., and DUQUE, E. (1975). *Am. J. clin. Nutr.*, **28,** 894.
——, TRIPATHY, K., GARCIA, F. T., BOLAÑOS, O. and GHITIS, J. (1968). *Am. J. clin. Nutr.*, **21,** 1053.
——, ——, ——, and GHITIS, J. (1966). *Gastroenterology*, **50,** 856.
——, ——, ——, and —— (1967). *Gastroenterology*, **53,** 507.
MEGAW, J. W. D. and GUPTA, J. C. (1927). *Indian med. Gaz.*, **62,** 299.
MEHTA, S. K., KAUR, S., AVASTHI, G., WIG, N. N., and CHHUTTANI, P. N. (1972). *Am. J. clin. Nutr.*, **25,** 545.
——, NAIK, S. R., KRISHNAN, S., NAIN, C. K., and SEHGAL, S. (1978). *J. trop. Med. Hyg.*, **81,** 131.
MEISEL, J. L., PERERA, D. R., MELIGRO, C., and RUBIN, C. E. (1976). *Gastroenterology*, **70,** 1156.
MENZIES, I. S. (1972). *Gut*, **13,** 847.
MERSON, M. H., MORRIS, G. K., SACK, D. A., WELLS, J. G., FEELEY, J. C., BRADLEY SACK, R., CREECH, W. B., KAPIKIAN, A. Z., and GANGAROSA, E. J. (1976). *New Engl. J. Med.*, **294,** 1299.
MEUWISSEN, J. H. E. T., TONGEREN, J. H. M. V., and WERKMAN, H. P. T. (1977). *Lancet*, **2,** 33.
MILLER, J. R. M. (1964). *E. Afr. med. J.*, **41,** 194.
MILNER, P. F., IRVINE, R. A., BARTON, C. J., BRAS, G., and RICHARDS, R. (1965). *Gut*, **6,** 574.
MISRA, R. C., KASTHURI, D., and CHUTTANI, H. K. (1966). *Br. med. J.*, **2,** 1230.
MOLLIN, D. L. (1967). In *Tropical Medicine Conference, 1967* (ed. J. H. Walters). p. 96. Pitman Medical Publishing Co. Ltd., London.

—— and Booth, C. C. (1971). In *Tropical sprue and megaloblastic anaemia.* p. 61. Churchill Livingstone, Edinburgh and London.

Montgomery, R. D., Beale, D. J., Sammons, H. G., and Schneider, R. (1973). *Br. med. J.*, **2,** 265.

——, Haeney, M. R., Ross, I. N., Sammons, H. G., Barford, A. V., Balakrishnan, S., Mayer, P. P., Culank, L. S., Field, J., and Gosling, P. (1978). *Q. Jl. Med.*, **47,** 197.

Moore, G. T., Cross, W. M., McGuire, D., Mollohan, C. S., Gleason, N. N., Healy, G. R., and Newton, L. H. (1969). *New Engl. J. Med.*, **281,** 402.

Moore, W. J. (1886). *A manual of the diseases of India.* 2nd ed. p. 162. Churchill, London.

Morecki, R. and Parker, J. G. (1967). *Gastroenterology*, **52,** 151.

Morehead, C. (1860). *Clinical Researches on disease in India.* 2nd ed. p. 316. Longman, Green, Longman and Roberts, London.

Moshal, M. G. (1970). *Lancet*, **2,** 827.

——, Hift, W., Kallichurum, S., and Pillay, K. (1973). *S. Afr. med. J.*, **47,** 1093.

Nalin, D. R., Levine, R. J., Levine, M. M., Hoover, D., Bergquist, E., McLaughlin, J., Libonati, J., Alam, J., and Hornick, R. B. (1978). *Lancet*, **2,** 856.

——, Levine, M. M., Rhead, J., Bergquist, E., Rennels, M., Hughes, T., O'Donnell, S., and Hornick, R. B. (1978). *Lancet*, **2,** 859.

Napier, L. E. (1949). *J. trop. Med. Hyg.*, **52,** 25.

Nicholls, L. (1919). *J. trop. Med. Hyg.*, **22,** 21.

Nwokolo, C. and Imohiosen, E. A. E. (1973). *Br. med. J.*, **2,** 153.

O'Brien, W. (1967). In *Tropical Medicine Conference, 1967* (ed. J. H. Walters). p. 86. Pitman Medical Publishing Co. Ltd., London.

—— (1975). *Trans. R. Soc. trop. Med. Hyg.*, **69,** 69.

—— and England, N. W. J. (1966). *Br. med. J.*, **2,** 1157.

—— and —— (1971). In *Tropical sprue and megaloblastic anaemia.* p. 25. Churchill Livingstone, Edinburgh and London.

Olsson, R. A. and Johnston, E. H. (1969). *Am. J. trop. Med. Hyg.*, **18,** 335.

Ophüls, W. (1929). *Archs Path.*, **8,** 1.

Paola, D. de Dias, L. B., and da Silva, R. J. (1962). *Am. J. dig. Dis.*, **7,** 1086.

Perea, V. D., Fernan-Zegarra, L., Cruz, V. M., Ballon, R., and Picoaga, J. L. (1978). *Lancet*, **2,** 550.

Peters, T. J., Jones, P. E., Wells, G., and Cook, G. C. (1979). *Clin. Sci. molec. Med.*, **56,** 479.

Petersen, H. (1972). *Scand. J. Gastroent.*, 7, Suppl. **14,** 1.

Pettersson, T. (1975). *Br. med. J.*, **1,** 395.

Pitney, W. R. and Jones, P. B. (1966). *Papua New Guin. med. J.*, **9,** 79.

Poltera, A. A. (1972). *Trans. R. Soc. trop. Med. Hyg.*, **66,** 520.

—— (1974). *Ann. trop. Med. Parasit.*, **68,** 81.

Porter, A. (1916). *Lancet*, **1,** 1166.

Poskitt, E. M. E. (1972). *Trans. R. Soc. trop. Med. Hyg.*, **66,** 931.

Pout, D. D. (1967). *Nature, Lond.*, **213,** 306.

Powell, K. C., Soatt, M., and Booth, K. (1970). *Papua New Guin. med. J.*, **13,** 56.

Pringle, J. (1764). *Observations on the diseases of the Army.* 4th ed. p. 224. Millar, Wilson and Durham, London.

Purtilo, D. T., Meyers, W. M., and Connor, D. H. (1974). *Am. J. Med.*, **56,** 488.

Reynolds, E. H., Hallpike, J. F., Phillips, B. M., and Matthews, D. M. (1965). *J. clin. Path.*, **18,** 593.

Ridley, M. J. and Ridley, D. S. (1976). *J. clin. Path.*, **29,** 30.

Rivera, E., Maldonado, N., Vélez-García, E. Grillo, A. J., and Malaret, G. (1970). *Ann. intern. Med.*, **72,** 199.

Rogers, L. (1913). *Dysenteries. Their differentiation and treatment.* p. 303. Oxford University Press, London.

ROSENBERG, I. H. (1969). *Am. J. clin. Nutr.*, **22,** 284.
ROWE, B., TAYLOR, J., and BETTELHEIM, K. A. (1970). *Lancet*, **1,** 1.
RUSSELL, P. K., AZIZ, M. A., AHMAD, N., KENT, T. H., and GANGAROSA, E. J. (1966). *Am. J. dig. Dis.*, **11,** 296.
SACK, R. B. (1976). *New Engl. J. Med.*, **295,** 893.
SAHA, T. K. and GHOSH, T. K. (1977). *Gastroenterology*, **72,** 402.
SALIH, S. Y. and ABDALLA, R. E. (1977). *J. trop. Med. Hyg.*, **80,** 11.
SCHREIBER, D. S., BLACKLOW, N. R., and TRIER, J. S. (1973). *New Engl. J. Med.*, **288,** 1318.
SCHULTZ, M. G. (1975). *J. Am. med. Ass.*, **233,** 1383.
SHEEHY, T. W., COHEN, W. C., and BRODSKY, J. P. (1963). *Am. J. dig. Dis.*, **8,** 826.
——, ——, WALLACE, D. K., and LEGTERS, L. J. (1965). *J. Am. med. Ass.*, **194,** 1069.
——, MERONEY, W. H., COX, R. S., and SOLER, J. E. (1962). *Gastroenterology*, **42,** 148.
SHINGLETON, W. W. and DOBBINS, W. O. (1968). *Malabsorption syndromes.* C. C. Thomas, Illinois.
SIANG, S. C., ENGLAND, N. W. J., and O'BRIEN, W. (1966). *Trans. R. Soc. trop. Med. Hyg.*, **60,** 668.
SIMPSON, G. E. C. (1975). *Med. J. Aust.*, **1,** 601.
SINGSON, C. N., BANZON, T. C., and CROSS, J. H. (1975). *Am. J. trop. Med. Hyg.*, **24,** 932.
SMITSKAMP, H. and OEY-MULLER, E. (1966). *Trop. geogr. Med.*, **18,** 133.
SPRINZ, H., SRIBHIBHADH, R., GANGAROSA, E. J., BENYAJATI, C., KUNDEL, D., and HALSTEAD, S. (1962). *Am. J. clin. Path.*, **38,** 43.
STANFIELD, J. P., HUTT, M. S. R., and TUNNICLIFFE, R. (1965). *Lancet*, **2,** 519.
STANNUS, H. S. (1942). *Trans. R. Soc. trop. Med. Hyg.*, **36,** 123.
STEFANINI, M. (1948). *Medicine, Baltimore*, **27,** 379.
STEMMERMANN, G. N. and NAKASONE, N. (1960). *J. Am. med. Ass.*, **174,** 1250.
STERNER, G., LANTORP, K., and LIDMAN, K. (1971). *Nord. med.*, **86,** 1343.
SUAREZ, R. M. (1938). *Ann. intern. Med.*, **121,** 529.
SULIMAN, G. I. (1978). *Gut*, **19,** 121.
TANDON, B. N., DAS, B. C., SARAYA, A. K., and DEO, M. G. (1966). *Br. med. J.*, **1,** 714.
——, MAGOTRA, M. L., SARAYA, A. K., and RAMALINGASWAMI, V. (1968). *Am. J. clin. Nutr.*, **21,** 813.
——, SARAYA, A. K., RAMACHANDRAN, K. and SAMA, S. K. (1969). *Gut*, **10,** 360.
——, TANDON, R. K., SATPATHY, B. K. and SHRINIWAS (1977). *Gut*, **18,** 176.
TASKER, P. W. G. (1961) *Trans. R. Soc. trop. Med. Hyg.*, **55,** 272.
TAUTE, M. (1919). *Arch. Schiffs- u. Tropenhyg.*, **23,** 523.
THIN, G. (1890). *Br. med. J.*, 1357.
—— (1897)). *Psilosis or 'sprue'. Its nature and treatment.* 2nd ed. Churchill, London.
THOMAS, G. and CLAIN, D. J. (1976). *Gut*, **17,** 877.
——, ——, and WICKS, A. C. B. (1976). *Gut*, **17,** 888.
TOH, C. C. S. and CHOW, K. W. (1969). *Ann. trop. Med. Parasit.*, **63,** 493.
TOMKINS, A. M., DRASAR, B. S., and JAMES, W. P. T. (1975). *Lancet*, **1,** 59.
——, JAMES, W. P. T., WALTERS, J. H., and COLE, A. C. E. (1974). *Br. med. J.*, **3,** 380.
——, MADI, K., and OGILVIE, B. M. (1978). *Proc. Nutr. Soc.*, **37,** 10A.
——, WRIGHT, S. G., DRASAR, B. S. and JAMES, W. P. T. (1976). *Gut*, **17,** 397.
TRIPATHY, K., DUQUE, E., BOLAÑOS, O., LOTERO, H., and MAYORAL, L. G. (1972). *Am. J. clin. Nutr.*, **25,** 1276.
TRONCALE, F. J., MILLER, L. H. KEUSCH, G. T., COMER, D. S., CHITTAYASOTHORN, K., PETCHKIT, W., and NYE, S. W. (1968). *Gastroenterology*, **54,** 1122.
TROWELL, H. C. (1960). In *Non-infective disease in Africa.* p. 213. Edward Arnold, London.
TWINING, W. (1835). *Clinical illustrations of the more important diseases of Bengal with*

the result of an inquiry into their pathology and treatment. 2nd ed. **1,** p. 177 and 203. Baptist Mission Press, Calcutta.

Van Heerden, P. D. R., Grieve, R., and Metz, J. (1966). *Trans. R. Soc. trop. Med. Hyg.*, **60,** 241.

Walia, B. N. S., Sidhu, J. K., Tandon, B. N., Ghai, O. P., and Bhargava, S. (1966). *Br. med. J.*, **2,** 1233.

Walters, J. H. (1947). *Lancet*, **1,** 861.

Walzer, P. D., Wolfe, M. S., and Schultz, M. G. (1971). *J. infect. Dis.*, **124,** 235.

Warren, P. M., Pepperman, M. A., and Montgomery, R. D. (1978). *Lancet*, **2,** 849.

Warwick, R. and Williams, P. L. (1973). eds. *Gray's Anatomy.* 35th ed. p. 1281. Longman Group Ltd., Edinburgh.

Watten, R. H., Beckner, W. M., Cross, J. H., Gunning, J-J., and Jarimillo, J. (1972). *Trans. R. Soc. trop. Med. Hyg.*, **66,** 828.

Weir, K., Bank, S., Novis, B., and Marks, I. N. (1972). *S. Afr. med. J.*, **46,** 505.

Wells, R. (1958). *Trans. R. Soc. trop. Med. Hyg.*, **52,** 431.

Whalen, G. E., Rosenberg, E. B., Gutman, R. A., Cross, J., Fresh, J. W., Strickland, T., and Uylangco, C. (1971). *Am. J. trop. Med. Hyg.*, **20.** 95.

——, ——, Strickland, G. T., Gutman, R. A., Cross, J. H., Watten, R. H., Uylangco, C., and Dizon, J. J. (1969). *Lancet*, **1,** 13.

Wharton, B., Howells, G., and Phillips, I. (1968). *Br. med. J.*, **4,** 608.

Willcox, M. (1975). *Br. med. J.*, **3,** 101.

Williams, A. O. and Osotimehin, B. (1970). *Ghana med. J.*, **9,** 23.

Willis, A. J. P. and Nwokolo, C. (1966). *Lancet*, **1,** 1396.

Wilson, S. and Thompson, A. E. (1964). *J. Path. Bact.*, **87,** 169.

Winawer, S. J., Sullivan, L. W., Herbert, V., and Zamcheck, N. (1965). *New Engl. J. Med.*, **272,** 892.

Wokes, F., Badenoch, J. and Sinclair, H. M. (1955). *Am. J. clin. Nutr.*, **3,** 375.

Wolfe, M. S. (1975). *J. Am. med. Ass.*, **233,** 1362.

Woodruff, A. W. (1949). *Trans. R. Soc. trop. Med. Hyg.*, **42,** 605.

Wright, S. G., Tomkins, A. M., and Ridley, D. S. (1977). *Gut*, **18,** 343.

Yale, L. E., Baligh, L. E., and Wu, J. P. (1974). *Archs Surg.*, **109,** 89.

Yardley, J. H., Takano, J., and Hendrix, T. R. (1964). *Bull. Johns Hopkins Hosp.*, **115,** 389.

21

Primary and secondary hypolactasia (lactase-deficiency)

Low intestinal lactase activity may be specific (*primary*); in that case all other disaccharidases are present at normal concentration and the small-intestinal mucosa is morphologically normal. However, low activity may also be *secondary* to damage of the brush-border of the enterocyte and loss of mucosal integrity; that sometimes occurs in postinfective tropical malabsorption ('tropical sprue') (Chapter 20) and after other small-intestinal infections (Chapter 17).

21.1. Specific (primary) adult hypolactasia

During the last few years it has become clear that the vast majority of the world's *adult* population, and that includes nearly all of those people indigenous to tropical countries, has a low concentration of jejunal lactase; that results in the incomplete hydrolysis of lactose at the brush-border of the enterocyte (Cook, 1973; 1974; 1978a); absorption of lactose is therefore incomplete. A minority of human adults retains a high concentration of lactase throughout life. Persistence of a high concentration of intestinal lactase into adult life (PL) is rarely found in the animal kingdom (Cook, 1969; 1973; Morris, Trudell, and Pencovic, 1977), and is confined to a small proportion of *Homo sapiens*. That conclusion is contrary to opinion held two decades ago, when low lactase activity in man was thought to be very unusual. Adult hypolactasia is therefore the normal state for the mammalian kingdom; the exception is the minority with PL.

It is now clear that the adult lactase concentration is not influenced by milk or lactose intake, but is under genetic control (Cook, 1973).

Working in Uganda, Cook and Kajubi (1966) demonstrated that whereas lactase was absent in most African adults (adult hypolactasia), those with an Hamitic ancestry (Fig 21.1) had PL. They also produced evidence that PL was not substrate related (i.e. dependent upon milk-drinking); neither was it related to any other environmental factor examined. It seemed therefore to have a genetic basis, and they suggested that it might not only be important in human nutrition, but could also be a valuable ethnological marker (Cook, 1968; 1969). McMichael, Webb, and Dawson (1965) had previously formed an impression that a genetic factor might be involved from limited studies on Greek Cypriots in London. The report from Uganda was closely followed by one from Bayless and Rosensweig (1966) working in the USA, who confirmed an earlier observation of Cuatrecasas, Lockwood, and Caldwell (1965) of a

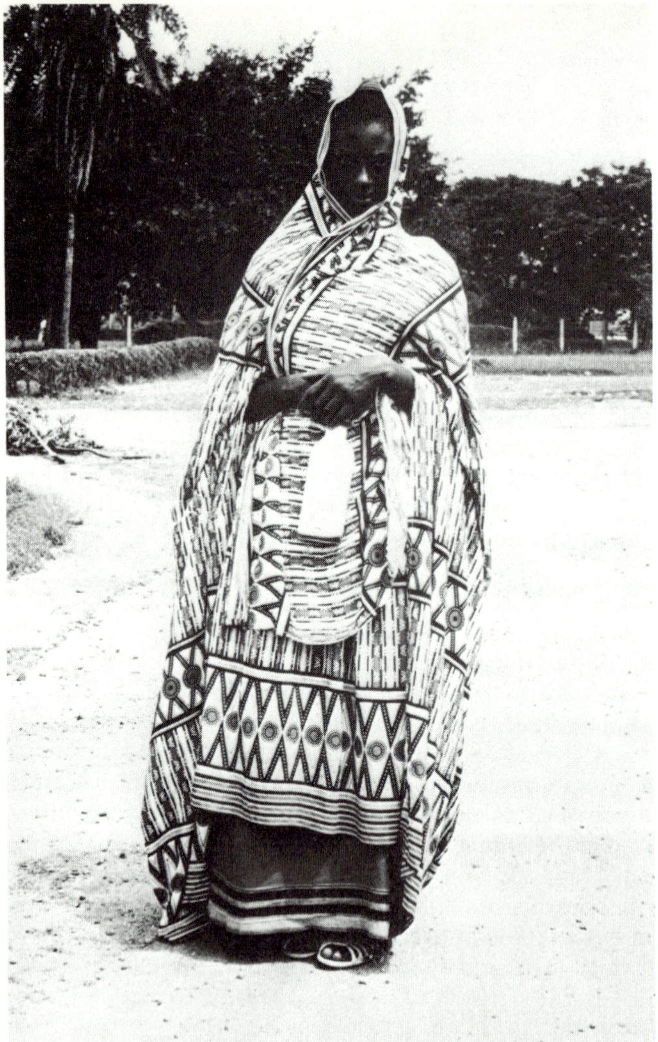

Fig. 21.1. A woman from the Hima tribe of western Uganda. The Hima are Hamites and retain a high jejunal lactase concentration into adult life (PL); they are thus able to drink large quantities of milk without getting symptoms, in contrast to the majority of Africans. The photograph was taken at Mbarara, Ankole.

significantly higher incidence of PL in white Americans than in American negroes. They also considered that genetic rather than environmental factors were responsible for that difference.

At one, or possibly several foci in the world, the gene for PL originated in *Homo sapiens*. Reports of differing incidence rates in population groups suggest that a likely site, and one from which the gene in African Hamites originated, was the Arabian peninsula (Cook, 1978a). If the high prevalence of PL in Pakistan can be confirmed (see below), the Arabian peninsula might also have been the original focus for a high incidence of the gene there. A more conjectural possibility is that the high gene frequency in northern Europeans also had its origin in Arabia, although it is possible that a further focus (foci) of PL occurred somewhere in Europe.

21.1.1. Physiology of hypolactasia

Lactose provides about 50 per cent of the calorie value of breast milk.

Lactase is located in the brush-border of the enterocyte; it is required for the hydrolysis of lactose prior to the absorption of its individual monosaccharides, glucose and galactose.

In the absence of lactase, two events give rise to abdominal colic and diarrhoea: (i) unabsorbed lactose in the lower small intestine draws, by osmosis, a large volume of water into the lumen, and that precipitates colic and diarrhoea, and (ii) bacterial lactases in the large intestine ferment lactose to lactic acid (which causes colonic irritation), with a similar result.

In most people (i.e. those who do not have PL), lactase falls from its high concentration at birth, to reach a very low concentration in adult life; the timing of that event was first investigated by Cook (1967a) in Uganda. Further reports relevant to that (Caskey, Payne-Bose, Welsh, Gearhart, Nance, and Morrison, 1977; Newcomer, Thomas, McGill, and Hofmann, 1977), and also the time of appearance of lactase in foetal life (Antonowicz and Lebenthal, 1977) are still being made.

21.1.2. Clinical aspects of hypolactasia

A history of colic and diarrhoea after drinking milk is often, but not always, obtained; frequently it is only after milk has been removed from the diet that an unexplained diarrhoea subsides. The stool following milk ingestion is fluid. Those symptoms after lactose constitute *lactose-intolerance*, a term which should not be confused with hypolactasia which refers to the lactase concentration in the brush-border of the enterocyte; only some hypolactasic subjects suffer from lactose-intolerance.

If adults with hypolactasia continue to drink milk for two weeks or more, a 'tolerance' is acquired. That is probably due to a change in the bacterial flora of the large intestine where adaptation occurs. However, gastric emptying time is reduced in hypolactasic individuals and the adaptation might be partly a result of that mechanism (Foster, 1974; Welsh and Hall, 1977).

21.1.3. Genetic regulation of lactase concentration in adult life

Several investigators have studied the mechanism of inheritance of adult hypolactasia (Sahi, Isokoski, Jussila, Launiala, and Pyorala, 1973; Lisker, Gonzalez, and Daltabuit, 1975; Newcomer, Gordon, Thomas, and McGill, 1977; Sahi and Launiala, 1977). However, because that condition is now known to be the normal state for the mammalian kingdom, a more meaningful approach involves determination of the genetic mechanism behind transmission of PL (Cook, 1973). Working along those lines, Ransome-Kuti, Kretchmer, Johnson, and Gribble (1975) concluded that the ability to digest lactose (PL) is transmitted as an *autosomal dominant* and represents either a mutated gene or a polymorphism. That investigation was carried out on the basis of Yoruba-European marriages and their progeny in Lagos, Nigeria; most Europeans have PL and most Yorubas adult hypolactasia.

The mechanism for the usual decline in lactase (hypolactasia) might be the same whether the fall is congenital (Holzel, Schwartz and Sutcliffe, 1959) or occurs, as it usually does, in childhood (Asp, Dahlqvist, Kuitunen, Launiala, and Visakorpi, 1973; Freiburghaus, Schmitz, Schindler, Rotthauwe, Kuitunen, Launiala, and Hadorn, 1976).

Persistence of lactase (PL) is possibly a comparable situation to the continuation of foetal haemoglobin into adult life (Fessas and Stamatoyannopoulos, 1964; Seigel, Cox, Schroeder, Huisman, Penner, and Rowley, 1970); there seems, however, to be only one human lactase (Freiburghaus, *et al.*, 1976). The 'high F' gene is inherited as a Mendelian dominant (Edington and Gilles, 1976); homozygotes have foetal haemoglobin only (Baglioni, 1963). Hereditary persistence of foetal haemoglobin occurs in approximately 0·1 per cent of American negroes and west Africans, and also exists in east Africa, Greece, Switzerland, and Jamaica.

21.1.4. Investigation of hypolactasia

The ideal method of determining hypolactasia in an individual is to obtain a jejunal-biopsy and undertake a direct estimation of the lactase concentration. It is also important to examine the morphology of the biopsy-specimen; in specific, *primary* hypolactasia, the villi are basically normal, together with the other disaccharidase concentrations.

A method frequently used in screening for hypolactasia, both in individuals and population groups, is the oral lactose loading test. 50g lactose, dissolved in 400 or 500 ml water, is given by mouth after an overnight fast. In children the amount given is usually 2g per kg bodyweight. Before lactose is ingested, two fasting capillary-blood specimens are obtained at a 10-minute interval; subsequent samples should be obtained at 15, 30, 60, 90, and 120 min. If lactase is present in low concentration, in the enterocyte, the blood glucose rise is less than 1·1 mmol per litre (Cook and Kajubi, 1966); at birth, during the first few years, and in adults with PL, the glucose rise is greater than 1·3 mmol per litre. During and for 24 hours after the loading-dose, symptoms should be sought; if hypolactasia is present, colic and diarrhoea (*lactose-intolerance*) may occur.

The hydrogen-breath method has recently been introduced to detect hypolactasia (Chapter 20) (Calloway and Murphy, 1968; Levitt and Donaldson, 1970; Metz, Jenkins, Peters, Newman, and Blendis, 1975; Cook, 1978b). After ingestion of lactose, expired breath-samples are collected into a syringe and analysed with a gas-chromatogram for their hydrogen concentration. On reaching the caecum any unabsorbed lactose is fermented by bacterial activity; liberation of various gases, including hydrogen, takes place and they enter the portal circulation and are ultimately expired in the breath. This technique has the advantage of being noninvasive.

In an investigation in Uganda, adults with hypolactasia were found to have a significant lactosuria (Cook and Howells, 1968); that observation may have a value in population studies because it is also a noninvasive technique.

Barium meals incorporating lactose give a characteristic 'malabsorption-pattern' radiologically (Laws and Neale, 1966); they are of limited value however in diagnosing hypolactasia.

In children, stool-acidity is of value in diagnosing both primary and secondary hypolactasia; commercially available 'Clinitest' tablets can be used. In adults, however, that simple test has no value.

The kinetics of lactose absorption, studied by a double-lumen tube jejunal system, have been investigated in adult Zambian Africans (Cook, Asp, and Dahlqvist, 1973a) all of whom have adult hypolactasia; lactose absorption rates were very low, and at all concentrations of lactose tested there was net water movement towards the small-intestinal lumen.

21.1.5. Treatment of hypolactasia

In primary hypolactasia, treatment is aimed at relieving symptoms; milk and all products containing lactose should be eliminated from the diet. A complete cure can easily be obtained. Aspirin has been given on the basis that it inhibits prostaglandin production and therefore diminishes peristalsis (Buisseret, Youlten, Heinzelmann, and Lessof, 1978; Lieb, 1978); preliminary results have been encouraging.

Many people in tropical countries with hypolactasia are familiar with the association between milk ingestion and diarrhoea; some in fact regulate bowel function by that means.

21.1.6. Practical importance of hypolactasia

At birth, jejunal lactase is present at high concentration (Cook, 1967a) and that applies to all ethnic groups, whatever the status of the enzyme in adult life; in those with adult hypolactasia, a fall takes place in the first four or five years of life, but at a variable age. In some, an early fall, within the first six to twelve months, has been recorded (Cook, 1967a); that doubtless accounts for many cases of marasmus, because lactose from breast milk is not absorbed and the rapid intestinal transit rate which accompanies that gives rise to an energy loss (Cook, 1967b). The overall importance of that event in the production of marasmus has not so far received adequate attention. King (1972) has reported that in Zambia, where there is an almost 100 per cent incidence of adult hypolactasia, diarrhoea during the breast feeding period is common, and that that is usually cured by weaning.

By the time adult life is reached lactase concentrations are low, and may in fact be down to zero (Cook, Asp, and Dahlqvist, 1973b); only extremely small amounts of lactose can be hydrolysed. Two-thirds to three-quarters of African and Asian adults experience diarrhoea and abdominal colic after lactose or milk; in them lactose is a valuable purgative. If given in large amounts, for example in the treatment of peptic ulcer, milk produces a torrential diarrhoea. It is clear that lactose-intolerant subjects are also milk-intolerant (Lisker and Aguilar, 1978); the frequency of symptoms is directly proportional to the lactose content of the milk. There seems no doubt, therefore, that hypolactasia has a clinical relevance when nutritional supplementation with milk is carried out, as it is in many third world countries (Lisker, Aguilar, and Zavala, 1978).

Milk is deficient in folic acid; in areas where folate deficiency is, for other reasons, a considerable problem, milk would seem to be an unsatisfactory foodstuff for adults.

Colonic pH is acid in people with hypolactasia, who drink milk; it seems possible that that prevents the growth of bacteria and possibly parasites also, e.g. *Entamoeba histolytica* (Elsdon-Dew, 1978). The probability of a protective action of hypolactasia against intestinal infections has not been adequately investigated.

Although PL is probably not associated with a significant elevation of serum cholesterol and bile acid concentrations (Cook, 1976; Wostmann, Bruckner-Kardoss, Beaver, Chang, and Madsen, 1976; Mann, 1977), there is evidence that subjects with PL have a higher mean serum triglyceride concentration than those with hypolactasia (Sahi, Jussila, Penttila, Sarna, and Isokoski, 1977). That would render people with adult hypolactasia relatively immune from the high incidence rate of arterial disease which is very common in some population groups.

21.1.7. Practical importance of lactase persistence

Persistence of lactase (PL) must presumably have conveyed a survival advantage, at some time in evolution, in one or more groups of the world's population. However the basis for that is unknown. If milk from the cow, camel, or another mammal was the only available nutrient, the ability to digest and absorb lactose, and the subsequent avoidance of colic and diarrhoea following its ingestion, would have been a distinct advantage. It has been suggested that lactase might have had a more subtle significance in human nutrition (Anderson, 1977; Hirschhorn, 1977; Mitchell, Brand, and Halbisch, 1977).

Flatz and Rotthauwe (1973) have suggested that the advantage of PL was associated with a lactose-induced enhancement of calcium absorption (Schaafsma and de Waard, 1978) from the intestine in areas, such as northern Europe, with a low ultraviolet radiation and a low dietary intake of vitamin D; that hypothesis is untenable, however, because some areas where the PL gene is very common are not, and seem never to have been, ones where there is a low level of ultraviolet radiation, e.g. the Arabian peninsula (see below) (Cook and Al-Torki, 1975). PL seems to have a protective influence against osteoporosis (Newcomer, Hodgson, McGill, and Thomas 1978; *Lancet*, 1979); the mechanism is probably via an increased calcium intake, and possibly an effect on calcium absorption.

Milk seems to exert a protective effect against the growth of intestinal bacteria in the human small intestine (Bullen, 1977); that would presumably be more marked in children, and adults with PL, who can tolerate milk. Milk contains lactoferrin, which has a bacteriostatic effect on *Escherichia coli*; it also favours the growth of anaerobic lactobacilli and is associated with a low pH, which discourages various pathogens. Reliance on milk, which is low in iron, as a calorie source, produces a chronic iron-deficiency state (Murray, Murray, Murray, and Murray, 1978a); because iron-deficiency produces a resistance to infections, including malaria, tuberculosis, and brucellosis, to which nomadic populations are continuously exposed, that offers a further explanation for the advantage of PL.The incidence of cerebral malaria is significantly lower in malnourished children on a milk, compared with a grain, diet (Murray, Murray, Murray, and Murray, 1978b); that effect is probably due to an inhibitory effect of milk on division of parasites (combined with a delayed recovery of T-cell function after malnutrition). It is thus possible that the advantage of PL is associated with a protective action of milk against fatal *Plasmodium falciparum* infections. A further hypothesis associates PL with intestinal rotavirus infections (Holmes, Rodger, Schnagl, Ruck, Gust, Bishop, and Barnes, 1976), but that would not seem to constitute a genetic advantage.

21.1.8. Geographical distribution of lactase in adults

Numerous reports have given incidence rates for PL in population groups throughout the world (Cook, 1973). Others, in the original inhabitants, have recently appeared from Trinidad (Bartholomew and Pong, 1976), Vietnam (Anh, Thuc, and Welsh, 1977), Sri Lanka (Senewiratne, Shanthi, and Perera (1977), Canada (Ellestad-Sayed and Haworth, 1977), Arizona (Johnson, Simoons, Hurwitz, Grange, Mitchell, Sinatra, Sunshine, Robertson, Bennett, and Kretchmer, 1977), Mexico (Woteki, Weser and Young, 1977), and the USA (Newcomer and McGill, 1977; Newcomer, McGill, Thomas, and Hofmann, 1978). Much information has therefore accumulated on the frequency of PL in different parts of the world.

Tables 21.1 to 21.4 summarize incidence rates for PL in some of the major studies in the Middle east, Africa, Asia, and Europe. In most series, results are based predominantly on the blood-glucose response to oral lactose; in some, lactase activity in jejunal-biopsy samples was estimated also.

Middle east. A minority of adults on the Mediterranean littoral has PL (Cook, 1973); that applies to arabs and sephardic, ashkenazi, and oriental jews at the eastern end of the Mediterranean. However, in Riyadh, Saudi Arabia, Cook and Al-Torki (1975), found a high incidence of PL in adults of Bedouin, urban Saudi, and Yemeni stock; a much lower incidence was found in a *Khadiry* group (who have a mixed ancestry, which is partly derived from Somalian and Ethiopian stock). Bedouin in Riyadh have apparently undergone only minor degrees of admixture with African stock (Field, 1956). The available studies from the Middle east also suggest a significant difference in the incidence of PL between jews and arabs of the Arabian peninsula; they are all semites (Hitti, 1960) but that is a linguistic and not an ethnic term.

Africa. The first population group to be shown to have an approximately 90 per cent incidence of hypolactasia in adult life was the Bantu population of Uganda (Cook and Kajubi, 1966); however, like the majority of northern Europeans and white Americans and their descendants, the Hamites of Uganda, Rwanda and Burundi (the Hima and Tutsi) have high concentrations (PL) (Cook and Kajubi, 1966; Cook and Dahlqvist, 1968). A study in Nigeria suggested a similar ethnic variation within that country (Kretchmer, Ransome-Kuti, Hurwitz, Dungy, and Alakija, 1971); the Yoruba and Ibo have a very high incidence of hypolactasia, while most Hausa and Fulani have PL. A third investigation in the lake Kivu region of Rwanda has confirmed that Hamites usually

Table 21.1. Incidence rates for PL in Middle-Eastern Populations.

Location of investigation	Group studied	No. Tested	Incidence of PL No.	Incidence of PL Percentage	Investigator(s)
Israel	Arabs (local)	67	13	19	Gilat, Malachi and Shochet (1971)
Israel	Arabs (Syria, Jordan, Libya, Saudi Arabia, Egypt, Iraq and Tunisia)	26	6	23	Rotthauwe, El-Schallah, and Flatz (1971)
Saudi Arabia	Bedouin	14	12	86	Cook and Al-Torki (1975)
	Urban Saudi	8	7	87	"
	Yemeni	8	6	75	"
	Khadiry	9	2	22	"
Jordan	Arabs (local)	56	13	23	Snook, Mahmoud, and Chang (1976)
Israel (Jews)	Jews (local)	93	36	39	Rozen and Shafrir (1968).
Israel (Jews)	Yemeni	36	20	56	Gilat, Kuhn, Gelman, and Mizrahy (1970)
	North African Sephardic	32	12	38	"
	Other Sephardic	36	10	28	"
	Ashkenazi	55	12	21	"
	Iraqi	38	6	16	"
	Orientals	20	3	15	"

have PL (Cox and Elliott, 1974). Investigations in Zambia (Cook, Asp, and Dahlqvist, 1973b), Zimbabwe Rhodesia (Bayless and Huang, 1969), South Africa (Jersky and Kinsley, 1967; Jenkins, Lehmann, and Nurse, 1974; Currie, Nurse, and Jenkins, 1978) and Kenya (Watson, Ferguson, and MacKay, 1968) have indicated a 90 to 100 per cent incidence of hypolactasia in the indigenous people of those countries.

The only Africans, therefore, to have high lactase concentrations in adult life (PL) are the Hamites, who are derived from a northern stock and are unrelated to the indigenous people of the continent (Cook, 1973). They are thought to have been derived in antiquity from Ethiopian and southern Arabian stock (Haddon, 1929).

Asia. Most reports from Asia give a very low incidence of PL, which is zero in many areas (Cook, 1973); however, two recent reports are at variance with them. In a large study in Afghanistan, a 17 per cent incidence of PL was recorded (Rahimi, Delbrück, Haeckel, Goedde, and Flatz, 1976). In a further investigation at Karachi, Pakistan, a 95 per cent incidence of PL was discovered (Rab and Baseer, 1976); that study gives one of the highest rates for PL so far reported; more evidence from there is required because Pakistani people in London usually have adult hypolactasia (Neale, 1968).

Europe. With the exception of the study by McMichael, Webb, and Dawson

Table 21.2. Incidence rates for PL in African Populations

Location of investigation	Group studied	No. Tested	Incidence of PL No.	Incidence of PL Percentage	Investigator(s)
Uganda	'Bantu' (mainly Ganda)	35	4	11	Cook and Kajubi (1966)
	Tutsi and Hima	23	20	87	"
	Hutu and Iru	28	18	64	"
	Nilotic	9	5	56	"
	'Bantu' (mainly Ganda)	12	0	0	Cook and Dahlqvist (1968)
	Tutsi and Hima	6	5	84	"
Nigeria	Yoruba	41	1	3	Kretchmer, Ransome-Kuti, Hurwitz, Dungy, and Alakija (1971)
	Hausa	17	4	24	"
	Fulani (Nomadic)	9	7	78	"
	Fulani (Urban)	24	7	30	"
	Yoruba	11	0	0	Ransome-Kuti, Kretchmer, Johnson, and Gribble (1975)
Rwanda	Tutsi	27	25	92	Cox and Elliott (1974)
	Hutu	36	15	42	"
	Twa	22	5	23	"
	Shi	28	1	4	"
	Hutu/Tutsi	11	5	45	"
Zambia	Many central African tribes	26	1	4	Cook, Asp, and Dahlqvist (1973b)
Namibia (south-west Africa)	Herero-speaking people	58	2	3	Currie, Nurse, and Jenkins (1978)
South Africa	San (! Kung)	40	0	0	Jenkins, Lehmann, and Nurse (1974)

(1965), in which the ethnic origin of the subjects is not stated, all surveys have given very high incidence rates of PL.

21.1.9. Anthropological implications of lactase

The true basis of the selective advantage of lactase in adult life (PL) is at present unknown. Milking of domestic sheep and goats in south-west Asia began between 5000 and 8000 years ago (Perkins, 1969; Cook, 1973; *Lancet*, 1975a). If, in fact, the Arabian peninsula was the site of origin of the PL gene, it seems likely that camels' milk, which has been widely consumed by desert nomads for many thousands of years, might be relevant. Domestication of camels for milk-production took place many thousands of years ago in the southern Arabian peninsula (Bulliet, 1975). From early times, the camel was also a beast of burden and was used for long journeys across the deserts of Arabia. Clearly, camels' milk during such journeys would both form a valuable nutrient and also provide vital fluid. People with PL would have been at a distinct advantage, and would have absorbed not only lactose but also water; in those with adult hypolactasia, failure to absorb lactose, a rapid intestinal transit-rate, and colic and diarrhoea would result. Increased survival of a group with PL would thus be anticipated. In severe gastrointestinal infections, including cholera, active absorption of monosaccharides is coupled to water absorption (*Lancet*, 1975b). Survival from epidemics of diarrhoeal diseases, such as cholera, which have for long been common in the Middle east, Asia, and to a lesser extent Africa (Chapter 18), would also be more likely in subjects with PL if milk formed a major source of water (Cook and Al-Torki, 1975). The selective advantage might in fact have been more directly related to water and electrolytes than to a nutritional factor.

The reasons behind the movements of nomadic pastoralists are complex (Guilliver, 1975), but availability of food for camels, cows, and other domestic animals is obviously an important factor. That factor has doubtless been, in part, responsible for the Hamitic migrations, with associated dispersal of the PL gene, into Africa, and to some extent for population movements into north-west Asia and northern Europe.

21.2. Secondary hypolactasia

21.2.1. Aetiology of secondary hypolactasia

Secondary depression of small-intestinal disaccharidases occurs when there is

Table 21.3. Incidence rates for PL in Asian and Pacific Populations

Location of investigation	Group studied	No. Tested	Incidence of PL: No.	Incidence of PL: Percentage	Investigator(s)
Singapore	Chinese	22	0	0	Bolin, Davis, Seah, Chua, Yong, Kho, Siak, and Jacob (1970)
Thailand	Bangkok Thais	39	0	0	Troncale, Keusch, Miller, Olsson, and Buchanan (1967)
	Northern Thais	75	0	0	Flatz, Saengudom, and Sanguanbhokhai (1969)
	Northern Thais	140	4	3	Keusch, Troncale, Thavaramara, Prinyanont, Anderson, and Bhamarapravathi (1969)
India	South Indians	38	0	0	Swaminathan, Mathan, Baker, and Radhakrishnan (1970)
Afghanistan	Tajik, Pashtun, Pasha-i, Uzbek, Hazara and mixed urban people	270	47	17	Rahimi, Delbrück, Haeckel, Goedde, and Flatz (1976)
Pakistan	Punjabis, Sindhis, Baluchis, Pathans and Mohajirs	55	52	95	Rab and Baseer (1976)
Papua New Guinea	Groups in various parts of the country	50	1	2	Cook (1979)

severe damage to the enterocyte. That sometimes takes place in tropical malabsorption ('tropical sprue') (Chapter 20), and in viral and bacterial infections of the small intestine (Chapter 17). It also occurs in severe kwashiorkor when there is severe jejunal mucosal damage (Cook, Lakin, and Whitehead, 1967); diarrhoea after lactose and other dissaccharides occasionally proves troublesome in that condition (Dean, 1952; Wharton, Howells, and Phillips, 1968). Although morphological recovery of the jejunal mucosa occurs after treatment of kwashiorkor, lactase can be decreased long after recovery (Cook and Lee, 1966); the explanation for that observation is not clear. Also, in any severe bacterial or viral infection of the small intestine, including rotavirus gastroenteritis (Walker-Smith, Manuel, and Hutchins, 1978), a transient secondary hypolactasia may ensue with the production of symptoms, which continue *after* the infection has been eliminated. That is often of considerable importance in children.

Table 21.4. Incidence rates for PL in European Populations

Location of investigation	Group studied	No. Tested	Incidence of PL: No.	Incidence of PL: Percentage	Investigator(s)
England	(not stated)	44	30	68	McMichael, Webb, and Dawson (1965)
	English	50	47	94	Neale (1968)
Denmark	Danish	700	665	95	Gudmand-Høyer, Dahlqvist, and Jarnum (1969)
Finland	Finnish	159	132	83	Jussila, Isokoski, and Launiala (1970)
Switzerland	Swiss	18	15	83	Auricchio, Rubino, Landolt, Semenza, and Prader (1963)
	Swiss	17	14	82	Haemmerli, Kistler, Ammann, Marthaler, Semenza, Auricchio, and Prader (1965)
Canada	Czechs	17	14	82	Leichter (1972)
Canada	Poles	21	15	72	Leichter (1972)

Candida albicans which has been implicated in chronic diarrhoea in adults (Kane, Chretien and Garagusi, 1976) has been shown to depress mucosal disaccharidase concentrations (Barnes, Bishop, and Townley, 1974). Systemic infection can also produce a secondary hypolactasia. Severe morphological damage of the mucosa is common in measles. Viral hepatitis (Chapter 7) also produces severe damage to the jejunum (Conrad, Schwartz, and Young, 1964).

Wharton *et al.* (1968) have shown that in very severe kwashiorkor, monosaccharide as well as disaccharide absorption may also be depressed.

21.2.2. Investigation of secondary hypolactasia

Investigations are similar to those used in primary hypolactasia. The main differences are that (i) the jejunal-mucosal specimen shows significant morphological changes (Chapter 20) and (ii) other disaccharidases, in addition to lactase and peptidases, are reduced.

21.2.3. Treatment of secondary hypolactasia

Treatment consists of: (i) symptomatic measures similar to the procedures used in primary hypolactasia, and (ii) measures aimed at the primary disease, e.g. in tropical malabsorption, tetracycline or folic acid supplements should be given.

21.3. Cows' milk allergy (cows' milk-sensitive enteropathy)

Cows' milk allergy, which is basically an allergy to the protein in cows' milk, should be distinguished from primary hypolactasia. The abnormal intolerance to cows' milk occurs in infants, and usually disappears by the age of two years. There is a jejunal-mucosal lesion, which ranges from a flat mucosa to a mild degree of 'partial villous atrophy' (Lamy, Nezelof, Jos, Frèzal, and Rey, 1963; Walker-Smith, Harrison, Kilby, Phillips, and France, 1978). Routine histological examination of intestinal-biopsy specimens, before and after a cows' milk challenge, is the best way of diagnosing the entity (Walker-Smith *et al.*, 1978); in that study, of five infants reported, two were Indian and a third West Indian. A secondary disaccharidase depression may be associated with the mucosal damage; in one study, 23 of 25 children with cows' milk protein intolerance had a secondary lactose intolerance (Harrison, Kilby, Walker-Smith, France, and Wood, 1976). The disease presents with an illness indistinguishable from infantile gastroenteritis; in two of the cases reported by Harrison *et al.* (1976), an enteropathogenic *E. coli* was isolated. Eight of 20 were partly deficient in IgA.

The disease can occur in breastfed infants whose mothers are drinking cows' milk (Jakobsson and Lindberg, 1978); symptoms disappear when the mother discontinues drinking cows' milk.

The condition is easily diagnosed on clinical grounds, and routine jejunal biopsy is probably not justified (Sumithran and Iyngkaran, 1977); there do not seem however to be any rigid criteria for diagnosis at present (Iyngkaran, Robinson, Prathap, Sumithran, and Yadav, 1978).

21.4. Sucrase-isomaltase deficiency

This genetically controlled condition is an important cause of sugar intolerance in infancy and childhood (Antonowicz, Lloyd-Still, Khaw, and Schwachman, 1972). It was first described by Weijers, Van de Kamer, Mossel and Dicke (1960). The condition is common in the Eskimo (Bell, Draper, and Bergan, 1973). However, there is no evidence that the incidence of this primary disaccharidase deficiency is high in any tropical population. A secondary deficiency of the enzyme may occur in the presence of severe jejunal mucosal damage (Wharton *et al.*, 1968).

References

Anderson, C. M. (1977). *Lancet*, **1**, 954.

Anh, N. T., Thuc, T. K., and Welsh, J. D. (1977). *Am. J. clin. Nutr.*, **30**, 468.

Antonowicz, I. and Lebenthal, E. (1977). *Gastroenterology*, **72**, 1299.

——, Lloyd-Still, J. D., Khaw, K. T., and Schwachman, H. (1972). *Pediatrics, Springfield*, **49**, 847.

Asp, N.-G., Dahlqvist, A., Kuitunen, P., Launiala, K., and Visakorpi, J. K. (1973). *Lancet*, **2,** 329.
Auricchio, S., Rubino, A., Landolt, M., Semenza, G., and Prader, A. (1963). *Lancet*, **2,** 324.
Baglioni, C. (1963). *Nature, Lond.*, **198,** 1177.
Barnes, G., Bishop, R., and Townley, R. (1974). *Acta paediat., Stockh.*, **63,** 423.
Bartholomew, C. and Pong, O. Y. (1976). *Trop. geogr. Med.*, **28,** 336.
Bayless, T. M. and Huang, S. S. (1969). *Am. J. clin. Nutr.*, **22,** 250.
—— and Rosensweig, N. S. (1966). *J. Am. med. Ass.*, **197,** 968.
Bell, R. R., Draper, H. H., and Bergan, J. G. (1973). *Am. J. clin. Nutr.*, **26,** 1185.
Bolin, T. D., Davis, A. E., Seah, C. S., Chua, K. L., Yong, V., Kho, K. M., Siak, C. L., and Jacob, E. (1970). *Gastroenterology*, **59,** 76.
Buisseret, P. D., Youlten, L. J. F., Heinzelmann, D. I., and Lessof, M. H. (1978). *Lancet*, **1,** 906.
Bullen, J. J. (1977). *Br. J. hosp. Med.*, **18,** 220.
Bulliet, R. W. (1975). In *The camel and the wheel.* p. 49. Harvard University Press, Cambridge, Mass.
Calloway, D. H. and Murphy, E. L. (1968). *Ann. N. Y. Acad. Sci.*, **150,** 82.
Caskey, D. A., Payne-Bose, D., Welsh, J. D., Gearhart, H. L., Nance, M. K., and Morrison, R. D. (1977). *Am. J. dig. Dis.*, **22,** 113.
Conrad, M. E., Schwartz, F. D., and Young, A. A. (1964). *Am. J. Med.*, **37,** 789.
Cook, G. C. (1967a). *Br. med. J.*, **1,** 527.
—— (1967b). *J. trop. Pediat.*, **13,** 85.
—— (1968). *Proc. R. Soc. Med.*, **61,** 1102.
—— (1969). *Man, N. S.*, **4,** 265.
—— (1973). In *Intestinal enzyme deficiencies and their nutritional implications* (ed. B. Borgström, A. Dahlqvist and L. Hambraeus) p. 52. Almqvist and Wiksell, Uppsala.
—— (1974). *Trans. R. Soc. trop. Med. Hyg.*, **68,** 419.
—— (1976). *Trop. geogr. Med.*, **28,** 339.
—— (1978a). *Man, N. S.*, **13,** 418.
—— (1978b). *Trans. R. Soc. trop. Med. Hyg.*, **72,** 277.
—— (1979). *Ann. Hum. Biol.*, **6,** 55.
—— and Al-Torki, M. T. (1975). *Br. med. J.*, **3,** 135.
——, Asp, N.-G., and Dahlqvist, A. (1973a). *Br. J. Nutr.*, **30,** 519.
——, ——, and —— (1973b). *Gastroenterology*, **64,** 405.
—— and Dahlqvist, A. (1968). *Gastroenterology*, **55,** 328.
—— and Howells, G. R. (1968). *Am. J. dig. Dis.*, **13,** 634.
—— and Kajubi, S. K. (1966). *Lancet*, **1,** 725.
——, Lakin, A., and Whitehead, R. G. (1967). *Gut*, **8,** 622.
—— and Lee, F. D. (1966). *Lancet*, **2,** 1263.
Cox, J. A. and Elliott, F. G. (1974). *Am. J. dig. Dis.*, **19,** 714.
Cuatrecasas, P., Lockwood, D. H., and Caldwell, J. R. (1965). *Lancet*, **1,** 14.
Currie, B., Nurse, G. T., and Jenkins, T. (1978). *S. Afr. J. Sci.*, **74,** 227.
Dean, R. F. A. (1952). *Br. med. J.*, **2,** 791.
Edington, G. M. and Gilles, H. M. (1976). *Pathology in the tropics.* 2nd ed. p. 426. Edward Arnold, London.
Ellestad-Sayed, J. J. and Haworth, J. C. (1977). *Am. J. clin. Nutr.*, **30,** 698.
Elsdon-Dew, R. (1978). *Trans. R. Soc. trop. Med. Hyg.*, **72,** 442.
Fessas, P. and Stamatoyannopoulos, G. (1964). *Blood*, **24,** 223.
Field, H. (1956). *Ancient and modern man in south western Asia*. p. 97. University of Miami Press, Florida.
Flatz, G. and Rotthauwe, H. W. (1973). *Lancet*, **2,** 76.
——, Saengudom, C., and Sanguanbhokhai, T. (1969). *Nature, Lond.*, **221,** 758.
Foster, D N. (1974). *E. Afr. med. J.*, 51, 26.

FREIBURGHAUS, A. U., SCHMITZ, J., SCHINDLER, M., ROTTHAUWE, H. W., KUITUNEN, P., LAUNIALA, K., and HADORN, B. (1976). *New. Engl. J. Med.*, **294,** 1030.
GILAT, T., KUHN, R., GELMAN, E., and MIZRAHY, O. (1970). *Am. J. dig. Dis.*, **15,** 895.
——, MALACHI, E. G., and SHOCHET, S. B. (1971). *Am. J. dig. Dis.*, **16,** 203.
GUDMAND-HØYER, E., DAHLQVIST, A., and JARNUM, S. (1969). *Scand. J. Gastroent.*, **4,** 377.
GULLIVER, P. H. (1975). In *Pastoralism in Tropical Africa* (ed. T. Monod) p. 369. Oxford University Press, London, Ibadan, and Nairobi.
HADDON, A. C. (1929). *The races of man*. p. 39. Cambridge University Press.
HAEMMERLI, U. P., KISTLER, H., AMMANN, R., MARTHALER, T., SEMENZA, G., AURICCHIO, S., and PRADER, A. (1965). *Am. J. Med.*, **38,** 7.
HARRISON, M., KILBY, A., WALKER-SMITH, J. A., FRANCE, N. E., and WOOD, C. B. S. (1976). *Br. med. J.*, **1,** 1501.
HIRSCHHORN, N. (1977). *Lancet*, **1,** 810.
HITTI, P. K. (1960). *History of the Arabs.* p. 10. Macmillan, London.
HOLMES, I. H., RODGER, S. M., SCHNAGL, R. D., RUCK, B. J., GUST, I. D., BISHOP, R. F., and BARNES, G. L. (1976). *Lancet*, **1,** 1387.
HOLZEL, A., SCHWARTZ, V., and SUTCLIFFE, K. W. (1959). *Lancet*, **1,** 1126.
IYNGKARAN, N., ROBINSON, M. J., PRATHAP, K., SUMITHRAN, E., and YADAV, M. (1978). *Archs Dis. Childh.*, **53,** 20.
JAKOBSSON, I. and LINDBERG, T. (1978). *Lancet*, **2,** 437.
JENKINS, T., LEHMANN, H., and NURSE, G. T. (1974). *Br. med. J.*, **2,** 23.
JERSKY, J. and KINSLEY, R. H. (1967). *S. Afr. med. J.*, **41,** 1194.
JOHNSON, J. D., SIMOONS, F. J., HURWITZ, R., GRANGE, A., MITCHELL, C. H., SINATRA, F. R., SUNSHINE, P., ROBERTSON, W. V., BENNETT, P. H., and KRETCHMER, N. (1977). *Gastroenterology*, **73,** 1299.
JUSSILA, J., ISOKOSKI, M. and LAUNIALA, K. (1970). *Scand. J. Gastroent.*, **5,** 49.
KANE, J. G., CHRETIEN, J. H., and GARAGUSI, V. F. (1976). *Lancet*, **1,** 335.
KEUSH, G. T., TRONCALE, F. J., THAVARAMARA, B., PRINYANONT, P., ANDERSON, P., and BHAMARAPRAVATHI, N. (1969). *Am J. clin. Nutr.*, **22,** 638.
KING, F. (1972). *Lancet*, **2,** 335.
KRETCHMER, N., RANSOME-KUTI, O., HURWITZ, R., DUNGY, C., and ALAKIJA, W. (1971). *Lancet*, **2,** 392.
LAMY, M., NEZELOF, C., JOS, J., FRÈZAL, J., and REY, J. (1963). *Presse méd.*, **71,** 1267.
Lancet (1975a). *Lancet*, **2,** 910.
—— (1975b). **1,** 79.
—— (1979). **1,** 86.
LAWS, J. W. and NEALE, G. (1966). *Lancet*, **2,** 139.
LEICHTER, J. (1972). *Am. J. dig. Dis.*, **17,** 73.
LEVITT, M. D. and DONALDSON, R. M. (1970). *J. Lab. clin. Med.*, **75,** 937.
LIEB, J. (1978). *Lancet*, **2,** 157.
LISKER, R. and AGUILAR, L. (1978). *Gastroenterology*, **74,** 1283.
——, AGUILAR, L., and ZAVALA, C. (1978). *Am. J. clin. Nutr.*, **31,** 1499.
——, GONZALEZ, B., and DALTABUIT, M. (1975). *Am. J. hum. Genet.*, **27,** 662.
MANN, G. V. (1977). *Lancet*, **2,** 556.
MCMICHAEL, H. B., WEBB, J., and DAWSON, A. M. (1965). *Lancet*, **1,** 717.
METZ, G., JENKINS, D. J. A., PETERS, T. J., NEWMAN, A., and BLENDIS, L. M. (1975). *Lancet*, **1,** 1155.
MITCHELL, J. D., BRAND, J., and HALBISCH, J. (1977). *Lancet*, **1,** 500.
MORRIS, J. G., TRUDELL, J., and PENCOVIC, T. (1977). *Br. J. Nutr.*, **37,** 365.
MURRAY, M. J., MURRAY, A. B., MURRAY, M. B. and MURRAY, C. J. (1978a). *Br. med. J.*, **2,** 1113.
——, ——, MURRAY, N. J. and MURRAY, M. B. (1978b). *Am. J. clin. Nutr.*, **31,** 57.
NEALE, G. (1968). *Proc. R. Soc. Med.*, **61,** 1099.

NEWCOMER, A. D., GORDON, H., THOMAS, P. J., and MCGILL, D. B. (1977). *Gastroenterology*, **73,** 985.

——, HODGSON, S. F., MCGILL, D. B., and THOMAS, P. J. (1978). *Ann. intern. Med.*, **89,** 218.

——, THOMAS, P. J., MCGILL, D. B., and HOFMANN, A. F. (1977). *Gastroenterology*, **72,** 234.

——, ——, THOMAS, P. J., and HOFMANN, A. F. (1978). *Gastroenterology*, **74,** 44.

—— and MCGILL, D. B. (1977). *Am. J. dig. Dis.*, **22,** 745.

PERKINS, D. (1969). *Science, N. Y.*, **164,** 177.

RAB, S. M. and BASEER, A. (1976). *Brit. med. J.*, **1,** 436.

RAHIMI, A. G., DELBRÜCK, H., HAECKEL, R., GOEDDE, H. W., and FLATZ, G. (1976). *Hum. Genet.*, **34,** 57.

RANSOME-KUTI, O., KRETCHMER, N., JOHNSON, J. D., and GRIBBLE, J. T. (1975). *Gastroenterology*, **68,** 431.

ROTTHAUWE, H. W., EL-SCHALLAH, M. O., and FLATZ, G. (1971). *Hum. genetik*, **13,** 344.

——, EMONS, D., KAEOPLUNG, M., TANTACHAMROON, T., and FLATZ, G. (1971). *Klin. Wschr.*, **49,** 503.

ROZEN, P. and SHAFRIR, E. (1968). *Israel J. Med. Sci.*, **4,** 100.

SAHI, T., ISOKOSKI, M., JUSSILA, J., LAUNIALA, K., and PYORALA, K. (1973). *Lancet*, **2,** 823.

——, JUSSILA, J., PENTTILA, I. M. SARNA, S., and ISOKOSKI, M. (1977). *Am. J. clin. Nutr.*, **30,** 476.

—— and LAUNIALA, K. (1977). *Gastroenterology*, **73,** 231.

SCHAAFSMA, G. and DE WAARD, H. (1978). *Am. J. clin. Nutr.*, **31,** 4.

SENEWIRATNE, B., SHANTHI, T., and PERERA, H. (1977). *Gastroenterology*, **72,** 1257.

SIEGEL, W., COX, R., SCHROEDER, W., HUISMAN, T. H. J., PENNER, O., and ROWLEY, P. T. (1970). *Ann. intern. Med.*, **72,** 533.

SNOOK, C. R., MAHMOUD, J. N., and CHANG, W. P. (1976). *Trop. geogr. Med.*, **28,** 333.

SUMITHRAN, E. and IYNGKAREN, N. (1977). *Lancet*, **2,** 1122.

SWAMINATHAN, N., MATHAN, V. I., BAKER, S. J., and RADHAKRISHNAN, A. N. (1970). *Clinica chim. Acta*, **30,** 707.

TRONCALE, F. J., KEUSCH, G. T., MILLER, L. H., OLSSON, R. A., and BUCHANAN, R. D. (1967). *Br. med. J.*, **4,** 578.

WALKER-SMITH, J., HARRISON, M., KILBY, A., PHILLIPS, A., and FRANCE, N., (1978). *Archs Dis. Childh.*, **53,** 375.

——, MANUEL, P., and HUTCHINS, P. (1978). *Lancet*, **2,** 470.

WATSON, W. C., FERGUSON, J. C., and MACKAY, N. (1968). *J. trop. Med. Hyg.*, **71,** 235.

WEIJERS, H. A., VAN DE KAMER, J. H., MOSSEL, D. A. A., and DICKE, W. K. (1960). *Lancet*, **2,** 296.

WELSH, J. D. and HALL, W. H. (1977). *Am. J. dig. Dis.*, **22,** 1060.

WHARTON, B., HOWELLS, G., and PHILLIPS, I. (1968). *Br. med. J.*, **4,** 608.

WOSTMANN, B., BRUCKNER-KARDOSS, E., BEAVER, M., CHANG, L., and MADSEN, D. (1976). *J. Nutr.*, **106,** 1782.

WOTEKI, C. E., WESER, E., and YOUNG, E. A. (1977). *Am. J. clin. Nutr.*, **30,** 470.

22

Salmonellosis (Typhoid fever)

VIEWED in the context of intestinal bacterial infections, typhoid fever falls between the upper small-intestinal group in which the mechanism of diarrhoea is predominantly by enterotoxin production, and the large-intestinal infections which exert their effect mainly by mucosal invasion. Typhoid fever affects the ileum, primarily, and is invasive, but only within the lymphoid aggregations (Peyer's patches).

Typhoid fever is the most severe of the illnesses produced by organisms of the salmonella group. A similar but less severe illness is produced by *S. paratyphi A, B,* and *C.* The taxonomy of the group is complex. There are three main species: *Salmonella cholera-suis* (whose natural host is the pig), *S. typhi* (which is the causative organism of typhoid fever), and *S. enteritidis* (*S. paratyphi A* and *S. typhimurium* are examples).

The salmonelloses still tend to be covered in texts of general medicine, and are underemphasized in many standard works devoted to tropical medicine. Typhoid fever is, in fact, unusual in northern Europe and north America today, but extremely common in tropical countries, where it carries very high morbidity and mortality rates (Mulligan, 1971). That has little to do with the tropics *per se*, but reflects the appalling public health standards of many developing countries. The overall mortality rate for the disease is probably of the order of two per cent of treated cases. Severity undoubtedly varies, however, in different areas (Ramachandran, Godfrey, and Lionel, 1978). There are marked differences, for example, in complication rates in different parts of Africa; whereas they are unusual in Zambia, in Uganda and Nigeria they account for a very substantial mortality. The disease is possibly more common, and is probably more severe, in bearers of the sickle-cell trait (AS) (Vandepitte, Colaert, Lambotte-Legrand, Lambotte-Legrand, and Perin, 1953); however, not all work supports that conclusion.

22.1. Bacteriology and pathology of salmonellosis

The bacterium responsible for the disease, typhoid fever, is named after Doctor D. E. Salmon, director of the Bureau of Animal Industry in Washington in the late nineteenth century (Grady and Keusch, 1971); his assistant Theobald Smith had in fact identified the organism, but had erroneously associated it with hog 'cholera'.

The responsible organisms are Gram-negative, actively motile bacilli, which can be differentiated from nonpathogenic Gram-negative bacilli by appropriate bacteriological techniques. Salmonellae can only grow between 4 and 36°C; outside that range growth stops, but survival is possible. They are killed when exposed for 15 min to 60°C, and rapidly by boiling. Growth is inhibited by acidity. The organisms invade the mucosa to a deep level, but do not produce significant amounts of enterotoxins, as do most bacteria associated with diarrhoea which is predominantly of small-intestinal origin (Grady and Keusch, 1971).

The disease is endemic in most parts of the tropics (Wicks, Holmes, and Davidson, 1971); large epidemics may however also occur (*Lancet*, 1975) due especially to contamination of water supplies (Budd, 1856). In both east and west Africa the disease is common at the end of the dry season when rivers are polluted. In Zimbabwe Rhodesia there is a rise in the incidence rate as water supplies become limited at the end of the dry season, and that reaches a peak when early rains have resulted in the downstream contamination of water supplies (Wicks *et al.*, 1971). Infected food, milk, shellfish, and watercress are responsible for some outbreaks. Prepared foods, poultry, and egg products are frequently incriminated. After thawing for an inadequate length of time, poultry are only too frequently roasted for too short a period, and then left at room temperature; heavy colonization of a carcase will then ensue within a few hours (*Br. med. J.*, 1978a). Human faeces are sometimes used for vegetable crop manure; vegetables imported from the subtropics and tropics to temperate zones may therefore be infected with *S. typhi* (*Br. med. J.*, 1978b). However, vegetables are fortunately not nearly as good a culture medium as meat, milk, and eggs. *S. paratyphi* infections, on the contrary, are usually caused by contaminated food rather than water supplies.

Carriers can excrete the organism in the stool or urine for long periods; the organisms can survive in the gall-bladder or urinary tract for months or years after clinical recovery. The disease is abnormally common following gastrectomy, presumably as a result of a low gastric acidity (Waddell and Kunz, 1956), and may be more severe (Axon and Poole, 1973). Antibiotic resistance of the causative organism is important in some epidemics. Following ingestion, *S. typhi* multiplies in the second part of the duodenum; bile forms a good culture medium. There may be an inflammatory reaction in the jejunum (Chapter 17). The disease starts with a septicaemia, the portal of entry probably being the lymphoid (Peyer's) patches in the terminal ileum, which the bacilli have already invaded, and in which they have multiplied. That explains the early symptoms of the disease and the wide variety of complications. There is widespread dissemination, especially to the liver, spleen, and reticuloendothelial system. After a few days, the organisms, which by then are being excreted at high concentration in the bile, are present at greatest concentration in lymphoid tissue, especially the Peyer's patches, where they produce ulcers which may later perforate or bleed (see below). Although the brunt of the insult is to the distal ileum, lesions may be as high as the jejunum and as low as the large intestine, where the ascending colon is not infrequently involved. In paratyphoid B infection, ulcers have been reported as far afield as the stomach and rectum (Edington and Gilles, 1976). Neighbouring lymph-glands become enlarged and there is usually splenomegaly.

The pathological changes in the intestine can be divided into four stages (Edington and Gilles, 1976): (i) hyperaemia, (ii) necrosis, (iii) ulceration, and (iv) healing, which correspond in crude terms to the chronological stages of the disease in weeks. At stage (i), large phagocytic monocytes (pale eosinophilic cells with an eccentric nucleus, 'typhoid fever' cells) derived from the reticuloendothial system, produce congestion and elevation of lymphoid tissue, so that it projects into the ileal lumen. Monocytes, lymphocytes, and plasma cells are also present. Toxins released from dead bacilli produce necrosis which extends into the mucosa and submucosa (ii); thrombosis of small blood vessels contributes to that process. Ulceration (iii) accompanied by sloughing, takes place on the antimesenteric border; the ulcers are oval (up to three or four cm in length) and lie on the long axis of the intestine (Morson and Dawson, 1972). They are usually separate, but may be confluent in the ileocaecal region. Ulcer edges are soft, raised and undermined; the floor contains necrotic green-black slough, and the muscularis may be visible. Healing (iv), rather surprisingly, is not followed by fibrosis and stricture formation; scarring is minimal. A fibrinous exudate may be found on the peritoneal surface; ileus is a complication of that (Bohrer, 1966).

There may be very extensive large-intestinal involvement, similar to that in shigellosis (Chapter 24) (Mandal and Mani, 1976).

22.2. Presentation of salmonellosis

Typhoid fever has a peak incidence at between 10 and 35 years of age. The disease has an incubation period of five to 21 days; in most cases that is 10 to 14 days. It is notifiable. Although contacts are not notifiable, they should be kept under surveillance for three weeks.

The onset is insidious; the temperature rises in 'stepladder' fashion over four or five days, and is usually higher at night than day. The pulse shows a relative bradycardia, when the height of the body-temperature is taken into account. Malaise, headache, drowsiness, and aching limbs and backache are prominent features. The patient is usually constipated at that stage, although occasionally there is diarrhoea; abdominal discomfort is common. Cough and epistaxes also frequently occur. At that stage, and also later in the disease, leucopenia is characteristic (see below). At the end of the first week a rash may appear on the upper abdomen and back; it cannot usually be recognized on a pigmented skin. It consists of 'rose spots' which fade on pressure; there may be a fresh crop of spots after two or three days, as the first batch is fading. At about seven to 10 days, splenomegaly is present; the organ is soft, and enlarged to one or two cm below the costal margin. However, because most people in tropical countries have splenomegaly that sign is of very limited value. At that time also, diarrhoea with peasoup stools starts; there is often tenderness in the right iliac fossa. Although the diarrhoea is usually of the small-intestinal type, small bloody stools occur more frequently than is generally recognized (Mandal and Mani, 1976). The patient may now lie motionless—the 'typhoid state'—with his eyes half closed—the 'typhoid facies'. Bronchitis and delirium may complicate the disease at that stage.

If untreated, by 14 days the patient will probably be severely ill, although the illness contains a wide spectrum of clinical courses. In the third week severe toxaemia, coma, and death may supervene. Haemorrhage or perforation from Peyer's patches (see below) may occur during the third week, although Davey (1968) considers that perforation in west Africa often takes place at the end of the first week of illness. If recovery is to occur, the temperature slowly falls, and anorexia and abdominal distension disappear. A rebound of the clinical illness may occur up to one or two weeks after the temperature has become normal; the secondary illness is less severe than the primary one. Mortality is highest is the young and old.

The disease must be distinguished clinically from other fevers associated with a depressed white blood-cell count: viral pneumonia, psittacosis, Q-fever, tuberculosis, brucellosis, and bacterial endocarditis, should all be considered. *Yersinia enterocolitica* can produce a similar clinical picture of enteritis, fever, diarrhoea, vomiting, abdominal pain, and mesenteric adenitis (Gutman, Ottesen, Quan, Noce, and Katz, 1973).

There is an interesting association between typhoid fever and glucose-6-phosphate dehydrogenase deficiency. A high incidence of the deficiency in patients with typhoid fever has been described in Ghana (Owusu, 1972). Also, typhoid fever can act as a trigger in the production of haemolysis in patients with glucose-6-phosphate dehydrogenase deficiency; that has been reported from a number of countries including South Africa, Malaysia, and Israel (Charmot, Dodin, Kauffmann, Voelckel, Auger, and Mailloux, 1966; Hersko and Vardy, 1967; Levin, 1967; Chan, Chesterman, McFadzean, and Todd, 1971), but in some cases it is undoubtedly related to the chemotherapy and not the disease.

If schistosomal hepatic fibrosis is present, the clinical picture may differ from that in an otherwise normal patient (Hathout, El-Ghaffar, and Awny, 1967).

Paratyphoid fever, and disease caused by other salmonella species are usually of lesser severity, with a slightly shorter incubation period (see below); complications are much less frequent.

22.3. Complications of salmonellosis

Haemorrhage and perforation, which classically occur at the end of the second week or during the third week of the disease, are the most important complications. Bleeding may be very severe, and there is often no previous warning. Perforation is usually from ulcerated Peyer's patches near the ileocaecal valve, in the second or third week (Jobson, 1978), and may be single or multiple. Those ulcers are deepest in the terminal 45 cm of ileum, are usually oval and longitudinal, and are situated on the antimesenteric aspect of the gut. Poor nutritional status and inadequate treatment are important predisposing factors. Other factors are: (i) late admission to hospital, (ii) extremely virulent strains of *S. typhi*, and (iii) lowered host resistance (Edington and Gilles, 1976). Small perforations, which are often asymptomatic, are certainly more common than is generally recognized; I have seen several cases in Zambia in which symptoms were minimal, but there was gas under the diaphragm. The signs and symptoms are due to a combination of peritonitis and obstruction; all grades of peritonitis are seen. There is loss of liver dullness. Rapid deterioration is usual.

Chloramphenicol may distort the classical clinical picture of peritonitis. Although perforation usually occurs at the classical time (see above), it is not uncommon during the first week of the disease in Nigeria (Davey, 1968) and Ghana (Archampong, 1969). A late typhoid perforation is often indistinguishable from perforated appendicitis, perforated amoebic abscess, tuberculous peritonitis, an infected ruptured ectopic pregnancy, and internal strangulation. In a series of 270 cases of 'enteric fever' in India, 30 (11 per cent) suffered a perforation (Khosla, 1977), and of those 18 died. Despite present day antibiotic treatment, perforation is still therefore a significant problem in this disease. A rare complication is intussusception (Leach and Wright, 1944).

Neuropsychiatric complications of the disease have probably been underestimated. In a study in India, Khosla, Srivastava, and Gupta (1977) found evidence of a confusional state, delirium, coma, generalized myoclonus, Parkinsonian rigidity, or psychoses in 124 of 246 cases. A relationship between psychiatric complications and severity of the anaemia has been suggested (Abu-Asha and Kaballo, 1976); folate deficiency and a high 'salmonella load' may be important.

The septicaemia present during the first week can give rise to complications in virtually all systems and organs. Thus, bronchitis, pneumonia and lung abscess, thrombophlebitis in the lower limbs, myocarditis and pericarditis, myositis (Zenker's degeneration), parotitis, arthritis, periostitis, osteomyelitis, spondylitis (typhoid spine), meningitis, peripheral neuropathy, orchitis, and cholecystitis may all occur; acute cholecystitis seems to be unusual in tropical countries.

Sickle-cell (haemoglobin SS and SC) disease favours the development of a salmonella osteomyelitis (Vandepitte, *et al.*, 1953; Hook, Campbell, Weens, and Cooper, 1957; Roberts and Hilburg, 1958; Hendrickse and Collard, 1960). It has been suggested that in patients with sickle-cell (SS and SC) disease there is a diminished resistance to invasion of the gastrointestinal tract by salmonellae; after crossing the enterocyte, they invade necrotic foci in bone-marrow with the production of osteitis and osteomyelitis.

Hepatocellular jaundice may be a complication (Chapter 5); the frequency of that event varies, however, in different areas. In Zambia, for example, it is common. In a study of 15 patients with typhoid fever in Vietnam, four were reported to be jaundiced, and six had hepatomegaly; in 14 of them, at least one liver-function-test was abnormal (Diem, My, Chi, Nhon, and Thuc, 1976). All 15 of those patients had liver-biopsy abnormalities; in eight there was spotty necrosis, and that was more common in those with hepatomegaly and jaundice. Other histological abnormalities were: swelling and fatty change in the hepatocytes, Kupffer cell hyperplasia, and monocytic infiltration of the perisinusoidal and portal spaces (Chapter 5). There is also a considerable variation in different reports from the same region; thus Ramachandran, Godfrey, and Perera (1974) reported an eight per cent, and Singh, Nair, Krishnasamy, Aurora, Chandrasekar, and Bisht (1978) a one per cent incidence of jaundice in Sri Lanka and south India. Acute haemolysis has been reported in glucose-6-phosphate deficient patients (Constantopoulos, Economopoulos, and Kandylas, 1973); fulminant diarrhoea was also a problem in that situation. There is occasionally massive haemolysis (Lwanga and Wing, 1970).

A haemolytic-uraemic syndrome may also complicate the disease (Kaplan and Drummond, 1978).

A toxic nephrosis, acute nephritis, pyelonephritis, pyelitis, and perinephric abscess (Belzer, 1965) have all been described following this disease.

Approximately two to four per cent of patients with the disease become chronic carriers; in most faecal carriers. There is a higher incidence of typhoid carriers amongst people infected with *Clonorchis sinensis* (Chapter 14) (McFadzean and Ong, 1966). In areas of the world where *Schistosoma haematobium* infections are common, a chronic urinary carrier state may result (Weir, Wasif, Hassan, Attia, and Kadu, 1952; Hathout, El-Ghaffar, Awny, and Hassan, 1966); these carriers have intermittent attacks of bacteraemia. Salmonella septicaemia has been described in *S. mansoni* infections in both Egypt and Brazil (Rocha, Kirk, and Hearey, 1971).

22.4. Investigation of salmonellosis

22.4.1. Routine investigations

During the first week, blood-culture (using bile-salt broth) is extremely important; at that time the organism is absent from the faeces and often the urine also. In a study involving 62 patients, *S. typhi* was isolated from bone-marrow culture in 90 per cent; corresponding percentages of positive results from blood, stool and urine were 40, 37, and 4 (Gilman, Terminel, Levine, Hernandez-Mendoza, and Hornick, 1975). The low rate for positive blood cultures in that investigation was , obably partly explained by previous chemotherapy (Watson, 1975). A leucopenia with a relative lymphocytosis suggests the diagnosis. During the second week, stool and urine cultures may reveal *S. typhi*. There may be haemolysis (McFadzean and Choa, 1953) and the Coomb's test is sometimes positive; occasionally that is superimposed on a deficiency of glucose-6-phosphate dehydrogenase (Meyer, 1973).

The *diazo* test is positive in 90 per cent of cases between the fifth and fourteenth day (Huckstep, 1962); that seems to be of great value in typhoid epidemics.*

Following perforation, erect and supine X-rays of the abdomen show signs of intestinal obstruction, and free intraperitoneal gas in 50 per cent of cases (Fig. 22.1); the large amount of gas present is due principally to the fact that the small intestine is greatly distended at the time of perforation (Bohrer, 1966).

22.4.2. Serology

The earliest serological response is a rise in the titre of the 0 (somatic) antibody; H (flagella) antibody develops more slowly and persists longer (*Br. med. J.*, 1978c). During the second week (at about the tenth day), the Widal

* The diazo reagent consists of 40 parts of solution A (sulphanilic acid 0·5g; concentrated hydrochloric acid 5·0 ml; distilled water 100 ml) and one part of solution B (sodium nitrite 0·5 g; distilled water 100 ml). 5 ml are added to 5 ml urine, and followed by the addition of a few drops of 30 per cent ammonia. After shaking, a pink or red colouration of the froth denotes a positive result. [N.B. the diazo reagent keeps for three days in a refrigerator].

reaction (agglutination test) (Widal, 1896) becomes positive, but often at a low titre. An 0 antibody of 1:60 is highly suggestive of the diagnosis, but a rising titre is of much greater significance. However, previous TAB immunization and earlier infections with salmonellae sharing common 0 antigens, can stimulate antibody production. Also, patients from communities with endemic typhoid often have higher H-antibody titres than those not exposed to the antigen; in them a single Widal test is of no value whatsoever (Levine, 1979).

Experience in a large outbreak of *S. typhi* infection in Aberdeen, Scotland, in 1964 has cast much doubt on the value of serology as a means of diagnosis of typhoid fever (Brodie, 1977a and b). A second Widal reaction in the second week may show a higher titre; that is of value in indicating that an increase in agglutination was not due to a previous TAB vaccination.

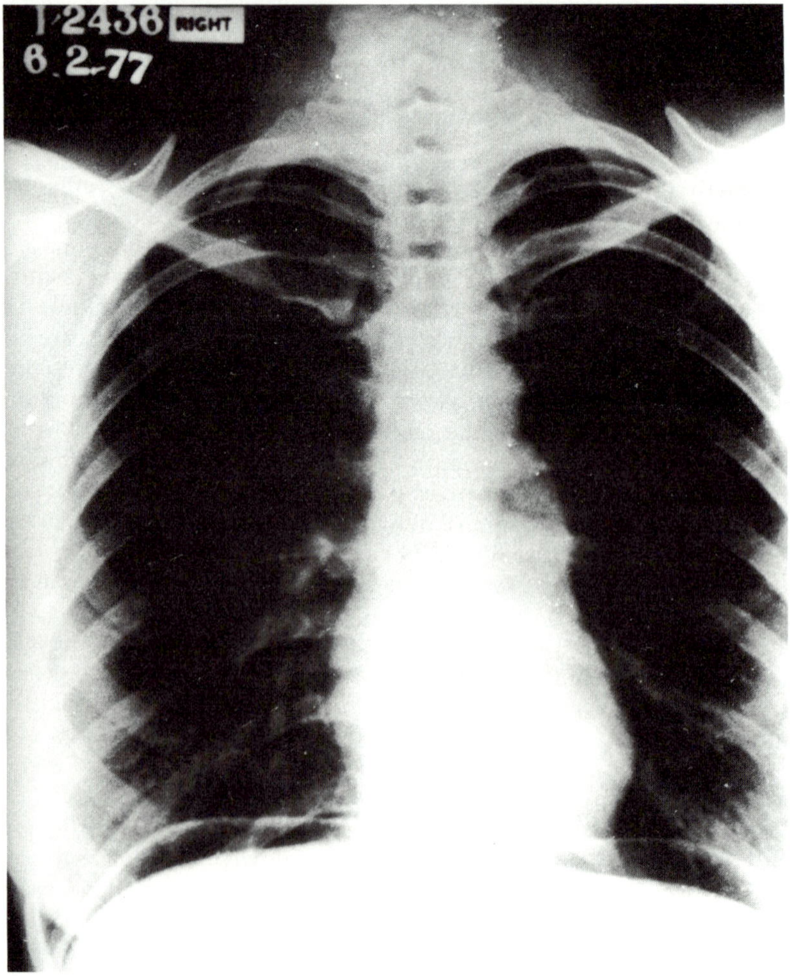

FIG. 22.1. Chest radiograph in a 32-year-old Papua New Guinean man with salmonellosis (typhoid fever). Gas is shown under both domes of the diaphragm following perforation of the ileum during the second week of the disease.

Detection of Vi antibody is of no value in diagnosing an acute attack or a clinical relapse; however, it is of value in the detection of carriers (Forrest, Matthews, Robertson, and Hanley, 1967). Seventy per cent of carriers of *S. typhi* have Vi (virulence) antibodies at a titre of 1:5 or more (*Public Health Laboratory Service Report*, 1961). Phage typing is of value in tracing the source of carriers.

22.4.3. Salmonella agglutinins in chronic liver disease

In patients with active chronic hepatitis and cirrhosis, serum antisalmonella agglutinins are sometimes raised. Thus 11 of 40 (27 per cent) of a group of patients in the USA with active chronic hepatitis had raised agglutinins (Protell, Soloway, Martin, Schoenfield, and Summerskill, 1971); bacteriological cultures for salmonella were negative in all of them. Because the annual incidence of salmonellosis in the USA is only 0·01 per cent, that high occurrence was considered to be significant. It may be that patients with active chronic hepatitis are unduly susceptible to typhoid; there is however no evidence for that. Chronic liver disease is therefore a source of false positive typhoid serology. That is probably due to disordered globulin formation in active chronic hepatitis, resulting from impaired sequestration of antigens by the Kupffer cells in the liver sinusoids (Chapter 8) (Triger and Wright, 1973).

22.5. Treatment of salmonellosis

Prophylactic treatment is with TAB, a vaccine prepared from typhoid and paratyphoid bacilli, which is given by the subcutaneous route; 0·5 ml should be followed by 1·0 ml after 2 weeks. That provides moderate protection (*Bull. Wld Hlth Org*., 1962; 1964) for about two years; where typhoid is a common disease, a booster dose of 0·5 to 1·0 ml should be given every two or three years. Close contacts of a carrier should be immunized. Travellers to third-world countries where the disease is common should take precautions with drinking water and foodstuffs likely to be affected (see above). For treatment of a suspected case of typhoid fever, bed rest and barrier nursing are necessary; provision of gowns and adequate washing facilities, sterilization of all personal articles, and disinfection of excreta are all important.

In the acute disease, fluid balance must be carefully maintained; parenteral fluids may be necessary (Chapter 17).

The antibiotic of choice is chloramphenicol (Woodward, Smadel, Ley, Green, and Mankikar, 1948); in adults 4 g should be given daily for two weeks. The response is usually dramatic. It may however produce haemolysis in glucose-6-phosphate dehydrogenase deficient individuals. Bone-marrow depression and sideroblastic anaemia (Foster, Obineche, and Traub, 1974) are possible complications. Fatal hypothermia following chloramphenicol treatment has been reported (Mulligan, 1971). Co-trimoxazole ('Septrin') has recently been used with good results (2 tablets twice daily for 2 weeks) (Akinkugbe, Lewis, Montefiore, and Okubadejo, 1968; Kamat, 1970; Farid, Hassan, Wahab, Sanborn, Kent, Yassa, and Hathout, 1970; Geddes, Fothergill, Goodall, and Dorken, 1971; Scragg and Rubidge, 1971; Sardesai, Karandikar, and Harshe, 1973; Obineche and Traub, 1976; Ramachandran, *et al.*,

1978) but its role in the treatment of typhoid fever is not yet established. Alternatively, ampicillin ('Penbritin') lg six hourly for two weeks may be used (Robertson, Wahab, and Raasch, 1968). Working in Hong Kong, Chan and Mak (1976) considered that ampicillin was undoubtedly inferior to chloramphenicol and co-trimoxazole, and should be used only: (i) in pregnancy, when both chloramphenicol and co-trimoxazole are harmful to the foetus, and (ii) in glucose-6-phosphate dehydrogenase deficiency, when co-trimoxazole is clearly contraindicated, due to its ability to produce acute haemolysis (Owusu, 1972; Chan and McFadzean, 1974). The Stevens-Johnson syndrome may also be a complication of co-trimoxazole therapy (Kikuchi and Okazaki, 1978). In many countries, including those of central and south America, reports have been made of strains of *S. typhi* which are resistant to chloramphenicol and ampicillin (Overturf, Marton, and Mathies, 1973; *Lancet*, 1975).

Typhoid fever resistant to chloramphenicol has become a very widespread problem throughout the tropics (*Lancet*, 1973; Butler, Linh, Arnold, and Pollack, 1973). A water-borne outbreak of *S. typhi* which was resistant to chloramphenicol has been reported from Mexico (Gonzalez-Cortes, Bessudo, Sanchez-Leyva, Fragoso, Hinojosa, and Becerril, 1973). Sensitivity tests should be carried out when possible.

In a report by Ramachandran, *et al*. (1978), 10 per cent of 42 patients with either typhoid or paratyphoid fever who were treated with co-trimoxazole, and none of 49 treated with chloramphenicol, were unresponsive to treatment; however the continued excretion of organisms after treatment was more common after chloramphenicol than after co-trimoxazole.

The serious complications, haemorrhage and perforation, must always be borne in mind. Haemorrhage is treated by blood transfusion; surgery is not indicated. Perforation occurs in from two to four per cent and accounts for 20 to 40 per cent of deaths in this disease (Davey, 1968). It should normally be treated conservatively; the patient is frequently too ill for surgery (Khosla, 1977). Intravenous fluids should be given cautiously due to the toxic state of the myocardium; the stomach should be aspirated with a nasogastric tube. Davey (1968) recommends that the patient should be nursed flat due to the 'parlous state of the circulatory system'. If laparotomy is undertaken, the ileal wall is found to be 'paper-thin' and apt to perforate further at operation; it is not unusual to find an adult *ascaris* within the abdominal cavity which has escaped from the typhoid perforation (Davey, 1968). Huckstep (1960;1962) has indicated that surgical treatment should be undertaken for: (i) a sudden perforation in an otherwise fairly fit patient, and (ii) a perforation leading to complications, i.e. intestinal obstruction and abscess formation. Davey (1968) considers, furthermore, that if the patient is moribund surgery should always be undertaken if there is any doubt at all of the diagnosis. If the patient is unfit for laparotomy, drainage of the right lower quadrant of the abdomen can be performed under local anaesthesia. In fact, surgery may be extremely difficult; suturing of the ragged ileum resulting from perforation of the Peyer's patches may be virtually impossible. Welch and Martin (1975) have recommended, from experience of typhoid perforation of the ileum in 50 patients, that either wedge excision (if there is a single area of diseased ileum), or segmental ileal resection (if the disease is more widespread) are the correct operations. Furthermore, surgery is often complicated by peripheral vascular failure, wound sepsis, abscess formation, burst abdomen, and intestinal obstruction. Healing of the perforation takes place by granulation and little scarring results. Reports of large series of patients with perforated typhoid ulcers have been made from Ibadan, Nigeria (Dickson and Cole, 1964) and Accra, Ghana (Badoe, 1966). Mortality rates with and without operation are high (Khosla, 1977); without an antibiotic cover, rates as high as 87 per cent have been reported (Baliga, 1949); with chloramphenicol a 60 per cent mortality rate has been recorded (Khosla, 1977).

After recovery the patient must be followed up carefully for three weeks. Relapses occur at different frequencies in different series, and range from 11 (*Br. med. J.*, 1963) to 41 (Huckstep, 1962) per cent. In the event of relapse a second course of antibiotic may be necessary. Six stool and three urine specimens must be negative before a patient can be declared free of the disease.

Antibiotics are overall of limited value, but should nevertheless be tried, in the carrier state; cholecystectomy may be necessary. Amoxycillin trihydrate ('Amoxil'), which is absorbed more rapidly and thus achieves a higher blood concentration than other oral penicillins, has given encouraging results in the treatment of carriers, in a limited therapeutic trial (Nolan and White, 1978); nine of 10 carriers who received 2 g amoxycillin three times daily for 28 days were cured of the disease, as opposed to two of five patients who were treated with smaller doses. The mean serum amoxycillin trihydrate concentration was higher in those who were cured. The only problem seemed to be gastrointestinal intolerance to the high doses used.

If a *S. mansoni* or *S. haematobium* infection is present (Farid, Higashi, Bassily, Young, and Sparks, 1972). It is important to eliminate that before treating chronic salmonellosis. Carriers must not be allowed to work as food handlers.

22.6. Food-poisoning caused by salmonella species

These organisms, which are closely related to *S. typhi*, produce food-poisoning. *S. typhimurium* is the most common of many salmonella serotypes; other examples are *S. poona*, *S. heidelberg*, *S. infantis*, *S. newport*, and *S. enteritidis*. They are frequently present in water supplies in developing countries throughout the world. In Trinidad, a large epidemic of salmonellosis was traced to contaminated powdered milk (Weissman, Doug Deen, Williams, Swanston, and Ali, 1977). Many species of animals and birds act as reservoirs of infection (Levine, 1979). Patients with Oroya fever (Bartonellosis) (Chapter 7) are especially susceptible to septicaemic infection with *S. typhimurium* (Cuadra, 1956), which may prove fatal. The organisms multiply in the intestine; most do not produce a toxin, and although there is superficial infection there is little invasion.

The incubation period is 8–48 hours. Onset is either abrupt or gradual, with diarrhoea, and often a low grade fever; there may be some vomiting. The disease should be differentiated from other causes of food-poisoning (Chapter 17); viral gastroenteritis, shigellosis, and amoebic and bacillary dysentery.

There is not usually a leucocytosis. Stool cultures are positive. A prolonged carrier state is common.

Fluid and electrolyte replacement may be necessary. Antibiotics should not be given unless systemic dissemination is suspected; recent reports indicate multiple antibiotic resistance in some salmonella strains. A *S. typhimurium* strain, resistant to not only chloramphenicol and ampicillin, but also trimethoprim has been reported (Finlayson and Jackson, 1978). An investigation into antibiotic sensitivities of salmonellae in Uganda has been made (Phillips and Tindimwebwa, 1972); multiple resistance was common there.

References

ABU-ASHA, H. and KABALLO, A. (1976). *E. Afr. med. J.*, **53,** 516.

AKINKUGBE, O. O., LEWIS, E. A., MONTEFIORE, D., and OKUBADEJO, O. A. (1968). *Br. med. J.*, **3,** 721.

ARCHAMPONG, E. Q. (1969). *Br. med. J.*, **3,** 273.

AXON, A. T. R. and POOLE, D. (1973). *Lancet*, **1,** 745.

BADOE, A. E. (1966). *Ghana med. J.*, **5,** 83.

BALIGA, A. V. (1949). *Indian J. Surg.*, **11,** 165.

BELZER, M. (1965). *J. Urol.*, **94,** 23.

BOHRER, S. P. (1966). *Br. J. Radiol.*, **39,** 37.

Br. med. J. (1963). **1,** 1041.

—— (1978a). **2,** 1385.

—— (1978b). **1,** 1008.

—— (1978c). **1,** 389.

BRODIE, J. (1977a). *J. Hyg., Camb.*, **79,** 161.

—— (1977b). *J. Hyg., Camb.*, **79,** 181.

BUDD, W. (1856). *Lancet*, **2,** 618.

Bull. Wld Hlth Org., (1962). **26,** 357.

—— (1964). **30,** 623.

BUTLER, T., LINH, N. N., ARNOLD, K., and POLLACK, M. (1973). *Lancet*, **2,** 983.

CHAN, A. C. H. and MAK, M. H. H. (1976). *Tropical Doctor*, **6,** 53.

CHAN, T. K., CHESTERMAN, C. N., MCFADZEAN A. J. S., and TODD, D. (1971). *J. Lab. clin. Med.*, **77,** 177.

—— and MCFADZEAN, A. J. S. (1974). *Trans. R. Soc. trop. Med. Hyg.*, **68,** 61.

CHARMOT, G., DODIN, A., KAUFFMANN, J. M., VOELCKEL, J., AUGER, C., and MAILLOUX, C. (1966). *Bull. Soc. Path. exot.*, **59,** 400.

CONSTANTOPOULOS, A., ECONOMOPOULOS, P., and KANDYLAS, J. (1973). *Lancet*, **1,** 1522.

CUADRA, C. M. (1956). *Tex. Rep. Biol. Med.*, **14,** 97.

DAVEY, W. W. (1968). *Companion to surgery in Africa.* p. 214. E. and S. Livingstone, Edinburgh and London.

DICKSON, J. A. S. and COLE, G. J. (1964). *Br. J. Surg.*, **51,** 893.

DIEM, L. V., MY T. Q., CHI, N. V., NHON, N. T., and THUC, T. K. (1976). *J. trop. Med. Hyg.*, **79,** 25.

EDINGTON, G. M. and GILLES, H. M. (1976). *Pathology in the tropics.* 2nd ed. p. 321. Edward Arnold, London.

FARID, Z., HASSAN, A., WAHAB, M. F. A., SANBORN, W. R., KENT, D. C., YASSA, A., and HATHOUT, S. E. (1970). *Br. med. J.*, **3,** 323.

——, HIGASHI, G. I., BASSILY, S., YOUNG, S. W., and SPARKS, H. A. (1972). *Am. J. trop. Med. Hyg.*, **21,** 578.

FINLAYSON, M. C. and JACKSON, F. L. (1978). *Lancet*, **2,** 375.

FORREST, C. R., MATTHEWS, R. N., ROBERTSON, M. J., and HANLEY, W. P. (1967). *Br. med. J.*, **2,** 472.

FOSTER, D. N., OBINECHE, E. N., and TRAUB, N. E. (1974). *E. Afr. med. J.*, **51,** 20.
GEDDES, A. M., FOTHERGILL, R., GOODALL, J. A. D., and DORKEN, P. R. (1971). *Br. med. J.*, **3,** 451.
GILMAN, R. H., TERMINEL, M., LEVINE, M. M., HERNANDEZ-MENDOZA, P., and HORNICK, R. B. (1975). *Lancet*, **1,** 1211.
GONZALEZ-CORTES, A., BESSUDO, D., SANCHEZ-LEYVA, R., FRAGOSO, R., HINOJOSA, M., and BECERRIL, P. (1973). *Lancet*, **2,** 605.
GRADY, G. F. and KEUSCH, G. T. (1971). *New Engl. J. Med.*, **285,** 831.
GUTMAN, L. T., OTTESEN, E. A., QUAN, T. J., NOCE, P. S., and KATZ, S. L. (1973). *New Engl. J. Med.*, **288,** 1372.
HATHOUT, S. E., EL-GHAFFAR, Y. A., And AWNY, A. Y. (1967). *Am. J. trop. Med. Hyg.*, **16,** 462.
——, ——, ——, and HASSAN, K. (1966). *Am. J. trop. Med. Hyg.*, **15,** 156.
HENDRICKSE, R. G. and COLLARD, P. (1960). *Lancet*, **1,** 80.
HERSKO, C. and VARDY, P. A. (1967). *Br. med. J.*, **1,** 214.
HOOK, E. W., CAMPBELL, C. G., WEENS, H. S., and COOPER, G. R. (1957). *New Engl. J. Med.*, **257,** 403.
HUCKSTEP, R. L. (1960). *Ann. R. Coll. Surg.*, **26,** 207.
—— (1962). *Typhoid fever and other salmonella infections.* E. and S. Livingstone, Edinburgh and London.
JOBSON, K. F. (1978). *Tropical Doctor*, **8,** 76.
KAMAT, S. A. (1970). *Br. med. J.*, **3,** 320.
KAPLAN, B. S. and DRUMMOND, K. N. (1978). *New Engl. J. Med.*, **298,** 964.
KHOSLA, S. N. (1977). *J. trop. Med. Hyg.*, **80,** 83.
KHOSLA, S. N., SRIVASTAVA, S. C., and GUPTA, S. (1977). *J. trop. Med. Hyg.*, **80,** 95.
KIKUCHI, S. and OKAZAKI, T. (1978). *Lancet*, **2,** 580.
Lancet (1973). **2,** 1008.
—— (1975). **1,** 1230.
LEECH, R. B. and WRIGHT, F. J. (1944). *E. Afr. med. J.*, **21,** 340.
LEVIN, S. E. (1967). *Br. med. J.*, **2,** 175.
LEVINE, M. M. (1979). *Tropical Doctor*, **9,** 4.
LWANGA, D. and WING, A. J. (1970). *E. Afr. med. J.*, **47,** 146.
MCFADZEAN, A. J. S. and CHOA, G. H. (1953). *Br. med. J.*, **2,** 360.
—— and ONG, G. B. (1966). *Br. med. J.*, **1,** 1567.
MANDAL, B. K. and MANI, V. (1976). *Lancet*, **1,** 887.
MEYER, H. A. (1973). *Lancet*, **1,** 729.
MORSON, B. C. and DAWSON, I. M. P. (1972). *Gastrointestinal pathology*. p. 251. Blackwell, Oxford, London, Edinburgh, and Melbourne.
MULLIGAN, T. O. (1971). *W. Afr. med. J.*, **20,** 358.
NOLAN, C. M. and WHITE, P. C. (1978). *J. Am. med. Ass.*, **239,** 2352.
OBINECHE, E. N. and TRAUB, N. E. (1976). *E. Afr. Med. J.*, **53,** 484.
OVERTURF, G., MARTON, K. I., and MATHIES, A. W. (1973). *New Engl. J. Med.*, **289,** 463.
OWUSU, S. K. (1972). *Lancet*, **2,** 819.
PHILLIPS, I. and TINDIMWEBWA, G. (1972). *E. Afr. med. J.*, **49,** 658.
PROTELL, R. L., SOLOWAY, R. D., MARTIN, W. J., SCHOENFIELD, L. J., and SUMMERSKILL, W. H. J. (1971). *Lancet*, **2,** 330.
Public Health Laboratory Service Report (1961). *J. Hyg., Camb.*, **59,** 231.
RAMACHANDRAN, S., GODFREY, J. J., and LIONEL, N. D. W. (1978). *J. trop. Med. Hyg.*, **81,** 36.
——, ——, and PERERA, M. V. F. (1974). *J. Am. med. Ass.*, **230,** 236.
ROBERTS, A. R. and HILBURG, L. E. (1958). *J. Pediat.*, **52,** 170.
ROBERTSON, R. P., WAHAB, M. F. A., and RAASCH, F. O. (1968). *New Engl. J. Med.*, **278,** 171.
ROCHA, H., KIRK, J. W., and HEAREY, C. D. (1971). *Archs intern. Med.*, **128,** 254.

Sardesai, H. V., Karandikar, R. S., and Harshe, R. G. (1973). *Br. med. J.*, **1,** 82.
Scragg, J. N. and Rubidge, C. J. (1971). *Br. med. J.*, **3,** 738.
Singh, D. S., Nair, P. N. R., Krishnasamy, S., Aurora, A. L., Chandrasekar, S., and Bisht, D. B. (1978). *J. trop. Med. Hyg.*, **81,** 68.
Triger, D. R. and Wright, R. (1973). *Lancet*, **1,** 1494.
Vandepitte, J., Colaert, J., Lambotte-Legrand, J., Lambotte-Legrand, C., and Perin, F. (1953). *Annls Soc. belge Méd. trop.*, **33,** 511.
Waddell, W. R. and Kunz, L. J. (1956). *New Engl. J. Med.*, **255,** 555.
Watson, K. C. (1975). *Lancet*, **1,** 1377.
Weir, J. M., Wasif, I. M., Hassan, F. R., Attia, S. M., and Kadu, M. A. (1952). *J. Egypt. publ. Hlth Ass.*, **27,** 55.
Weissman, J. B., Doug Deen, R. M. A., Williams, M., Swanston, N., and Ali, S. (1977). *W. Indian med. J.*, **26,** 135.
Welch, T. P. and Martin, N. C. (1975). *Lancet*, **1,** 1078.
Wicks, A. C. B., Holmes, G. S., and Davidson, L. (1971). *Q. Jl. Med.*, **40,** 341.
Widal, G. F. I. (1896). *Bull. Soc. méd. Hôp. Paris*, **13,** 561.
Woodward, T. E., Smadel, J. E., Ley, H. L., Green, R., and Mankikar, D. S. (1948). *Ann. intern. Med.*, **29,** 131.

23

Chronic infections, tumours, and trauma involving the small intestine and peritoneum

23.1. Abdominal tuberculosis

THE clinical spectrum of intra-abdominal tuberculosis is broad. It includes upper gastrointestinal lesions, small-intestinal ulceration which is usually in the ileum, infection of the omentum and mesenteric lymph nodes, hyperplastic ileocaecal disease, tuberculous peritonitis, anorectal lesions, miliary tuberculosis, and hepatitis.

Abdominal tuberculosis may be primary or secondary and is very common not only in the tropics, but also in immigrants from Africa and Asia in European and other non-tropical countries. In Manchester, England, 15 cases of abdominal tuberculosis were diagnosed in a five-year period; all except one were in immigrants, of whom 11 were from the Indian subcontinent and one was from Africa (Mandal and Schofield, 1976). Eleven had been in England for several years. In another review of the condition in Britain, 14 cases were documented by Bentley and Webster (1967); only 50 per cent of those were secondary to tuberculosis elsewhere.

Francis (1972) has reviewed 106 cases of abdominal tuberculosis seen at Ibadan, Nigeria; they were drawn from 1583 consecutive post-mortems on individuals of 10 years of age and more. That constituted 10·6 per cent of those examined. The disease affected all age groups, from 10 to 62 years, and was more common in females. Diarrhoea was a symptom in 60 of them; 46 complained of abdominal swelling. Only 20 had had febrile episodes. Most were malnourished. Twenty-one had hepatomegaly and 33 per cent of those had splenomegaly. Forty had ascites, and in six an abdominal mass could be felt. Of those with ascites, 54 per cent had enlarged abdominal glands and peritoneal nodes, 17 per cent abdominal glands alone, and 15 per cent glands and perforated tuberculous intestinal ulcerations, which were usually ileal. Seventy per cent of 45 patients tested, had a negative Heaf result. Forty had straight abdominal radiographs; none showed calcified abdominal glands. A report of 65 cases of abdominal tuberculosis has been made from Khartoum, Sudan (El Masri, Boulos, and Malick, 1977).

Abdominal tuberculosis is probably more common in patients receiving corticosteroids and immunosuppressive agents. Diagnosis at post-mortem is all too common.

23.1.1. Glandular tuberculosis

Numerically this is the most common type of abdominal tuberculosis in tropical countries (Edington and Gilles, 1976). There is not usually a pulmonary parenchymal lesion, but there may be significant lymphadenopathy in the neck, groins, and axillae, and also the mesenteric, para-aortic, and upper abdominal groups of glands. When a gland ruptures, the whole of the mesenteric and peritoneal surfaces are studded with tubercles; tuberculous peritonitis is a sequel (see below). That form of tuberculosis may also be secondary to infection of the Fallopian tubes.

Massive caseation of the mesenteric lymph glands can occur in children (Jelliffe, 1949) and adults (Ball, 1968); in most that ultimately calcifies, and opacities are obvious on straight abdominal radiographs in later life (Fig. 23.1).

The onset is usually insidious with loss of weight and progressive ill-health, followed by swelling of the abdomen and legs. Abdominal pain is either mild and transient, or may be absent altogether, especially in the elderly. On examination oedema involving the legs, and sometimes the face and trunk also, together with painless ascites, anaemia, and depigmented skin may be present; there may also be a low-grade fever and peripheral vasoconstriction. Enlarged glands may be palpated in the neck, axillae, or groins. If there is hepatosplenomegaly, miliary disease should be suspected. Dinner (1965) has given his experience of the disease at Johannesburg, South Africa.

Histological examination of a superficial lymph node frequently clinches the diagnosis; cervical glands are most likely to be positive. A parenchymal lesion on chest radiography is rare; there may be enlarged hilar glands, however. Sputum does not often contain acid-fast bacilli; Heaf and Mantoux reactions are usually positive, and are of little help. If there is no clinical evidence of peritonitis, the ascitic fluid is yellow, with flakes of fibrin; it may occasionally be haemorrhagic. If a transudate, the fluid contains less than 20 g per l protein, and a few cells; however the protein concentration is often 25 g per l or more and numerous lymphocytes and bacilli can be seen on stained smears. Culture or animal inoculation may be necessary. There is usually a normochromic anaemia. Hypoalbuminaemia is present and is often severe; that is due to impaired albumin synthesis and also increased catabolism. Lymphoedema of the intestinal mucosa, due to lymphatic obstruction, is probably the main cause of albumin loss from the intestine.

A laparotomy may be necessary to clinch the diagnosis, but frequently the patient is too ill, and a therapeutic trial of anti-tuberculous agents usually establishes the diagnosis.

Other causes of fluid retention, associated with anaemia, should be excluded. In severe hookworm anaemia, there is often hypoproteinaemia. The nephrotic syndrome, frequently associated with *Plasmodium malariae* infection, is common in many tropical countries. Cirrhosis of the liver, which is very common in most parts of the tropics (Chapter 8), also produces hypoalbuminaemia; a small firm liver, and splenomegaly are usually demonstrable.

Antituberculous agents should be given and improvement occurs over weeks or months (Fox, 1977). Occasionally hypoalbuminaemia, anaemia, and malab-

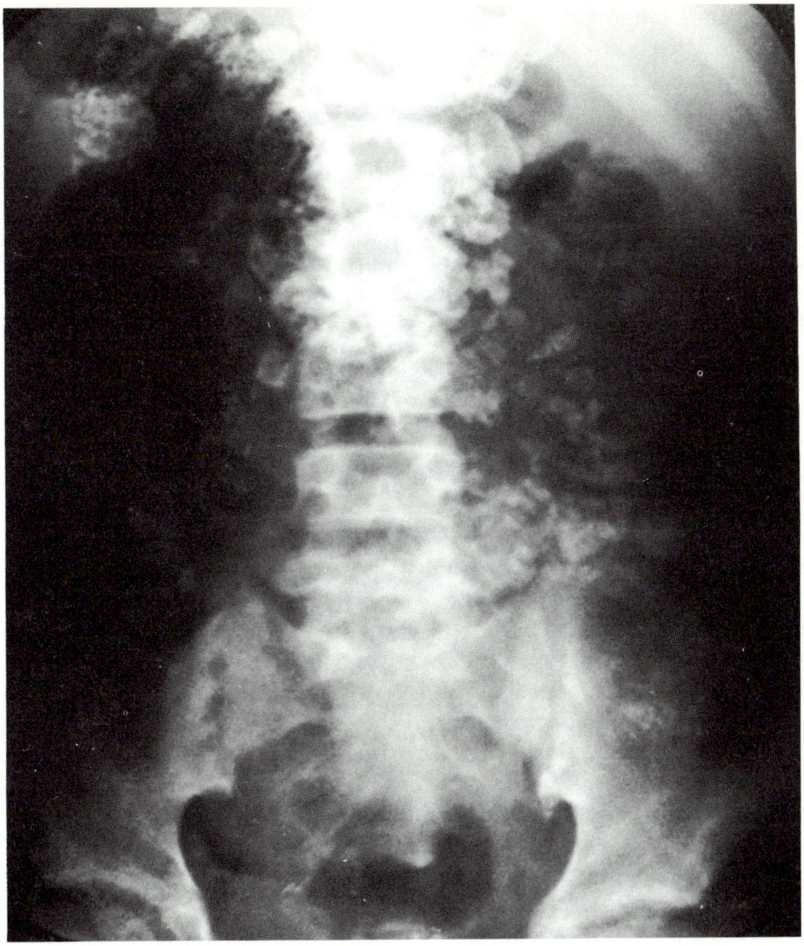

FIG. 23.1. Straight abdominal radiograph in a 13-year-old Papua New Guinean boy. He had previously been admitted, and treated, for glandular tuberculosis involving the cervical and mediastinal glands. Gross calcification of the mesenteric glands is shown; the cervical, axillary and mediastinal glands were also calcified.

sorption which is due to a bile-salt deficiency, may occur. Barium meal should be performed; and may show ileal strictures (ileocaecal tuberculosis) (see below); in that case surgery is indicated.

23.1.2. Ileocaecal tuberculosis

Throughout tropical countries, tuberculosis of the ileocaecal region is an important and underdiagnosed cause of intestinal disease, including intestinal malabsorption. It is probable that that disease, as well as various intestinal parasitic infections (Chapter 20), contributed to many of the cases designated as *tropical sprue* since Manson's description of that entity in 1880.

The condition should be suspected in all immigrants from Africa and Asia with symptoms suggesting malabsorption, even after several years residence in for example, the UK or USA, and in all indigenous people in tropical countries.

The disease is either a sequel to miliary tuberculosis, or follows ulceration of the ileum following ingestion of infected sputum. Following involvement of the Peyer's patches and the formation of transverse ulcers, which have undermined edges, fibrosis of the muscular coat and stenosis occurs; perforation is unusual. This results in hypertrophic ileocaecal disease (Morson and Dawson, 1972) which clinically may simulate carcinoma of the caecum (Anand, 1956); the appendix also may be involved. That condition must be excluded in every case of overt malabsorption in a tropical country. The resulting malabsorption and steatorrhoea are due largely to a chronic loss of bile salts, which are normally reabsorbed in the terminal ileum (Chapter 20). The diarrhoea is made worse by a direct effect of bile salts, which have not been reabsorbed, on the colon; water absorption is depressed.

Lewis and Kolawole (1972) described 20 cases of ileocaecal tuberculosis at Ibadan, Nigeria, in a clinicopathological study. Fever, abdominal pain, anorexia, weight loss, and diarrhoea were common presenting symptoms. Two presented with 'adult kwashiorkor' and three with generalized lymphadenopathy. Eleven had an abdominal mass, and two serous, lymphocytic ascites. On radiological grounds those authors defined five types: (i) hyperplastic disease, with long constricted regions and narrowing of the lumen, (ii) ulcerative disease, (iii) mixed hyperplastic and ulcerative types, (iv) carcinoma-like lesions, with short annular filling defects, and (v) a mixed group with fistula formation, appendicular mass, and extensive diverticula. Only five of those cases had demonstrable steatorrhoea. The disease is often complicated by miliary spread, dissemination within the peritoneal cavity, and granulomas in the ileum and colon, and rarely the abdominal wall (Ball, 1968).

Although severe diarrhoea in a patient with known tuberculosis must always be investigated for ileocaecal disease, an acute bacterial cause is in practice statistically more likely.

The clinical picture is dominated by diarrhoea and weight loss, often with symptoms caused by malabsorption (Fig. 23.2). A low grade pyrexia and anaemia are common. Lymphadenopathy is unusual. A mass is sometimes felt in the right iliac fossa.

The Mantoux test is nearly always positive. Barium meal and follow-through, or barium enema, will often show multiple ileal strictures (Fig. 23.3 shows multiple ileal strictures, associated with ileocaecal tuberculosis, in a Zambian African woman); there may also be shortening of the ascending colon and caecum, with loss of the normal ileocaecal angle. Chest radiography is normal. Acid-fast bacilli are rarely identified in the stool. Anaemia and hypoalbuminaemia are usually present. Absorption tests often show evidence of fat and vitamin B_{12} malabsorption. There may be a protein-losing enteropathy. If there is significant malabsorption, a megaloblastic anaemia may be present. The diagnosis is often difficult (Croker, Record, and Wright, 1978) and diagnostic laparotomy is frequently necessary. Resected specimens and regional lymph nodes usually show evidence of caseation and acid-fast bacilli.

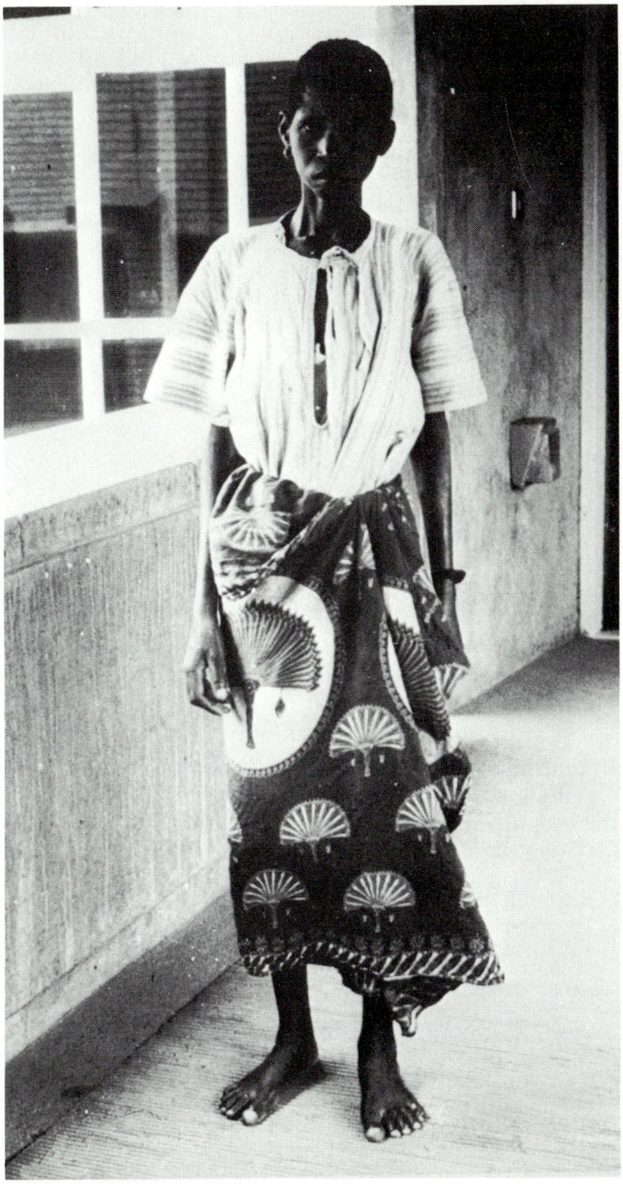

FIG. 23.2. A 30-year-old Zambian woman from the Chewa tribe, at the University Teaching Hospital, Lusaka. Presentation was with severe weight loss and fevers. Serum albumin and gammaglobulin concentrations were 17 and 17 g per l respectively. There was evidence of malabsorption, and barium meal showed ileal strictures. At laparotomy, nine ileal strictures were demonstrated; an ileal resection was performed. Histology of a mesenteric gland showed caseation; acid-fast bacilli were present.

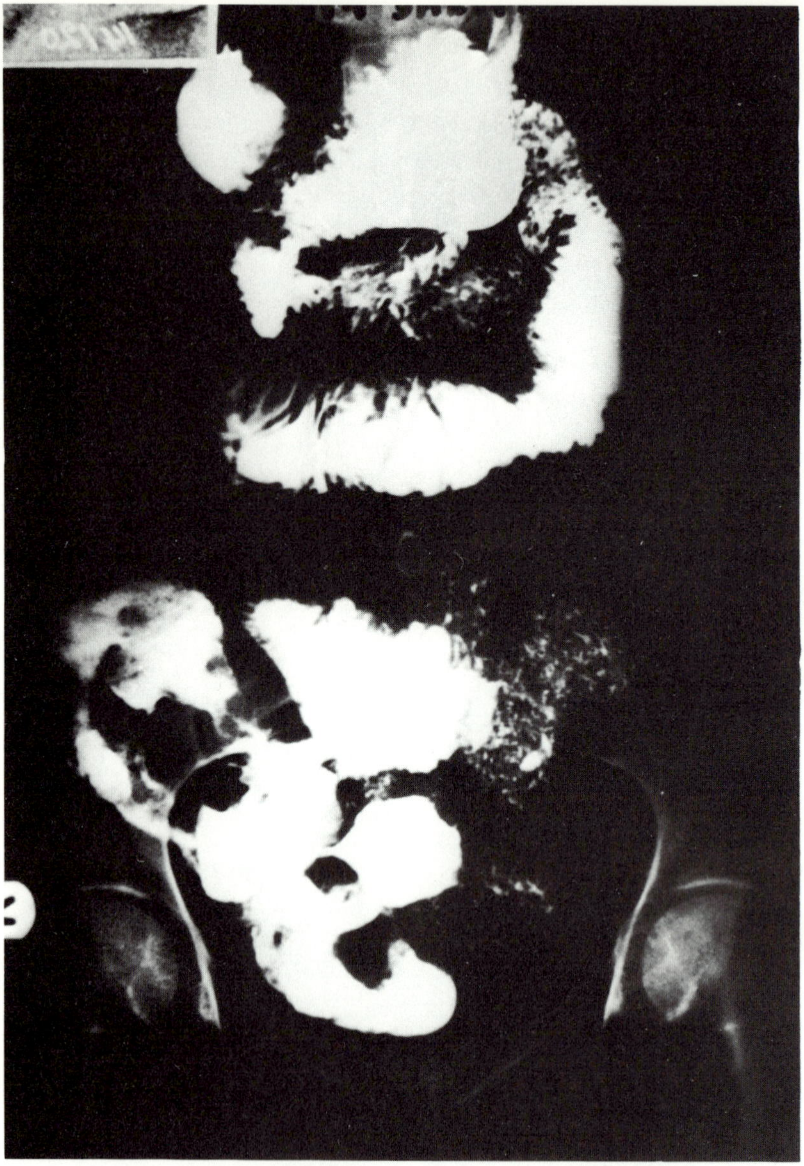

FIG. 23.3. Barium meal in the 30-year-old Zambian woman shown in Fig. 23. 2. Multiple ileal strictures are shown.

Crohn's disease is an important differential diagnosis (*Br. med. J.*, 1977) (Chapter 29). Ileocaecal tuberculosis should in fact be suspected in every case of Crohn's disease, before corticosteroids are started. Vomiting, fever, and menstrual disorders are more common in tuberculosis than in Crohn's disease. Diarrhoea is apparently much more common in Crohn's disease than tuberculosis. Clinical signs are usually unhelpful. A peripheral lymphocytosis, a postive Mantoux, and a lymphocytosis and high protein in the ascitic fluid (if present), together with granulomas in a liver-biopsy specimen strongly suggest tuberculosis. Random peritoneal biopsy may be of value (Das and Shukla, 1975).

An ileocaecal infection with *Yersinia enterocolitica* (Chapter 27) may give a similar clinical picture to that of ileocaecal tuberculosis.

Treatment is with anti-tuberculous agents, and a rapid recovery is usual. If there is doubt about the diagnosis a diagnostic laparotomy is mandatory; that has been the only proof of diagnosis in several cases that I have seen in Zambia and Papua New Guinea. Resection of ileal strictures is frequently necessary. Right hemicolectomy may be required (Hoon, Dockerty, and Pemberton, 1950; Anand, 1956; Singh, Roy, and Vaidya, 1973), and is possibly the correct operation (Croker, *et al.*, 1978). Chemotherapy should be started before surgical intervention.

23.1.3. Tuberculous peritonitis

A generalized peritonitis, often of fairly acute onset, may be caused by tuberculosis. Nwokolo (1967) has reported that that condition accounts for 24 per cent of adults presenting with ascites in Ibadan, Nigeria; it may be either primary, or secondary to pulmonary tuberculosis (Francis, 1972).

The history may reveal an insidious onset of ill-health before abdominal pain was experienced. Fever is usual. Peripheral oedema is unusual unless lymph glands are also involved. Ileus occurs as a late sequel to small-intestinal obstruction, and is caused by adhesive bands.

The ascitic fluid is usually clear, but it may occasionally be bloody or even chylous (Calder and Norredam, 1972); there is often a lymphocytosis and a reduction in the polymorphonuclear leucocyte count, but that is certainly not always the case. The total white blood-cell count is usually greater than 400 per cu mm. Protein content of the fluid is usually high, from 30–60 g per l. Tubercle bacilli are rarely seen on a direct film; culture is usually positive.

When the peritonitis is generalized, the diagnosis is usually straightforward; with disease localized to the pelvis, it is often difficult without laparotomy. A slow leak from a perforated typhoid ulcer may make diagnosis difficult (Chapter 22). Similarly a leak from a chronic amoebic abscess may be difficult to distinguish clinically (Chapter 25). Perforated duodenal ulcer and a primary pyogenic peritonitis should be excluded; the ascitic fluid usually contains an excess of polymorphonuclear leucocytes.

Constrictive pericarditis (often, but by no means always, caused by tuberculosis), which is common throughout the tropics, and endomyocardial fibrosis (EMF) of the right ventricle (a common disease in tropical Africa) (Abrahams, 1962), can cause ascites without breathlessness and oedema; the ascites is a consequence of the high central venous pressure. In that condition the liver is enlarged; the ascitic fluid may contain a high protein concentration.

Tuberculous peritonitis responds rapidly to treatment with antituberculous agents; there is limited evidence that corticosteroids in addition to chemotherapy are of value (Singh, Bhargava, and Jain, 1969). Laparotomy is not indicated.

23.1.4. Other conditions associated with mesenteric adenitis and ileal ulceration

Yersinia enterocolitica. This frequently involves the ileocaecal region, but usually produces an acute illness (Vantrappen, Agg, Ponette, Geboes, and Bertrand, 1977); it is dealt with in Chapter 27.

Pasteurella pseudotuberculosis. This produces a mesenteric lymphadenitis, usually in boys between five and 15 years old (Mair, 1968). Lymph glands contain small abscesses; palisading of histiocytes may be reminiscent of cat scratch fever and lymphogranuloma venereum (Chapter 30). Apart from isolation of the organism, specific antibodies are present in the serum and there is a specific skin test antigen.

Primary non-specific ileal ulcers have been reported in children (Grosfeld, Schiller, Weinberger, and Clatworthy, 1970). Presentation is with anaemia and often acute and chronic rectal bleeding. The aetiology is obscure.

23.2. Leprosy involving the small intestine

The literature on this subject (Mitsuda and Ogawa, 1937; Kean and Childress, 1942; Powell and Swann, 1955; Desikan and Job, 1968; Bernard and Vazquez, 1973) is difficult to interpret. There is experimental evidence in the armadillo, in which leprosy which resembles that in man can be produced, that extensive involvement of the gastrointestinal tract can occur (Kirchheimer, Storrs, and Binford, 1972). Twenty-five patients with leprosy, 15 of whom had lepromatous, 5 borderline, and 5 tuberculoid disease, were studied at Chandigarh, India (Kaur, Mehta, Kumar, Chakravarty, and Sidhu, 1978); although mild morphological and functional small-intestinal changes were demonstrated, they were almost certainly those of *tropical enteropathy* (Chapter 20). It was concluded, in that study, that the small intestine is not affected by leprosy.

23.3. Other causes of chronic peritonitis

23.3.1. Histoplasmosis

Perforation of the intestine, leading to peritonitis, which results from a *Histoplasma duboisii* infection has been described (Camain, Berteim, Klefstad-Sillonville, Mafart, Vilasco, and Drouchet, 1958). A case of primary infection of the jejunum by *H. duboisii* has been documented at Ibadan, Nigeria (Adekunle, Sudhakaran, and Timeyin, 1978); tubercles were scattered over the surface of the bowel and mesentery, and there was stricture formation and enlarged mesenteric glands. That disease is difficult to distinguish from tuberculosis, carcinoma, and lymphoma of the jejunum.

23.3.2. Ascariasis

A granulomatous peritonitis, due to *Ascaris lumbricoides* ova, has been recorded. A giant-cell response can be demonstrated histologically, with a chronic inflammatory reaction. Presence of adult worms in the peritoneal cavity has also been reported (Qassab and Al-Khateeb, 1966), and they too may set up a granulomatous peritonitis (Areán, 1958). Rarely, adult worms are discharged from a peri-umbilical abscess, or from umbilical fistulae (Jelliffe, 1952).

23.3.3. *Filariasis*

In some forms of filariasis, i.e. those caused by *Wuchereria bancrofti* and *Brugia malayi*, there may be severe lymphatic blockage within the abdomen, and that may produce involvement of abdominal glands with the production of ascites which is usually chylous. In *Mansonella ozzardi* infections, present in south America and the Caribbean, adult worms have been identified in the mesentery and peritoneum.

23.3.4. *Schistosomiasis*

In severe *Schistosoma mansoni* and *S. japonicum* infections, the muscular layer and serosa of the intestine may be involved with pseudotubercle formation; a focal exudative peritonitis, and intestinal adhesions may result. Intestinal obstruction may be a consequence.

23.3.5. *Paragonimiasis*

The lung fluke, *Paragonimus westermani*, which passes through the peritoneal cavity during its migratory phase, is occasionally associated with a fibrinous exudate containing ova and eosinophils. Adhesions and subsequent intestinal obstruction are occasional accompaniments.

23.4. Small-intestinal tumours

There are areas in Africa and the Middle east where small-intestinal lymphoma is common. Burkitt's lymphoma involving the small intestine is frequently seen in children in many tropical countries.

Carcinoma of the small intestine is a rarity in the tropics as it is in temperate zones; several explanations have been suggested for that (Bone and Wright, 1973; Lowenfels, 1973; Renshaw and McCrae, 1973). Apart from rapid passage of its liquid contents, and its relative sterility, a protective action of small-intestinal enzymes, and the very high rate of cellular proliferation have been suggested as being important.

23.4.1. *Mediterranean lymphoma*

In this condition, there is a diffuse lymphoplasmacytic proliferation, which may be associated with alpha heavy chains in the serum and other biological fluids (Eidelman, Parkins, and Rubin, 1966; Rappaport, Ramot, Hulu, and Park, 1972; Al-Saleem, 1978).

This is a relatively common tumour in the Middle east, and northern (Rambaud and Seligmann, 1976) and southern Africa (Lewin, Kahn, and Novis, 1976). The disease is less common in the Mediterranean part of Europe (Bonomo, Dammacco, Marano, and Bonomo, 1972; Pittman, Tripathy, Isobe, Bolaños, Osserman, Pittman, Lotero, and Duque, 1975) and south-east Asia (Rambaud and Seligmann, 1976); it is rare in south America (Dutz, Asvadi, Sadri, and Kohout, 1971). In Iraq, small-intestinal primary tumours account for 50 to 60 per cent of all non-Hodgkin's lymphomas; 90 per cent of all malignant small-intestinal tumours are lymphomas (Al-Saleem, 1978).

Young adults in low socioeconomic groups are especially affected (Rambaud and Seligmann, 1976); the sex incidence is close to unity. There is chronic diarrhoea, abdominal pain, clubbing of the fingers, and late in the disease, small-intestinal obstruction (Rambaud and Seligmann, 1976; Al-Saleem and Zardawi, 1978). There is often no clinical evidence of a frank neoplasm.

Immunoglobulin IgG and IgM concentrations are abnormally low (Al-Saleem, 1978). There is usually hypoalbuminaemia and hypokalaemia. Alkaline phosphatase concentration may be elevated (Al-Saleem and Zardawi, 1978). Radiologically and pathologically there is evidence in the upper small intestine of a mucosal abnormality, with thickening and polypoid changes; superimposed multicentric tumour masses are sometimes present.

Lymphoplasmacytic proliferation is usually limited to the lamina propria. The enterocytes are intact but there is frequently villous atrophy (Eidelman *et al.*, 1966; Rappaport *et al.*, 1972). In advanced cases, immature plasma cells appear, which cross the muscularis mucosae; frank lymphoplasmacytic neoplasms are thus formed (Tabbane, Tabbane, and Cammoun, 1976; Galian, Lecestre, Scotto, Bognel, Matuchansky, and Rambaud, 1977). Mesenteric lymph gland involvement is common, but the liver, spleen and peripheral lymph-nodes are not affected until very late (Salem, Nassar, Shahid, Hajj, Alami, Balikian, and Salem, 1977; Al-Bahrani, Al-Saleem, Al-Mondhiry, Bakir, Yahia, Taha, and King, 1978).

Taking geographical distribution and the involvement of low socioeconomic groups into account, it has been suggested that chronic infections or genetic factors might be important aetiologically (Rambaud and Seligmann, 1976). Chronic diarrhoea in infancy and impairment of immune processes have also been postulated (Dutz *et al.*, 1971). Because this tumour involves particularly the upper small intestine, an area where bacterial infections are uncommon, and because there has probably been a recent spread of the tumour in the Middle east and Africa, exposure to the enterotoxin of *Vibrio cholerae* has been suggested as being aetiologically important, by depressing local immunity (Al-Saleem, 1978); the high incidence areas of the tumour are usually endemic for cholera and there must be frequent exposures to the enterotoxin of *V. cholerae*, which is known to have potent effects on immune reactions (Lichtenstein, Henney, Bourne, and Greenough, 1973).

Clinical and immunological remissions occur frequently after tetracycline treatment (Rambaud and Seligmann, 1976; Al-Bahrani, *et al.*, 1978). If diagnosed early, the prognosis is good.

23.4.2. Burkitt's lymphoma

This lymphoma has a characteristic geographical distribution in the tropics, and usually involves children (Chapter 1). Although presentation is usually with jaw tumours, abdominal symptoms herald its appearance in many cases. Abdominal masses may be palpated per abdomen. It may appear at one or multiple sites in the small-intestinal wall. Haemorrhage and occasionally intussusception may result. Ileal and jejunal tumours may give rise to intestinal obstruction. Abdominal lymph glands may be involved. Ascites may occasionally be present, but it is not usually gross; tumour cells may be identified in ascitic fluid using a phase-contrast technique.

The tumour is soft and yellowish-white in colour, and sometimes with areas of necrosis and haemorrhage. It may involve the whole thickness of the intestine and appear as an umbilicated deposit (Fig. 23.4).

23.4.3. Carcinoid tumour

Throughout the gastrointestinal tract there are chromaffin or argentaffin cells in the mucosa (Kultchitsky cells). The highest concentrations of these cells are in the ileum and the appendix; they produce serotonin (5-hydroxytryptamine). Tumours composed of those cells readily metastasize to many sites, including the liver. Although these tumours occur in tropical populations there is no evidence of a different incidence rate from temperate areas.

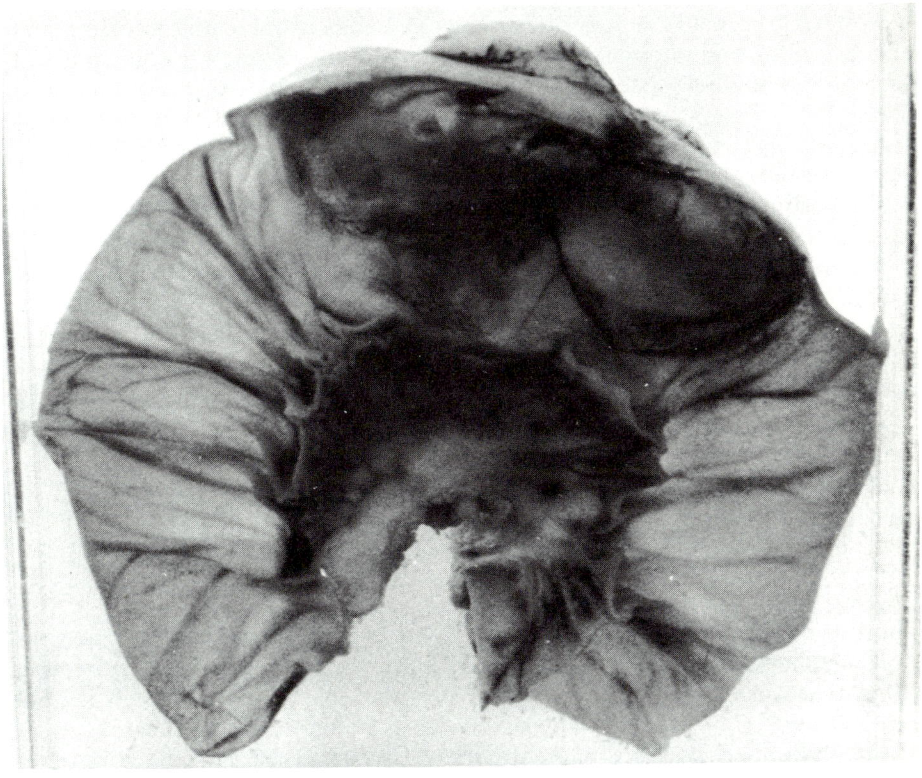

FIG. 23.4. Post-mortem specimen of small intestine from a five-year-old Papua New Guinean girl from the Gulf Province. Presentation was with severe weight loss; an abdominal tumour was palpated per abdomen. At laparotomy extensive tumour deposits were demonstrated, involving the small intestine, abdominal lymph-glands, ovaries, and kidneys. The intestinal deposits involved the full thickness of the wall. Histology showed the classical appearances of Burkitt's lymphoma. She died soon after the laparotomy.

23.4.4. Other malignancies

Other tumours also cause small-intestinal obstruction and occasional perforation. In Papua New Guinea, lymphosarcoma of the small intestine, sometimes producing pathology from the duodenum to ileum, seems to be more common than expected. Such cases may present with small-intestinal obstruction; at laparotomy, a number of strictures throughout the small intestine, caused by multiple tumours up to two or three cm in diameter, are found. Owor (1977) has reported 40 cases of non-Burkitt's lymphoma involving the gastrointestinal tract, from Uganda; 10 of them involved the small intestine.

23.5. Small-intestinal obstruction

Intestinal obstruction accounts for a very large proportion of cases admitted to tropical hospitals with an 'acute abdomen'; in one series 49·3 per cent of 'acute abdomens' were caused by obstruction, at Lusaka, Zambia (Umerah and Obadike, 1978).

Strangulated inguinal hernia is the commonest cause; strangulated femoral and internal herniae are less often seen. Volvulus of the small intestine and sigmoid colon, and intussusception seem to be more common in some parts of Africa than in the western world (see below) (Chapter 27). *Ascaris lumbricoides* causes obstruction, especially in children (Chapter 19). Rarely a mass of tapeworms (Chapter 19) may be responsible, and perforation with secondary peritonitis has been recorded.

Schistosomiasis is a rare cause of obstruction (Malik, Satir, Veress, and El Hassan, 1975) (see above).

Tuberculosis is a further cause (see above), due either to stenosis of the lumen, or to pressure of enlarged glands on the third part of the duodenum and jejunum (Anand and Pathak, 1961; Davey and Pearson, 1965). In children, Burkitt's lymphoma is sometimes responsible. In the Middle east, and north and southern Africa, the Mediterranean lymphoma (see above) accounts for some cases. Lymphosarcoma causes obstruction of the small intestine in Papua New Guinea. Ileus following peritonitis is a not uncommon event.

In Botswana, an overall mortality rate of 23·2 per cent has been reported in intestinal obstruction (Johnson, 1975); that was thought to be largely due to delay in seeking medical attention.

23.5.1. Hernia

The true incidence of hernia in tropical countries is difficult to assess. Nine per cent of young Africans seeking work in Zimbabwe Rhodesia have been found to have external hernias (Evans, 1961); a comparable figure for the UK is 2 per cent (Davey, 1968). In an analysis of causes of hernia at the Goroka Base Hospital, Papua New Guinea over a three-year period, 56, 50, and 24 were reported to be epigastric, para-umbilical, and inguinal, respectively (Wagner and Shepherd, 1976); the total number of hernias during that period was 137.

Umbilical hernia is usually asymptomatic and therefore medical attention is not often sought. Such hernias, although often of enormous proportions, rarely in fact give rise to obstruction and strangulation. They are present in up to 66 per cent of preschool children in western Nigeria (Wyatt and Matthew, 1972); there is a marked fall in prevalence with age there, which is not the case in South Africa. It is more common in the lower socioeconomic groups; malnutrition, a bulky carbohydrate diet, heavy intestinal parasite infections, and splenomegaly have all been suggested to be important aetiological factors. Strangulated inguinal hernia accounts for over three-quarters of obstructions in Accra (Badoe, 1965) and for more than one-third in Bulawayo (White, 1961; 1962) and Ibadan, Nigeria (Cole, 1964; 1965); there are however local differences in incidence rates (Burkitt, Nelson, and Williams, 1963). Direct inguinal hernia seems to be relatively more common in Africans than in other groups, and to strangulate more often (Davey, 1968). Femoral hernia is overall less common in Africa than in Europe; however there is a high incidence rate in Uganda in the Kampala and Jinja regions (Eckhart, 1964). A lower overall incidence of femoral hernia might be due, in part, to the fact that the femoral canal is often blocked by an enlarged lymph-gland resulting from chronic leg and foot sepsis. Giant hernias are common in Africa and to a lesser extent in Asia; they are occasionally filled with omentum, small and large bowel, stomach, and sometimes bladder also; they rarely strangulate, but repair can be difficult.

In sickle-cell (SS) disease, straight abdominal radiographs during a 'crisis' may reveal dilated loops of gut with fluid levels strongly suggesting organic obstruction.

Due to delay in arrival at hospital, and consequent fluid and electrolyte loss, associated with toxaemia, blood loss, gangrene, and faecal fistula, the mortality rate is high; Cole (1964) gives a figure as high as 50 per cent when presentation is as late as the fifth day. The type of hernia is of little prognostic importance. Davey (1968) has summarized the principles of management of a strangulated hernia in Africa; (i) antibiotic treatment should be started at once, (ii) the extracellular fluid deficit should be assessed and half of the estimated loss replaced in 2 hours, (iii) if there is no response to repletion, hydrocortisone should be given, and (iv) when the heart rate is less than 100 per min and the systolic blood pressure greater than 90 mm of mercury, operation should be undertaken.

Strangulated hernias may perforate; an acute faecal fistula may form, and that is often a result of interference by a local 'practitioner'; the prognosis is bad, and a chronic fistula may result.

23.5.2. Volvulus of the small intestine

This condition is relatively more common in Africans than Europeans; that probably applies especially to east and South Africa.

In Kampala, small-intestinal volvulus accounts for 2·5 per cent of cases of intestinal obstruction (Burkitt, 1952); it seems to be more common in other parts of Uganda. Five to seven cases are seen annually at the Kenyatta National Hospital, Nairobi (Kerr and Kirkaldy-Willis, 1946; Miller, 1961). At the University Hospital, Ibadan, it accounted for 3·4 per cent of cases of intestinal obstruction during a six-year period and was more common than colonic obstruction (Cole, 1965). At the Korle Bu Hospital, Accra, it only accounted for 0·5 per cent of cases of intestinal obstruction in a five-year period (Badoe, 1965). In Zimbabwe Rhodesia it accounted for 2·5 per cent of cases of intestinal obstruction at the Mpilo Hospital, Bulawayo during a four-year period (White, 1961; White and Palmer, 1963).

For primary small-intestinal volvulus, a narrow elongated mesentery is essential; in secondary volvulus, which is the more common variety, an additional predisposing lesion, for example, adhesions, a Meckel's diverticulum, or ascariasis must be present. Diet has been suggested as being important in primary volvulus in Africa; it often occurs after the harvest, when large meals of maize are eaten in a semi-solid form, and are then washed down with many pints of fluid, frequently locally brewed beer. During Ramadan, in Islamic countries, large meals are eaten after sunset.

Although such factors might be important, the explanation for most cases is obscure. In some, congenital bands fixing the terminal ileum to the posterior abdominal wall have been noted. The pedicle of tortion is formed by the terminal ileum, its related bands, and most of the mesentery of the small intestine. Maximum tortion occurs in the terminal ileal mesentery, which is supplied by the ileocolic branch of the superior mesenteric artery, with axial tortion of the ileal wall about seven or eight cm proximal to the caecum. Secondary volvulus is more common in African women due to the high prevalence of adhesions following pelvic inflammatory disease; frequent intestinal infections, and mesenteric glandular enlargement may also play a part.

The condition should be differentiated from (i) simple volvulus of the pelvic colon, (ii) compound volvulus ('knotting of the bowel') (Chapter 27), and (iii) internal hernia. All of those conditions can produce massive intestinal strangulation, and frequently they cannot be distinguished before operation; the history, clinical features, and a knowledge of geographical pathology and likelihood of the condition occurring in that area, are important. Radiology may help (White and Palmer, 1963). The less common form of 'knotting' is of the ileo-ileal type (Weinberg, 1958); unless treated with great urgency, the outlook is bad. Internal hernia of the small intestine (see above), which is so highly mobile in Africans, is a considerable problem in differential diagnosis; the small intestine herniates into various peritoneal fossae and foraminae. In addition there is a high frequency of herniation of the small intestine through defects in the ileal and pelvic mesenteries. The bowel is always tightly strangulated and the strangulated loop can become the site of a secondary volvulus. Urgent surgical attention is vital.

Acute fulminating and slowly progressive forms of small-intestinal volvulus are recognized. The fulminating form has an acute onset and occurs more often in men than women; most patients are in the third or fourth decade. An account has been given by Warambo (1971) in Nairobi, Kenya; it is apparently common in pregnancy (Roles, 1965). Severe pain, often radiating to the back, gives way to diffuse pain, secondary to peritoneal irritation and strangulation; vomiting is common. The abdominal muscles are rigid. Distension is common in less severe cases; respiratory movements may be restricted in a severe case. As a large quantity of blood is trapped in the engorged bowel and mesentery, oligaemic circulatory collapse may occur. The slowly progressive form cannot be distinguished on clinical grounds from other causes of ileal obstruction.

Plain abdominal radiographs show a relatively empty large intestine in the supine view, and a series of gas-fluid levels in the distended ileum and jejunum; they extend in a 'stepladder' pattern from the right iliac fossa to the left hypochondrium, in the erect view.

Resuscitation and urgent surgery are necessary. Although the bowel may be viable, operation is urgently required to prevent extensive venous thrombosis; if that occurs, only a few cm of small intestine proximal to, and distal to, the fixed parts of the ileum and jejunum, respectively, may survive.

23.6. Meckel's diverticulum

During the period 1966–72, 30 instances of Meckel's diverticulum were discovered during 592 appendicectomies and laparotomies in Kenyan African patients at Nairobi (Kamdar and Knight, 1973); the sex incidence was equal. That incidence is higher than in most reported series and suggests that that congenital anomaly might be unusually common in Africans.

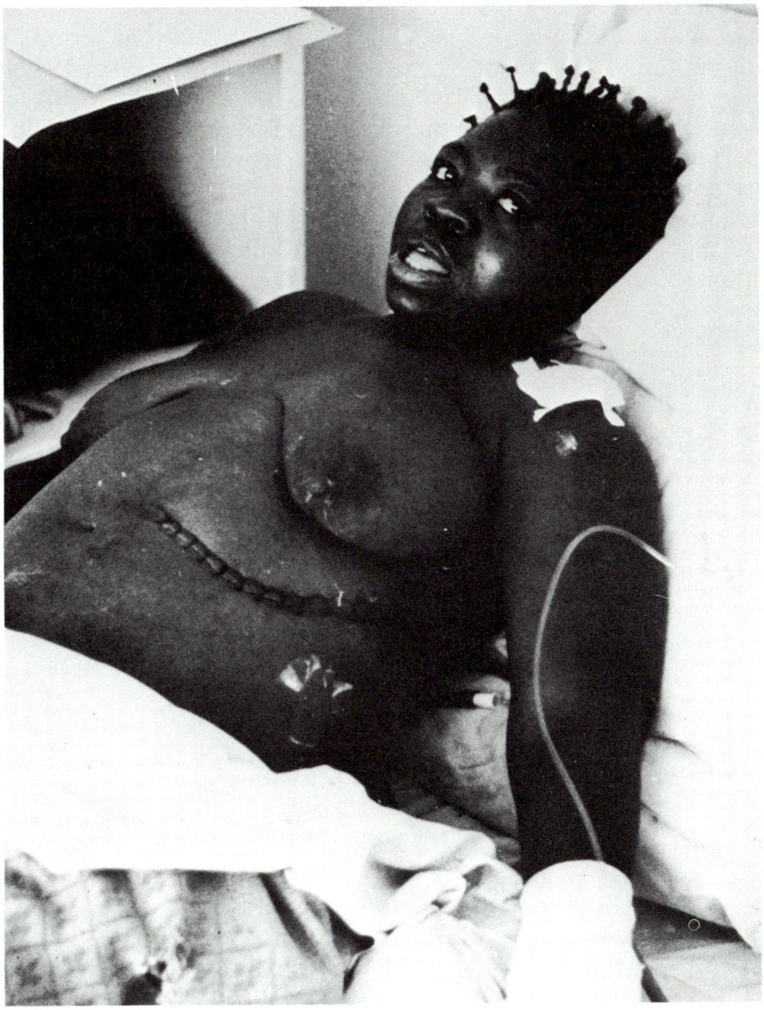

FIG. 23.5. A Zambian woman who had been involved in a fight in a beer-hall a few days before. She had been stabbed in the left hypochondrium, and a ruptured spleen was diagnosed. At laparotomy, splenectomy was carried out, together with resection of a considerable length of small intestine which was also severely damaged.

23.7 Trauma to the small intestine

In many parts of Africa small intestinal injury is caused by either knife or gunshot wounds (Fig. 23.5) (Chapter 27). Gunshot wounds usually produce much more severe damage to the intestine and lead to a greater length of gut resection. In the highlands of Papua New Guinea arrow wounds are still a considerable problem and not infrequently lead to severe abdominal trauma. Road traffic accidents, common in most third-world countries, do not usually necessitate intestinal resection. Road accidents were responsible for 60 per cent of 75 cases of abdominal injury treated at the University College Hospital, Ibadan, between 1967 and 1975 (Adekunle and Ajayi, 1977); the small intestine was involved in only 12 cases. In a series from Lusaka, Zambia, 12·9 per cent of admissions with an 'acute abdomen' over a one-year period were for traumatic rupture of abdominal viscera (Umerah and Obadike, 1978).

Because it has certain specialized functions, i.e. absorption of B_{12} and bile salts, the ileum should clearly be preserved if possible. Jejunal resection is far less important as the ileum adapts and demonstrates a compensatory hypertrophy. The consequences of resection of considerable lengths of small intestine have been reviewed (Compston and Creamer, 1977; *Lancet*, 1978). Following extensive small-intestinal resection, long-term follow-up is extremely important, although very difficult in many parts of the third world.

References

ABRAHAMS, D. G. (1962). *Q. Jl. Med.*, **31,** 1.

ADEKUNLE, O. O. and AJAYI, O. O. (1977). *E. Afr. med. J.*, **54,** 380.

——, SUDHAKARAN, P., and TIMEYIN, E. D. (1978). *J. trop. Med. Hyg.*, **81,** 88.

AL-BAHRANI, Z., AL-SALEEM, T., AL-MONDHIRY, H., BAKIR, F., YAHIA, H., TAHA, I., and KING, J. (1978). *Gut*, **19,** 627.

AL-SALEEM, T. I. (1978). *Lancet*, **2,** 709.

—— and ZARDAWI, I. M. (1978). *Lancet*, **1,** 775.

ANAND, S. S. (1956). *Ann. R. Coll. Surg.*, **19,** 205.

—— and PATHAK, K. (1961). *J. Indian med. Ass.*, **37,** 423.

AREÁN, V. M. (1958). *Archs Path.*, **66,** 427.

BADOE, E. A. (1965). *Ghana med. J.*, **4,** 128.

BALL, P. A. J. (1968). In *Companion to surgery in Africa* (by W. W. Davey). p. 267. E. and S. Livingstone, Edinburgh and London.

BENTLEY, G. and WEBSTER, J. H. H. (1967). *Br. J. Surg.*, **54,** 90.

BERNARD, J. C. and VAZQUEZ, C. A. J. (1973). *Int. J. Lepr.*, **41,** 94.

BONE, G. and WRIGHT, N. A. (1973). *Lancet*, **1,** 618.

BONOMO, L., DAMMACCO, F., MARANO, R., and BONOMO, G. M. (1972). *Am. J. Med.*, **52,** 73.

Br. med. J. (1977). **1,** 1557.

BURKITT, D. P. (1952). *E. Afr. med. J.*, **29,** 189.

——, NELSON, C. L., and WILLIAMS, E. H. (1963). *E. Afr. med. J.*, **40,** 1.

CALDER, J. F. and NORREDAM, K. (1972). *E. Afr. med. J.*, **49,** 684.

CAMAIN, R., BERTEIM, KLEFSTAD-SILLONVILLE, F., MAFART, J., VILASCO, J. A., and DROUCHET, E. (1958). *Bull. Soc. Path. exot.*, **51,** 83.

CROKER, J., RECORD, C. O., and WRIGHT, J. T. (1978). *Postgrad. med. J.*, **54,** 410.

COLE, G. J. (1964). *Trans. R. Soc. trop. Med. Hyg.*, **58,** 441.

—— (1965). *Gut*, **6,** 151.

COMPSTON, J. E. and CREAMER, B. (1977). *Q. Jl. Med.*, **46,** 485.

DAS, P. and SHUKLA, H. S. (1975). *Br. J. Surg.*, **62,** 610.
DAVEY, W. W. (1968). *Companion to surgery in Africa.* p. 241 and 280. E. and S. Livingstone. Edinburgh and London.
—— and PEARSON, J. B. (1965). *Br. J. Surg.*, **52,** 189.
DESIKAN, K. V. and JOB, C. K. (1968). *Int. J. Lepr.*, **36,** 32.
DINNER, M. (1965). *S. Afr. J. Surg.*, **3,** 97.
DUTZ, W., ASVADI, S., SADRI, S., and KOHOUT, E. (1971). *Gut*, **12,** 804.
ECKHART, P. (1964). *E. Afr. med. J.*, **41,** 59.
EDINGTON, G. M. and GILLES, H. M. (1976). *Pathology in the tropics.* 2nd ed. p. 396. Edward Arnold, London.
EIDELMAN, S., PARKINS, R. A., and RUBIN, C. E. (1966). *Medicine, Baltimore*, **45,** 111.
EL MASRI, S. H., BOULOS, P., and MALICK, M. O. A. (1977). *E. Afr. med. J.*, **54,** 319.
EVANS, P. A. S. (1961). *Cent. Afr. J. Med.*, **7,** 55.
FOX, W. (1977). *Proc. R. Soc. Med.*, **70,** 4.
FRANCIS, T. I. (1972). *Trop. geogr. Med.*, **24,** 232.
GALIAN, A., LECESTRE, M-J., SCOTTO, J., BOGNEL, C., MATUCHANSKY, C., and RAMBAUD, J-C. (1977). *Cancer, N. Y.*, **39,** 2081.
GROSFELD, J. L., SCHILLER, M., WEINBERGER, M., and CLATWORTHY, H. W. (1970). *Am. J. Dis. Child.*, **120,** 447.
HOON, J. R., DOCKERTY, M. B., and PEMBERTON, J. DE J. (1950). *Int. Abstr. Surg.*, **91,** 417.
JELLIFFE, D. B. (1949). *J. trop. Med. Hyg.*, **52,** 251.
—— (1952). *W. Afr. med. J.*, **1,** 183.
JOHNSON, R. H. (1975). *E. Afr. med. J.*, **52,** 319.
KAMDAR, H. H. and KNIGHT, E. O. W. (1973). *E. Afr. med. J.*, **50,** 426.
KAUR, S., MEHTA, S. K., KUMAR, B., CHAKRAVARTY, R. N., and SIDHU, H. K. (1978). *Int. J. Lepr.*, **46,** 35.
KEAN, B. H. and CHILDRESS, M. E. (1942). *Int. J. Lepr.*, **10,** 51.
KERR, W. G. and KIRKALDY-WILLIS, W. H. (1946). *Br. med. J.*, **1,** 799.
KIRSCHHEIMER, W. F., STORRS, E. E., and BINFORD, C. H. (1972). *Int. J. Lepr.*, **40,** 229.
Lancet (1978). **1,** 424.
LEWIN, K. J., KAHN, L. B., and NOVIS, B. H. (1976). *Cancer, N.Y.*, **38,** 2511.
LEWIS, E. A. and KOLAWOLE, T. M. (1972). *Gut*, **13,** 646.
LICHTENSTEIN, L. M., HENNEY, C. S., BOURNE, H. R., and GREENOUGH, W. B. (1973). *J. clin. Invest.*, **52,** 691.
LOWENFELS, A. B. (1973). *Lancet*, **1,** 24.
MAIR, N. S. (1968), *Recent advances in Clinical Pathology*. p. 35. J. and A. Churchill, London.
MALIK, M. O. A., SATIR, A. A., VERESS, B., and EL HASSAN, A. M. (1975). *E. Afr. med. J.*, **52,** 183.
MANDAL, B. K. and SCHOFIELD, P. F. (1976). *Practitioner*, **216,** 683.
MILLER, J. R. M. (1961). *E. Afr. med. J.*, **38,** 543.
MITSUDER, K. and OGAWA, M. A. (1937). *Int. J. Lepr.*, **5,** 53.
MORSON, B. C. and DAWSON, I. M. P. (1972). *Gastrointestinal Pathology.* p. 246. Blackwell, Oxford, London, Edinburgh, and Melbourne.
NWOKOLO, C. (1967). *Br. med. J.*, **1,** 33.
OWOR, R. (1977). *E. Afr. med. J.*, **54,** 666.
PITTMAN, F. E., TRIPATHY, K., ISOBE, T., BOLAÑOS, O. M., OSSERMAN, E. F., PITTMAN, J. C., LOTERO, H. R., and DUQUE, E. E. (1975). *Am. J. Med.*, **58,** 424.
POWELL, C. S. and SWANN, L. L. (1955). *Am. J. Path.*, **31,** 1131.
QASSAB, K. and AL-KHATEEB, A. K. (1966). *J. Fac. Med. Baghdad*, **8,** 62.
RAMBAUD, J. C. and SELIGMANN, M. (1976). *Clins Gastroent.*, **5,** 341.
RAPPAPORT, H., RAMOT, B., HULU, N., and PARK, J. K. (1972). *Cancer, N.Y.*, **29,** 1502.
RENSHAW, A. and MCCRAE, J. S. (1973). *Lancet*, **1,** 425.
ROLES, N. C. (1965). *E. Afr. med. J.*, **42,** 340.

SALEM, P. A., NASSAR, V. H., SHAHID, M., HAJJ, A., ALAMI, S. Y., BALIKIAN, J., and SALEM, A. (1977). *Cancer, N.Y.*, **40,** 2941.
SINGH, H. N., ROY, S. K., and VAIDYA, M. P. (1973). *Am. Surg.*, **39,** 706.
SINGH, M. M., BHARGAVA, A. N., and JAIN, K. P. (1969). *New Engl. J. Med.*, **281,** 1091.
TABBANE, S., TABBANE, F., and CAMMOUN, M. (1976). *Cancer, N.Y.*, **38,** 1989.
UMERAH, B. C. and OBADIKE, G. (1978). *E. Afr. med. J.*, **55,** 77.
VANTRAPPEN, G., AGG, H. O., PONETTE, E., GEBOES, K., and BERTRAND, P. (1977). *Gastroenterology*, **72,** 220.
WAGNER, F. B. and SHEPHERD, A. (1976). *Papua New Guin. med. J.*, **19,** 156.
WARAMBO, M. W. (1971). *E. Afr. med. J.*, **48,** 209.
WEINBERG, N. J. (1958). *Proc. Mine med. Offrs' Ass.*, **38,** 57.
WHITE, A. (1961). *E. Afr. med. J.*, **38,** 525.
—— (1962). *Cent. Afr. J. Med.*, **8,** 1.
—— and PALMER, P. E. S. (1963). *Clin. Radiol.*, **14,** 211.
WYATT, G. B. and MATTHEW, G. K. (1972). *Trans. R. Soc. trop. Med. Hyg.*, **66,** 508.

Section 6: The large intestine

24

Shigellosis (Bacillary dysentery)

THIS is an acute, usually self-limiting, disease characterized by severe diarrhoea and fever; the stool often contains blood and pus. There is a high mortality rate with some infections, especially in children. Bacillary dysentery is always a major problem in times of war; that was the case in both world wars (Fairley and Boyd, 1943; Boyd, 1957). The large intestine is involved to a much greater extent than the small intestine.

The disease exemplifies classical dysentery (Pringle, 1764; Twining, 1835; Rogers, 1913; Manson-Bahr, 1943; Grady and Keusch, 1971) and separates it from the basically small-bowel syndromes of which cholera is the best example; however there is some overlap, because some at least of these organisms both penetrate the mucosa and also produce an enterotoxin. Thus the toxin of *Shigella dysenteriae-l* (Shiga's bacillus) induces ileal hypersecretion to nearly the same extent as cholera enterotoxin (Keusch, Mata, and Grady, 1970), in addition to causing direct mucosal injury. The causative organisms are confined to the intestinal tract, chiefly the colon, and are excreted at high concentration in the faeces. Only rarely do they pass into the bloodstream (Graber, Browning, and Davis, 1966). Human carriers constitute the only significant reservoir of infection (Levine, 1979). The disease is highly contagious and is spread by food-handlers and contaminated objects including bed-linen; the organism is readily destroyed by direct sunlight.

Dysentery was first considered to be caused by shigellae by Chantemesse and Widal (1888); the organism was described in detail by Shiga during a massive epidemic in Japan in 1898. Strong and Musgrave (1900) working in the Philippines confirmed that finding. In 1901, Flexner isolated a new organism; other major observations were by Sonne in Denmark and Boyd in India.

24.1. Distribution of shigellosis

Like many so-called 'tropical diseases', this is an illness which also occurs in temperate climates. Like many other tropical diseases, it has become localized to the tropics due principally to the poorer socioeconomic conditions and lower standards of public and personal hygiene (Moore, de la Cruz, and Vargas-Mendez, 1965) in those areas.

Infection can be derived from patients with the disease, healthy convalescents, and symptomless carriers. Contaminated food, especially milk and ice-cream, and water-borne infections are important. Some water-borne outbreaks have been associated with viral hepatitis epidemics. Flies play a part in transmission but that might have been exaggerated (Wolff and Van Zijl, 1969). Young children and the elderly are more liable to severe infections. In a large study at Karachi, Pakistan, shigellae were found to be the commonest bacterial pathogens in children of less than two years old (Ingram, Rights, Ali Khan, Hashimi, and Ansari, 1966); 12·4 per cent of 655 children under two years with diarrhoeal disease had that organism in the stool.

24.2. Presentation of shigellosis

The incubation period is from one to seven days; in most cases it is one or two days. That is followed by an abrupt onset of fever (up to 40°C) and tachycardia. Within 24 hours diarrhoea, tenesmus, and colic follow; the stools (often 20 or more in 24 hours) are watery and contain blood and mucus; later, pieces of necrotic mucosa and pus may be passed per rectum. Frank bleeding is unusual. Tenesmus is often severe. Abdominal pain and tenderness, and vomiting, may become worse, and an acute abdomen may be mimicked. If the diarrhoea is severe, dehydration and vascular collapse dominate the picture. The spectrum of disease is wide. In a prospective study, using infected volunteers, one-quarter had a high fever with minimal enteric symptoms, and a further one-quarter had severe watery diarrhoea with evidence of small-intestinal involvement (Du Pont, Hornick, and Dawkins, 1969); the remaining half had a disease of intermediate severity with fever after an incubation period of one or two days, diarrhoea and colic after a further two days, and dysentery two or three days after that.

In children especially, the mortality rate is substantial if correct management is not implemented early. Due to so many variable factors it is impossible to give an overall mortality rate. Untreated, the condition is usually self-limiting after a period lasting up to three weeks.

Inflammatory lesions involving the eyes (conjunctivitis, iridocyclitis, and corneal ulceration), joints (polyarthropathy), peripheral nerves, myocardium, and spleen may complicate an otherwise straightforward attack; such lesions are bacteriologically sterile. An arthropathy is fairly common and usually follows some two to five weeks after the acute illness; joint fluid is sterile and the process is considered to be a hypersensitivity reaction.

Differential diagnosis is from other causes of bloody diarrhoea, especially those which are common in tropical countries, i.e., amoebic dysentery (Chapter 25) and schistosomiasis (*Schistosoma mansoni* and *S. japonicum*) (Chapter 26). Mesenteric thrombosis and, in children, intussusception are important differential diagnoses. Travellers' diarrhoea is usually less severe and of shorter duration. Small-intestinal diarrhoea does not normally produce bloody stools, although that occasionally occurs in salmonellosis. Tropical malabsorption (*tropical sprue*) with or without a *Giardia lamblia* infection (Chapter 20), and diarrhoea and abdominal pain associated with *Plasmodium falciparum* infections must also be borne in mind. Chronic cases may be confused with non-specific ulcerative colitis, colonic carcinoma and diverticulitis (Chapter 29).

24.3. Severe complications of shigellosis

Local complications consist of perforation, which is unusual, and haemorrhage.

Prolapsed haemorrhoids sometimes prove troublesome. There may be a secondary depression of disaccharidases.

Renal and circulatory failure may complicate the picture if dehydration is severe. In addition to the distant complications mentioned above, Reiter's syndrome (nonspecific urethritis, conjunctivitis, and arthritis) is an occasional sequel. Development of Reiter's syndrome after dysentery occurs significantly more often if the major histocompatibility complex (HLA) (Bodmer, 1978) is B27 (Brewerton, 1978; Hochberg, Bias, and Arnett, 1978).

In severe shigellosis, circulating endotoxin from the colon may produce a coagulopathy, thrombocytopenia, renal microangiopathy, and haemolytic anaemia (haemolytic-uraemic syndrome). In a prospective study in Bangladesh, 207 children and 34 adults with shigellosis were investigated (Koster, Levin, Walker, Tung, Gilman, Rahaman, Majid, Islam, and Williams, 1978); 19 children had an acute haemolytic anaemia, a leukaemoid reaction, thrombocytopenia and oliguria, and nine others had in addition a raised serum urea concentration. Eight of those nine had a pseudomembranous colitis, of whom six died. Circulating immune complexes were found in 10 of 20 patients with uncomplicated shigellosis and in four of six with a severe haemolytic-uraemic syndrome. The limulus assay for endotoxaemia was positive in nine of 18 with haemolysis, and in three of 61 with uncomplicated shigellosis ($P < 0{\cdot}001$).

Cerebral oedema with atrophy of glial tissue may rarely occur in children; that has been reported from Japan (Suwa, 1966). Convulsions, pyelonephritis, pneumonitis, and myocarditis have also been recorded (Barrett-Connor and Connor, 1970). *S. dysenteriae-l* produces a neurotoxin (Van Heynigen and Gladstone, 1953); prostration, meningismus, and seizures may occur in children infected with that organism.

Portal pyaemia with multiple liver abscess formation is a rare complication.

Occasionally a chronic state associated with severe emaciation and postinfective malabsorption results (Chapter 20). The overall role of colonic infections in the pathogenesis of postinfective tropical malabsorption (TM) is difficult to evaluate. Most early reports of the disease stressed colonic changes including ulceration following the onset of severe diarrhoea (Chapter 20) (Cook, 1978). It seems possible that that predisposes to bacterial colonization of the small intestine, which is the ultimate cause of TM.

A chronic course, with postdysenteric colitis similar to that occurring after amoebic dysentery, is a well-recognized entity (Hurst, 1943; Felsen, 1945; Steward, 1950; Powell and Wilmot, 1966).

24.4. Bacteriology and pathology of shigellosis

The shigellae are Gram-negative, non-motile facultative anaerobes. They are lactose fermenters. Although they can survive in alkaline faeces for days, they die in a few hours in acid faeces (Christie, 1968). They are killed in one hour at 55°C. There are four species: *S. dysenteriae, flexneri, boydii,* and *sonnei*. The original Shiga bacillus is now designated *S. dysenteriae-1* (i.e. the first antigenically determined subtype of *dysenteriae*); it produces a powerful exotoxin with a molecular weight of 60 000 and a pH optimum of 8·0, and is usually responsible for the most severe disease. That enterotoxin causes severe ileal hypersecretion (see above), and in addition the organism is capable of deep penetration of the mucosa. *S. sonnei* usually produces the mildest disease, and is often seen in temperate climates.

S. dysenteria, S. flexneri, and *S. boydii* possess 10, 6, and 15 antigenically separate subtypes, respectively. It is probably intraepithelial multiplication after penetration, rather than penetration alone, which characterizes the virulent strains.

Identification of the species and serotype is useful in tracing epidemiological patterns and for obtaining information on antibiotic sensitivities.

The disease affects the whole colon, but especially the distal part (Gonzalez-Licea and Yardley, 1966). The organisms after being swallowed multiply in the colon with great speed, where they largely take the place of the normal bacterial flora. They penetrate the intact epithelium and pass through the mucous membrane within a few hours (Takeuchi, Sprinz, La Brec, and Formal, 1965). A rapidly developing hyperaemia of the mucosa is followed by oedema and haemorrhage. Infiltration with leucocytes, macrophages, and plasma cells extends down to the submucosa. Necrosis and desquamation of the epithelium with formation of a membrane are followed by the formation of shallow ulcers, a few millimetres in diameter, which may extend deeply into the muscularis mucosae as secondary infection occurs. The intervening mucosa is hypertrophic and polypoid. The ileum also is usually involved to some extent, a fact which was well recognized in early writings but which has been underemphasized in recent accounts of the disease. Perforation is rare, but extensive fibrosis of the mucosa and submucosa, forming cyst-like lesions which harbour the bacteria, may ensue in a chronic case. In a fatal case, extensive necrosis of the intestine occurs. Extensive fibrosis may lead to a postdysenteric colitis (Morson and Dawson, 1972). Subepithelial cysts may arise from the submucosal foci of epithelium isolated by the inflammatory process. The bacilli remain localized in the intestine and mesenteric lymph nodes; there is no haematogenous spread.

24.5. Investigation of shigellosis

Diagnosis is made easy if there is a contact history; the disease is often epidemic. In family outbreaks, the index case is usually a child. Stool microscopy shows a polymorphonuclear leucocytosis, which may be most impressive, with red blood-cells and macrophages.

Ultimate diagnosis is dependent on the isolation of the causative shigella from the stool. Several fresh stool specimens or rectal swabs should be examined for the organism and its sensitivities as soon as possible after the diagnosis has been suspected. Shigellae survive for only a short time in faeces. There may be a polymorph leucocytosis in the peripheral blood. Proctoscopy or sigmoidoscopy shows a diffusely reddened mucosa, usually with a purulent and bloody exudate. Those procedures are however exquisitely painful, and may even be dangerous, in acute shigellosis. Serology is of very limited value in diagnosis.

24.6. Treatment of shigellosis

Prophylaxis depends on the prevention of faecal contamination of food and water, and bed-linen; flies are one source of infection. Avoidance of foodstuffs likely to be contaminated, and sterilization of water, are essential; foods to be avoided are listed in Chapter 17 under 'travellers' diarrhoea'. The objectives of treatment of an attack are: (i) replacement of fluid-loss, which may be considerable, (ii) symptomatic treatment, and (iii) eradication of the infecting organism. The role of immune mechanisms in shigellosis is at present impossible to delineate; immunization does not currently play a part in prophylaxis.

Fluid replacement can usually be accomplished orally as it is in cholera; dilute normal saline (saline diluted four times) mixed with fruit juice, with added potassium chloride (2g four-hourly), is of great value. Alternatively, an oral solution, such as that used in the rehydration of cholera patients, may be used:

Glucose	20·0 g
Sodium chloride	3·5 g
Sodium bicarbonate	2·5 g
Potassium chloride	1.5 g

made up to one litre. That formula is produced in the form of a sachet by UNICEF (15-611-00) and can be dissolved, when required, in one litre of drinking water. It is virtually impossible to overload the circulation in an otherwise fit person by the oral route. When vomiting is severe, intravenous fluid replacement is often necessary, and in children especially, rehydration by that route is sometimes of great urgency as in cholera (Chapter 18). Intravenous calcium gluconate is occasionally required if tetany complicates the clinical picture.

Symptomatic measures consist of oral propantheline bromide ('Probanthine') (15 mg four hourly), or diphenoxylate hydrochloride ('Lomotil') (2·5 to 5·0 mg, p.r.n.); the latter agent should however be used with caution, because by slowing peristalsis it probably allows increased bacterial proliferation in the intestine, with the production of small-intestinal colonization and malabsorption. Shigellae are excreted for a greater length of time, also, and there is probably an increased risk of severe colonic ulceration.

In most cases specific treatment should be reserved until a clear diagnosis has been made; indiscriminate use of antibiotics can be responsible for the production of resistant strains of shigellae (Levine, 1979). Most shigella infections are self-limiting and without specific treatment death is unusual. In a case of average severity caused by *S. sonnei*, specific treatment is not required. In a severely ill patient, on the other hand, such treatment may have to be started before bacteriological proof of the diagnosis. For many years, sulphonamides have been the main standby; they are still of great value, especially in the third world, where their low cost is a great advantage. The main risk is of crystalluria in a dehydrated patient, and that is made more likely by a hot climate. However, non-absorbable compounds, e.g. sulphaguanidine (3g four-hourly, for five to seven days) and phthalylsulphathiazole ('Thalazole') (2g four-hourly for five to seven days), are relatively safe because they are poorly absorbed. Mixtures of sulphonamides (e.g. sulphadiazine, sulphathiazole, and sulphamerazine), some of which are absorbed, are advocated by some physicians, the rationale being that an attack on bacteria via the bloodstream, in addition to that via the lumen of the intestine, produces a more rapid cure; the mixture of sulphonamides also reduces the risk of crystalluria. Antibiotics may be used as an alternative and are clearly indicated where there is resistance of the causative organism to sulphonamides. Thus, oral tetracycline (500 mg four times daily for five to seven days), ampicillin or chloramphenicol (500 mg four times daily for five days), or streptomycin (2g twice daily for five to seven days) are also used. Neomycin (1 g six-hourly for five days), and combinations of antibiotics and sulphonamides have also proved of value. Nalidixic acid (1 g six hourly) has also been used; that agent should not be given during the first trimester of pregnancy. Reports of antibiotic sensitivities of the organism must be carefully taken into account, as soon as they are available, and if necessary the specific treatment changed. Unlike experience with salmonellae, laboratory sensitivity reports correlate well with clinical results (Christie, 1968). In recent years resistance to therapeutic agents has become a real problem. In one outbreak of shigellosis in the USA the causative organism was resistant to several antibiotics (Mata, Gangarosa, and Cáceres, 1969). In London, ampicillin resistance has been reported in up to 90 per cent of Shigellae (Davies, Farrant, and Uttley, 1970). In fact, so great is the difference in antibiotic sensitivity in different parts of the world, that it is impossible to make clear recommendations on therapy. Generally speaking the more conservative approaches seem to be the most desirable.

24.7. Food-poisoning by shigella species

Closely resembling the more pathogenic shigellae, these organisms are responsible for some cases of 'food-poisoning'. They grow in the superficial gut epithelium as well as the lumen of the intestine, and produce a toxin which produces hypersecretion in the small intestine, via the cyclic AMP system. There is large-intestinal involvement with shedding of the epithelium, also. In field studies of diarrhoeal disease, shigella species are the most common bacterial pathogens to be identified (Gordon, 1964; Gordon, Ascoli, Pierce, Guzmán, and Mata, 1965; Levine, 1979). In the war in Vietnam, of approximately 1000 US Marines to be admitted to hospital, about one-third were infected with *Shigella* spp. (Forman, Tong, Murrell, and Cross, 1971). The faecal-oral route is the usual one for infection (Christie, 1968). As with the more pathogenic strains, they can survive on a wooden lavatory seat for as long as 17 days (Hutchinson, 1956); shade, coolness, and relatively high humidity favour survival outside the gastrointestinal tract (Christie, 1968).

The incubation period is from 24 to 72 hours. The onset of diarrhoea is usually abrupt, with blood, mucus, and pus in the stool; there may also be cramps, tenesmus, and lethargy. Vomiting is not a dominant feature. There may be a mild fever. The disease is usually mild and self-limiting. In children there may be prostration, meningismus, and seizures.

Stool cultures are positive.

Maintenance of fluid and electrolyte balance is important. In severe cases it is necessary to give antibiotics as for severe shigellosis, e.g. tetracycline, ampicillin, chloramphenicol, or neomycin (see above).

References

Barrett-Connor, E. and Connor, J. D. (1970). *Am. J. Gastroent.*, **53,** 234.
Bodmer, W. F. (1978). *Br. med. Bull.*, **34,** 213.
Boyd, J. S. K. (1957). *Trans. R. Soc. trop. Med. Hyg.*, **51,** 471.
Brewerton, D. A. (1978). *Jl. R. Soc. Med.*, **71,** 331.
Chantemesse, A. and Widal, F. (1888). *Bull. Acad. Méd.*, **19,** 522.
Christie, A. B. (1968). *Br. med. J.*, **2,** 285.
Cook, G. C. (1978). *Jl. R. Coll. Phycns*, **12,** 329.
Davies, J. R., Farrant, W. N., and Uttley, A. H. C. (1970). *Lancet*, **2,** 1157.
Du Pont, H. L., Hornick, R. B., and Dawkins, A. T. (1969). *J. infect. Dis.*, **119,** 296.
Fairley, N. H. and Boyd, J. S. K. (1943). *Trans. R. Soc. trop. Med. Hyg.*, **36,** 253.
Felsen, J. (1945). *Bacillary dysentery, Colitis and Enteritis*, W. B. Saunders Co., Philadelphia.
Flexner, S. (1901). *J. Am. med. Ass.*, **36,** 6.
Forman, D. W., Tong, M. J., Murrell, K. D., and Cross, J. H. (1971). *Am. J. trop. Med. Hyg.*, **20,** 598.
Gonzalez-Licea, A. and Yardley, J. H. (1966). *Bull. Johns Hopkins Hosp.*, **118,** 444.
Gordon, J. E. (1964). *Am. J. med. Sci.*, **248,** 345.
——, Ascoli, W., Pierce, V., Guzmán, M. A., and Mata, L. J. (1965). *Am. J. trop. Med. Hyg.*, **14,** 404.
Graber, C. D., Browning, D., and Davis, J. S. (1966). *Am. J. clin. Path.*, **46,** 221.
Grady, G. F. and Keusch, G. T. (1971). *New Engl. J. Med.*, **285,** 831 and 891.
Hochberg, M. C., Bias, W. B., and Arnett, F. C. (1978). *Medicine, Baltimore*, **57,** 463.
Hurst, A. F. (1943). *Medical diseases of war*, 3rd ed. Arnold, London.
Hutchinson, R. I. (1956). *Mon. Bull. Minist. Hlth*, **15,** 110.
Ingram, V. G., Rights, F. L., Ali Khan, H., Hashimi, K., and Ansari, K. (1966). *Am. J. trop. Med. Hyg.*, **15,** 743.
Keusch, G. T., Mata, L. J., and Grady, G. F. (1970). *Clin. Res.*, **18,** 442.
Koster, F., Levin, J., Walker, L., Tung, K. S. K., Gilman, R. H., Rahaman, M. M., Majid, M. A., Islam, S., and Williams, R. C. (1978). *New Engl. J. Med.*, **298,** 927.
Levine, M. M. (1979). *Tropical Doctor*, **9,** 4.
Manson-Bahr, P. H. (1943). *The dysenteric disorders: the diagnosis and treatment of dysentery, sprue, colitis and other diarrhoeas in general practice*. 2nd ed. p. 168. Cassell and Co. Ltd., London.
Mata, L. J., Gangarosa, E. J., and Cáceres, A. (1969). *J. infect. Dis.*, **122,** 170.
Moore, H. A., De La Cruz, E., and Vargas-Mendez, O. (1965). *Am. J. Epidemiol.*, **82,** 162.
Morson, B. C. and Dawson, I. M. P. (1972). *Gastrointestinal pathology*. p. 448. Blackwell, Oxford, London, Edinburgh, and Melbourne.
Powell, S. J. and Wilmot, A. J. (1966). *Gut*, **7,** 438.
Pringle, J. (1764). *Observations on the diseases of the army*. 4th ed. Millar, Wilson and Durham, London.
Rogers, L. (1913). *Dysenteries. Their differentiation and treatment*. Oxford University Press, London.
Shiga, K. (1898). *Zentbl. Bakt. ParasitKde*, **24,** 913.
Stewart, G. T. (1950). *Br. med. J.*, **1,** 405.
Strong, R. P. and Musgrave, W. E. (1900). *J. Am. med. Ass.*, **35,** 498.
Suwa, N. (1966). *Pathological anatomy of bacillary dysentery in Japan*. Internat. Acad. Path. Kyoto.

TAKEUCHI, A., SPRINZ, H., LA BREC, E. H., and FORMAL, S. B. (1965). *Am. J. Path.*, **47,** 1011.

TWINING, W. (1835). *Clinical illustrations of the more important diseases of Bengal with the result of an inquiry into their pathology and treatment*. 2nd ed. **1,** Baptist Mission Press, Calcutta.

VAN HEYNIGEN, W. E. and GLADSTONE, G. P. (1953). *Br. J. exp. Path.*, **34,** 202, 221 and 230.

WOLFF, H. L. and VAN ZIJL, W. J. (1969). *Bull. Wld Hlth Org.*, **41,** 952.

25

Intestinal amoebiasis

ALTHOUGH reported incidence rates are often strikingly different, most diseases of the large intestine which are common in the western world also exist in developing countries and *vice versa*. Present evidence suggests that nonspecific ulcerative colitis is less common in tropical Africa, and that Crohn's disease is rare in large areas of the third world, compared with the respective incidence rates in the UK (Chapter 29). Similarly, colonic and rectal carcinomas are unusual in most third world countries. The reasons for those differences are not yet clear, although several hypotheses have been advanced. Altered bowel function associated with blood in the stool in an African or Arab undergoing investigations either in his home country or in the UK, will probably be due to bacillary or amoebic dysentery, or schistosomiasis. However, other lesions, such as ulcerative colitis and colonic carcinoma, must also be carefully considered in the differential diagnosis, and must under no circumstance be ruled out on probability grounds. The finding of amoebic cysts or even trophozoites, although indicating amoebiasis, does not positively exclude other organic disease. The reverse situation is however equally, if not more, important. People from the UK or another western country, especially those who have travelled in tropical areas at some stage of their lives, must be properly and adequately investigated for amoebiasis (Stamm, 1976) and schistosomiasis, before a confident diagnosis of nonspecific ulcerative colitis is made. I have personal knowledge of three cases of amoebic colitis misdiagnosed as ulcerative colitis, over an approximately six-month period, in reputable hospitals in southern England. Treatment consisted of colectomy and/or corticosteroids with resultant death in all three; a course of metronidazole would almost certainly have resulted in a permanent cure in all of them. The widow of one of those patients was subsquently awarded £51 000 damages (*The Times*, 1978; *Br. med. J.*, 1978). Examination of the case-notes of 30 patients who had died of amoebiasis revealed that 12 had been diagnosed at post-mortem (Stamm, 1975b). The importance of early diagnosis of that disease has also been stressed at Southampton, England (Triger, 1978).

Amoebic disease should be suspected in all patients with diarrhoea of two or more weeks standing, and in all patients with liver disease of unknown aetiology, especially when there is a history of tropical exposure (Stamm, 1975, 1976). Problems in diagnosis in the UK have been outlined by Wright (1966).

Although common in all parts of the tropics and third world, numerous cases of amoebiasis are on record in patients who have never left the UK or other temperate areas. Severe infections occur most commonly in tropical and subtropical countries. The disease is characteristically endemic and epidemics are very unusual. It is hyperendemic in some cities e.g. Durban (Wilmot, 1962), Ibadan, and Kampala (Poltera and Owor, 1973).

25.1. Distribution of amoebic colitis

The disease is extremely common throughout the tropics and subtropics. In 1958, 52 (3·6 per cent) medical admissions to University Hospital, Ibadan, Nigeria, were for amoebiasis (Lauckner, Rankin, and Adi, 1961); 21 had fulminating dysentery and 10 died (one with a colonic perforation). In Lagos, 14 children died from amoebiasis during a seven-month period; 13 had fulminant intestinal changes, and in four perforation had occurred (Nnochiri, 1965; Olatunbosun, 1965). In Kenya, 17 children were treated at the Kenyatta National hospital, Nairobi, over a two-year period; over 50 per cent died, most of them however also had an hepatic abscess (MacDougall, 1960). In Durban, South Africa, 3 per cent of 13 700 admissions to the King Edward VIII hospital were admitted for amoebiasis; 6 per cent died (Wilmot, 1962).

There can be no doubt that morbidity and mortality from the disease varies from area to area. It is certainly much more severe in some countries than others. In Zambia and Papua New Guinea for example it is a mild disease with little in the way of complications, whereas in Uganda and Nigeria, the severity of the disease and high complication rate are very serious medical problems.

25.2. Presentation of amoebic colitis

The disease affects all age groups; the maximum number of cases occur between 20 and 50 years of age; men seem to get severe amoebic dysentery more often than women. The incubation period is extremely variable and only very rarely can it be delineated. Intestinal disease is characterized by either severe diarrhoea, which is often bloody, and which may alternate with normal bowel function, or even constipation, or it may be entirely asymptomatic (the cyst-carrier state). Most diagnostic difficulties arise when the disease is in its mild and insidious form.

With acute amoebic dysentery, the incubation period may be as short as eight to 10 days, and in about half of them the onset is sudden. Frank amoebic dysentery, which occurs during the active invasive stage in the large intestine, seems to be more common in the tropics than in temperate countries; in the latter it is more common in summer than winter.

Acute or intermittent diarrhoea, with blood and mucus are the usual initial symptoms. Headache, nausea, chills, fever, and colic may accompany the diarrhoea. Between bouts the patient may be entirely free of symptoms. Severe fulminating infections are said to be more common in pregnancy and the puerperium. In childhood also, amoebiasis may be especially severe if it is associated with malnutrition or follows measles (Lewis and Antia, 1969). Experimentally, protein-deficient rats are more susceptible to infection and caecal ulceration compared with controls (Ross and Knight, 1973). Fatal necrotizing amoebic enterocolitis has been described in a patient with severe cutaneous burns (Panke, Teegarden, and Lescher, 1978); it was felt that impaired immunity, nutritional imbalance, and coexistent bacterial infections predisposed to that event.

Chronic dysentery may result from untreated cases of the acute disease (see below). That is associated with progressive scarring and deformity of the colon, and with intermittent attacks of fever, and bloody diarrhoea with mucus and pus in the stools.

Amoebic colitis must be differentiated from nonspecific ulcerative colitis, with which it may be clinically indistinguishable, carcinoma of the large intestine, and other large bowel disorders. Necrotizing colitis (Chapter 27) and antibiotic-induced colitis (Chapter 28) should also be excluded. Amoebic appendicitis and amoeboma (see below) may complicate the disease.

Rectal amoeboma may closely mimic carcinoma. There may be ulceration of the anus or abdominal wall. Amoebic infection of the genitalia may be a result of normal or abnormal sexual intercourse. An arthritis has been reported (Rappaport, Rossien, and Rosenblum, 1951).

The commonest clinical type, however, is the cyst-carrier state. Patients with that condition may either have acquired an infection and not experienced the active disease, or be convalescent from amoebic dysentery, but continue to excrete cysts in the stool. Only a minority of cyst-carriers experience symptoms. Carrier rates of *E. histolytica* amongst symptomless people vary between 20 and 80 per cent in some communities (Stamm, 1966; *Lancet*, 1968).

There is no evidence that a previous bout of amoebiasis confers any degree of immunity.

25.3. Parasitology and pathology of amoebic colitis

Amoebic dysentery is caused by the protozoan *Entamoeba histolytica*. It seems probable that there are two variants of *E. histolytica*: one which causes tissue invasion and the acute symptoms of amoebic dysentery, and one which is relatively benign (Godfrey, 1978); isoenzyme characterizations are different, and distinct, for those two types (Sargeaunt, Williams, and Grene, 1978; *Lancet*, 1979). *E. histolytica*, in its cystic stage, infects man in his food or drink (usually contaminated water or raw fruit and vegetables) via the gastro-intestinal tract. Food-handlers may be cyst-carriers. Enzymes in the gastro-intestinal tract destroy the cyst-wall, and trophozoites emerge as four-nucleated amoebae which divide to form uninucleate trophozoites. The trophozoites actively invade the large intestinal tissues, producing colonies in the intestinal wall and subsequently ulcerative lesions. Some trophozoites pass towards the rectum, cyst formation takes place, and the life-cycle is completed by further orofaecal infection. The cysts are rapidly destroyed by drying and are killed if heated to 50°C for five minutes; chlorination does not kill cysts in water, however. They will survive for as long as a month at 10°C.

Invasion of the host tissues by the trophozoite is the basis for the pathological changes. In order to establish itself in the colon, *E. histolytica* requires an association with bacteria such as *Escherichia coli* and *Enterobacteria aerogenes*; it is still not clear how the amoebae invade the mucosa (Neal, 1960; 1972; Rao and Padma, 1971). The entire large intestine from caecum to rectum may be involved; the most common sites, probably due to faecal stasis, are the caecum and descending colon (Fig. 25.1). Widespread ulceration and granulomatous formation can sometimes be seen, with a sigmoidoscope, in the upper rectum. The appendix and rarely the ileum may also be invaded.

Early on, lysis of the epithelium produces superficial erosions. Microscopically they appear initially as shallow ulcers with overhanging edges, a necrotic

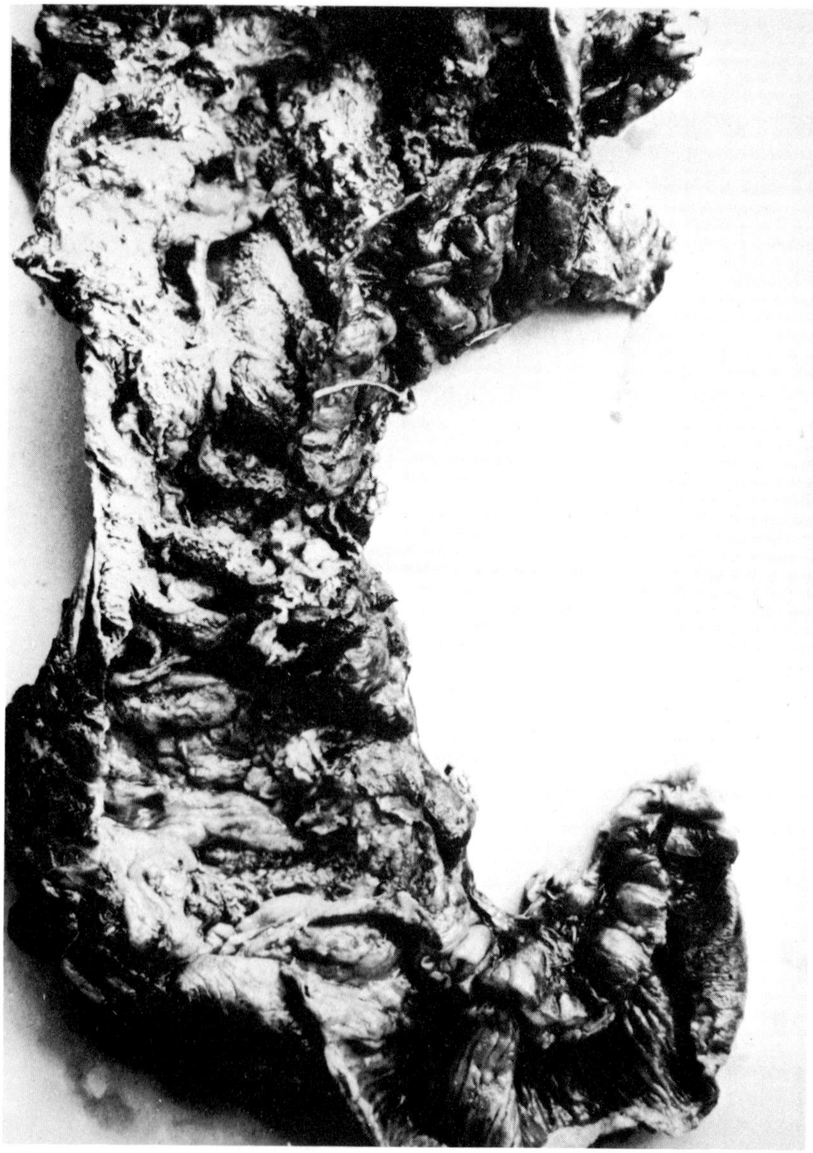

FIG. 25.1. Amoebiasis of the caecum and colon. A hemi-colectomy specimen is shown which had been removed from an Australian nurse several weeks after her arrival in Port Moresby, Papua New Guinea. A diagnosis of nonspecific ulcerative colitis had been made. The specimen shows multiple large ulcers with overhanging edges.

base, and a surrounding zone of hyperaemia (Morson and Dawson, 1972). Extension occurs to the submucosa, and deeper lesions are formed ('vertical ulcers'). The ulcers spread laterally in the submucosa and may become confluent. Although there is virtually no leucocyte response, and little oedema initially, secondary bacterial infection rapidly occurs. Rarely, extreme and rapid invasion may produce severe haemorrhage from the large intestine. In patients receiving corticosteroids, and in pregnancy, the whole mucosa may slough, and appear dark and gangrenous.

Entry of the trophozoites into the portal vein radicles leads to liver metastases (Chapter 12). It has been suggested, but not proved, that alcohol and malnutrition predispose to tissue invasion by *E. histolytica*.

Other amoebae may infect the large intestine: *Entamoeba coli, Dientamoeba fragilis, Endolimax nana*, and *Iodamoeba bütschlii*. There is no concrete evidence however that any of them is pathogenic to man; one report suggests that a very heavy infection with *I. bütschlii* might have serious consequences (Derrick, 1948). *Entamoeba polecki* is common in Papua New Guinea (McMillan and Kelly, 1970). It is a parasite of pigs, and it is unusual for it to invade man (Levin and Armstrong, 1970). It is difficult to differentiate the trophozoite from that of *E. histolytica*; however the cysts are always uninucleate and the nucleus is smaller than that of *E. histolytica*. Furthermore, the cyst of *E. polecki* contains up to 30 chromatid bars, and that of *E. histolytica* fewer than 10.

25.4. Investigation of amoebic colitis

Diagnosis depends on finding amoebae, either cysts or trophozoites, in stool specimens. In dysentery, motile trophozoites are usually found. The fact that the stools must be fresh should be emphasized; it is impossible to detect a motile trophozoite in a specimen more than a few minutes old. The trophozoite contains ingested red blood-cells, if they are available, and that is an important point in differentiating *E. histolytica* from nonpathogenic amoebae. The stool may also be cultured if facilities are available. If the stools are formed, only cysts are likely to be found. Iodine staining reveals one to four nuclei and a glycogen mass; one or more barshaped chromatin bodies are present. Concentration techniques make identification easier.
make identification easier.

Identification of amoebae in faeces, pus, or tissue depends on the skill and diligence of the physician or microbiologist. In an investigation in the USA, three laboratories were found to be reporting false-positive identifications of *E. histolytica*; in most cases that was due to the mistaking of leucocytes for amoebae. In four other cases the diagnosis of amoebic colitis was missed either by laboratory failure to detect amoebae, or clinical failure even to consider the condition (Krogstad, Spencer, Healy, Gleason, Sexton, and Herron, 1978). Faecal specimens (preserved in 10 per cent formalin for cysts, and in polyvinyl alcohol for trophozoites) can be kept for many years and a positive identification still made (*Br. med. J.*, 1978). Amoebae are easily missed in routine histological sections; whenever amoebiasis is suspected, biopsy-specimens should be examined by an expert using an immunofluorescent technique

(Parelkar, Stamm, and Hill, 1971). That procedure should be applied to all patients with a clinical diagnosis of ulcerative colitis or Crohn's disease.

Proctoscopic and sigmoidoscopic examinations, during which scrapings or biopsy of the mucosa are taken (McAllister, 1962; Doxiades and Yiotsas, 1965), are also important in diagnosis (Fig. 25.2). Small yellow ulcers with surrounding hyperaemia are present. It should again be stressed that demonstration of amoebae in fresh stools, or faecal samples obtained by proctoscopy, is the main standby in diagnosis. Radiology is of limited value; however it may help to differentiate other lesions such as nonspecific ulcerative colitis (Figs. 25.3 and 25.4). A barium enema showing colonic ulceration, a contracted caecum, or multiple tumours, or constricted areas, should suggest amoebiasis (Hill and Goldberg, 1967); if any of those features is present, that disease should be positively excluded. Radiology is also of value in the assessment of response to treatment of an amoeboma.

In the *invasive* stage, serology is of value (*Br. med. J.*, 1978), but is much more likely to be positive if there is extraintestinal involvement (Chapter 12). The indirect haemagglutination test is positive in 98 per cent of cases of dysentery and 66 per cent of asymptomatic carriers (Kessel, Lewis, Pasquel, and Turner, 1965). The complement-fixation test is positive in 16 per cent of patients with intestinal amoebiasis (Robinson, 1972); controls give negative results. Titres are usually much lower in intestinal disease than in hepatic disease, and fall more rapidly than haemagglutination titres. The indirect fluorescent antibody test (FAT) (Parelkar and Stamm, 1973) is more often positive in acute than chronic cases of intestinal amoebiasis; however false positive results also occur. In the FAT, fluorescence of cultured *E. histolytica* takes place on exposure to serum from a patient with invasive amoebic disease. The FAT, as well as the other serological tests, remains positive for long after successful treatment and is of no value in assessing a cure (Krupp and Powell, 1971). The gel-diffusion test (Powell, Maddison, Wilmot, and Elsdon-Dew, 1965) is a better guide than the FAT in assessing the efficacy of treatment. A simple latex agglutination test (Morris, Powell, and Elsdon-Dew, 1970), which is presented as a commercial kit ('Serameba'), has recently been evaluated (Stamm, Ashley, and Parelkar, 1973) and seems to be reliable.

White blood-count may show a mild or moderate polymorphonuclear leucocytosis.

25.5. Treatment of amoebic colitis

Treatment has been revolutionized by the discovery that metronidazole ('Flagyl') is an effective and seemingly safe antiamoebic agent (Lewis and Cole, 1971; Powell, 1970; 71; Cohen and Reynolds, 1975; Krogstad, Spencer, and Healy, 1978). Reports of carcinogenicity in rats and mutagenicity in bacteria (Voogd, Van der Stel, and Jacobs, 1974), led to initial doubts about safety (*Med. Lett. Drugs Ther.*, 1975), but neither of those toxic effects has yet been documented in man. In India, however, a 35 per cent failure of response to metronidazole has been reported (Datta, Singh, and Chhuttani, 1974). A disturbingly high incidence of failure using metronidazole in extraintestinal disease has also been reported in Southampton, England (Triger, 1978); four

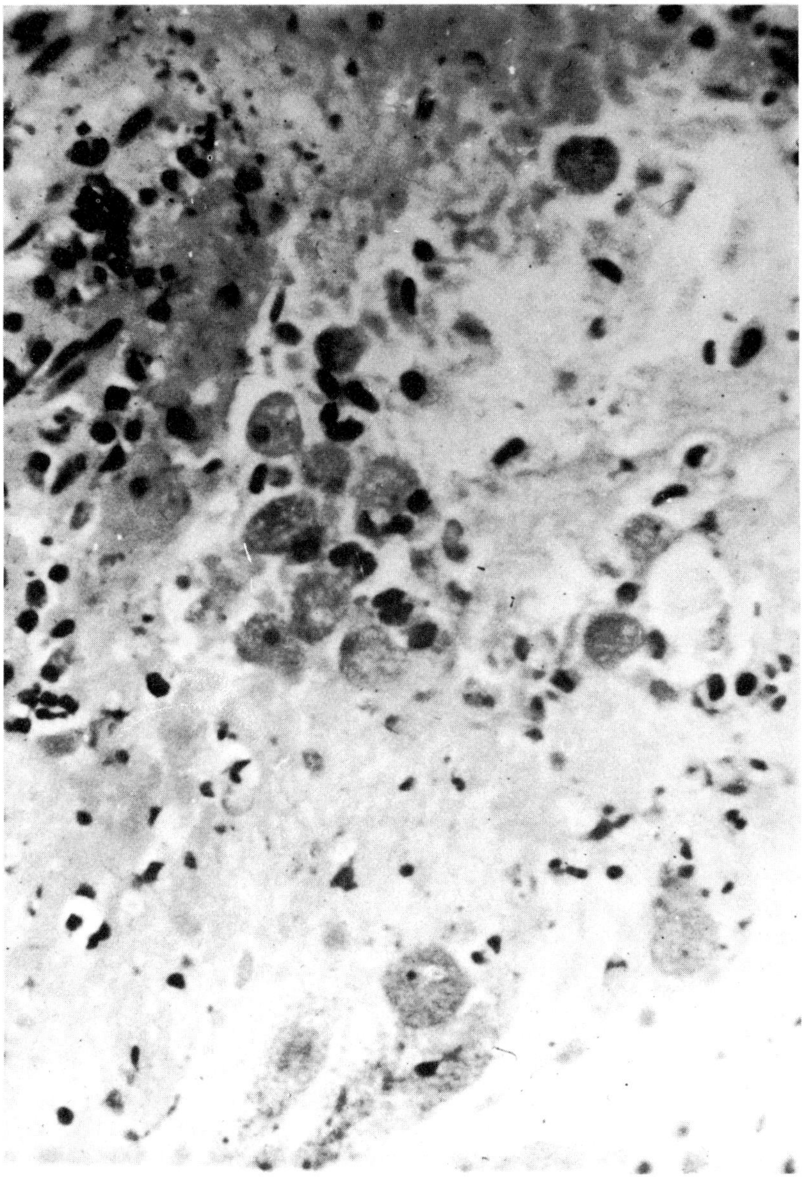

Fig. 25.2. Rectal biopsy (haematoxylin and eosin) showing numerous trophozoites of *Entamoeba histolytica.*

of five failures occurred in patients from India and the Far east. A straightforward attack of amoebic dysentery should respond to 800 mg metronidazole three times daily for five days (Powell, 1970). Mild side-effects such as nausea and lethargy are common. The drug has an antabuse action and the patient should be warned not to take alcohol while the treatment is taking place. In a particularly severe attack of dysentery in, for example, a child, a debilitated adult, or a patient on immunosuppressive therapy, the metronidazole regime should be combined with tetracycline (250 mg orally six-hourly for 10 days, together with a course of diloxanide furoate ('Furamide')* (see below). Tinidazole (Miller, Howes, and English, 1969), given in a dose of 2·0g daily for three days, has given promising results in 50 patients with chronic intestinal amoebiasis (Islam and Hasan, 1975).

If intestinal amoebiasis persists after treatment, an infection with *Entamoeba polecki* (see above) should be considered.

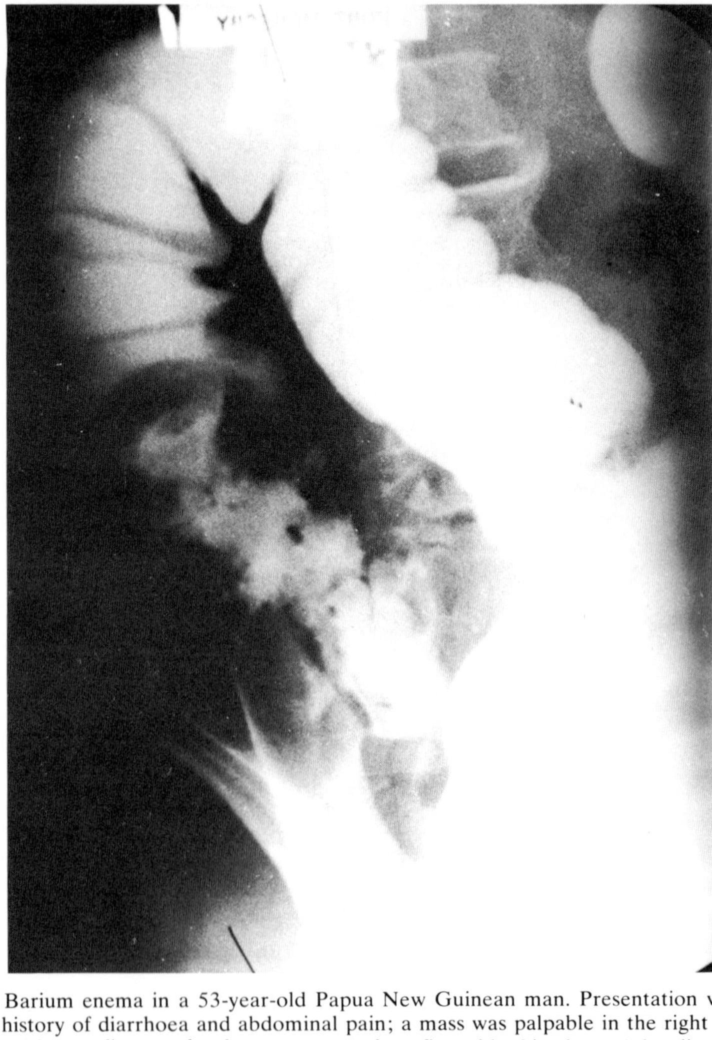

FIG. 25.3. Barium enema in a 53-year-old Papua New Guinean man. Presentation was with a two-week history of diarrhoea and abdominal pain; a mass was palpable in the right abdomen. Amoebic colitis was diagnosed at laparotomy, and confirmed by histology. A localized segment of the ascending colon was involved.

* Diloxanide furoate has not been approved by the FDA for use in the USA.

For the cyst-carrier state, diloxanide furoate, 500 mg three times daily for 10 days, is used (Krogstad, Spencer, and Healy, 1978). Neither metronidazole nor tinidazole is of value for treating the carrier-state (Spillmann, Ayala, and de Sanchez, 1976); after treatment, cysts of *E. histolytica* were found in 37 per cent of 30 patients given metronidazole, 62 per cent of 34 given tinidazole, and 70 per cent of 31 given a placebo. At least six stools should be clear before a cure can be documented.

Older therapeutic regimes involving emetine hydrochloride or iodide, combined with chloroquine and other antiamoebic agents are now rarely used. That is largely due to the toxicity of emetine (Reynolds, 1971), which has in fact probably been grossly overemphasized. Emetine is not now produced in the United Kingdom.

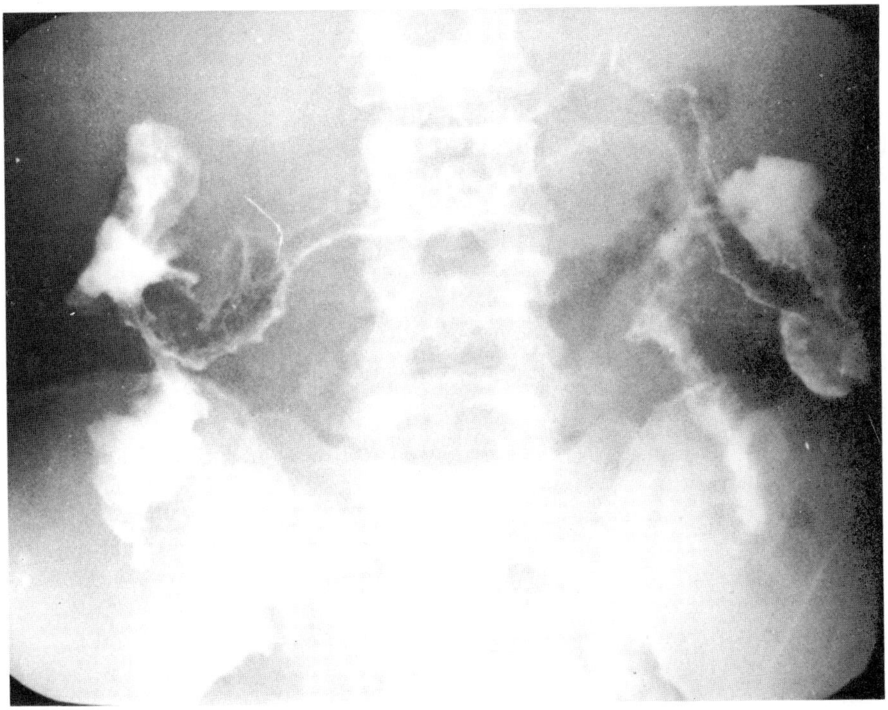

FIG. 25.4. Barium meal in a 34-year-old Papua New Guinean woman. There was a short history of bloody diarrhoea. Trophozoites of *E. histolytica* were demonstrated in fresh stool-specimens. Amoebiasis of the transverse and descending colon was diagnosed. The symptoms rapidly improved after a course of oral metronidazole.

25.6. Complications of intestinal amoebiasis

25.6.1. Amoebic peritonitis

Peritonitis is an uncommon complication of amoebic disease (Turner, Millikan, Carter, Thompson, and Hinshaw, 1965); it is nevertheless an extremely important one and the most common local complication of amoebic disease of the colon in Durban (Wilmot, 1962). Kapoor, Nathwani, and Joshi (1972) have described 73 cases of amoebic peritonitis seen in Bombay, India. Peritonitis may result (Davey, 1968) from: (i) diffusion of organisms from a 'blotting-paper'-like colon (Powell and Wilmot, 1966), (ii) perforation of the large intestine (Peláez, Villazón, and Sieres Zaraboso, 1966), especially in the rectosigmoid or caecal areas, which is followed by gross faecal flooding, (iii) perforation of the colon into the retroperitoneal tissues, through areas uncovered with peritoneum, and (iv) a local perforation or leak into a confined space caused by previous adhesions; that may result in a pericolic abscess or an internal intestinal fistula.

There is usually minimal pain, and tenderness along the length of the colon; perforation is usually insidious and is followed by generalized distension and loss of bowel sounds. Some patients pursue a chronic course and develop signs suggesting tuberculosis of the abdomen.

Appendicitis may be simulated. Typhoid and other causes of perforation, and large intestinal obstruction (Chapter 27) must be excluded.

A straight abdominal radiograph in the erect position shows free intraperitoneal gas; the findings are similar to those in a typhoid perforation. Paracentesis and examination of the fluid may assist diagnosis.

Intravenous fluids and gastric suction must be instituted immediately. Metronidazole and a broad-spectrum antibiotic should be given. Owing to the wet 'blotting-paper' colon, surgery is best avoided (Davey, 1968); overall mortality is of the order of 50 per cent and after surgery that is nearer 100 per cent! Occasionally, with a short clearcut history of perforation similar to that of peptic ulcer, in a patient who is not too ill, surgical closure with an omental patch gives a good result.

25.6.2. Amoeboma

An amoeboma is caused by an intense localized granulomatous reaction following ulceration or penetration of tissues by *E. histolytica.* An amoeboma may arise at the site of an amoebic ulcer (Powell, 1974). The amoebae are present in the central zone of fibrosis, or necrotic tissue. A variable length of bowel is involved; there may be multiple amoebomas.

A painful tender mass is present which varies in its degree of mobility; it may involve the overlying abdominal wall. The most common site is the rectosigmoid or caecal region; the rectum is certainly not an uncommon site. Regional lymph nodes may be enlarged and hyperplastic. Projection into the bowel, or the formation of a stricture, may cause an intestinal obstruction, or may produce a starting point for an intussusception (Chapter 27) of the ileocaecal or caecocolic type.

An appendix mass, and carcinoma of the colon or rectum should always be considered in the differential diagnosis. Carcinoma of the colon and rectum are uncommon in most parts of the third world (Chapter 29); there is no reason why they should not coexist with amoebiasis.

Stool examination may be negative. Rectal examination may reveal a firm tender swelling; usually there is no ulceration, which is common with a rectal carcinoma. There may be changes in the perianal skin, due to spread outside the rectum. Sigmoidoscopy may reveal ulcers in the adjacent colon. Barium enema may show a smooth stricture which is virtually diagnostic. Because it is invasive (Recio, 1965) serology is usually positive.

Metronidazole should be given as for amoebic colitis. Resolution is usually rapid and within one week; however occasionally a longer period is required. If there is no decrease in the size of a suspected amoeboma after 72 hours of metronidazole, the diagnosis should be critically reassessed.

25.6.3. Rectal haemorrhage

This is uncommon but can be severe; it is caused by bleeding from colonic or rectal ulcers. Treatment is with blood transfusion and the outlook is usually good.

25.6.4. Other complications

Postdysenteric colitis. This usually follows a severe acute attack of amoebic dysentery. Although there is residual colonic damage, amoebae are absent following treatment. The mucosa appears red and oedematous and there is usually no ulceration, although superficial erosions may exist. Serological tests are usually positive. Appendicitis and an appendix abscess are unusual complications. Massive necrosis (Essenhigh and Carter, 1966) of the colon is a rare complication. Toxic megacolon has been reported (Faegenburg, Chiat, Mandel, and Ross, 1967).

Stricture of the colon, intussusception, rectal, enterocolic (Shaff and Wolfowitz, 1962), and anal fistulae, and ulceration of the anus and abdominal wall have all been described (Wilmot, 1962). Spread to cervical, vaginal and inguinal regions, and urethral amoebiasis are rarely seen.

Hepatic amoebiasis is the commonest extraintestinal complication of intestinal amoebiasis (Ochsner and De Bakey, 1943; Wilmot, 1962) (Chapter 12). In most cases intestinal symptoms are not present; presentation is with a large tender liver in a sick patient.

References

Br. med. J. (1978). **2,** 379.

Cohen, H. G. and Reynolds, T. B. (1975). *Gastroenterology*, **69,** 35.

Datta, D. V., Singh, S. A. K., and Chhuttani, P. N. (1974). *Am. J. trop. Med. Hyg.*, **23,** 586.

Davey, W. W. (1968). *Companion to Surgery in Africa*. p. 247. E. and S. Livingstone. Edinburgh and London.

Derrick, E. H. (1948). *Trans. R. Soc. trop. Med. Hyg.*, **42,** 191.

Doxiades, T. H. and Yiotsas, Z. (1965). *Am. J. Gastroent., N.Y.*, **43,** 229.

Essenhigh, D. M. and Carter, R. L. (1966). *Gut*, **7,** 444.

Faegenburg, D., Chiat, H., Mandel, P. R., and Ross, S. T. (1967). *Am. J. Roentg.*, **99,** 74.

Godfrey, D. G. (1978). *Nature, Lond.*, **273,** 600.

Hill, M. C. and Goldberg, H. I. (1967). *Am. J. Roentg.*, **99,** 77.

Islam, N. and Hasan, M. (1975). *Curr. ther. Res.*, **17,** 161.

Kapoor, O. P., Nathwani, B. N., and Joshi, V. R. (1972). *J. trop. Med. Hyg.*, **75,** 11.

Kessel, J. F., Lewis, W. P., Pasquel, C. M., and Turner, J. A. (1965). *Am. J. trop. Med. Hyg.*, **14,** 540.

Krogstad, D. J., Spencer, H. C., and Healy, G. R. (1978). *New Engl. J. Med.*, **298,** 262.

——, ——, ——, GLEASON, N. N., SEXTON, D. J., and HERRON, C. A. (1978). *Ann. intern. Med.*, **88,** 89.
KRUPP, I. M. and POWELL, S. J. (1971). *Am. J. trop. Med. Hyg.*, **20,** 421.
Lancet (1968). **1,** 77.
—— (1979). **1,** 303.
LAUKHNER, J. R., RANKIN, A. M., and ADI, F. C. (1961). *W. Afr. med. J.*, **10,** 3.
LEVIN, R. L. and ARMSTRONG, D. E. (1970). *Am. J. clin. Path.*, **54,** 611.
LEWIS, E. A. and ANITA, A. U. (1969). *Trans. R. Soc. trop. Med. Hyg.*, **63,** 633.
—— and COLE, T. O. (1971). *W. Afr. med. J.*, **20,** 253.
MCALLISTER, T. A. (1962). *Br. med. J.*, **1,** 362.
MACDOUGALL, L. G. (1960). *E. Afr. med. J.*, **37,** 279.
MCMILLAN, B. and KELLY, A. (1970). *Trans. R. Soc. trop. Med. Hyg.*, **64,** 792.
Med. Lett. Drugs Ther. (1975). **17,** 53.
MILLER, M. W., HOWES, H. L., and ENGLISH, A. R. (1969). *Antimicrob. Agents Chemother.*, **9,** 257.
MORRIS, M. N., POWELL, S. J., and ELSDON-DEW, R. (1970). *Lancet*, **1,** 1362.
MORSON, B. C. and DAWSON, I. M. P. (1972). *Gastrointestinal pathology.* p. 453. Blackwell, Oxford, London, Edinburgh, and Melbourne.
NEAL, R. A. (1960). *Parasitology*, **50,** 531.
—— (1972). *Trans. R. Soc. trop. Med. Hyg.*, **66,** 514.
NNOCHIRI, E. (1965). *J. trop. Med. Hyg.*, **68,** 231.
OCHSNER, A. and DE BAKEY, M. (1943). *Surgery, St. Louis*, **13,** 460 and 612.
OLATUNBOSUN, D. A. (1965). *Trans. R. Soc. trop. Med. Hyg.*, **59,** 72.
PANKE, T. W., TEEGARDEN, D. K., and LESCHER, T. J. (1978). *Am. J. trop. Med. Hyg.*, **27,** 766.
PARELKAR, S. N. and STAMM, W. P. (1973). *Trans. R. Soc. trop. Med. Hyg.*, **67,** 659.
——, ——, and HILL, K. R. (1971). *Lancet*, **1,** 212.
PELÁEZ, M., VILLAZÓN, A., and SIERES ZARABOSO, R. (1966). *Dis. Colon Rectum*, **9,** 356.
POLTERA, A. A. and OWOR, R. (1973). *E. Afr. med. J.*, **50,** 344.
POWELL, S. J. (1970). *Gut*, **11,** 967.
—— (1971). *Bull. N. Y. Acad. Med.*, **47,** 469.
—— (1974). *Medicine*, **26,** 1544.
——, MADDISON, S. E., WILMOT, A. J. and ELSDON-DEW, R. (1965). *Lancet*, **2,** 602.
—— and WILMOT, A. J. (1966). *Trans. R. Soc. trop. Med. Hyg.*, **60,** 544.
RAO, V. G. and PADMA, M. C. (1971). *Trans. R. Soc. trop. Med. Hyg.*, **65,** 606.
RAPPAPORT, E. M., ROSSIEN, A. X., and ROSENBLUM, L. A. (1951). *Ann. intern. Med.*, **34,** 1224.
RECIO, P. M. R. (1965). *Dis. Colon Rectum*, **8,** 205.
REYNOLDS, T. B. (1971). *Gastroenterology*, **60,** 952.
ROBINSON, G. L. (1972). *Trans. R. Soc. trop. Med. Hyg.*, **66,** 435.
ROSS, G. W. and KNIGHT, R. (1973). *Trans. R. Soc. trop. Med. Hyg.*, **67,** 560.
SARGEAUNT, P. G., WILLIAMS, J. E., and GRENE, J. D. (1978). *Trans. R. Soc. trop. Med. Hyg.*, **72,** 519.
SHAFF, B. L. and WOLFOWITZ, J. (1962). *Br. J. Surg.*, **49,** 535.
SPILLMANN, R., AYALA, S. C., and DE SANCHEZ, C. E. (1976). *Am. J. trop. Med. Hyg.*, **25,** 549.
STAMM, W. P. (1966). In *The pathology of parasitic diseases* (ed. A. E. R. Taylor). p. 1. Blackwell, Oxford.
—— (1975). *Br. med. J.*, **2,** 452.
—— (1976). *Jl. R. Coll. Phycns*, **10,** 294.
——, ASHLEY, M. J., and PARELKAR, S. N. (1973). *Trans. R. Soc. trop. Med. Hyg.*, **67,** 211.
The Times, London (1978). 15th March 1978. p. 4.
TRIGER, D. R. (1978). *J. trop. Med. Hyg.*, **81,** 54.

Turner, G. R., Millikan, M., Carter, R., Thompson, R. J., and Hinshaw, D. B. (1965). *Am. Surg.*, **31,** 759.

Voogd, C. E., van der Stel, J. J., and Jacobs, J. J. A. (1974). *Mutat. Res.*, **26,** 483.

Wilmot, A. J. (1962). *Clinical Amoebiasis.* Blackwell, Oxford.

Wright, R. (1966). *Br. med. J.*, **1,** 957.

26

Intestinal schistosomiasis

SCHISTOSOMIASIS was first described by the German pathologist, Bilharz, in 1852; he noted the adult worms while performing a post-mortem on a young Egyptian in Egypt. Sambon (1907) was responsible for naming *Schistosoma mansoni*, and in 1904, Katsurada described *S. japonicum* (Katsurada, 1922).

Three species of schistosomes (trematodes or blood-flukes) commonly produce intestinal disease: *Schistosoma mansoni, S. japonicum*, and *S. intercalatum* (Wright, Southgate, and Knowles, 1972). Although other species occasionally affect man they are of minor importance. The various species can be recognized by their characteristic ova. There are significant infraspecific variations among schistosomes (Godfrey, 1978); infectivity, growth-rate, maturation time, ova production, and tissue ova deposition vary with different strains. Acid phosphatase and malate dehydrogenase are of value in differentiating the morphologically similar ova of *S. intercalatum* from *S. haematobium* (the schistosome responsible for urinary tract disease).

Distribution of these organisms depends on the presence of susceptible snail hosts, and on human sanitary habits; indiscriminate defaecation constitutes the most important factor in continued transmission. There is a marked seasonal fluctuation in snail numbers; during the rainy seasons they decrease and then multiply at a great rate as the dryer, warmer months approach (Webbe, 1965).

This group of diseases affects many millions of people in the tropics (from 36°N to 34°S), especially in Africa, and is one of the greatest unconquered parasitic diseases (Weller, 1976). It has been estimated that some 200 million people in the world suffer from schistosomiasis (Jordon and Webbe, 1969). Furthermore, the world incidence is at present increasing, because the extent of the habitat of the intermediate hosts, various freshwater snail species, is increasing, as new dams, e.g. the Aswan High Dam, and irrigation schemes (Brown, 1975; Choudhry, 1975) are constructed. A recent survey in the Sudan for example suggests that there has been a great increase in the incidence of *S. mansoni* infection over a 25-year period (Omer, Hamilton, Marshall, and Draper, 1976).

Pathological manifestations depend on (i) species of parasite, (ii) intensity of infection (Edington, Von Lichtenberg, Nwabuebo, Taylor, and Smith, 1970), (iii) frequency and severity of exposure (Cheever, Kamel, Elwi, Mosimann, Danner, and Sippel, 1978), (iv) the immunological status (Warren, 1972; Massoud and Nelson, 1972), and probably (v) the nutritional status of the individual (de Witt, Oliver-González, and Medina, 1964; Bell, 1964). There are undoubtedly geographical differences in severity of infection; to what extent those depend on strain difference, acquired resistance to infection, and nutritional status of the host is unknown.

Even if clinical morbidity is not apparent, it seems likely that physical activity and working capacity are impaired by the disease, and that it is important in an economic context (Hiatt and Gebre-Medhin, 1977); morbidity, as would be expected, is dependent on intensity of infection (Siongok, Mahmoud, Ouma, Warren, Muller, Handa, and Houser, 1976; Hiatt, 1976). Physiological studies designed to assess work capacity are difficult to perform (Collins, Brotherhood, Davies, Doré, Hackett, Imms, Musgrove, Weiner, Amin, Karim, Ismail, Omer, and Sukkar, 1976); however there is evidence that lung function is diminished in infected individuals (Omer and El Din Ahmed, 1974), and that would clearly lead to impaired physical performance.

26.1 Parasitology and pathology of intestinal schistosomiasis

Man acquires infection when fresh water containing cercariae comes into contact with his skin and mucous membranes. Whenever he is exposed to infected water, during paddling, swimming, fishing or sailing, even very briefly, he is in danger of infection. Drinking infected water is also hazardous. Infect with *S. mansoni* has been demonstrated at as early as six months of age in the West Nile district of Uganda (Ongom, 1973). The cercariae penetrate intact skin and as they do so lose their tails and become schistosomules which reach the liver via the circulation (the exact route is unknown); from there they enter the portal system and develop into adult worms. They can live there for up to 20 to 30 years. The females (14–26 mm in length), after fertilization by males (10–15 mm long), migrate against the direction of blood-flow to the terminal tributaries of the portal venous system, and the veins draining the large intestine, the mesenteric plexus; eggs are deposited, extruded into the intestine and ultimately excreted in the faeces. Assuming the ova enter fresh water, a larva (miracidium) emerges, and swims around until a suitable species of snail is found. Within the snail, the life cycle is completed by the production and liberation of many new cercariae. A heavily infected snail may shed 1500 to 2000 cercariae daily for up to 200 days.

Viable ova lodge in human tissues and produce an inflammatory reaction, and granuloma formation (Morson and Dawson, 1972); subsequently fibrosis, and sometimes calcification, give rise to the longterm sequelae of the disease.

Lesions develop in the walls of the large intestine. Granulomatous reactions give rise to ulceration, bleeding papillomata, and fibrosis; carcinomatous change is rare (El-Sabai, 1961). Embolization of ova to the liver gives rise to the main complication (Chapter 10).

Granulomas precede periportal fibrous formation, upon which portal hypertension becomes superimposed (Chapter 11); an enlarged spleen, ascites and bleeding oesophageal varices result. *S. haematobium* can also give rise to liver granulomata (Ragheb, 1956; Carter and Shaldon, 1959). Ova sometimes embolize to the lungs, giving rise ultimately to pulmonary hypertension. They may also reach the spinal cord and occasionally the brain, giving rise to space-occupying lesions.

26.2 *Schistosoma mansoni* and *S. intercalatum* infections

26.2.1. Distribution and characteristics of S. mansoni *and* S. intercalatum

Africa, the Middle east, particularly the Arabian peninsula, including Saudi Arabia (Arfaa, 1976), and the Yemen, south and central America, and the Caribbean are the main areas in which *S. mansoni* is common. The disease is common in Puerto Rico (Díaz-Rivera, Ramos-Morales, Sotomayor, Lichtenberg, García-Palmieri, Cintrón-Rivera, and Marchand, 1957). Although baboons can harbour *S. mansoni*, the practical significance of that reservoir is unknown. The intermediate snail hosts are various species of *Biomphalaria, Australorbis*, and *Tropicorbis*. Infection with *S. intercalatum* occurs in Zaire and Gabon and although the ova resemble those of *S. haematobium*, the schistosome which produces urinary tract disease, the clinical course is similar to that of *S. mansoni.* The snail host is *Bulinus forskali.*

26.2.2. Presentation of S. mansoni *and* S. intercalatum *infections*

The clinical features of schistosomiasis, as seen in Zimbabwe Rhodesia, have been described by Gelfand (1963). Clinically, the disease may begin with a local erythematous reaction ('swimmers' itch') following penetration of the cercariae; that reaction lasts a few days only, and often does not occur at all. After four to six weeks, a generalized allergic reaction, accompanied by an eosinophilia, is usual and that may last for several weeks; fever, malaise, muscle pains, and urticaria may occur. There may be anorexia and weight-loss. Children complain of tiredness, listlessness, and lack of energy; they tend to fall behind with their studies and games. At that stage, and also after months or years, intestinal symptoms, diarrhoea with blood and mucus, and tenesmus, appear. Exacerbations occur every few weeks and they may resemble amoebic colitis. Severe dysentery with blood and mucus seem to be confined to Egypt and the Sudan; in one investigation in Zimbabwe Rhodesia, 58 per cent had mild diarrhoea, 40 per cent had no change in bowel habit, and 2 per cent had noted some blood and mucus (Gelfand, 1963). Epigastric discomfort is a common complaint.

In most parts of Africa visible lesions of the large intestine are unusual, despite the fact that ova are widely distributed in the submucosa and muscle. The colon may become thickened and tender. It may be reddened and granular, with pinpoint yellowish elevations, surrounded by a hyperaemic zone; there may be shallow ulcers, but they are more common in *S. japonicum* infections (see below). In Egypt, gross lesions in the rectosigmoid region are common; ulcerations of the mucosa become secondarily infected, with polyp formation; the lesions are up to 2·0 cm in diameter. In Egypt, 17 to 20 per cent of patients with *S. mansoni* infections develop polyposis of the colon, from which there may be excessive protein loss (Lehman, Farid, Bassily, Haxton, Wahab, and Kent, 1970; Farid, Miner, Higashi, and Hassan, 1976); fortunately that responds to niridazole treatment. The mode of action of the drug on the polyps is unknown; its main effect is on adult schistosomes. Polyposis does not seem to occur in Brazil (Cheever and Andrade, 1967); there was no evidence of that entity in 502 people with *S. mansoni* infections. Massive polyposis can be associated with fatal intestinal haemorrhage. Such lesions are not usually premalignant (Dimmette, Elwi, and Sproat, 1956; El-Sabai, 1961). Intestinal adhesions and exudative peritonitis with progressive fibrosis can give rise to a rigid colon with stenosis; the mesentery is infected and thickened and venous thromboses may occur. Masses in the lymph-glands may simulate a malignancy. Colonic disease, with stenosis and intestinal obstruction has also been reported in *S. haematobium* infection (Gelfand and Hammar, 1966).

The appendix may be involved and frequently contains ova of *S. mansoni*, and also *S. haematobium*; it may be involved in several ways (Barsoum, 1934; Elwi and El Tiraei, 1955; El Gazaverli and Khalil, 1954; Lovett-Campbell, 1935; Lovett-Campbell and Rose, 1936; Stewart, 1930). There may be diffuse lesions throughout the wall, sometimes in the absence of symptoms; that is seen in specimens following appendectomy, or occasionally at post-mortem. Alternatively subserosal nodules, which consist of ova encapsulated with fibrous tissue, may be seen macroscopically; they may also occur on the serosal aspect of the neighbouring caecum, paracolic gutter, pelvic floor, and omentum. Such lesions occasionally coalesce to form a localized 'tumour' of the appendix and rarely produce obstructive appendicitis by causing stenosis.

Rectal involvement occurs in approximately 70 per cent of *S. haematobium* infections; it is not uncommon for lesions to be found in other parts of the colon and appendix, and they may be polypoid in type (Gelfand and Hammar, 1966).

Acute large-intestinal obstruction following intussusception, due to granulomatous lesions in the colon, has been described. In *S. mansoni* (and also *S. japonicum*) infections, fibrosis may produce a pseudotumour; caecocolic intussusception and obstruction have been reported. Abdominal lymphadenopathy may be present.

Inflammatory masses in the intestinal wall (bilharziomata) may be formed. Owor and Madda (1977) have stressed that schistosomiasis in Uganda may often present with tumour-like masses, which are frequently misdiagnosed clinically as intra-abdominal Burkitt's lymphomas; the masses are granulomatous and often fibrous. Presentation of *S. mansoni* infections with abdominal masses ('bilharziomas'), causing intestinal obstruction, which mimic intestinal tumours, has also been reported from the Sudan (Malik, Satir, Veress, and El Hassan, 1975). In the south-eastern corner of Lake Victoria, Uganda, a group of patients has been described in whom firm, nodular, painless masses are present in the small intestine; obstruction is an occasional sequel. At operation conglomerations of granulomata are present on the antimesenteric border of the ileum, and occasionally the jejunum (Wydell, 1958); the condition resolves on specific schistosomal treatment.

As hepatic involvement occurs, hepatosplenomegaly and evidence of portal hypertension appears (Chapter 11). Ascites and bleeding from oesophageal varices occur late in the course of the disease. Pulmonary involvement is heralded by haemoptyses, and signs of *cor pulmonale* (De Leon and Tavera, 1968; Briers, 1974). The presence of ova in the lungs produces a periarteritis, and fibrosis of the pulmonary arterioles.

Renal involvement is probably far more common than has been hitherto recognized (Rocha, Cruz, Brito, and Susin, 1976); of 100 patients with *S. mansoni* infections in Brazil, 15 had persistent proteinuria, and in 9 there was a nephrotic syndrome. Membrano-proliferative glomerulonephritis was the most common histological lesion. An association between schistosomal infections and renal amyloidosis has been suggested (Gold, 1978); evidence is however limited at present.

The spinal cord lesion produced by *S. mansoni* is usually a transverse myelitis (Abbot and Spencer, 1953; Marcial-Rojas and Fiol, 1963).* Salmonella septicaemia has been reported in the presence of *S. mansoni* infections (Rocha, Kirk, and Hearey, 1971; Rocha, Oliveira, Oliveira, and Prata, 1971); the typhoid carrier state may be a sequel.

26.3 *Schistosoma japonicum* infections

26.3.1. Distribution and characteristics of S. japonicum

South-eastern China, Japan, Taiwan, the Philippines, and parts of Burma and Thailand are the main areas involved. The disease has also been described in Malaysia (Murugasu and Dissanaike, 1973). There is no schistosomiasis in Papua New Guinea. A reservoir of *S. japonicum* exists in various mammals: the dog, cow, cat, rat, pig, water-buffalo, and goat; it is thus a zoonosis. However it is estimated that 75 per cent of transmission is from man himself. Infection is common in farm-workers. The snail intermediate hosts are various species of *Oncomelania, Katayama*, and *Schistosomophora*. One worm pair of *S. japonicum* may produce 3000 ova daily. As with *S. mansoni* infections, the disease is primarily an intestinal one. The superior, as well as inferior mesenteric vein, and thus the small intestine and proximal colon, are involved. Liver pathology and portal hypertension are similar to those in *S. mansoni* infections. It is more common to find ova in ectopic sites than with other species of schistosomes. Pulmonary involvement is less common. Central nervous system involvement (mainly the brain) is associated with lesions containing large numbers of ova in necrotic material, often surrounded by eosinophils, and is much more common than in *S. mansoni* infections; epilepsy is a result.

26.3.2. Presentation of S. japonicum *infections*

'Swimmers' itch' is unusual. A severe dermatitis ('Kabure itch') seen in Japan is apparently caused by an avian schistosome. The allergic phase ('Katayama syndrome') occurring two to three weeks after infection may be severe, and is followed more rapidly by symptoms of intestinal involvement than with *S. mansoni*. The clinical manifestations are undoubtedly more severe than with any of the other schistosomal infections. The mucosa may be reddened and granular and there may be shallow ulcers which are more marked than in *S. mansoni* infections. Acute colonic obstruction has been reported (Nai-Kuang and Pen-Ching, 1957). Chronic colitis in *S. japonicum* infections is probably a premalignant condition; uni- or multifocal adenocarcinomas may arise from polyps (Ch'en, Hu, Chang, Chuang, Ts'ao, Chang, Wang, Ch'en, and Chou, 1965; Ming-Chai, Jen-Chun, P'ei-Yu, Ch'i-Yuan, P'eng-Fei, Shen-Hsing, Fu-P'an, Ts'u-Ling, and Shun-Ch'uan, 1965).

* Anterior spinal artery occlusion has been recorded (Siddorn, 1978).

The nephrotic syndrome has been reported in a *S. japonicum* infection in Malaysia (Murugasu, Wang, and Dissanaike, 1978).

26.4. Investigation of intestinal schistosomiasis

Diagnosis depends on finding the ova (either a lateral spine for *S. mansoni,* a lateral knob for *S. japonicum*, or terminal spine for *S. intercalatum*) in the stool; numerous stools may have to be examined before a positive diagnosis can be made. Concentration techniques may be required. *S. mansoni* ova are occasionally found in the urine. There is usually an eosinophilia in the early invasive stage of the disease, and a study in Khartoum indicated that patients with an eosinophilia (of 400 per cu mm or more) excrete significantly more *S. mansoni* ova than those without an eosinophilia (Salih, Sabaa, and Ali, 1977). Sigmoidoscopy might show ulcerations and polyps and is of particular value in *S. japonicum* infections. In *S. japonicum* infections, granulomas, scars, discrete depressions in the mucosa, and polypoid growths may be present; the latter occasionally produce intestinal obstruction at the rectal or sigmoid level, and also undergo carcinomatous change. Rectal biopsy and aspiration liver-biopsy are of great value in diagnosis in both *S. mansoni* and *S. japonicum* infections (Kruatrachue, Bhaibulaya, and Harinasuta, 1964). *S. haematobium* may also be found in biopsy-specimens from those two sites. *S. mansoni* ova calcify much less often than those of *S. japonicum.* Adult worms are occasionally found in rectal polyps. Barium enema shows an immobile colon with irregular constrictions; polyps may be outlined. Portal venography, and a liver 'scan' will give additional information if there is chronic liver involvement (Chapter 10); there may be haematological evidence of hypersplenism. When the lungs are affected, typical ova may appear in the sputum. Chest radiography, if pulmonary involvement is present, shows right ventricular hypertrophy, an increased pulmonary artery component to the cardiac outline, and mottling of the lung parenchyma. The lesions contain large numbers of ova and necrotic material surrounded by eosinophils and multinucleated giant cells. The cerebrospinal fluid shows an increase in protein and cells, especially eosinophils. Chronic salmonellosis may complicate the disease in patients with chronic *S. mansoni* infections; there are reports of that from Egypt (Hathout, El-Ghaffar, Awny, and Hassan, 1966; Hathout, El-Ghaffar, and Awny, 1967; Farid, Higashi, Bassily, Young, and Sparks, 1972; Higashi, Farid, Bassily, and Miner, 1975), south America (Neves and Lobo Martins, 1967; Neves, Marinho, Lobo Martins, de Araujo, and Lucciola, 1969) and the Sudan (Salih, Abu Subaa, Abu Asha, and Abdel Stair, 1977). In the latter study, 21 patients were reported; in 16, *S. typhi* or *S. paratyphi A* were isolated from blood cultures. They had chronic pyrexias, and most had severe anaemia. Serum alkaline phosphatase was raised in 16 of them. Three patients also had a nephrotic syndrome. All recovered after chloramphenicol treatment.

Intradermal and serological diagnosis. In all forms of schistosomiasis, serodiagnosis is of value approximately four weeks after infection, but that is no substitute for finding the ova. Immunodiagnosis has been reviewed by Draper (1978) and Lehman (1978). Complement fixation, florescent-antibody, and precipitin techniques are of value; the antigens are prepared from adult schistosomes or from viable ova. Intradermal tests with suitable antigens are also of value, although there are some false positive reactions. None of the reactions is species specific.

The *intradermal test* gives positive results in about 90 per cent of infected patients (Pellegrino, Memoria, and Macedo, 1957; Kagan and Pellegrino, 1961); there are about five per cent false positive results. It is of value in diagnosing early infections. The *complement-fixation* test is positive in 90 to 95 per cent of cases (Chaffee, Bauman, and Shapilo, 1954). The *immunofluorescence test* (Sadun, Anderson, and Williams, 1961) is positive in approximately 85 per cent of infected patients; there are about five per cent false positive results. Because capillary blood can be used it is of use in survey work. A *slide flocculation test* (Anderson, 1960) gives positive results in about 95 per cent of cases, with six per cent false positives. *A plasma-card test* (Sadun, Anderson, and Schoenbechler, 1963) is positive in approximately 86 per cent of infected patients and gives a false-positive result in about six per cent. Enzyme-linked immunosorbent assay (ELISA) and radioimmunoassays have been used with encouraging results to detect antischistosome antibodies (Schinski, Clutter, and Murrell, 1976).

26.5. Treatment of intestinal schistosomiasis

The present status of treatment of severe disease has been reviewed by McMahon (1976) and Omer (1978a). The major difficulty is to decide which patients with this disease should be treated, for in endemic areas the majority of people will rapidly become reinfected; there seems to be no clear answer to that enigma. There is no doubt, on the contrary, that people who will not be re-exposed should undergo treatment aimed at complete eradication of the disease.

Development of shistosomicides has been slow. That is largely due to (i) marked interspecies variation in susceptibility, and (ii) a very poor correlation between *in-vitro* and *in-vivo* tests (McMahon, 1976). The most widely used treatment at present is niridazole ('Ambilhar') (Mahmoud, 1978) which is given orally at a dose of either 25 mg per kg daily for seven days, or 20 mg for 10 days; the least successful results with that compound are in *S. japonicum* infections. Niridazole inhibits glucose uptake and reduces the glycogen stores; it is extensively metabolized in both the host liver and in schistosomes. In addition, niridazole can profoundly suppress cell-mediated hypersensitivity, which is important in schistosome granuloma formation. A metabolite of niridazole, rather than the compound itself, may very well be the active component (Van den Bossche, 1978). Toxic effects, though usually mild, preclude the drug from being of use in *mass* treatment. Such effects are most marked in the presence of portal-systemic anastomoses, when the unmetabolized compound has a direct effect on cerebral metabolism; mental confusion, hallucinations, and convulsions result. Niridazole is thus contraindicated in the presence of severe hepatocellular disease and known portal-systemic shunting, and also in psychotic patients. It may give rise to haemolysis in glucose-6-phosphate dehydrogenase deficiency.

Promising results have recently been obtained with oral oxamniquine ('Vansil'), a hydroxytetrahydroquinoline derivative: up to 60 mg per kg bodyweight over two days. In the Sudan, results are very satisfactory (Omer, 1978b); viable ova were absent from the stools six months after treatment in 95 per cent of those who received 60 mg per kg bodyweight, in 79 per cent of those who had 40 mg per kg, and in 69 per cent after 30 per kg. In those patients who were not cured, the ova count was diminished. Dizziness was the only significant side effect; abdominal pain and diarrhoea also occurred. Those who received the high dose had a transient rise in the blood eosinophil count and alanine aminotransferase concentration. In Brazil also, oxamniquine has given good results (Katz, Zicker, and Pereira, 1977). Effective treatment of *S. mansoni* infections with oxamniquine has also been reported from South Africa (Pitchford and Lewis, 1978); there, too, the incidence of side effects was low. Electroencephalographic changes after oxamniquine, and the production of *grand mal* fits in patients with idiopathic epilepsy have however been reported (Keystone, 1978). It should be noted however that there are probably marked differences in response in different geographical areas (Omer, 1978b). It may well be that oxamniquine will be of greater value than niridazole in *S. japonicum* infections, although animal experiments with that parasite have given disappointing results.

Praziquantel, a broad spectrum antischistosomal compound (a pyrozinoisoquinolinone), has given promising results in preliminary clinical studies in Zambia, Brazil, Japan, and the Philippines, and seems effective against *S. mansoni, S. intercalatum* and *S. japonicum* (Van den Bosshe, 1978). Its effect is on the membrane potential of the muscle cells of the schistosome.

A further compound worthy of trial is 4-isothiocyanato-4′-nitrodiphenylamine, which is effective against both *S. mansoni* and *S. japonicum*; unlike hycanthone (see below) and niridazole, this compound is devoid of mutagenic activity, although it gives rise to a mutagenic metabolite in the urine—probably as a result of intestinal bacterial action (Van den Bossche, 1978). Metrifonate ('Bilarcil') seems effective in *S. mansoni* infection involving the urinary bladder (Omer and Teesdale, 1978); that is a relatively unusual event however. Sodium antimony tartrate, stibocaptate ('Astiban') and stibophen ('Fantorin') are alternative therapeutic agents, but with troublesome side effects.

Hycanthone ('Etrenol') given as a single intramuscular injection (3 mg per kg bodyweight) has given good results; however, hepatocellular toxicity can be severe. Overt hepatitis and acute hepatic necrosis can occur (Cohen, 1978) Chapter 7); although the incidence of such complications is low they must constantly be borne in mind. The mechanism of the therapeutic action of hycanthone is not yet fully understood. In St. Lucia, Cook and Jordan (1971) reported a reduction in the excretion of ova in 81 per cent of patients after hycanthone; in a further study (Cook, Jordan, and Armitage, 1976) those workers showed that a dose of 1·5 to 2·0 mg per kg is as effective as one of 3·0 mg per kg, and much less likely to produce side effects. In another investigation (Cook, Jordan, and Bartholomew, 1977) they attempted to control the disease by *mass* treatment; following that, the incidence of new infections in children fell from 21 to 4 per cent after two years. Similar findings have been reported by Clarke, Blair, and Weber (1969) from Zimbabwe Rhodesia, and Figueiredo and Prata (1969) from Brazil. In a study in Puerto Rico, however, 20 patients with *S. mansoni* infections were given intramuscular hycanthone, and a further 20 a placebo injection (Sotomayor, Febles, Ramos Morales, Sanchez, and Rivera, 1976); 14 of the hycanthone group had symptoms: nausea, vomiting, anorexia, abdominal pain, and diarrhoea. About one third developed hepatosplenomegaly. The placebo group was asymptomatic. Ten of the hycanthone group had a rise in serum SGOT; four weeks after treatment they were all free of ova on stool examination. In Kenya, Warren, Arap Siongok, Ouma, and Houser (1978) have assessed the effectiveness of three different doses of hycanthone (1·5, 0·75, and 0·375 mg per kg) on *S. mansoni* infections; a decrease in egg output was achieved in 96 per cent, 85 per cent, and 11 per cent respectively, at one month after treatment. There were no side effects with the lower doses. Those workers claimed on the basis of that study that 100 per cent lethal doses of antischistosomal agents are not required, especially in endemic areas, because (i) *S. mansoni* does not multiply in the human host and (ii) the disease is closely associated with intensity of infection; toxic side effects of treatment (and cost) are thus reduced. Resistance of *S. mansoni* to hycanthone has been reported, and that is cross-resistant with related drugs such as oxamniquine, but not with niridazole (Jansma, Rogers, Liu, and Bueding, 1977). Hycanthone has been shown to be of less use, however, in *S. japonicum* infections (Hillman, Gibler, and Anderson, 1977); in that study, although the integument of *S. mansoni* was destroyed by hycanthone, that of *S. japonicum* was unchanged. Hycanthone binds to acetylcholine sites—that is much less easily reversed in *S. mansoni* than in *S. japonicum* infections. Hycanthone has no protective effect when given orally; in an investigation in hamsters it was ineffective when given by that route (Girgis, Mansour, and Henry, 1973).

A protective vaccine for schistosomiasis may be on the distant horizon (Lehman, 1978).

Assessment of cure in schistosomiasis is difficult; survival of a few adult worms can give rise to a recurrent output of ova. Continued absence of viable ova three months after treatment suggests cure. Dead ova in urine, stool or biopsies after treatment are of no pathological significance.

Breaking the transmission cycle by controlling cerariae has been attempted with many different agents. Treatment of water with niclosamine (0·5 mg per l) has given promising results in the Volta lake in Ghana (Chu, 1978).

Treatment of liver disease and portal hypertension may require portacaval anastomosis and other measures for arresting bleeding from oesophageal varices (Chapter 11). Brain and spinal-cord involvement may require surgery, and respiratory and cardiac complications appropriate therapeutic regimes.

References

Abbot, P. H. and Spencer, H. (1953). *Trans. R. Soc. trop. Med. Hyg.*, **47,** 221.
Anderson, R. I. (1960). *Am. J. trop. Med. Hyg.*, **9,** 299.
Arfaa, F. (1976). *Am. J. trop. Med. Hyg.*, **25,** 295.
Barsoum, H. (1934). *J. trop. Med. Hyg.*, **37,** 387.

BELL, D. R. (1964). *Lancet*, **1,** 643.
BILHARZ, T. (1852). *Z. wiss. Zool.*, **4,** 53,
BRIERS, P. J. (1974). *Proc. R. Soc. Med.*, **67,** 861.
BROWN, D. S. (1975). *E. Afr. med. J.*, **52,** 42.
CARTER, R. A. and SHALDON, S. (1959). *Lancet*, **2,** 1003.
CHAFFEE, E. F., BAUMANN, P. M., and SHAPILO, J. J. (1954). *Am. J. trop. Med. Hyg.*, **3,** 905.
CHEEVER, A. W. and ANDRADE, Z. A. (1967) *Trans. R. Soc. trop. Med. Hyg.*, **61,** 626.
——, KAMEL, I. A., ELWI, A. M., MOSIMANN, J. E., DANNER, R., and SIPPEL, J. E. (1978). *Am. J. trop. Med. Hyg.*, **27,** 55.
J. E. (1978). *Am. J. trop. Med. Hyg.*, **27,** 55.
CH'EN, M. C., HU, J. C., CHANG, P. Y., CHUANG, C. Y., TS'AO, P. F. CHANG, S. H., WANG, F. P., CH'EN, T. L., and CHOU, S. C. (1965). *China med. J.*, **84,** 513.
CHOUDHRY, A. W. (1975). *E. Afr. med. J.*, **52,** 120.
CHU, K. Y. (1978). *Bull. Wld Hlth Org.*, **56,** 313.
CLARKE, V. DE V., BLAIR, D. M., and WEBER, M. C. (1969). *Cent. Afr. J. Med.*, **15,** 1.
COHEN, C. (1978). *Gastroenterology*, **75,** 103.
COLLINS, K. J., BROTHERHOOD, R. J., DAVIES, C. T. M., DORÉ, C., HACKETT, A. J., IMMS, F. J., MUSGROVE, J., WEINER, J. S., AMIN, M. A., EL KARIM, M., ISMAIL, H. M., OMER, A. H. S., and SUKKAR, M. Y. (1976). *Am. J. trop. Med. Hyg.*, **25,** 410.
COOK, J. A. and JORDAN, P. (1971). *Amer. J. trop. Med. Hyg.*, **20,** 84.
——, ——, and ARMITAGE, P. (1976). *Am. J. trop. Med. Hyg.*, **25,** 602.
——, ——, and BARTHOLOMEW, R. K. (1977). *Am. J. trop. Med. Hyg.*, **26,** 887.
DELEON, E. P. and TAVERA, P. M. (1968). *Dis. Chest*, **53,** 154.
DEWITT, W. B., OLIVER-GONZÁLEZ, J., and MEDINA, E. (1964). *Am. J. trop. Med. Hyg.*, **13,** 25.
DÍAZ-RIVERA, R. S., RAMOS-MORALES, F., SOTOMAYOR, Z. R., LICHTENBERG, F. GARCÍA-PALMIERI, M. R., CINTRÓN-RIVERA, A. A., and MARCHAND, E. J. (1957). *Ann. intern. Med.*, **47,** 1082.
DIMMETTE, R. M., ELWI, A. M., and SPROAT, H. F. (1956). *Am. J. clin. Path.*, **26,** 266.
DRAPER, C. C. (1978). *Tropical Doctor*, **8,** 19.
EDINGTON, G. M., VON LICHTENBERG, F., NWABUEBO, I., TAYLOR, J. R. and SMITH, J. H. (1970). *Am. J. trop. Med. Hyg.*, **19,** 982.
ELWI, A. M. and EL TIRAEI, L. (1955). *J. Egypt Med. Ass.*, **38,** 311.
EL GAZAVERLI, M. and KHALIL, H. A. (1954). *J. Egypt med. Ass.*, **37,** 1068.
EL-SABAI, I. (1961). *Kasr-el-Aini J. Surg.*, **2,** 905.
FARID, Z., HIGASHI, G. I., BASSILY, S., YOUNG, S. W., and SPARKS, H. A. (1972). *Am. J. trop. Med. Hyg.*, **21,** 578.
——, MINER, W. F., HIGASHI, G. I., and HASSAN, A. (1976). *J. trop. Med. Hyg.*, **79,** 164.
FIGUEIREDO, J. F. M. and PRATA, A. (1969). *Gaz. med. Bahia*, **69,** 16.
GELFAND, M. (1963). *Cent. Afr. J. Med.*, **9,** 319.
—— and HAMMAR, B. (1966). *Trans. R. Soc. trop. Med. Hyg.*, **60,** 231.
GIRGIS, N. I., MANSOUR, N. S., and HENRY, W. (1973). *E. Afr. med. J.*, **50,** 105.
GODFREY, D. G. (1978). *Nature, Lond.*, **273,** 600.
GOLD, C. H. (1978). *S. Afr. med. J.*, **53,** 681.
HATHOUT, S. E., EL-GHAFFAR, Y. A., and AWNY, A. Y. (1967). *Am. J. trop. Med. Hyg.*, **16,** 462.
——, ——, ——, and HASSAN, K. (1966). *Am. J. trop. Med. Hyg.*, **15,** 156.
HIATT, R. A. (1976). *Am. J. trop. Med. Hyg.*, **25,** 808.
—— and GEBRE-MEDHIN, M. (1977). *Am. J. trop. Med. Hyg.*, **26,** 473.
HIGASHI, G. I., FARID, Z., BASSILY, S., and MINER, W. F. (1975). *Am. J. trop. Med. Hyg.*, **24,** 713.
HILLMAN, G. R., GIBLER, W. B., and ANDERSON, J. B. (1977). *Am. J. trop. Med. Hyg.*, **26,** 238.

Jansma, W. B., Rogers, S. H., Liu, C. L., and Bueding, E. (1977). *Am. J. trop. Med. Hyg.*, **26,** 926.
Jordan, P. and Webbe, G. (1969). *Human schistosomiasis*. p. l. Heinemann, London.
Kagan, I. G. and Pellegrino, J. (1961). *Bull. Wld Hlth Org.*, **25,** 611.
Katsurada, F. (1922). *Nisshin Igaku*, suppl. 1.
Katz, N., Zicker, F., and Pereira, J. P. (1977). *Am. J. trop. Med. Hyg.*, **26,** 234.
Keystone, J. S. (1978). *Am. J. trop. Med. Hyg.*, **27,** 360.
Kruatrachue, M., Bhaibulaya, M., and Harinasuta, C. (1964). *Ann. trop. Med. Parasit.*, **58,** 276.
Lehman, J. S. (1978). *Tropical Doctor*, **8,** 21.
——, Farid, Z., Bassily, S., Haxton, J., Wahab, M. F. A., and Kent, D. C. (1970). *Gastroenterology*, **59,** 433.
Lovett-Campbell, A. C. (1935). *W. Afr. med. J.*, **8,** 15.
—— and Rose, A. W. (1936). *Trans. R. Soc. trop. Med. Hyg.*, **30,** 335.
McMahon, J. E. (1976). *E. Afr. med. J.*, **53,** 295.
Mahmoud, A. A. (1978). *New Engl. J. Med.*, **297,** 1329.
Malik, M. O. A., Satir, A. A., Veress, B., and El Hassan, A. M. (1975). *E. Afr. med. J.*, **52,** 183.
Marcial-Rojas, R. A. and Fiol, R. E. (1963). *Ann. intern. Med.*, **59,** 215.
Massoud, J. and Nelson, G. S. (1972). *Bull. Wld Hlth Org.*, **47,** 591.
Ming-Chai, C., Jen-Chun, H., P'ei-yu, C., Ch'i-Yuan, C., P'eng-Fei, T., Shen-Hsing, C., Fu-P'an, W., Ts'u-Ling, C., and Shun-Ch'uan, C. (1965). *China med. J.*, **84,** 513.
Morson, B. C. and Dawson, I. M. P. (1972). *Gastrointestinal pathology*, p. 456. Blackwell, Oxford, London, Edinburgh, and Melbourne.
Murugasu, R. and Dissanaike, A. S. (1973). *Trans. R. Soc. trop. Med. Hyg.*, **67,** 880.
——, Wang, F., and Dissanaike, A. S. (1978). *Trans. R. Soc. trop. Med. Hyg.*, **72,** 389.
Nai-Kuang, C. and Pen-Ching, C. (1957) *China med. J.*, **75,** 324.
Neves, J. and Lobo Martins, N. R. daL. (1967). *Trans. R. Soc. trop. Med. Hyg.*, **61,** 541.
——, Marinho, R. P., Lobo Martins, N. R. daL., de Araujo, P. K., and Lucciola, J. (1969). *Trans. R. Soc. trop. Med. Hyg.*, **63,** 79.
Omer, A. H. S. (1978a). *Tropical Doctor*, **8,** 3.
—— (1978b). *Br. med. J.*, **2,** 163.
—— and El DinAhmed, N. (1974). *E. Afr. med. J.*, **51,** 217.
——, Hamilton, P. J. S., Marshall, T. F. deC., and Draper, C. C. (1976). *J. trop. Med. Hyg.*, **79,** 151.
—— and Teesdale, C. H. (1978). *Ann. trop. Med. Parasit.*, **72,** 145.
Ongom, V. L. (1973). *E. Afr. med. J.*, **50,** 581.
Owor, R. and Madda, J. P. (1977). *E. Afr. med. J.*, **54,** 137.
Pellegrino, J., Memoria, J. M. P., and Macedo, D. G. (1957). *J. Parasit.*, **43,** 304.
Pitchford, R. J. and Lewis, M. (1978). *S. Afr. med. J.*, **53,** 677.
Ragheb, M. (1956). *Gastroenterology*, **30,** 631.
Rocha, H., Cruz, T., Brito, E., and Susin, M. (1976). *Am. J. trop. Med. Hyg.*, **25,** 108.
——, Kirk, J. W., and Hearey, C. D. (1971). *Archs intern. Med.*, **128,** 254.
——, Oliveira, M. M. C., Oliveira, V. S., and Prata, A. (1971). *Revta Inst. Med. trop. S. Paulo*, **13,** 399.
Sadun, E. H., Anderson, R. I., and Schoenbechler, M. J. (1963). *Proc. Soc. exp. Biol. Med.*, **112,** 280.
——, ——, and Williams, J. S. (1961). *Expl Parasit.*, **11,** 117.
Salih, S. Y., Abu Sabaa, H., Abu Asha, H., and Abdel Satir, A. (1977). *J. trop. Med. Hyg.*, **80,** 14.
——, Sabaa, H. M. A., and Ali, M. S. (1977). *E. Afr. med. J.*, **54,** 421.
Sambon, M. F. (1907). *J. trop. Med. Hyg.*, **11,** 3 and 44.
Schinski, V. D., Clutter, W. C. and Murrell, K. D. (1976). *Am. J. trop. Med. Hyg.*, **25,** 824.

Siddorn, J. A. (1978). *Am. J. trop. Med. Hyg.*, **27,** 532.
Siongok, T. K. A., Mahmoud, A. A. F., Ouma, J. H., Warren, K. S., Muller, A. S., Handa, A. K., and Houser, H. B. (1976). *Am. J. trop. Med. Hyg.*, **25,** 273.
Sotomayor, Z. R., Febles, F., Ramos Morales, F., Sanchez, G., and Rivera, M. (1976). *J. trop. Med. Hyg.*, **79,** 18.
Stewart, Q. (1930). *W. Afr. med. J.*, **4,** 3.
*V*an den Bosshe, H. (1978). *Nature, Lond.*, **273,** 626.
Warren, K. S. (1972). *Trans. R. Soc. trop. Med. Hyg.*, **66,** 417.
——, Arap Siongok, T. K., Ouma, J. H., and Houser, H. B. (1978). *Lancet*, **1,** 352.
Webbe, G. (1965). *E. Afr. med. J.*, **42,** 605.
Weller, T. H. (1976). *Am. J. trop. Med. Hyg.*, **25,** 208.
Wright, C. A., Southgate, V. R., and Knowles, R. J. (1972). *Trans. R. Soc. trop. Med. Hyg.*, **66,** 28.
Wydell, S. H. (1958). *E. Afr. med. J.*, **35,** 413.

27

Other conditions involving the large intestine in the tropics

27.1. Colonic infections

27.1.1. Viral and bacterial infections

Lymphogranuloma venereum. This disease is usually confined to the anal, anorectal, and genital regions (Chapter 30). However, the distal colon may occasionally be involved.

Salmonellosis (typhoid fever). Although the distal ileum bears the brunt of this disease, the large intestine, usually the ascending colon, may be affected (Mandal and Mani, 1976). In paratyphoid B infections, the large intestine, including the rectum, may be involved (Edington and Gilles, 1976).

Tuberculosis of the colon. This is unusual (El Masri, Boulos, and Malick, 1977); the clinical presentation and barium enema appearances may be confused with amoebiasis (Fig. 27.1). There are reports of the disease involving principally the distal colon (Rhoades, Klein, and Welsh, 1960; Need and Behnke, 1963) and rectum (Walker Davis, 1957; Hawley, Wolfe, and Fullerton, 1968).

Tuberculous disease of the intestinal tract is usually localized to the ileocaecal region (Chapter 23).

Yersinia infection of the colon. This infection is caused by small Gram-positive coccobacilli (*Yersinia enterocolitica*) which are common in birds, hares, pigs, and dogs. Over the past two decades it has become clear that the disease is by no means uncommon in man and usually presents with acute disease of the ileocaecal region (Winblad, Niléhn, and Sternby, 1966; Vantrappen, Agg, Ponette, Geboes, and Bertrand, 1977). In one recent outbreak in the USA, 36 children were infected by drinking contaminated chocolate milk (Black, Jackson, Tsai, Medvesky, Shayegani, Feeley, MacLeod, and Wakelee, 1978); 16 subsequently had appendicectomies.

The infection produces white nodules, closely resembling tubercles, in the ileocaecal region; there is regional lymph-node involvement.

Serology is of value in diagnosis and has given positive results in patients with symptoms suggestive of acute appendicitis.

Parenteral streptomycin, or oral sulphonamides, are the therapeutic agents of choice. Good results have also been reported with tetracycline and chloramphenicol (Vantrappen, *et al.*, 1978).

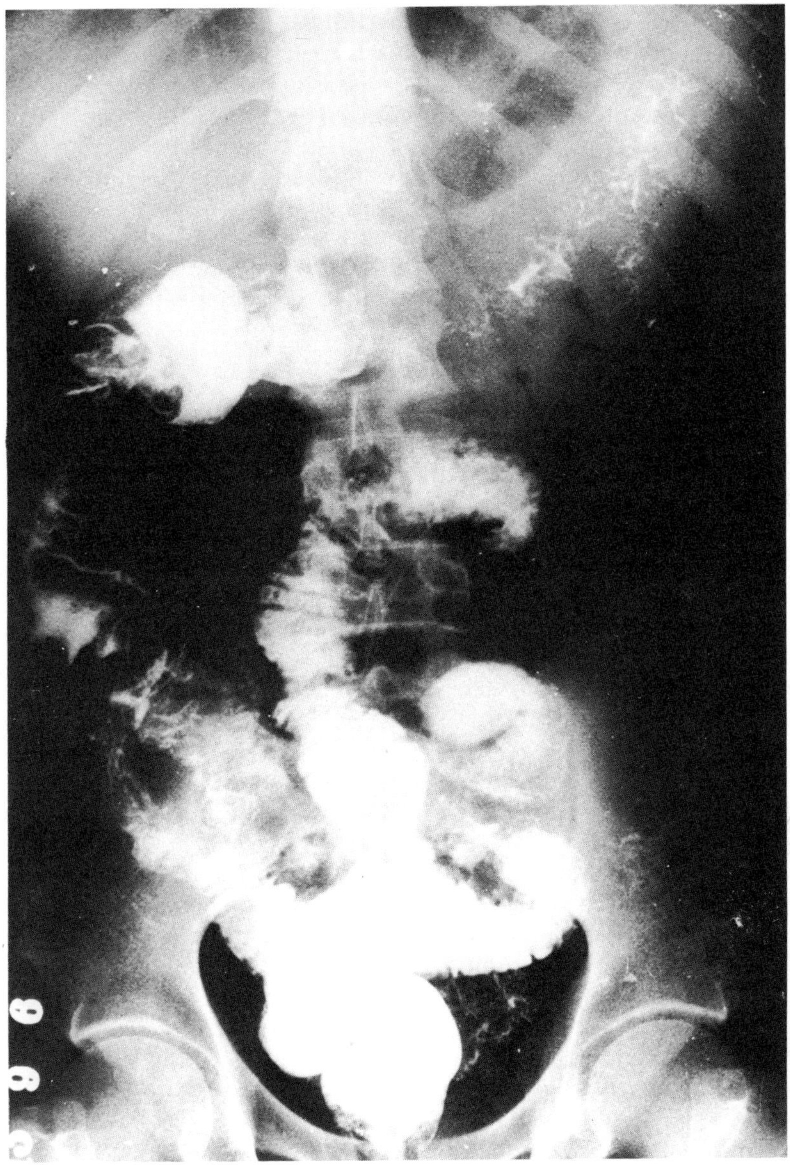

FIG. 27.1. Barium meal in a Papua New Guinean man who presented with a short history of abdominal pain, diarrhoea, and anaemia. A diagnosis of amoebiasis of the ascending colon was made, but there was no response to anti amoebic treatment. At subsequent laparotomy, tuberculosis, with four strictures of the ascending colon, was demonstrated; a diagnosis of tuberculosis was confirmed by finding caseation with acid-fast bacilli in a mesenteric gland biopsy.

27.1.2. *Mycotic infections*

Actinomycosis. This is an uncommon mycotic disease of the colon (Powers, Kramer, and Drake, 1961) and rectum (Morson, 1961); the ileocaecal region and rectum are most frequently involved. It is caused by *Actinomyces israelii* or *A. bovis*. It is a chronic suppurative disease; induration without mucosal ulceration is seen initially, and that is followed by fistula formation. The disease should be considered in smooth submucous strictures of the rectum. It seems likely that the organism is frequently a secondary invader, following the primary ulcerating lesions. Pus-filled tracks and abscesses are constant findings. The lesions spread locally. Diagnosis is from a biopsy; characteristic colonies of actinomyces can often be identified. 'Sulphur granules', which consist of tangled masses of filaments, and can be demonstrated with Gram's stain, can often be recognized in pus from an abscess; the organism can be cultured. The best antibiotic is penicillin.

Other mycotic infections. These have been reviewed by Morson and Dawson (1972). Primary infections with mucormycosis (De Feo, 1961), cryptococcus (Unat, Pars, and Kosyak, 1960), and histoplasma (Cole, Ridley, and Wolfe, 1965) have been reported, but all are rare.

Mucormycosis, caused by fungi of the genera *Rhizopus, Absidia*, and *Mucor* can produce ulceration of the colon, especially in malnourished children. Amphotericin B is of proven efficacy in those infections.

Candidiasis or 'thrush' may invade the colon, especially in debilitated and undernourished patients, and after antibiotics, corticosteroids, and immunosuppressives. It is caused by the yeast *Candida albicans*. The hyphae stain densely and are readily identified.

27.1.3. *Protozoal infections*

Balantidiasis. This is a relatively uncommon condition, but one which may produce severe dysentery (Miller and Peck, 1948; Areán and Koppisch, 1956). It is caused by the large ciliated protozoan *Balantidium coli*, which is a common parasite of pigs, wild boars, sheep, horses, rats, frogs, guinea-pigs, and monkeys; man may also be a host. It is encountered mainly in areas where pigs are kept in poor hygienic surroundings; the disease is apparently common in the Papua New Guinean highlands (Van der Hoeven and Rijpstra, 1957; Radford, 1973). It is seen also in southern Iran (McCarey, 1952).

Balantidiasis is contracted by swallowing cysts of *B. coli*, which has a similar life cycle to that of *Entamoeba histolytica*. The cysts are large and ovoid; details of the life cycle of this parasite are not well known. The organism can be cultured (Areán and Koppisch, 1956). Food, drinking water, and green vegetables grown in soil fertilized with pig faeces are sources of infection. The trophozoite can exist for long periods in the terminal ileum and colon without producing symptoms. However, when invasion occurs, irregular rounded ulcers, with a base of necrotic material and undermined edges, are produced; they tend to be larger than those in amoebic dysentery. The extent of the ulcerative lesions can be great, from caecum to rectum; the rectosigmoid colon is most commonly, and severely, involved. Rarely, the disease affects the terminal ileum (Areán and Koppisch, 1956). Macroscopically, the ulcers are similar to those of amoebic dysentery (Chapter 25). Perforation, with peritonitis, and acute and chronic appendicitis are unusual complications. *B. coli* has been found in lymph nodes, but extra-intestinal involvement, which is such a problem with *E. histolytica*, does not usually occur; however, the organism has been demonstrated in the heart (Edington and Gilles, 1976). Microscopically, necrosis and lymphocytic infiltration of the submucosa is present; neutrophils are abundant. *B. coli* are found at the periphery of the lesions and also in the muscular coat.

As with *E. histolytica* infections there is a wide spectrum of disease; the condition may be asymptomatic, or there may be dysentery, with blood and mucus in the stool. In the majority of cases there is no history of contact with pigs. Tenesmus and colic occur intermittently. There may be tenderness over the caecum or colon. During attacks of diarrhoea the trophozoites, and between attacks the cysts, of the organism are found in the stool.

Examination of the stool, which is usually mucoid and bloody, shows large ovoid cysts of 45–60 μm in length; in fresh samples, the trophozoites, which are 30–200 μm in breadth, may also be seen. Direct and indirect antibody techniques are available to assist in diagnosis (Zaman, 1965). Treatment is with tetracycline, or one of its derivatives; 500 mg should be given six hourly for 10 days. Ampicillin is also effective. Metronidazole has been used in this infection with success (Garcia-Laverde and De Bonilla, 1975).

Trichomonas hominis. This protozoan parasite, which measures 10–15 μm in length, is an inhabitant of the caecum and colon. There are three flagella and a single ovoid nucleus is present at the more rounded end. There is no cystic phase. Presence of the organism in a diarrhoeic stool has no pathological significance.

Chilomastix mesnili and Trichomonas vaginalis. These two protozoan parasites are occasionally identified in stool specimens. Although they produce vaginitis and anterior urethritis in women, and occasionally urethritis in men, they do not produce large-intestinal symptoms or pathology.

South American Trypanosomiasis (Chagas' disease). This infection is caused by *Trypanosoma cruzi*, which is transmitted to man in the faeces of the reduviid bug, in which it has a cycle of development. Dogs, cats, and many wild animals, including the armadillo and opossum, harbour the infection and act as reservoirs.

The importance of the infection in the context of the colon is that in the chronic state, Auerbach's plexus is destroyed, with resulting denervation and muscular degeneration. There is subsequent dilatation of the colon (megacolon), caecum, and appendix (Ferreira-Santos, 1961; Köberle, 1963).

Diagnosis is based largely on a geographical history. Exposure in a rural area of south America, the West Indies or the southern USA is a prerequisite for diagnosis. There may be a history of an acute illness in the past, in either infancy or childhood.

Trypanosomes are present at low concentration in the peripheral blood. The complement-fixation test is of very limited diagnostic value in chronic cases.

Xenodiagnosis, i.e. demonstration that the patient can infect the vector, is of value.

No effective treatment is available. Prophylaxis is therefore of paramount importance.

27.1.4. Nematode infections

Trichuriasis of the caecum. This is a common, worldwide nematode infection which is caused by *Trichuris trichiura*, the 'whipworm' (Mathan and Baker, 1970). Adult worms are 30–50 mm in length. The disease is acquired by ingestion of ova; the worms hatch out in the upper small intestine and pass to the caecum and upper colon, anchoring themselves to the mucosa by their whip-like anterior portion. Ova are passed in the stool about four weeks after infection. The life cycle is thus simple, unlike that of the small-intestinal nematodes (Chapters 19 and 20). After passage in the faeces, the ova require two to five weeks of larval development before they are infective.

The disease is usually asymptomatic, and ova are discovered on a routine stool examination. Blood loss in minimal. Heavy infection, with a load exceeding 1000 worms, in children, especially if they are malnourished, occasionally produces abdominal pain and distension, growth retardation, rectal bleeding and prolapse (Jung and Jelliffe, 1952; Ramsay, 1962), and anaemia. Severe infections in children may be associated with finger-clubbing (Bowie, Morison, Ireland, and Duys, 1978); resolution takes place within about three months after treatment. The higher prevalence of the infection in children is probably a result of greater exposure; it seems probable that malnutrition predisposes to increased pathogenicity (Marques, Snitikowski, and Sobral, 1962).

Ova are found on direct smear examination of a stool specimen; concentration and quantitative techniques are available. Eosinophils and Charcot-Leyden crystals may also be found. On sigmoidoscopic examination, the worms can be visualized, attached to the mucosa, which is hyperaemic, friable and bleeds easily; there is an excess of mucus. A mild eosinophilia (5–20 per cent) is sometimes found in the peripheral blood; in very heavy infections there is sometimes a hypochromic anaemia with bone-marrow hyperplasia.

Treatment has been reviewed by Davis (1973). If it is decided to attempt eradication of the parasite, the benzimidazole carbamate derivative, *mebendazole* ('Vermox') in a dose of 100 mg thrice daily for three days should be given (Maqbool, Lawrence, and Katz, 1975). Alternatively, 100 mg twice daily for six days gives satisfactory results. Using that regime, an 88 per cent cure rate was claimed by Scragg and Proctor (1978); the efficiency of treatment was enhanced by adding loperamine hydrochloride ('Imodium') to the therapeutic regime. No toxic effects were reported. In Malaysia, however, treatment with one three-day course was found to be unsatisfactory (Nagalingam, Lam, Robinson, and Dissanaike, 1976); in that study, two and three three-day courses gave 80 and 100 per cent cure rates, respectively. Oxantel embonate (a meta-oxyphenol analog of pyrantel) seems to be of value in treating trichuriasis. Light to moderate infections were treated with that agent in 24 children and 37 adults with single doses (Garcia, 1976); at 10, 15, and 20 mg per kg bodyweight, cure rates of 77, 92, and 100 per cent were reported. There were no side effects. In severe clinical infections, also, results are encouraging (Lee, Inygkaran, Grieve, Robinson, and Dissanaike, 1976); of 25 children treated with a 20 mg per kg dose for three days, 17 were cured after one course and the remaining eight after two courses. There were no side effects.

Dithiazanine iodide is an effective agent, but it is too toxic and manufacture has had to be discontinued. Thiabendazole is ineffective. Levamisole, although of value in treating ascariasis, is also of no value in *T. trichiura* infections (Wagner and Rexinger, 1978).

Strongyloides stercoralis. Small ulcers have been described in the large intestine in strongyloidiasis (Rivas Gomez and Aleman, 1967); focal abscesses have also been attributed to that parasite. The colon and appendix are sites of larval reinvasion. Tuberculoid foci can be seen in all coats of the intestine, with necrosis at the centre; degenerating larvae may be seen at the centre of some of them. A granulomatous colitis may be present (Edington and Gilles, 1976).

Anisakis and Terranova infections. Larvae of these two ascarid parasites, which are about two cm in length, ay infect man by the ingestion of raw fish ('herring-worm disease'). Eosinophilic granuloma of the colon is a rare possibility (see below). They can also involve the stomach and small intestine. Although human disease is uncommon, arine fish are frequently infected; human infection only takes place after eating raw or undercooked fish (Hadidjaja, Ilahude, Mahfudin, Burhanuddin, and Hutomo, 1978).

Oesophagostoma. Infection with this nematode occurs in east Africa. It causes colonic and appendix abscesses (Marshall and Deneka, 1969), usually in children; abdominal abscesses containing sterile cloudy fluid have also been reported.

27.1.5. Eosinophilic granuloma of the caecum and colon

Eosinophilic granuloma, which is thought to be of parasitic origin (Chapter 4), occasionally involves the caecum and colon in many parts of the world.

In many cases, the nematode *Eustoma rotundatum* seems to be responsible, but that organism is not present in all cases of the disease; other parasites may be involved (Ashby, Appleton, and Dawson, 1964).

There is a diffuse eosinophilic infiltration of the caecum and colon. The lesions may be diffuse or localized. Eosinophils are present in large numbers in the submucosa, and sometimes the muscular coat; fragments of larvae may also be present. There may be a peripheral eosinophilia.

Corticosteroids are apparently of value in treatment.

27.2. Acute appendicitis

Appendicitis occurs throughout the tropics; in many countries there is evidence of a marked increase in frequency over the last few decades, and that applies especially to urban areas (Janssens and Muynck, 1966; Kakande, Kavuma, and Kayondo, 1978).

At the Mulago Hospital, Uganda, 23 cases of appendicitis were admitted in 1964 (Kiryabwire, 1965), and there was evidence of a steady increase in the 1970–5 period (Kakande *et al.*, 1978). In Kenya, there were over 100 cases in

1964; the condition was the major abdominal emergency (Miller, 1964). In Nigeria, Ghana, and Sierra Leone, appendicitis is similarly a common condition (Davey, 1968); in Lagos, 158 proven cases were seen in 1963–4 (Omo-Daré and Thomas, 1966) and in Ibadan 55 cases in 1959–60 (Udeh, 1962). The condition accounts for about 14 per cent of abdominal emergencies in west Africa (Joly and Thomas, 1954; Badoe, 1967). At Salisbury, Zimbabwe Rhodesia, appendicitis is now common, and is more often seen in urban than rural areas (Gordon, 1963); 147 appendicectomies were carried out at the Harari Central Hospital between 1958 and 1961; however during the same period 2113 appendicectomies were performed at the Salisbury Central Hospital which deals only with Europeans. In Lusaka, Zambia, acute appendicitis accounted for 16·8 per cent of admission for 'acute abdomen' over a one-year period (Umerah and Obadike, 1978); only one condition, intestinal obstruction, was a more common cause. The disease still seems to be unusual, however, in the population of Papua New Guinea. During a three-year period, 12 cases were seen at the Goroka Base Hospital (Wagner and Shepherd, 1976), and during that same period there were 11 cases in expatriates; the ratio of expatriates to Papua New Guineans in that population is about 1:150.

There seems little doubt therefore that the condition becomes more frequent as the local lifestyle gives way to that of the western world, but the reason for that is so far obscure. Bowel transit rate, and fibre, meat, and vegetable content of the diet have all been suggested. There is some evidence that schistosomiasis (Chapter 26) and amoebiasis (Chapter 25) can occasionally predispose to appendicitis, but there is no evidence that either of those diseases has significantly increased. In a report from Khartoum, Sudan, 17 cases of schistosomiasis have been described in which the appendix was involved (Malik, Satir, Veress, and El Hassan, 1975); nine presented with acute appendicitis. *Strongyloides stercoralis* (Chapter 20) and *Trichuris trichiura* (see above) have both been associated with peritonitis; in the latter infection the adult worms have been identified in the peritoneal cavity.

Yersinia enterocolitica (see above) is probably an underdiagnosed cause of appendicitis in tropical countries.

The clinical history and presentation is similar to that in western countries. The main difference is that cases frequently present late in the disease; at Ibadan, 40 per cent of cases present as uncomplicated appendicitis, 40 per cent as peritonitis, and 20 per cent with an acute inflammatory mass in the right iliac fossa (Davey, 1968). Omo-Daré and Thomas (1966) have suggested that in Lagos, the frequent use of purgatives for abdominal pain, of any description, accounts for the high complication rate and also the high incidence of diarrhoea at presentation.

27.3. Volvulus of the large intestine

This is a common cause of intestinal obstruction in some parts of the tropics; however, it seems to have clear geographical differences in incidence rate. Whereas, for example, it is very common in some African countries, in others it is of little importance. It is also common in parts of India and south America.

There are two types of volvulus of the sigmoid colon in Africa. (i) The *common* type which accounts for 85 to 90 per cent of the Ugandan and Zimbabwe Rhodesian cases (Davey, 1968); that is usually slowly progressive. The pelvic colon is enlarged and thickened (megacolon); as the ileocaecal region and rectum are approached, a normal calibre is however resumed. The circular muscle is hypertrophied, and the longitudinal coat thinned over the surface of the tubular megacolon; normal haustration is completely lacking. The mesocolon is thickened, and that may be a result of recurrent tortion which precedes acute obstruction by many years; the blood supply is increased. As volvulus occurs, abdominal distension and fluid loss occur, but there is no interference with the vascular supply of the colon; that is late and unusual. (ii) The *unusual* type (which will not be dealt with in detail) accounts for 10–15 per cent of the Ugandan and Zimbabwe Rhodesian cases. The colon, including haustrations, mesentery, and blood supply is relatively normal; in fact the colon at operation is the same as that in sigmoid volvulus in elderly Europeans. A compound or an acute fulminating volvulus is produced in young patients. Blood-supply is interfered with, blood-stained ascites appears, and in approximately 10 per cent gangrene supervenes.

Sequestration of blood in the long loops of intestine produces oligaemic shock.

27.3.1. Distribution of sigmoid volvulus

In Uganda, 400 cases were seen at the Mulago hospital in a 16-year period (Burkitt, 1952; Hall-Craggs, 1960; McAdam, 1961). Burkitt (1952) reported that volvulus of the sigmoid colon was common in Uganda, especially in the Ganda tribe. Hall-Craggs (1960) recorded 104 cases of sigmoid volvulus at Mulago Hospital, seen in 1952–6; during the period 1961–3 over 120 cases were admitted. In that series, 80 per cent were Ganda, and 94 per cent male. In Lango, central Uganda, volvulus is the commonest cause of intestinal obstruction (de Souza, 1966); most involve the sigmoid colon. Shepherd (1967) also reported a high incidence in Uganda. The condition is also common in Ethiopia (Johnson, 1966) and Eritrea (Polivka, 1966). In Kenya an average of eight cases are seen each year at the Kenyatta National Hospital (Miller, 1961). In Ghana, in one year 27 patients with the condition were seen at the Korle Bu Hospital, Accra (Badoe, 1965), but in Ibadan, Nigeria only one case was detected in a five-year period during an analysis of 436 cases of intestinal obstruction (Cole, 1965). At Lusaka, Zambia sigmoid volvulus accounted for 11 cases of intestinal obstruction during one year (Umerah and Obadike, 1978); the only condition which accounted for more cases of obstruction was adhesions, which were usually pelvic. The condition is common in Zimbabwe Rhodesia (Gelfand, 1957). At Bulawayo, 20 patients were seen over a four-year period; the condition was responsible for 20 per cent of all intestinal obstructions (White, 1961). It is common in South Africa (Sartorius, 1947); at the Baragwanath hospital, Johannesburg, approximately 13 per cent of cases of intestinal obstruction are due to sigmoid volvulus. Skapinker (1953) also reported a 15 per cent incidence rate in intestinal obstruction in South Africa.

In western India and Pakistan (Ahsan and Rahman, 1967), it accounts for rates of 24 and 30 per cent of cases of intestinal obstruction. In Brazil a high incidence rate has been reported (de Oliveira, Cutait, Branco, Speranzini, Fujimura, and Campos, 1963), but that might be associated with Chagas' disease. In north America the condition is more common in Negroes than in white Americans (Pool and Dunavent, 1951).

27.3.2 Aetiology of sigmoid volvulus

Genetic factors have been considered to be important, but there is no concrete evidence to support that. It has been suggested that the two loops of the sigmoid colon in Africans are held together by a long loop with a short mesenteric base, and that that may have a genetic basis. A high residue diet may be important (Teubes, 1963), although that could not explain the geographical variation in incidence because such diets are common throughout Africa. Enemata which contain herbal extracts and other irritants, are frequently used in some parts of Africa and have been incriminated, but that hypothesis has not been proved. There seems to be a relative deficiency of ganglion cells in the intramural plexuses of the colon (Shepherd and Wright, 1965; Wright and Shepherd, 1966); that could be important. Vacuolization and chromatolysis of neurones without a reduction in the overall number has been reported (Böhn and Smith, 1966).

Shepherd and Wright (1965) have drawn attention to a high incidence of megacolon in Uganda; that may account for the high incidence of sigmoid volvulus in the Ganda of Uganda. They have drawn attention to: (i) dilatation of the pelvic part of the sigmoid colon; haustrations in that region are abnormal, after evacuation the colon does not contract down, and at laparotomy it appears flabby, (ii) the muscle coat of the same region is thickened; the longitudinal muscle is broad and widely spread out, instead of being collected into narrow bands, and (iii) the mesocolon is thickened and usually elongated; its blood vessels and lymphatics are enlarged.

27.3.3. Presentation of sigmoid volvulus

There is a marked male predominance. Ninety per cent are men, the majority of whom are between 30 and 50 years old. The general condition of the patient is usually good, unless gangrene has supervened. Recurrent attacks of abdominal distension, constipation, and mild colicky pain, with a sudden relief, are characteristic. If the pain is severe, gangrene of a compound volvulus rather than an uncomplicated sigmoid volvulus should be considered. Examination reveals a grossly distended abdomen, which is drum-like; respiratory movements may be embarrassed if the distension is extreme, and there may be hiccoughs. There is usually very little tenderness. Visible peristalsis is rarely seen, and it may be possible to palpate the entire distended colon. Rectal examination is normal.

Other conditions which produce massive strangulation must be considered in the differential diagnosis; in most it will not be possible to distinguish them before operation however. The following should be considered: (i) primary volvulus of the small intestine (Chapter 23), (ii) compound volvulus (see below), and (iii) internal herniae. The history, clinical features, and a knowledge of the local geographical pathology should assist in diagnosis.

27.3.4. Investigation of sigmoid volvulus

A straight abdominal radiograph often reveals a huge gas-shadow in the form of an inverted-U, in the absence of colonic haustrations; there may also be two fluid levels, due to liquid faeces in the lower parts of the ascending and descending limbs of the U. Radiology is sometimes of value in differentiating the condition from other causes of massive strangulation (White and Palmer, 1963).

27.3.5. Treatment of sigmoid volvulus

The first measure in the acute stage of the disease is to relieve the distension; that can be accomplished by passing a flatus tube through a sigmoidoscope, and at the same time valuable information about the presence or absence of gangrene can be obtained. Although perforation is very unusual, as a precaution the patient should be prepared for laparotomy before sigmoidoscopy. That measure is successful in 90 per cent of uncomplicated cases (Davey, 1968). Alternatively, the flatus tube can be inserted by manipulation at laparotomy. Abnormal bowel should be resected after the distension has subsided, and the bowel sterilized (Davey, 1968); the type of operation will depend on the length of gangrenous bowel. Blood transfusion may be necessary to counteract the shock.

With the simple form of volvulus, mortality rates of under two per cent are to be expected with competent treatment; however when the volvulus is a compound one and there is extensive gangrene, a high mortality, which may approach 50 per cent, should be expected.

27.3.6. Compound volvulus (knotting of the bowel)

This condition is seen wherever volvulus of the sigmoid colon is common: the condition was originally referred to as a 'double volvulus', but 'knotting' is a more accurate description. The common form is ileosigmoid (Shepherd, 1967), in which the pelvic colon becomes knotted with a loop of ileum. A much less common type is the ileoileal knot (Chapter 23). The symptoms are more acute, gangrene occurs more rapidly, and the mortality is considerably higher than with simple volvulus.

Seventy-three cases were reported from the Mulago Hospital, Uganda during a 16-year period (McAdam, 1961). At the Mpilo Hospital, Bulawayo, 15 cases were seen during a four-year period, and that constituted 30 per cent of cases of sigmoid volvulus seen during that time (White, 1962). In South Africa, nine cases were seen in a 10-year period (Weinberg, 1958; Visser, 1963).

Treatment is essentially the same as for simple sigmoid volvulus. It is absolutely vital that the most urgent treatment is given; blood transfusion, rehydration, and correction of electrolyte imbalance must be followed by emergency laparotomy and resection.

27.4. Intussusception of the large intestine

In temperate parts of the world, intussusception is primarily a disease of children (Peck, Lynn, and DuShane, 1963); in some parts of the tropics it is much more common however in adults (Davey, 1968). The common variety in most parts of Africa is the caecocolic variety, which was first described from west Africa by Majekodunmi (1948).

In children the well-known ileocaecal type occurs in all countries in which it has been looked for; however clinically, it may closely resemble acute gastroenteritis, and may thus be overlooked with disastrous consequences.

27.4.1. Distribution of intussusception

At Ibadan, Joly and Thomas (1954) found 33 patients with caecocolic intussusceptions during a three-year period; two were infants and 30 adults. In a review of 436 admissions for intestinal obstruction at University Hospital, Ibadan, during a five-year period, Cole (1965) found 119 cases of intussusception; 10 were in infants, and 76 (of the caecocolic type) were in adults and children; the condition accounted for over one fifth of abdominal emergencies. In Kampala, McAdam (1961) found 30 intussusceptions during a two-year period, in a series of 794 cases of intestinal obstruction, 16 of which were in adults and were of the caecocolic type. In Rwanda and Burundi, Burkitt (1966) considered that chronic ileocolic and colocolic intussusceptions in adults were the commonest cause of intestinal obstruction. In southern Africa, White (1961) reported 11 intussusceptions amongst 172 cases of intestinal obstruction in Bulawayo, Zimbabwe Rhodesia; two were adults with ileoileal and ileocolic types, respectively. In Durban, South Africa, in a nine-year period, 56 intussusceptions, 35 of which were of the ileocaecal variety, were reported by Kark and Rundle (1960); 39, 6, and 11 were in adults, children and infants, respectively.

The condition has also been reported to be common in adults in Korea (Dietrick and Lee, 1965). Caecocolic intussusception seems to be common in Papua New Guinea (McCullagh, 1956).

27.4.2. Aetiology of intussusception

Intussusception following amoeboma of the colon is a well-recognized complication of amoebiasis; it may be of the ileocaecal or caecocolic type (Chapter 25) (Kark and Rundle, 1960). Rarely it occurs after an abdominal operation (Petcher, 1955), or in association with Burkitt's lymphoma, when there are deposits in the bowel wall. However, in the majority of cases there is no obvious underlying cause.

In a small percentage there is an associated intestinal polyp (Awoliyi, 1960). An abnormally mobile caecum has been suggested to be an important cause (Davey, 1968). *Ascaris lumbricoides* has been incriminated but in most cases there is no convincing evidence of that (Cole, 1966). Kark and Rundle (1960) have suggested that amoebiasis might be involved; however in one study (Joly and Thomas, 1954) only two of 26 patients with the condition had evidence of that disease. Dietary factors may also be important.

In Ibadan, there is a seasonal variation in incidence of intussusception; most patients are admitted at the end of the dry season. The reason for that is obscure.

The adult intussusception which is seen commonly in west Africa begins in the anterolateral wall of the caecum; the terminal ileum, appendix, and related walls of the caecum are drawn into the ascending colon as it advances (Fig. 27.2). In 10 per cent of cases the apex either prolapses, or can be felt, rectally. The blood supply is not usually obliterated and gangrene is unusual. In the ileoileal and ileocaecal types, gangrene is three times more common than with the caecocolic type (Cole, 1965).

27.4.3. Presentation of intussusception

There is a slight male predominance; although the average age is in the late teens, it is not uncommon in infants and children. The mean length of history is two to three weeks on average but ranges from six hours to nine months (Davey, 1968). In three quarters the illness starts suddenly, and in one quarter insidiously. Pain is always present, it is colicky in type and is localized to the umbilical region and epigastrium. A palpable mass, which may be tender, and hardens on palpation, is present in the line of the transverse and descending parts of the colon in three quarters of cases; if distension is present the mass may be difficult to feel. Vomiting is usually present at some stage and may occur at the onset, during attacks of pain and when intestinal obstruction has developed. Diarrhoea is present in approximately 60 per cent of cases; in one third blood and mucus is present in the stool. Chronic cases may have suffered gross weight-loss; peristalsis in them may be visible through the anterior abdominal wall. The condition can occur on several occasions in the same individual (Parnis, 1960).

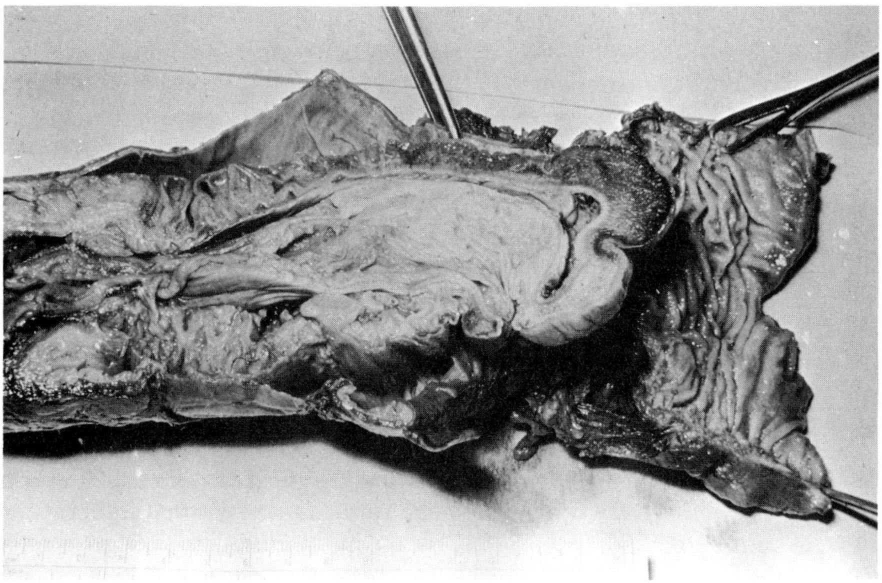

FIG. 27.2. Operative specimen from a 35-year-old Ugandan woman, showing an ileocolic intussusception.

27.4.4. Investigation of intussusception

Radiology is of value in confirming a diagnosis in about 95 per cent of cases. Straight abdominal radiographs may show (Davey, 1968): (i) emptiness in the right iliac fossa, with absence of a caecal gas shadow, (ii) a soft tissue mass which is the intussusception, (iii) a crescentic-shaped shadow of colonic gas outlining the apex, and (iv) a 'ground-glass' appearance of the right side of the abdomen due to an exudate, which is always present. Barium meal examination may be of value, and shows (i) an obstruction, which moves proximally, (ii) 'watch spring' spirals, and (iii) the characteristic outline of the intussusception and its apex. If obstruction has already supervened, multiple gas-fluid levels may obscure those signs.

27.4.5. Treatment of intussusception

Treatment of intussusception is surgical; reduction of the intussusception, or resection of a segment of bowel, are necessary in 80 and 20 per cent of cases, respectively (Davey, 1968). If there has been prolonged diarrhoea, fluid replacement and correction of hypokalaemia may be necessary before operation. Resection usually involves a right colectomy with end-to-end anastomosis; recurrence after surgery is unusual. Postoperative diarrhoea is common, but usually clears up spontaneously. Prognosis is good.

27.5. Miscellaneous colonic lesions

27.5.1. Injury involving the colon

Apart from road accidents, stab and gunshot wounds are important causes of colonic injury in many parts of the tropics; at the Baragwanath Hospital, Johannesburg, for example, an average of 2300 patients are admitted annually with stab wounds (Davey, 1968). In the Papua New Guinea highlands, spear wounds are still very common.

Davey (1968) has emphasized the importance of discovering the time of injury and the nature of the weapon; those are important factors which influence prognosis. Many patients are drunk on admission; the history is therefore often very unreliable. When an injury which has been caused by a knife, or animal horn (which is commonly used by the Fulani of Nigeria and the Hima and Tutsi of east Africa), is dealt with at under six hours, the mortality rate should be negligible; if more than 24 hours have passed, a 90 per cent mortality resulting from peritonitis should be anticipated. The track of a stab wound is a straight line, and there is injury to a definite part of the abdomen (Sorour and Bijlsma, 1966); however, bullet wounds are much more unpredictable and any part of the abdomen may be injured (Grattan, 1955). Perforation of a stomach distended with beer worsens the prognosis. In children, especially, the colon may be perforated while an enema is being given; alternatively, articles introduced into the rectum or vagina can result in a concealed injury.

Chest and abdominal radiographs should be routine. Pleural penetration may have given rise to a pneumothorax; free-gas under the diaphragm or a peritoneal effusion can result from abdominal penetration. Opaque foreign bodies will be obvious.

Resuscitation is the first priority in management; blood transfusion and antibiotics are often necessary. A formal laparotomy should be carried out (Davey, 1968) for: (i) bullet wounds, (ii) herniation of abdominal contents, (iii) evidence of internal haemorrhage, (iv) abdominothoracic wounds on the left side, and (v) haematemesis, bloody gastric-aspirate, and rectal bleeding. The extent of resection of intestine depends on the amount of damage. Injury to the spleen should be treated by splenectomy. Liver injuries must always be explored, and sutures applied if necessary.

27.5.2. Hirschprung's disease

This is not uncommon in the tropics. It usually presents in the first week of life with vomiting, abdominal distension, and abnormal bowel function. Caecal perforation is an occasional complication (Ajayi, Solanke, Seriki, and Bohrer, 1969).

27.5.3. Necrotizing colitis (necrosis of the colon)

A necrotizing colitis, probably associated with *Clostridium welchii* is occasionally encountered throughout the tropics; there may be extensive necrosis, and sloughing of the entire large intestine.

A minority of patients with 'pig-bel' disease (enteritis necroticans) (Chapter 17) has colonic involvement, and that disease is sometimes confined to the colon. In many respects this resembles other clostridial diseases of the intestinal tract: colitis of the newborn, and antibiotic-induced colitis (Chapter 28). The condition may resemble, clinically, ischaemic colitis; laparotomy and post-mortem appearances are however quite distinct.

27.5.4. Obstruction of the colon

In many parts of Africa, charcoal is used as a fuel and is occasionally ingested, especially by children. By impacting in the rectum this may give rise to colonic obstruction. Presentation is with abdominal colic and diarrhoea; on abdominal and rectal examination rock-like masses are found in the pelvic colon and rectum, respectively.

Foreign bodies introduced into the rectum may also produce colonic obstruction (Fig. 27.3).

27.5.5. Iliac adenitis

This is a common entity throughout tropical Africa (Pearson, 1965), and also other parts of the tropics. It is usually the result of trauma to the lower limbs. Most people in the third world walk around barefoot; an ascending lymphangitis, and either inguinal or iliac adenitis follow injuries to the feet. Lymphatics from the buttocks and anal canal also drain into the inguinal lymph nodes, and those areas should also be carefully examined for the site of infection. Frequently the 'portal of entry' on the foot or leg has already healed and there is little or no evidence of trauma.

Presentation is usually with a mass in the iliac fossa which can be mistaken for a carcinoma, or appendix-mass or abscess. Alternatively, an inflammatory mass in one iliac fossa, extending into the hypogastrium, may be palpable on rectal examination. The classical physical sign is a flexion deformity of the hip on the affected side; that is present in over 50 per cent of cases (Davey, 1968).

Pyomyositis of the psoas, iliacus, or one of the abdominal wall muscles can give rise to confusion in diagnosis; however, in that condition it is unusual to get inguinal lymphadenopathy.

Surgical drainage, through a para-inguinal incision, must be carried out and an appropriate antibiotic, which may have to be changed in the light of the results of culture should be given.

27.6. Lymphoma of the colon

Burkitt's lymphoma usually presents with deposits in the jaws, but involvement of abdominal viscera is not uncommon. The large intestine and appendix are occasionally involved; haemorrhage and rarely intussusception may result. Ascites is unusual. Owor (1977) has reported 40 cases of non-Burkitt's lymphoma of the gastrointestinal tract in Uganda; those were usually localized tumours and the most common sites, which accounted for 19 of them, were the caecum and colon.

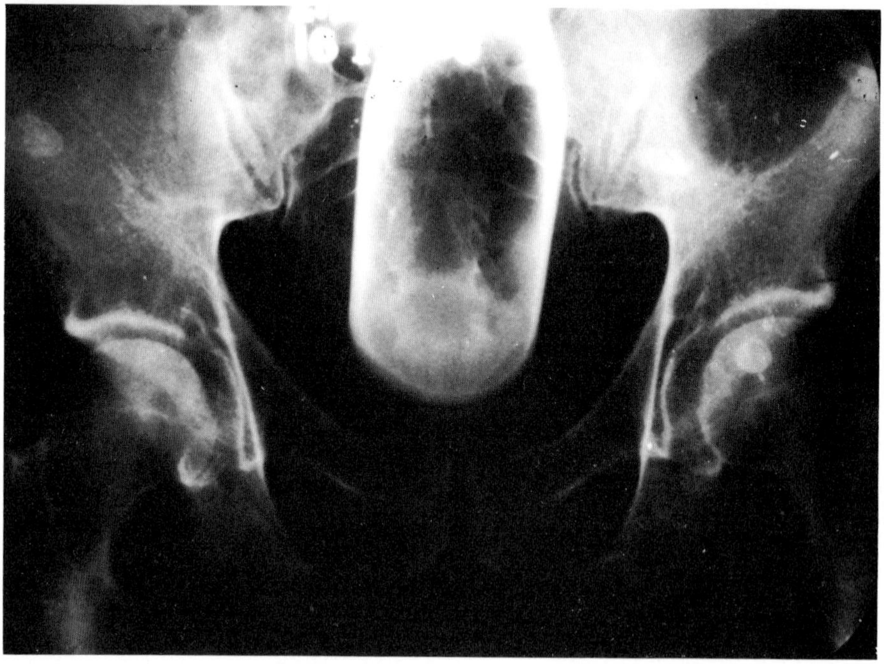

FIG. 27.3. Straight abdominal radiograph in a young Papua New Guinean man showing a large opaque foreign body. At laparotomy a beer-bottle was located, which had been introduced into the rectum.

References

AHSAN, I. and RAHMAN, H. (1967). *Br. med. J.*, **1,** 29.

AJAYI, O. O. A., SOLANKA, T. F., SERIKI, O., and BOHRER, S. P. (1969). *Pediatrics*, **43,** 102

AREÁN, V. M. and KOPPISCH, E. (1956). *Am. J. Path.*, **32,** 1089.

ASHBY, B. S., APPLETON, P. J., and DAWSON, I. (1964). *Br. med. J.*, **1,** 1141.

AWOLIYI, S. O. (1960). *W. Afr. med. J.*, **9,** 219.

BADOE, E. A. (1965). *Ghana med. J.*, **4,** 128.

—— (1967). *Ghana med. J.*, **6,** 69.

BLACK, R. E., JACKSON, R. J., TSAI, T., MEDVESKY, M., SHAYEGANI, M., FEELEY, J. C., MACLEOD, K. I. E., and WAKELEE, A. M. (1978). *New Engl. J. Med.*, **298,** 76.

Böhm, G. M. and Smith, B. (1966). *Gut*, **7**, 662.
Bowie, M. D., Morison, A., Ireland, J. D., and Duys, P. J. (1978). *Archs Dis. Childh.*, **53**, 411.
Burkitt, D. P. (1952). *E. Afr. med. J.*, **29**, 189.
—— (1966). *Ann. R. Coll. Surg.*, **39**, 236.
Cole, A. C. E., Ridley, D. S., and Wolfe, H. R. I. (1965). *J. trop. Med. Hyg.*, **68**, 92.
Cole, G. J. (1965). *Gut*, **6**, 151.
—— (1966). *Br. J. Surg.*, **53**, 415.
Davey, W. W. (1968). *Companion to surgery in Africa*. p. 228, 235, 257, and 270. Churchill Livingstone. Edinburgh, London and New York.
Davis, A. (1973). *Drug treatment in intestinal helminthiases*. p. 45. WHO Geneva.
De Feo, E. (1961). *Am. J. Roentg.*, **86**, 86.
De Oliveira, M. R., Cutait, D. E., Branco, P. D., Speranzini, M. B. Fujimura, I., and Campos, S. deM. (1963). *Revta Hosp. Clín. Fac. Med. Univ. S. Paulo*, **18**, 469.
De Souza, L. J. (1966). *E. Afr. med. J.*, **43**, 264.
Dietrick, R. B. and Lee, M. H. (1965). *Surgery, St. Louis*, **57**, 651.
Easman, C. O. and Lahiri, H. S. (1963). *Ghana med. J.*, **2**, 62.
Edington, G. M. and Gilles, H. M. (1976). *Pathology in the tropics*. 2nd ed. p. 88, 109 and 323. Edward Arnold, London.
Elebute, E. A. and Adesola, A. O. (1964). *Br. J. Surg.*, **51**, 440.
El Masri, S. H., Boulos, P., and Malick, M. O. A. (1977). *E. Afr. med. J.*, **54**, 319.
Ferreira-Santos, R. (1961). *Proc. R. Soc. Med.*, **54**, 1047.
Garcia, E. G. (1976). *Am. J. trop. Med. Hyg.*, **25**, 914.
Garcia-Laverde, A. and De Bonilla, L. (1975). *Am. J. trop. Med. Hyg.*, **24**, 781.
Gelfand, M. (1957). *The sick African*. 3rd ed. p. 726. Juta and Co. Ltd., Cape Town.
Gordon, J. A. (1963). *Cent. Afr. J. Med.*, **9**, 170.
Grattan, E. (1955). *Br. J. Surg.*, **43**, 279.
Hadidjaja, P., Ilahude, H. D., Mahfudin, H., Burhanuddin, and Hutomo, M. (1978). *Am. J. trop. Med. Hyg.*, **27**, 51.
Hall-Craggs, E. C. B. (1960). *Br. med. J.*, **1**, 1015.
Hawley, P. R., Wolfe, H. R. I., and Fullerton, J. M. (1968). *Gut*, **9**, 461.
Janssens, P. G. and Muynck, A. de (1966). *Trop. geogr. med.*, **18**, 81.
Johnson, L. P. (1966). *Ethiopian med. J.*, **4**, 197.
Joly, B. M. and Thomas, H. O. (1954). *W. Afr. med. J.*, **3**, 1.
Jung, R. C. and Jelliffe, D. B. (1952). *W. Afr. med. J.*, **1**, 11.
Kakande, I., Kavuma, J., and Kayondo, J. (1978). *E. Afr. med. J.*, **55**, 172.
Kark, A. E. and Rundle, W. J. (1960). *Br. J. Surg.*, **48**, 296.
Kiryabwire, J. W. M. (1965). *E. Afr. med. J.*, **42**, 524.
Köberle, F. (1963). *Gut*, **4**, 399.
Lee, E-L., Iyngkaran, N., Grieve, A. W., Robinson, M. J., and Dissanaike, A. S. (1976). *Am. J. trop. Med. Hyg.*, **25**, 563.
McAdam, I. W. J. (1961). *E. Afr. med. J.*, **38**, 536.
McCarey, A. G. (1952). *Br. med. J.*, **1**, 629.
McCullagh, S. F. (1956). *Papua New Guin. med. J.*, **1**, 114.
Majekodunmi, M. A. (1948). *Br. med. J.*, **2**, 224.
Malik, M. O. A., Satir, A. A., Veress, B., and El Hassan, A. M. (1975). *E. Afr. med. J.*, **52**, 183.
Mandall, B. K. and Mani, V. (1976). *Lancet*, **1**, 887.
Maqbool, S., Lawrence, D., and Katz, M. (1975). *J. Pediat.*, **86**, 463.
Marques, A. N., Snitikowski, N., and Sobral, M. T. C. (1962). *Hospital, Rio de J.*, **74**, 549.
Marshall, D. and Deneka, S. I. (1969). *Can. med. Ass. J.*, **100**, 913.
Mathan, V. I. and Baker, S. J. (1970). *Am. J. dig. Dis.*, **15**, 913.

MILLER, A. A. and PECK, C. R. (1948). *Br. med. J.*, **1,** 448.
MILLER, J. R. M. (1961). *E. Afr. med. J.*, **38,** 543.
—— (1964). *E. Afr. med. J.*, **41,** 419.
MORSON, B. C. (1961). *Proc. R. Soc. Med.*, **54,** 723.
—— and DAWSON, I. M. P. (1972). *Gastrointestinal pathology.* p. 452. Blackwell, Oxford.
NAGALINGHAM, I., LAM, L. E., ROBINSON, M. J., and DISSANAIKE, A. S. (1976). *Am. J. trop. Med. Hyg.*, **25,** 568.
NEED, R. L. and BEHNKE, R. H. (1963). *Am. Rev. resp. Dis.*, **88,** 69.
OMO-DARÉ, P. and THOMAS, H. O. (1966). *W. Afr. med. J.*, **15,** 217.
OWOR, R. (1977). *E. Afr. med. J.*, **54,** 666.
PARNIS. R. O. (1960). *Br. med. J.*, **2,** 308.
PEARSON, J. B. (1965). *W. Afr. med. J.*, **14,** 115.
PECK, D. A., LYNN, H. B., and DU SHANE, J. W.(1963). *Surgery Gynec. Obstet.*, **116,** 398.
PETCHER, P. (1955). *W. Afr. med. J.*, **4,** 208.
POLIVKA, J. (1966). *Ethiopian med. J.*, **4,** 205.
POOL, R. M. and DUNAVENT, W. D. (1951). *Ann. Surg.*, **133,** 719.
POWERS, P. W., KRAMER, S. G., and DRAKE, W. L. (1961). *Am. J. Surg.*, **102,** 713.
RADFORD, A. J. (1973). *Med. J. Aust.*, **1,** 238.
RAMSEY, F. C. (1962). *W. Indian med. J.*, **11,** 235.
RHOADES, E. R., KLEIN, L. J., and WELSH, J. D. (1960). *Gastroenterology*, **38,** 654.
RIVAS GOMEZ, A. and ALEMAN, C. (1967). *G.E.N.*, **21,** 253.
SARTORIUS, K. H. (1947). *Proc. Transv. Mine med. Offrs' Ass.*, **27,** 33.
SCRAGG, J. N. and PROCTOR, E. M. (1978). *Am. J. trop. Med. Hyg.*, **27,** 255.
SHEPHERD, J. J. (1967). *Br. J. Surg.*, **54,** 561.
—— and WRIGHT, P. G. (1965). *E. Afr. med. J.*, **42,** 401.
SKAPINKER, S. (1953). *S. Afr. med. J.*, **27,** 237.
SOROUR, V. E. and BIJLSMA, P. J. (1966). *S. Afr. J. Surg.*, **4,** 85.
TEUBES, M. N. (1963). *S. Afr. med. J.*, **37,** 1151.
UDEH, F. N. (1962). *Br. J. Surg.*, **50,** 39.
UMERAH, B. C. and OBADIKE, G. (1978). *E. Afr. med. J.*, **55,** 77.
UNAT, E. K., PARS, B., and KOSYAK, J. P. (1960). *Br. med. J.*, **2,** 1501.
VAN DER HOEVEN, J. A. and RIJPSTRA, A. C. (1957). *Trop. geogr. Med.*, **9,** 225.
VANTRAPPEN, G., AGG, H. O., PONETTE, E., GEBOES, K., and BERTRAND, P. (1977). *Gastroenterology*, **72,** 220.
VISSER, J. D. (1963). *S. Afr. med. J.*, **37,** 863.
WAGNER, E. D. and REXINGER, D. D. (1978). *Am. J. trop. Med. Hyg.*, **27,** 203.
WAGNER, F. B. and SHEPHERD, A. (1976). *Papua New Guin. med. J.*, **19,** 156.
WALKER DAVIS, J. (1957). *Am. J. Surg.*, **93,** 490.
WEINBERG, N. J. (1958). *Proc. Transv. Mine med. Offrs' Ass.*, **38,** 57.
WHITE, A. (1961). *E. Afr. med. J.*, **38,** 525.
—— (1962). *Jl. R. Coll. Surg. Edinb.*, **7,** 138.
—— (1963). *Jl. R. Coll. Surg. Edinb.*, **9,** 37.
—— and PALMER, P. E. S. (1963). *Clin. Radiol.*, **14,** 211.
WINBLAD, S., NILÉHN, B., and STERNBY, N. H. (1966). *Br. med. J.*, **2,** 1363.
WRIGHT, P. G. and SHEPHERD, J. J. (1966). *Gut*, **7,** 41.
ZAMAN, V. (1965). *Trans. R. Soc. trop. Med. Hyg.*, **59,** 80.

28

Antibiotic-associated colitis

ANTIBIOTICS are very widely prescribed in third world countries because many common diseases there are caused by bacterial infections. There are intestinal complications of such therapy of which the physician working in those countries should be aware.

Gastrointestinal symptoms associated with antibiotic therapy range from mild abdominal discomfort to a life-threatening colitis (Bartlett and Gorbach, 1977; Medline, Shin, and Medline, 1976). Clindamycin, lincomycin, tetracycline, chloramphenicol, cephalosporin, and penicillin have at various times been implicated (Ecker, Williams, and McKittrick, 1970; Tedesco, Barton, and Alpers, 1974; Tedesco, 1975; Tures, Townsend, and Rose, 1976). Although in the 1950s, tetracyclines were often incriminated in pseudomembranous colitis (see below), they do not seem to be nearly so important at present (Bartlett and Gorbach, 1978); the reason for that is obscure. However they are still associated with antibiotic-associated diarrhoea. Lethal diarrhoea can be induced in guinea-pigs with penicillin, chlortetracycline, bacitracin, and erythromycin (Eyssen, DeSomer, and Van Dijck, 1957).

28.1. Staphylococcal enterocolitis

Staphylococcal infection of the intestine may be associated with a fulminant enterocolitis (Dearing, Baggenstoss, and Weed, 1960; Speare, 1954); that disease involves principally the lower small intestine and is fortunately rare. There is an overgrowth of antibiotic-resistant bacteria in staphylococcal enterocolitis (Tom, Drake, Jacobson, and Van Prohaska, 1959; Khan and Hall, 1966); that has not been described in clindamycin-associated colitis, which is a separate entity.

28.2. Pseudomembranous colitis (PMC)

Pseudomembranous colitis (Kleckner, Bargen, and Baggenstoss, 1952; Goulston and McGovern, 1965) is a far more serious problem than straightforward overgrowth with resistant bacteria in the colon, and is particularly associated with lincomycin and clindamycin treatment, but also with other antibiotics, including ampicillin (*Br. med. J.*, 1978). Gorbach, Spanknebel, and Weinstein (1969) have demonstrated that lincomycin produces a striking overgrowth of enterobacter, proteus, and candida in the stool when given to man, but that is not usually associated with diarrhoea or any other symptoms. The aetiology of pseudomembranous colitis must therefore be different.

The disease has been recognized for nearly 30 years (Reiner, Schlesinger, and Miller, 1952), and seems usually to be caused by cytopathic toxins produced by *Clostridium sordellii* (Larson, Parry, Price, Davies, Dolby, and Tyrell, 1977; Rifkin, Fekety, Silva, and Sack, 1977; Larson and Price, 1977) and *Cl. difficile* (Bartlett, Chang, and Onderdonk, 1978a and b; George, Symonds, Dimock, Brown, Arabi, Shinagawa, Keighley, Alexander-Williams, and Burdon, 1978). The antibiotics seem to encourage growth of those clostridia, which secrete an exotoxin which has a necrotizing effect on the colonic mucosa. The toxin of *Staphylococcus aureus* has also been associated with pseudomembranous colitis. As well as having received an antibiotic, some patients have also undergone abdominal surgery (Pettet, Baggenstoss, Dearing, and Judd, 1954; van Prohaska, Mock, Baker, and Collins, 1961; Kappas, Shinagawa, Arabi, Thompson, Burdon, Dimock, George, Alexander-Williams, and Keighley, 1978). In a prospective study of 241 patients who underwent gastrointestinal surgery, postoperative diarrhoea was significantly more common after antibiotic therapy, and occurred in 24 per cent (Keighley, Burdon, Alexander-Williams, Shinagawa, Arabi, Thompson, Youngs, Bentley, and George, 1978); 9 patients had high titres of neutralizable faecal toxin characteristic of pseudomembranous colitis and in all of them *Cl. difficile* was isolated from the stool.

28.2.1. Aetiology of PMC

In man, pseudomembranous colitis has been associated with antibiotic therapy for a considerable time (Hale and Cosgriff, 1957; Pearce and Dineen, 1960; Cummins, 1961).

Small (1968) suggested that an alteration in bowel flora might be responsible for the fatal colitis induced by clindamycin is hamsters. A lethal enterocolitis can be produced in Syrian hamsters by oral or parenteral administration of clindamycin in doses comparable to those used in man (1–10 mg per kg) (Small, 1968; Humphrey, Pittman, and Pittman, 1975; Lusk, Fekety, Silva, Browne, Ringler, and Abrams, 1978). An acute inflammatory reaction with pseudomembrane formation results; concentrations of *Escherichia coli, Streptococcus faecalis*, and clindamycin resistant *Cl. sordellii* and *Cl. difficile* are increased. Bacteria or viruses are not seen in the intestinal lesions.

Entercolitis has been produced in hamsters with caecal content, and filtrates of caecal content (pore-size of filter, 0·02 μm), obtained from other animals after clindamycin administration (Bartlett, Onderdonk, Cisneros, and Kasper, 1977). Both cultures of a species of clostridium, and also the cell-free supernatant, also produce the disease. It seems clear, therefore, that a clindamycin-resistant, toxin-producing strain of clostridium produces clindamycin-associated colitis in hamsters.

In rabbits, whereas clindamycin produces a rapidly fatal enterocolitis, other antibiotics at similar dosage have no effect (Katz, La Mont, Trier, Sonnenblick, Rothman, Broitman, and Rieth, 1978). Simultaneous administration of vancomycin prevented that lesion occurring, and penicillin and neomycin were effective in that respect in three of five, and one of five animals.

In hamsters death is due to dehydration, reduced intravascular volume, and hypotension secondary to the diarrhoea. Bacteraemia is not responsible for death (Rifkin, Silva and Fekety, 1978); if vancomycin and clindamycin are both given, death can be prevented even though there is a bacteraemia (Browne, Fekety, Silva, Boyd, Work, and Abrams, 1977). Those observations support the hypothesis that the disease results from clostridial toxins, the production of which has been enhanced by the effect of clindamycin on the intestinal flora. Four patients with pseudomembranous colitis, which resulted from antibiotic therapy, all had a substance in the stool which produced cytotoxicity in tissue culture (Bartlett, Chang, Gurwith, Gorbach, and Onderdonk, 1978); only one of 54 patients with straightforward antibiotic-associated diarrhoea gave a positive response. In each case, cytotoxicity in tissue culture and enterocolitis in hamsters were neutralized by pretreatment with gas-gangrene serum.

Thus, although the pathogenesis of the syndrome is not completely established, it now seems clear that it is caused by clostridial toxins which are produced by organisms within the colon (Larsen and Price, 1977; Rifkind, Fekety, Silva, and Sack, 1977); furthermore, production of toxin is clearly enhanced by the effect of clindamycin on the bowel flora.

Gastrointestinal reactions to antibiotics require much more attention if the morbidity and mortality associated with the use of valuable therapeutic agents is to be prevented (*Br. med. J*., 1974). The importance of clostridial toxins in intestinal disease has for long been recognized in veterinary medicine (*Lancet*, 1977); this is thus another example of the medical profession's lack of interest in the animal literature.

The disease is therefore in some respects comparable to 'pig-bel' disease (necrotizing jejunitis), which is seen in several parts of the tropics including the Papua New Guinea highlands (Chapter 17).

28.2.2. Presentation of PMC

The disease can occur at any age. The clinical picture is very variable; it may consist of a mild diarrhoea, or the disease can present with a severe fulminant colitis. Symptoms usually start after 4–10 days of treatment, but in some not until one or two weeks after the antibiotic(s) have been stopped. Diarrhoea is usually severe; blood in the stool is however unusual. Protein-losing enteropathy, disorientation, and collapse may complicate the disease. Diagnosis is often difficult and is not infrequently made at post-mortem examination; it should however always be considered in patients who have had antibiotics and who deteriorate after surgery. The mortality rate is high.

Shigellosis (Chapter 24) may be simulated. Amoebic colitis should be excluded (Chapter 25). In the western world, ulcerative colitis is an important differential diagnosis (Goulston and McGovern, 1965). Necrotizing colitis due to *C. welchii*, which does not seem to be associated with antibiotic therapy, may also be difficult to differentiate on clinical grounds. In the newborn, clostridial colitis should also be excluded.

28.2.3. Pathology of PMC

The colon is dilated and has lost its mucosal pattern. The mucosal surface contains slightly raised yellowish-green foci, of variable size and appearance, ranging from bran-like particles to large areas of yellow friable membrane (Goulston and McGovern, 1965). Ulcers may form and occasionally perforate; death usually occurs however before ulceration is marked.

The exudate consists of fibrin, mucus, and usually many leucocytes; it forms on areas of fibrinoid necrosis on the surface of the mucosa. Adjacent exudates, together with the necrotic superficial zones of mucosa, coalesce to form an extensive membrane. Vasculitis is not a feature of the disease.

As the condition progresses, the whole mucosa undergoes coagulative necrosis, and the membrane may be sloughed off leaving an ulcer with a pyogenic surface which may penetrate the muscle coat.

28.2.4. Investigation of PMC

Sigmoidoscopy shows a grey, white, or yellow pseudomembrane; however there may be nonspecific changes only. A similar pseudomembrane may also be present in ischaemic colitis. Histology of a rectal biopsy is diagnostic. Barium enema should not be performed because it is not diagnostic and may be dangerous. A polymorphonuclear leucocytosis and hypoalbuminaemia are usually present.

28.2.5. Treatment of PMC

All antibiotics should be stopped immediately and substituted with vancomycin or a non-absorbable sulphonamide, to which the responsible clostridia are highly sensitive. Corticosteroids and intravenous fluids may also be given. A suggestion has been made that blood-transfusion may be dangerous in necrotizing enterocolitis, because several clostridia split off N-acetylneuraminic acid from the plasma membrane of the red cell (Seger, Joller, Kenny, Hitzig, Metaxas, and Metaxas-Bühler, 1979); the practical importance of that is not yet clear.

Vancomycin seems at present to be the antibiotic of choice (Barlett, Onderdonk, and Cisneros, 1977; Browne *et al*., 1977; Rifkind, Fekety, Silva, and Sack, 1977); in a study in hamsters, that antibiotic exerted a marked protective action, and in a patient treated with that agent a rapid clinical recovery was accompanied by the disappearance of toxin from the stool. Studies in man are sparse however. Khan and Hall (1966) showed that oral vancomycin was clinically effective in patients with suspected antibiotic-associated colitis. Because *Cl. difficile* is susceptible to tetracycline (Bartlett and Gorbach, 1978) it seems likely that that agent would be of value; there is limited evidence to support that (De Jesus and Peternel, 1978). Metronidazole is beneficial against anaerobes elsewhere, but has not yet been adequately evaluated in antibiotic-associated colitis. In a preliminary study, three patients were treated with that agent, and a dramatic response was recorded (Matuchansky, Aries, and Maire, 1978).

28.3. Allergy and transient ischaemic colitis

Bloody diarrhoea has been reported after penicillin and ampicillin (Toffler, Pingoud, and Burrell, 1978; Barrison and Kane, 1978); the disease is clinically distinct from pseudomembranous colitis and is thought to be an allergic reaction, possibly a vasculitis of the intestine which gives rise to a transient ischaemia. Bacterial toxins may have a strong affinity for sympathetic nervous tissue and that would explain the ischaemic nature of the lesions (Buxton Hopkin, 1978). Barium enema examination shows spasm, nodularity, and ulceration of the ascending colon, consistent with ischaemic disease. The lesion is transient and quite distinct from pseudomembranous colitis. Awareness of the condition, which is transient, should lead to a conservative approach and the avoidance of needless corticosteroid therapy, and laparotomy.

That disease is distinct from ischaemic enterocolitis (McGovern and Goulston, 1965); that is usually a result of hypotension, shock, or arterial disease.

References

Barrison, I. G. and Kane, S. P. (1978). *Lancet*, **2,** 843.

Bartlett, J. G., Chang, T. W., Gurwith, M., Gorbach, S. L., and Onderdonk, A. B. (1978). *New Engl. J. Med.*, **298,** 531.

——, ——, and Onderdonk, A. B. (1978a). *J. infect. Dis.*, **138,** 81.

——, ——, and —— (1978b). *Lancet*, **1,** 338.

—— and Gorbach, S. L. (1977). *Adv. internal Med.*, **22,** 455.

—— and —— (1978). *Gastroenterology*, **74,** 952.

——, Onderdonk, A. B., and Cisneros, R. L. (1977). *Gastroenterology*, **73,** 772.

——, ——, ——, and Kasper, D. L. (1977). *J. infect. Dis.*, **136,** 701.

Br. med. J. (1974). **4,** 65.

—— (1978). **1,** 669.

Browne, R. A., Fekety, R., Silva, J., Boyd, D. I., Work, C. O., and Abrams, G. D. (1977). *Johns Hopkins Hosp. Bull.*, **141,** 183.

Buxton Hopkin, D. A. (1978). *Lancet*, **2,** 1058.

Cummins, A. J. (1961). *Am. J. dig. Dis.*, **6,** 429.

Dearing, W. H., Baggenstoss, A. H., and Weed, L. A. (1960). *Gastroenterology*, **38,** 441.

De Jesus, R. and Peternel, W. W. (1978). *Gastroenterology*, **74,** 818.

Ecker, J. A., Williams, R. G., and McKittrick, J. E. (1970). *Am. J. Gastroent. N.Y.*, **54,** 214.

Eyssen, H., De Somer, P., and Van Dijck, P. (1957). *Antibiotics Chemother.*, **7,** 55.

George, R. H., Symonds, J. M., Dimock, F., Brown, J. D., Arabi, Y., Shinagawa, N., Keighley, M. R. B., Alexander-Williams, J., and Burdon, D. W. (1978). *Br. med. J.*, **1,** 695.

Gorbach, S. L., Spanknebel, G., and Weinstein, L. (1969). *J. infect. Dis.*, **120,** 298.

Goulston, S. J. M. and McGovern, V. J. (1965). *Gut*, **6,** 207.

Hale, H. W. and Cosgriff, H. J. (1957). *Am. J. Surg.*, **94,** 710.

Humphrey, C. D., Pittman, J. C., and Pittman, F. E. (1975). *Clin. Res.*, **23,** 27.

Kappas, A., Shinagawa, N., Arabi, Y., Thompson, H., Burdon, D. W. Dimock, F., George, R. H., Alexander-Williams, J., and Keighley, M. R. B. (1978). *Br. med. J.*, **1,** 675.

Katz, L., La Mont, J. T. Trier, J. S., Sonnenblick, E. B., Rothman, S. W., Broitman, S. A., and Rieth, S. (1978). *Gastroenterology*, **74,** 246.

Keighley, M. R. B., Burdon, D. W., Alexander-Williams, J., Shinagawa, N., Arabi, Y., Thompson, H., Youngs, D., Bentley, S., and George, R. H. (1978). *Lancet*, **2,** 1165.

Khan, M. Y. and Hall, W. H. (1966). *Ann. intern. Med.*, **65,** 1.

Kleckner, M. S., Bargen, J. A., and Baggenstoss, A. H. (1952). *Gastroenterology*, **21,** 212.

Lancet (1977). **2,** 1113.
LARSON, H. E., PARRY, J. V., PRICE, A. B., DAVIES, D. R., DOLBY, J., and TYRRELL, D. A. J. (1977). *Br. med. J.*, **1,** 1246.
—— and PRICE, A. B. (1977). *Lancet*, **2,** 1312.
LUSK, R. H., FEKETY, R., SILVA, J., BROWNE, R. A., RINGLER, D. H., and ABRAMS, G. D. (1978). *J. infect. Dis.*, **137,** 464.
MCGOVERN, V. J. and GOULSTON, S. J. M. (1965). *Gut*, **6,** 213.
MATUCHANSKY, C., ARIES, J., and MAIRE, P. (1978). *Lancet*, **2,** 580.
MEDLINE, A., SHIN, D. H., and MEDLINE, N. M. (1976). *Hum. Pathol.*, **7,** 693.
PEARCE, C. and DINEEN, P. (1960). *Am. J. Surg.*, **99,** 292.
PETTET, J. D., BAGGENSTOSS, A. H., DEARING, W. H., and JUDD, E. S. (1954). *Surgery Gynec. Obstet.*, **98,** 546.
REINER, L., SCHLESINGER, M. J., and MILLER, G. M. (1952). *Archs Path.*, **54,** 39.
RIFKIN, G. D., FEKETY, F. R., SILVA, J., and SACK, R. B. (1977). *Lancet*, **2,** 1103.
——, SILVA, J., and FEKETY, R. (1978). *Gastroenterology*, **74,** 52.
SEGER, R., JOLLER, P., KENNY, A., HITZIG, W., METAXAS, M., and METAXAS-BÜHLER, M. (1979). *Lancet*, **1,** 48.
SMALL, J. D. (1968). *Lab. Anim. Care*, **18,** 411.
SPEARE, G. S. (1954). *Am. J. Surg.*, **88,** 523.
TAN, T. L., DRAKE, C. T., JACOBSON, M. J., and VAN PROHASKA, J. (1959). *Surgery Gynec. Obstet.*, **108,** 415.
TEDESCO, F. J. (1975). *Am. J. dig. Dis.*, **20,** 295.
——, BARTON, R. W., and ALPERS, D. H. (1974). *Ann. intern. Med.*, **81,** 429.
TOFFLER, R. B., PINGOUD, E. G., and BURRELL, M. I. (1978). *Lancet*, **2,** 707.
TURES, J. F., TOWNSEND, W. F., and ROSE, H. D. (1976). *J. Am. med. Ass.*, **236,** 948.
VAN PROHASKA, J., MOCK, F., BAKER, W., and COLLINS, R. (1961). *Int. Abstr. Surg.*, **112,** 103.

29

Large-intestinal diseases which are uncommon in the third world

'I hav finally kum to the konklusion,
that a good reliable sett ov bowels iz
wurth more tu a man, than enny
quantity ov brains'
Josh Billings: his sayings (1818 to 1885).

THE four diseases dealt with in this chapter are either unusual or rare in most parts of the third world. For example, during a three-year period in which there were 1754 admissions for gastrointestinal disease to Goroka Base Hospital, Papua New Guinea, there were no cases of ulcerative colitis, Crohn's disease, or diverticular disease (Wagner and Shepherd, 1976). That is not to say that those diseases do not occur; they do indeed exist, and must always be kept in mind in the same way that diseases common in tropical countries must always be considered in the UK and USA in people who have been exposed to them. The physician who works on probabilities in the third world will usually prove to be correct, but his occasional patient will suffer as a result of that approach.

The great differences in incidence rates of these diseases must conceal important aetiological factors responsible for those conditions in the western world; many factors have been considered, but, to date, no clear cause-effect relationships have been established.

29.1. Colonic physiology

29.1.1. Bowel habit in the third world

Due to the large bulky meals taken by indigenous people in most parts of the tropics, together with repeated gastrointestinal and systemic infections, and to a lesser extent hypolactasia (Chapter 21), constipation is unusual. Studies from South Africa (Bremner, 1964; Van der Horst, 1964) indicate that two to three stools daily are usual, and that one is virtually abnormal. In an investigation of the bowel habits of 1245 rural Ugandans at Kasangati, 89 per cent had more than one stool daily (Ekwueme, 1978); there were no tribal differences. However, in a study in Nigeria, 48 per cent of 362 adults passed only one stool daily (Fakunle, Ajagbonna, Ani, and Awofeso, 1978); 30 per cent had two motions or more. Table 29·1 summarizes stool-weights in groups of people in Africa, India, and the UK; there can be no reasonable doubt that the mean weight is higher in the indigenous people of Africa and Asia when they are living on their normal diets. The part played by intestinal parasites on bowel function, including transit time, is difficult to evaluate at present (Crofts, 1977).

A simple method for measuring whole gastrointestinal transit involves ingesting radioopaque pellets; following stool collection their presence can be rapidly estimated from an X-ray of the stool specimen. Many other markers have been used, including barium sulphate, copper thiocyanate, polyethylene glycol, and chromium sesquioxide; however radioopaque pellets seem to be as good as any, and easy to estimate (Branch and Cummings, 1978).

Using radioopaque pellets, Burkitt, Walker, and Painter (1972) and Balasegaram and Burkitt (1976) investigated transit-rates in several ethnic groups; there seems to be little doubt that transit-rate, as well as stool-weight, is greater in people living on the local diets of much of Africa and Asia. Those authors have attributed that to a high dietary 'fibre' content. In Nigeria, 58 per cent of 50 healthy adults had a transit time of less than 24 hours (Fakunle, *et al.*, 1978).

Results of several studies suggest that an increase in dietary fibre—especially that of vegetable origin—increases stool bulk (Kelsay, 1978). In South Africa, African children and adults have a shorter intestinal transit time than white subjects (Walker and Walker, 1969). However, information in adults is, overall, conflicting at present (Kelsay, 1978).

Table 29.1. *Daily stool weights in the third world compared with those in the UK.*

Ethnic group	No. of observations	Age (years)	Mean stool weight (g per 24 hours)	Investigator(s)
North Indians	36	< 15	374	Tandon and Tandon (1975)
"	514	> 15	311	"
Africans (South Africa)	500	rural school children	275	Burkitt, Walker, and Painter (1972)
Rural Ugandan	15	adults	470	"
Malays	10	rural adults	465	Balasegaram and Burkitt (1976)
Malay Chinese	10	rural adults	489	"
Malay Indians	8	rural adults	385	"
English	6	adults	175	Burkitt, Walker and Painter (1972)
"	24	adult vegetarians	225	"
"	9	teenage children	110	"
"	15	adults	104	"

29.1.2. Purgatives and enemas

The use of purgatives and enemas is very common in many parts of the third world, especially in children. Some patients in west Africa, for example, give themselves up to 200 enemas annually (Davey, 1968). That may be part of a health routine.

The fruit, leaves, bark, and roots of *Cucumis africanus* are used extensively in purgatives and enemas in South and central Africa. Ginger, pepper, soap, water, undiluted 'Dettol', alum, turpentine, potassium permanganate, salt, mentholatum, tobacco, and finely ground ash and coal are also used (Davey, 1968). Cows' horns (Bremner, 1964), reeds (Van der Horst, 1964), hollowed-out narrow-necked gourds, and in more recent years rubber syringes can be used for administration of the enema; several enemas are sometimes given daily.

The diagnosis of purgative or enema-induced colitis is made from a history and proctoscopy; the mucosa shows friable granulations. Barium enema may show changes which could easily be mistaken for nonspecific ulcerative colitis or Crohn's disease—i.e. narrowing of the descending colon with loss of normal haustrations. A haemorrhagic proctocolitis, which may have a similar sigmoidoscopic appearance to that in other colonic lesions, including amoebic colitis, may also be produced. Severe pelvic peritonitis can occur; a slough protruding from the anus may resemble a gangrenous intussusception which is often followed by stricture formation. Hepatorenal failure and neurological complications have been reported following herbal enemas. If tobacco is used, shock and collapse may follow their use.

Sedation, intravenous therapy, antibiotics, and corticosteroids usually bring about resolution (Davey, 1968); surgery should be avoided.

29.1.3. Role of the colon in nutrition

There has been a tendency to regard the colon as a mere storage organ. It now seems clear however that it plays an important part in nutrition. Nitrogen absorption, after bacterial metabolism, can occur there (Bayley, Cho, and Holmes, 1974; Gibson, Sladen, and Dawson, 1976). Similarly it is clear that free fatty acids formed as breakdown products of carbohydrate fermentation and which have not been absorbed by the small intestine, may be absorbed there (McNeil, Cummings, and James, 1978). Adult hypolactasia is present in most inhabitants of the third world (Chapter 21); however after drinking milk for 10 to 14 days, there is little diarrhoea in people with that condition. It seems likely that much of that adaptation takes place in the colon; there may simply be adaptation of the colonic flora, or possibly absorption of the fermentation products of lactose takes place. In malabsorption states, undigested and unabsorbed nutrients reach the colon in considerable quantities (Chapter 20). It is important to know to what extent the colon can absorb those compounds; however at present there is no accurate information on that.

The extent to which the colon reabsorbs water and electrolytes in small-intestinal diarrhoea and malabsorption, and also in hot climates, has not been adequately investigated.

The colon is undoubtedly an important endocrine organ (Cristina, Lehy, Zeitoun, and Dufougeray, 1978; Moxey, 1978); the importance of that has not yet been evaluated in the western world, let alone the third world.

The effect of intraluminal pH, and oxygen concentration (Bond, Beggs, and Levitt, 1978), on the bacterial flora of the colon is clearly important; much work needs to be carried out in those areas.

29.2. Colonic cancer

29.2.1. Distribution

This tumour has for long been known to be unusual in Africans in Africa (Trowell, 1960; Oettlé, 1964). That observation also applies to most third world countries. During the period 1953–5, seven cases were reported in Africans in South Africa (Higginson and Oettlé, 1957). In Johannesburg the mortality rate is one tenth of that in Denmark. In a retrospective study, Turner (1962) found only two cases annually at Mombasa, Kenya. A series of patients with large-bowel carcinomas was reported from Nairobi, Kenya (Sande, 1975); however it is not clear how many of those patients, if any, were Africans. In Bulawayo, Zimbabwe Rhodesia, White (1961) reported three cases in three years. In a nine-year period (1952–60), 39 cases (1·3 per cent of all cancers) were reported in the Kampala cancer registry (Davies, Elmes, Mtimavalye, Owor, and Shaper, 1964). At the Mulago Hospital, Kampala, only 10 cases of carcinoma of the caecum were seen in the period 1952–64 (*E. Afr. med. J.*, 1966). In Papua New Guinea, this tumour is also unusual although certainly not unknown. In a three-year period, eight, 11, and three cases of colonic, rectal, and anal carcinoma were seen at the Goroka Base Hospital (Wagner and Shepherd, 1976); during that time there were 141 malignancies of the gastrointestinal tract including the liver. So rare is the condition that single case reports have been considered worthwhile in Africa (Kajubi, 1966).

Evidence is beginning to emerge that colonic carcinoma is becoming more common in Africans in Africa. In a study at Lusaka, Zambia, five cases were seen out of 38 patients presenting with intestinal obstruction over a one-year period (1975–6) (Umerah and Obadike, 1978).

29.2.2. Aetiology

There can be no doubt that environmental factors are of paramount importance in colorectal carcinoma (Jansson, 1978). The low incidence of colonic carcinoma in the tropics is perhaps surprising in view of the very high incidence of parasitic infections and other inflammatory conditions of the colon. Because amoebiasis and schistosomiasis are so common throughout Africa, they are obviously not involved. Although rarely colonic carcinoma has been reported in a patient with amoebic disease, there is no evidence to suggest a cause-effect relationship.

It seems possible that the diets of people living in tropical countries, especially Africa, contain very low concentrations of carcinogens. In the western world fats are frequently used for frying; in Africa total and saturated fat intake is usually very low. Alternatively, carcinogens may be diluted by the large faecal mass associated with the very high carbohydrate content of the diets; studies on colonic flora in Africans in Uganda have shown that there are marked differences when compared with a UK population. Intestinal bacteria might be able to produce carcinogens from dietary fats and bile steroids; different bacterial concentrations could account for different rates of carcinogen production (Hill, Crowther, Drasar, Hawksworth, Aries, and Williams, 1971). Faeces from countries with a low incidence of colonic cancer

(Uganda, south India, and Japan) have lower *Bacteroides* counts and higher counts of enterococci and other aerobic bacteria than a population in the western world. Bowel actions tend to be more frequent and stool volumes higher in the third world compared with western countries; that clearly leads to a relatively brief contact time between carcinogens and the colonic mucosa.

Whether or not a high 'fibre' diet protects against colonic cancer is still a controversial issue (Fleiszer, Murray, MacFarlane, and Brown, 1978; Cruse, Lewin, and Clark, 1978a). Burkitt (1975; 1977) has argued for a causal relationship between dietary fibre and colonic cancer; that is not supported by experimental studies on rats (Cruse, Lewin, and Clark, 1978b). Cleave (1974) has sought a correlation between the consumption of large amounts of refined sugar and colonic carcinoma.

Conditions associated with colonic carcinoma—ulcerative colitis, polyposis coli, and adenomatous polyps—are also unusual in most populations living in tropical countries.

The tumour, when it occurs, is similar to that in the western world; two-thirds are in the left half of the colon, usually in the rectosigmoid. The caecum is the other part which is frequently involved. The intermediate areas have a lower incidence rate; possibly that is because there is less faecal stasis there. The tumour is an adenocarcinoma; protuberant, ulcerative, and infiltrative growths occasionally occur, the latter being more common in Africa than in temperate areas (Edington and Gilles, 1976). Mucoid and anaplastic tumours are apparently more common in Africa; that is probably because a higher proportion is in young patients. Carcinoma is a very rare cause of intestinal obstruction in Africans; scanty reports have come from Nigeria, Ghana, Uganda, and Zimbabwe Rhodesia (Davey, 1968).

29.2.3. Clinical aspects

The clinical picture is similar to that in western countries (Avery Jones, Gummer, and Lennard-Jones, 1968). The mean age at presentation was lower however in a series of 42 patients seen in a 10-year period at the Baragwanath Hospital, Johannesburg (Bremner, 1965), and the history of the disease longer; in that series 21 per cent were colloid carcinomas which is a high figure and one which has also been noted in other parts of Africa (Awoliyi, 1961).

The most important differential diagnosis is amoeboma (Chapter 25). A mass in the right iliac fossa in a tropical country is likely to be caused by pyomyositis (in the ileopsoas muscle), an appendix mass or abscess, or possibly a helminthoma; carcinoma of the caecum is very low on the list of probabilities. In areas where schistosomiasis is common peritoneal granulomas, in association with an irregular hard liver, can be mistaken for abdominal and hepatic secondary deposits from a colonic carcinoma; those granulomas however tend to be of uniform size and are especially dense on the pelvic floor.

A course of metronidazole should be given initially on the supposition that the lesion is an amoeboma; if that is the correct diagnosis, some reduction in the size of the mass occurs in 72 hours. Colonic carcinoma and appendix abscess do not respond to that regime. The chemotherapy of colorectal cancer has been reviewed by Moertel (1978).

29.3. Non-specific ulcerative colitis

29.3.1. Distribution

The first report of the disease in tropical Africa, in four Ganda patients in Uganda, was by Billinghurst and Welchman (1966) at the Mulago Hospital, Kampala; the history, sigmoidoscopy, radiology, and response to corticosteroids were classical in three of them. Four cases have been reported in Africans at Durban, South Africa (Pillay, 1964). One was described at Ibadan, Nigeria (Greenwood and Larbi, 1966). Four further cases were reported from Nairobi, Kenya, by Awori, Rees, and Roy (1972). A further three cases were seen at Dar-es-Salaam, Tanzania (Spencer and Nhonoli, 1972), and a fourth reported by Jones, Bewes, and Hulme-Moir (1977). The disease seems to be extremely rare in south-east Asia (Tinckler, 1966). In India, however, the disease is seen but seems to be limited to the rectum, and sigmoid and descending colon (Chuttani, Nigam, Sama, Dhanda, and Gupta, 1967).

It is exceedingly difficult to know how common this disease really is in tropical countries. There is so much diarrhoeal disease and postdysenteric colitis, often with blood and mucus in the stool, that ulcerative colitis could well be submerged beneath a mass of other conditions, especially amoebic colitis. The disease may occur coincidentally with salmonella infections (Dronfield, Fletcher, and Langman, 1974).

29.3.2. Aetiology

The aetiology is unknown.

The pathology is chronic ulceration of the colonic mucosa and submucosa (Morson and Dawson, 1972); the infiltrate contains lymphocytes, plasma cells, and histiocytes, and occasionally eosinophils are present in considerable numbers. Polypoid hyperplasia and carcinomatous change in long-standing cases are complications of the disease.

29.3.3. Clinical aspects

The disease, when it occurs, behaves in a similar way to that in temperate climates (Avery Jones, Gummer, and Lennard-Jones, 1968). It is very important that amoebic disease of the colon is positively excluded before embarking on corticosteroid treatment, because those agents lead to a significant mortality from colonic (Chapter 25) and hepatic (Chapter 12) complications.

29.4. Crohn's disease

29.4.1. Distribution

Crohn's disease (Crohn, Ginzberg, and Oppenheimer, 1932) is probably very rare in most parts of the developing world. However there is a real possibility that the disease is masked by an enormous umbrella of tuberculous, and possibly *Yersinia enterocolitica*, disease of the ileocaecal region (Chapter 27). A report from Khartoum (El Masri and Satir, 1975) described three cases of the disease in Sudanese patients; in one the sigmoid colon and rectum, and in two the distal ileum were involved. Two recent reports have appeared of Crohn's disease in West Indian patients in the United Kingdom (O'Donoghue and Clark, 1976; O'Donoghue and Dawson, 1977); two were West Indian children who were born in the UK, and a third was a man in his twenties who had lived there for 12 years. Five cases have been reported from South Africa (Giraud, Luke, and Schmaman, 1969).

Recently, Das and Shukla (1976) reviewed 182 cases of abdominal tuberculosis in a teaching hospital in Allahabad, India, and were not able to find a definite case of Crohn's disease. However, in the past (Das and Shukla 1975) those investigators have emphasized the histological similarity between Crohn's disease and tuberculosis; the only clear distinction lies in finding caseation and/or acid-fact bacilli.

29.4.2. Aetiology

The aetiology is not understood. However, a filterable agent from Crohn's disease tissue can cause granulomata in animals (Michell and Rees, 1970; Sachar, Taub, and Janowitz, 1975; Cave, Mitchell, and Brooke, 1975). There is evidence that mycobacteria might be responsible (Golde, 1968; Burnham, Lennard-Jones, Stanford, and Bird, 1978); the latter workers suggested that cell-wall deficient mycobacteria might be the causative agents. Furthermore, they suggested possible analogies between Crohn's disease and *Mycobacterium leprae* and *M. ulcerans* infections.

The pathology consists of a chronic granulomatous reaction, usually involving the lower end of the colon; any part of the gastrointestinal tract may however be involved (Morson and Dawson, 1972). There is narrowing of the bowel lumen. Histologically there is necrosis and an infiltrate of polymorphs, lymphocytes, and plasma cells in the mucosa and muscular coat. As the disease progresses, histiocytes replace the polymorphs.

29.4.3. Clinical aspects

When it occurs, the condition is similar to that in western countries (Avery Jones, Gummer, and Lennard-Jones, 1968). The clinical signs and symptoms of Crohn's disease and intestinal tuberculosis tend to be different. Vomiting, fever, and menstrual disturbances are more common in tuberculosis, whereas abdominal pain and colic are present in both. Diarrhoea is unusual in tuberculosis, and constipation common, whereas diarrhoea is more common in Crohn's disease. Ascites is more often present in tuberculosis, but in both, an ileocaecal mass may be felt.

In tuberculosis, a lymphocytosis, positive Mantoux test, lymphocytosis and high protein content in the ascitic fluid, and granulomas in a needle liver-biopsy, provide valuable diagnostic assistance. Peritoneal biopsy may also be of value (Das and Shukla, 1975).

29.5. Diverticular disease

Although this disease, and its corollary diverticulitis, occasionally occurs in all parts of Africa, it is sufficiently rare to make it the subject of a clinical demonstration or clinicopathological conference when a case is diagnosed. A similar situation exists in Papua New Guinea. The sigmoid colon is usually most affected; muscle thickening is associated with the diverticula. However, there is evidence of an increasing incidence-rate of diverticular disease with urbanization in South Africa (Segal, Solomon, and Hunt, 1977); in that report, 16 cases were recorded in Africans, of whom five were in their fourth decade, and only four over the age of 60 years. Four, incidentally, also had haemorrhoids.

Increased pressure within the colon has been suggested to be important aetiologically. Dietary factors, especially lack of 'fibre' and low faecal bulk have been suggested to be important (Cleave, 1974; Painter and Burkitt, 1971; 1975). If that theory is correct, and there is certainly some evidence against it (Kelsay, 1978), the high 'fibre' diet which is usually taken in tropical countries acts as a preventive agent.

29.6. Haemorrhoids

In most parts of the third world haemorrhoids are less common than in the western world, despite the fact that chronic diarrhoeal disease is a frequent problem; that may be associated with higher 'fibre' diets (Cleave, 1974; Burkitt, 1975) but that has not been proved.

29.7. Maintenance of nutrition in chronic large-intestinal disease

Only in recent years has emphasis been placed on the importance of maintaining good nutritional status in patients with chronic large intestinal disease, e.g. intestinal malignancies, Crohn's disease, and ulcerative colitis (Calman, 1978; Russell, 1978). The importance of: (i) supplementary feeding, (ii) nasogastric feeding with a liquidized diet, (iii) elemental diets, and (iv) intravenous nutrition, have all been reported as providing important nutritional and metabolic support. The problems associated with prolonged intravenous feeding have been discussed by Powell-Tuck, Nielsen, Farwell, and Lennard-Jones (1978).

References

Avery Jones, F., Gummer, J. W. P., and Lennard-Jones, J. E. (1968). *Clinical gastroenterology*, 2nd ed. p. 389, 599 and 619. Blackwell, Oxford and Edinburgh.

Awoliyi, S. O. (1961). *W. Afr. med. J.*, **10,** 53.

Awori, N. W., Rees, P. H., and Roy, A. D. (1972). *E. Afr. med. J.*, **49,** 604.

Balasegaram, M. and Burkitt, D. P. (1976). *Lancet*, **1,** 152.

Bayley, H. S., Cho, C. Y., and Holmes, J. H. G. (1974). *Fedn Proc. Fedn Am. Socs exp. Biol.*, **33,** 94.

Billinghurst, J. R. and Welchman, J. M. (1966). *Br. med. J.*, **1,** 211.

Billings, Josh (Henry Wheeler Shaw): his sayings. Ch. 29 (1968). In *Familiar Medical Quotations* (ed. M. B. Strauss). p. 44. Little, Brown and Co., Boston.

Bond, J. H., Beggs, W. H., and Levitt, M. D. (1978). *Gastroenterology*, **75,** 419.

Branch, W. J. and Cummings, J. H. (1978). *Gut*, **19,** 371.

Bremner, C. G. (1964). *S. Afr. J. Surg.*, **2,** 119.

—— (1965). *S. Afr. J. Surg.*, **3,** 35.

Burkitt, D. P. (1975). In *Refined carbohydrate foods and disease* (ed. D. P. Burkitt and H. C. Trowell). p. 117, 143. Academic Press, London, New York, and San Francisco.

—— (1977). *Am. J. clin. Nutr.*, **30,** 262.

——, Walker, A. R. P., and Painter, N. S. (1972). *Lancet*, **2,** 1408.

Burnham, W. R., Lennard-Jones, J. E., Stanford, J. L., and Bird, R. G. (1978). *Lancet*, **2,** 693.

Calman, K. C. (1978). *Proc. Nutr. Soc.*, **37,** 87.

CAVE, D. R., MITCHELL, D. N., and BROOKE, B. N. (1975). *Gastroenterology*, **69,** 618.
CHUTTANI, H. K., NIGAM, S. P., SAMA, S. K., DHANDA, P. C., and GUPTA, P. S. (1967). *Br. med. J.*, **4,** 204.
CLEAVE, T. L. (1974). *The saccharine disease*. p. 29, 37 and 44. John Wright and Sons, Ltd., Bristol
CRISTINA, M. L., LEHY, T., ZEITOUN, P., and DUFOUGERAY, F. (1978). *Gastroenterology*, **75,** 20.
CROFTS, T. J. (1977). *Tropical Doctor*, **7,** 115.
CROHN, B. B., GINZBURG, L., and OPPENHEIMER, G. D. (1932). *J. Am. med. Ass.*, **99,** 1323.
CRUSE, J. P., LEWIN, M. R., and CLARK, C. G. (1978a). *Lancet*, **2,** 843.
——, ——, and —— (1978b). *Lancet*, **2,** 1278.
DAS, P. and SHUKLA, H. S. (1975). *Br. J. Surg.*, **62,** 610.
—— and —— (1976). *Br. J. Surg.*, **63,** 941.
DAVEY, W. W. (1968). *Companion to Surgery in Africa*. p. 257. E. and S. Livingstone, Edinburgh and London.
DAVIES, J. N. P., ELMES, S., HUTT, M. S. R., MTIMAVALYE, L. A. R., OWOR, R., and SHAPER, L. (1964). *Br. med. J.*, **1,** 259.
DRONFIELD, M. W., FLETCHER, J., and LANGMAN, M. J. S. (1974) *Br. med. J.*, **1,** 99.
E. Afr. med. J. (1966). **43,** 343.
EDINGTON, G. M. and GILLES, H. M. (1976). *Pathology in the tropics*. 2nd ed. p. 539. Edward Arnold, London.
EKWUEME, O. (1978). *Trop. geogr. Med.*, **30,** 247.
EL MASRI, S. H. and SATIR, A. A. (1975). *E. Afr. med. J.*, **52,** 284.
FAKUNLE, Y. M., AJAGBONNA, S. O., ANI, O. E. O., and AWOFESO, O. (1978). *J. trop. Med. Hyg.*, **81,** 137.
FLEISZER, D., MURRAY, D., MACFARLANE, J., and BROWN, R. A. (1978). *Lancet*, **2,** 552.
GIBSON, J. A., SLADEN, G. E., and DAWSON, A. M. (1976). *Br. J. Nutr.*, **35,** 61.
GIRAUD, R. M. A., LUKE, I., and SCHMAMAN, A. (1969). *S. Afr. med. J.*, **43,** 610.
GOLDE, D. W. (1968). *Lancet*, **1,** 1144.
GREENWOOD, B. M. and LARBI, E. B. (1966). *Br. med. J.*, **1,** 1300.
HIGGINSON, J. and OETTLÉ, A. G. (1957). *Final report, Cancer Research Unit.* South African Institute for Medical Research, Johannesburg.
HILL, M. J., CROWTHER, J. S., DRASAR, B. S., HAWKSWORTH, G., ARIES, V., and WILLIAMS, R. E. O. (1971). *Lancet*, **1,** 95.
JANSSON, B. (1978). *Gastroenterology*, **75,** 321.
JONES, M. E., BEWES, P. C., and HULME-MOIR, I. (1977). *E. Afr. med. J.*, **54,** 670.
KAJUBI, S. K. (1966). *E. Afr. med. J.*, **43,** 100.
KELSAY, J. L. (1978). *Am. J. clin. Nutr.*, **31,** 142.
MCNEIL, N. I., CUMMINGS, J. H., and JAMES, W. P. T. (1978). *Gut*, **19,** 819.
MITCHELL, D. N. and REES, R. J. W. (1970). *Lancet*, **2,** 168.
MOERTEL, C. G. (1978). *New Engl. J. Med.*, **299,** 1049.
MORSON, B. C. and DAWSON, I. M. P. (1972). *Gastrointestinal pathology*, p. 458 and 475. Blackwell, Oxford, London, Edinburgh and Melbourne.
MOXEY, P. C. (1978). *Gastroenterology*, **75,** 147.
O'DONOGHUE, D. P. and CLARK, M. L. (1976). *Br. med. J.*, **2,** 796.
—— and DAWSON, A. M. (1977). *Archs Dis. Childh.*, **52,** 627.
OETTLÉ, A. G. (1964). *J. natn. Cancer Inst.*, **33,** 404.
PAINTER, N. S. and BURKITT, D. P. (1971). *Br. med. J.*, **2,** 450.
—— and —— (1975). In *Refined carbohydrate foods and disease* (ed. D. P. Burkitt and H. C. Trowell). p. 99. Academic press, London, New York and San Francisco.
PILLAY, V. K. G. (1964). *Br. med. J.*, **2,** 689.
POWELL-TUCK, J., NIELSEN, T., FARWELL, J. A., and LENNARD-JONES, J. E. (1978). *Lancet*, **2,** 825.

RUSSELL, R. I. (1978). *Proc. Nutr. Soc.*, **37,** 79.
SACHAR, D. B., TAUB, R. N., and JANOWITZ, H. D. (1975). *New Engl. J. Med.*, **293,** 354.
SANDE, G. M. (1975). *E. Afr. med. J.*, **52,** 365.
SEGAL, I., SOLOMON, A. and HUNT, J. A. (1977). *Gastroenterology*, **72,** 215.
SPENCER, S. S. and NHONOLI, A. M. (1972). *E. Afr. med. J.*, **49,** 163.
TANDON, R. K. and TANDON, B. N. (1975). *Lancet*, **2,** 560.
TINCKLER, L. F. (1966). *Br. med. J.*, **1,** 734.
TROWELL, H. C. (1960). *Non-infective Disease in Africa*. p. 219. Edward Arnold, London.
TURNER, P. P. (1962). *E. Afr. med. J.*, **39,** 121.
UMERAH, B. C. and OBADIKE, G. (1978). *E. Afr. med. J.*, **55,** 77.
VAN DER HORST, R. L. (1964). *S. Afr. med. J.*, **38,** 465.
WAGNER, F. B. and SHEPHERD, A. (1976). *Papua New Guin. med. J.*, **19,** 156.
WALKER, A. R. P. and WALKER, B. F. (1969). *Br. med. J.*, **3,** 238.
WHITE, A. (1961). *E. Afr. med. J.*, **38,** 525.

30

Diseases involving the anal region

MANY colonic conditions described in other chapters of this section can involve the anal region. This chapter covers some diseases, most of a venereal nature (Marino, 1964; Morson, 1964), which have not previously been covered, and also emphasizes others that have already been mentioned, but have a more marked effect on the anal region than on the colon (Morson and Dawson, 1972).

30.1. Viral and bacterial infections of the anal region

30.1.1. Lymphogranuloma venereum (lymphogranuloma inguinale, tropical bubo, esthiomène, paradenitis nostras, Durand-Nicolas-Favre disease)

This is a specific venereal infection which is especially common amongst sexually promiscuous individuals (Abrams, 1968). It tends to be confined to lower socioeconomic groups. Lymphogranuloma venereum is caused by one of the chlamydia group of organisms, which can be seen as elementary bodies in Giemsa-stained leucocytes; it is related to the psittacosis-trachoma group of large viruses, and is an intermediate between viruses and rickettsiae. The virus does not live long outside the cell and is very sensitive to environmental changes; little immunity is developed. Complications often first occur late in life, i.e. well after the menopause; most patients present at approximately 40–50 years. In third world countries, patients often do not present for treatment until the disease is far advanced.

The disease is widespread throughout the world in both tropical and temperate climates. It is common in the Caribbean, where good accounts have been given in Jamaica (Miles, 1957; Annamunthodo, 1961), central and South America, south India, Indonesia, and tropical Africa. During 1951–61, 283 patients were admitted to the Mulago Hospital, Kampala with the disease; of 12 women admitted in 1961 two had rectal strictures (Davey, 1968). There has apparently been a steep decline in Kampala since then. In 1955–9, 26 patients were seen at the University Hospital, Ibadan; 11 of them had anorectal strictures. The disease has also been well described in Ghana (Bowesman, 1960). About 90 per cent of patients are women who usually present at gynaecological departments; only a minority of them get rectal strictures.

Although genital involvement is usual, the disease occasionally affects the anorectal region (Bensaude and Lambling, 1936) and distal colon only, in both sexes. In men the initial lesion is usually on the penis; in women it is usually in the vagina, is seldom seen, and frequently not detected. The transient primary lesion (a papule or shallow ulcer) is followed after about six weeks by superficial and deep lymphadenitis (bubo), and that is succeeded by suppuration and fistula formation. There are occasionally constitutional symptoms; typhoid fever may erroneously be diagnosed. Following that, a chronic proctocolitis develops which after months or years, especially if untreated, leads to an anorectal stricture. Infection of the rectum in women presumably takes place from the vagina. In male homosexuals the organism is directly implanted into the anal region, and the consequences may be similar, starting with diarrhoea, tenesmus, haemorrhage, and purulent discharge some six weeks after exposure. The chronic disease is usually most spectacular in women (Lawson, 1963); it produces a chronic proctitis, rectovaginal fistulae, and perirectal abscesses; rectal stricture and perianal elephantiasis may also ensue. Genital elephantiasis occurs in both sexes. The features of the proctocolitis are those of a colitis of varying severity and duration, with diarrhoea, constipation, and blood and pus in the discharge and stools. There is a coarse granular feeling on rectal examination, and proctoscopy shows intense inflammation with a friable mucosa which easily bleeds. Anorectal stricture is an important chronic manifestation (Hawe, 1951; Miles, 1957), with diarrhoea, constipation, and incontinence; later there may be symptoms of partial obstruction, abdominal colic, and difficulty in defaecation with pencil-like stools. Examination at that stage reveals thickened and oedematous perianal skin; buttonholing ('bridging-folds') which can be detected with a probe are pathognomonic. The lower edge of the stricture is nearly always within reach of the index finger, i.e. not more than about 10 cm from the anal margin. The strictures vary from a mild constriction to complete stenosis. The anal sphincter may be patulous or indurated and that accounts for incontinence. A rectovaginal fistula may be present, and incontinence of faeces occurs via the vagina. The fistula has a constant position, in the centre of the posterior vaginal wall distal to the stricture, and just above the anorectal ring. Perianal and perirectal fibrosis and abscesses are common, and they may result in fistula formation.

The most likely condition to be confused with lymphogranuloma venereum is a rectal carcinoma, which is uncommon in the third world (Levin, Romano, Steinberg, and Welsh, 1964). In that condition the history is usually shorter. Perianal skin is normal with a rectal carcinoma and the lesion which has a sharp edge, does not usually produce a stricture, and is usually in the middle one-third rather than the lower one-third of the rectum. Other clinical differential diagnoses include Donovanosis (see below), filarial adenitis, tularaemia, and femoral hernia.

The primary lesion is an ulcer surrounded by plasma cells and histiocytes; eosinophils may be prominent. In the secondary lesion, there is proliferation of monocytes, plasma cells, and eosinophils in the lymph glands; epithelioid cell transformation with central necrosis and giant-cell systems can be similar to the lesions of tuberculosis. In the abscesses, eosinophils and plasma cells predominate; intracytoplasmic inclusion bodies may be present. Fibrosis occurs later. Malignant change has been described (Levin *et al.*, 1964).

A Giemsa-stained smear from the primary lesion may show intracytoplasmic inclusion bodies. Virus isolation in a yolk-sac, or intracerebral inoculation into a monkey or mouse is possible.

A complement-fixation test and the Frei skin test are of value in diagnosis. The complement-fixation test is easier to perform than the Frei test and in the early stages of the disease may be of value in assessing the success of treatment; a titre of 1:40 is diagnostic. The Frei test is a delayed hypersensitivity reaction which utilizes fluid taken from a bubo, after preparation and sterilization. The intradermal injection gives a hyperaemic patch after 24–48 hours if it is positive and that often persists for two to three weeks; a strong positive result is diagnostic but a false weak positive response may occur. The test becomes positive 7–40 days after the onset of adenitis, and is irreversible; it is of no value in assessing treatment. Biopsy is often nonspecific, but of value in excluding Donovanosis (see below) and rectal carcinoma, which in fact rarely gives rise to a stricture. Barium enema gives valuable anatomical information about the length of the stricture; that usually extends into the rectosigmoid colon; occasionally there are multiple strictures, and pararectal sinuses may run at right angles to the bowel (Annamunthodo and Marryatt, 1961). Involvement of much of the descending colon, with lack of haustrations and spasm, may be detected. Serum globulin concentration is usually elevated. Treatment is with tetracycline or chloramphenicol, 2·0 g daily, and must be continued for three to six weeks in early cases and for several months in chronic cases; erythromycin is also effective. Symptomatic and sigmoidoscopic improvement is often dramatic and a permanent cure may ensue. Surgery is indicated in the following situations (Davey, 1968): (i) when there is gross destruction of the anal region, (ii) in the presence of a rectovaginal fistula, (iii) if there is evidence of intestinal obstruction, and (iv) when there is general ill-health from the infection, which has failed to improve with antibiotics. A colostomy alone will reduce the secondary infection, but if the disease is still active it may spread to involve the colostomy. Operations to conserve the anal sphincter are rarely satisfactory, because the lesion is usually too low. Dilatation is a dangerous procedure and tends to accentuate the incontinence. An abdominoperineal resection with a permanent colostomy is usually the operation of choice, especially if there has been gross destruction and fistula formation.

30.1.2. Donovanosis (granuloma inguinale, granuloma venereum, chancroid, soft sore)

This is usually a venereal infection, which produces chronic ulcerated and painful lesions around the genitalia, sometimes with extension to the anal region (Knight and Fowler, 1956; Lal and Nicholas, 1970). It occurs sporadically throughout the tropics. It is very common in many tropical countries including the Caribbean, East Indies, South America, Africa, and India, and is especially common in Papua New Guinea (Maddocks, 1967; Zigas, 1971). It is also common in immigrants to the United Kingdom from the West Indies and the Indian subcontinent. It is caused by the bacillus *Donovania granulomatis* (Ducrey's bacillus) which produces a granulomatous reaction and is accompanied by extensive fibrosis as healing occurs. It is an encapsulated, Gram-negative coccobacillus which is seen in lesions in man, within the phagocytes (the 'Donovan bodies') (Donovan, 1905). Secondary contact lesions are common. The incubation period is from a few days to several months. The disease may run a very chronic course, and formation of gross mutilating lesions with ulceration is common. Epidermoid carcinomas arise in approximately five per cent of cases with chronic anorectal granulomas. Diagnosis is by demonstration of Donovan bodies within large vacuolated histiocytes; the Giema stain or a silver impregnation method give the best results. Treatment is with intramuscular streptomycin, 4 g daily for five to 10 days, or oral chloramphenicol, 500 mg four times daily for five to 10 days. Ampicillin has also been used successfully (Thew, Swift, and Heaton, 1969).

30.1.3. Primary syphilis and gonorrhoea

Lesions due to these two venereally transmitted infections occur in the anal region of male homosexuals.

Primary chancre of the anal region (usually in the anal canal rather than the rectum) (Wells, Kierland, and Jackman, 1959; Smith, 1965; Samenius, 1968) may be difficult to distinguish from an epithelioma, a tuberculous ulcer, or Crohn's disease. Demonstration of spirochaetes is often difficult and serological tests should be carried out. The Kahn precipitation test and the Venereal Disease Research Laboratory's flocculation test (VDRL) may give false positive results in the presence of malaria, tuberculosis, leprosy, kala-azar and after smallpox vaccination. The *Treponema pallidum* immobilization test (TPI) distinguishes individuals with biologically false-positive Kahn or VDRL tests; it does not incidentally differentiate syphilis from yaws. Dermatitis of the perianal skin and condyloma lata in the anal region are manifestations of secondary syphilis. The condylomata should be distinguished from giant condylomata, which are probably of viral origin (Shah and Hertz, 1972).

Rectal gonorrhoea is a cause of proctitis in men; it may present with an acute superficial inflammatory lesion of the lower rectum. Gonococci can be detected in direct smears. In women, spread of gonococci from vagina to rectum can occur (Nicol, 1948) and abnormal sexual behaviour need not necessarily be suspected.

30.1.4. Tuberculosis

This is an unusual cause of disease of the anal region (Logan, 1969). However, it is occasionally seen as a manifestation of secondary tuberculosis in third world countries, and in Asians and Africans in the United Kingdom. There may be anal ulceration; tubercular bacilli can easily be demonstrated in smears from the ulcer, or in biopsy material. A rectovaginal fistula may result. Alternatively there may be chronic anorectal abscesses within fistulae; distinction from Crohn's disease (Chapter 29) even with satisfactory histology is sometimes difficult. Guinea-pig inoculation and culture of fresh tissue from the lesion may be necessary.

30.2. Mycotic infections of the anal region

30.2.1. Histoplasmosis

Although this infection has been recorded in the anal region (Earle, Highman, and Lockey, 1960), it is very rare. In that report a case of histoplasmosis occurring in an Englishman who had spent 30 years in India was recorded.

30.2.2. South American blastomycosis

This disease, which is caused by *Paracoccidioides brasiliensis*, is common in most countries in South America. Although it usually affects the nasal and oral mucosa (Chapter 1), the anorectal region may also be involved. It is characterized by slowly-spreading granulomatous ulcers, usually with regional lymphadenopathy.

30.3. Parasitic infections of the anal region

30.3.1. Amoebiasis

Amoebiasis of the perianal skin, often with papillomata, is an unusual complication of that disease (Chapter 25); it may be difficult to differentiate on clinical grounds from a carcinoma (Ten Seldam, 1970). Working in Papua New Guinea, that author considered that the condition is probably more common there, than is generally appreciated.

30.3.2. Enterobius vermicularis (oxyuriasis)

Enterobius vermicularis is also known as the threadworm or pinworm. This organism produces a very common infection, especially in children, and can involve whole families; it is also a problem in schools and mental institutions. It should not be designated a tropical disease because it is probably more common in temperate than tropical areas. *E. vermicularis* is a small nematode; the female is approximately 10 mm in length and the male 2·5 mm. Infection occurs when ova are ingested in contaminated food or drink, or from hands and fingernails contaminated with faeces; the ova are most viable in cool, moist surroundings. Larvae are liberated in the upper small intestine and pass to the ileal region. The females migrate to the caecum or colon where they attach loosely to the mucosa, and as their ova develop they pass through the anus showering sticky ova over the perianal skin. There may be up to 15 000 and they are infective within a few hours. Retroinfection can occur, when larvae having hatched outside the anus, re-enter the colon. The time interval between ingestion of an ovum and production of a mature female is approximately two months.

The infection presents with an intense *pruritis ani*, which is frequently nocturnal, and that usually leads to autoinfection (Mayers and Purvis, 1970). Loss of sleep and irritability are common. There may be mild gastrointestinal discomfort. Local dermatitis, eczema, secondary bacterial infections, and vulvovaginitis, with vaginal discharge, may result; prostatitis is a rare complication (Symmers, 1957). This infection is a rare cause of appendicitis (Richmond and Guthrie, 1964; McDonald and Hourihane, 1972) and even more rarely intestinal obstruction. The parasite sometimes migrates to ectopic sites (Chandrasoma and Mendis, 1977); in that report, the worms passed through pre-existing breaches in the intestinal mucosa in three cases, to the peritoneal cavity via the female genital tract in another (Beddoe, 1956), and in two others, male worms were found on the outer surface of the intestine, and that suggested active penetration of the intestinal wall. Secondary infection and abscess formation is an unusual complication (Croce, MacGillivray, and Murphy, 1956).

Diagnosis is by identifying ova in perianal skin, under the fingernails, or in faeces. The ova can often be obtained for identification by placing a piece of 'Sellotape' across the anus and then sticking it to a glass microscope slide; that should be carried out in the morning before bathing or defaecation. That procedure may have to be repeated on several occasions. There may be a mild eosinophilia.

Treatment has been reviewed by Davis (1973). Piperazine citrate ('Antepar'), 2g daily for six days, is given orally and is effective. Mebendazole ('Vermox') (a benzimidazole carbamate) given as a 100 mg oral dose is often effective; that gives better results if repeated after two weeks (Miller, Krupp, Little, and Santos, 1974). Pyrantel embonate, given as a single dose of 10 mg per kg bodyweight, is also effective; a similar dose should be given after two weeks. A further agent is viprynium embonate ('Vanquin'); 7·5 mg per kg bodyweight should be given on three occasions at 15-day intervals. Children's nails should be cut short to prevent autoinfection; the ova are resistant to household disinfectants and drying, and they may remain infective in dust for a long time. It is often advisable to treat all members of the family simultaneously.

30.3.3. Schistosomiasis

Fibroepithelial polyps are not uncommon in the anal region in *Schistosoma mansoni* and *S. japonicum* infections (Chapter 26). Following secondary infection, ischiorectal and anorectal abscesses, and fistulae may occur. Rectal prolapse is a rare complication.

30.4. Anorectal suppuration (perianal abscess and fistula-in-ano)

This disease is similar to that in the western world. Bremner (1964) has recorded his experience of the disease in Africans at Johannesburg, South Africa. The disease usually presents late, however, and extensive fistulae spreading into the buttocks and pelvis are frequently present. Tuberculosis, so common in all third world countries, must always be considered in the differential diagnosis.

30.5. Rectal prolapse

Rectal prolapse is common in malnourished children and in the elderly. It occasionally occurs in association with heavy *Trichuris trichiura* infections (Chapter 27). It has also been reported in Children with the 'swollen-belly' syndrome which is probably caused by a *Strongyloides fülleborni* infection (Chapter 20).

30.6. Other conditions involving the anal region

Haemorrhoids are on the whole uncommon in the indigenous people of most third world countries (Chapter 29); it seems likely that they become more common with urbanization (Segal, Solomon, and Hunt, 1977). They may however be troublesome after severe dysentery and tropical malabsorption, especially in expatriates.

Carcinoma and Crohn's disease, which not infrequently involve the anal region in the western world, are uncommon (Chapter 29). Other tumours of the anorectal region also seem to be uncommon and do not differ from those in temperate countries (Morson and Dawson, 1972).

References

Abrams, A. J. (1968). *J. Am. med. Ass.*, **205,** 199.

Annamunthodo, H. (1961). *Ann. R. Coll. Surg.*, **29,** 141.

—— and Marryatt, J. (1961). *Br. J. Radiol.*, **34,** 53.

Beddoe, H. L. (1956). *Am. J. Dis. Child.*, **91,** 577.

Bensaude, R. and Lambling, A. (1936). *Proc. R. Soc. Med.*, **29,** 1441.

Bowesman, C. (1960). *Surgery and Clinical Pathology in the Tropics*. Livingstone, Edinburgh.

Bremner, C. G. (1964). *S. Afr. J. Surg.*, **2,** 147.

Chandrasoma, P. T. and Mendis, K. N. (1977). *Am. J. trop. Med. Hyg.*, **26,** 644.

Croce, E. J., MacGillivray, W. F., and Murphy, C. J. (1956). *New Engl. J. Med.*, **254.** 67.

Davey, W. W. (1968). *Companion to Surgery in Africa.* p. 257. E. and S. Livingstone, Edinburgh and London.

Davis, A. (1973). *Drug treatment in intestinal helminthiases*. p. 37. W.H.O., Geneva.

Donovan, C. (1905). *Indian med. Gaz.*, **40,** 411.

Earle, J. H. O., Highman, J. H., and Lockey, E. (1960). *Br. med. J.*, **1,** 607.

Hawe, P. (1951). *Proc. R. Soc. Med.*, **44,** 426.

Knight, G. H. and Fowler, W. (1956). *Br. med. J.*, **2,** 980.

Lal, S. and Nicholas, C. (1970). *Br. J. vener. Dis.*, **46,** 461.

Lawson, J. B. (1963). *W. Afr. med. J.*, **12,** 89.

Levin, I., Romano, S., Steinberg, M., and Welsh, R. A. (1964). *Dis. Colon Rectum*, **7,** 129.

Logan, V. StC. D. (1969). *Proc. R. Soc. Med.*, **62,** 1227.

McDonald G. S. A. and Hourihane, D. O'B. (1972). *Gut*, **13,** 621.

Maddocks, I. (1967). *Papua New Guin. med. J.*, **10,** 49.

Marino, A. W. M. (1964). *Dis. Colon Rectum*, **7,** 121.

Mayers, C. P. and Purvis, R. J. (1970). *Can. med. Ass. J.*, **103,** 489.

Miles, R. P. M. (1957). *Br. J. Surg.*, **45,** 180

Miller, M. J., Krupp, I. M., Little, M. D., and Santos, C. (1974). *J. Am. med. Ass.*, **230,** 1412.

Morson, B. C. (1964). *Proc. R. Soc. Med.*, **57,** 179.

—— and Dawson, I. M. P. (1972). *Gastrointestinal pathology*. p. 601. Blackwell, Oxford, London, Edinburgh, and Melbourne.

Nicol, C. S. (1948). *Br. J. vener. Dis.*, **24,** 26.

Richmond, H. G. and Guthrie, W. (1964). *J. Path. Bact.*, **87,** 415.

Samenius, B. (1968). *Dis. Colon Rectum*, **11,** 462.

Segal, I., Solomon, A., and Hunt, J. A. (1977). *Gastroenterology*, **72,** 215.

Shah, I. C. and Hertz, R. E. (1972). *Dis. Colon Rectum*, **15,** 207.

Smith, D. (1965). *Dis. Colon Rectum*, **8,** 57.

Symmers, W. St. C. (1957). *J. Path. Bact.*, **73,** 549.

Ten Seldam, R. E. J. (1970). *Trop. geogr. Med.*, **22,** 142.

Thew, M. A., Swift, J. T., and Heaton, C. L. (1969). *J. Am. med. Ass.*, **210,** 866.

Wells, B. T., Kierland, R. R., and Jackman, R. J. (1959). *Archs Derm.*, **79,** 719.

Zigas, V. (1971). *Papua New Guin. med. J.*, **14,** 148.

Index

Important page references are given in bold type